The Complete Guide to Yoga Props

Jenny Clise

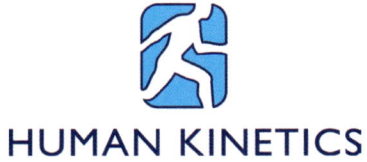

HUMAN KINETICS

Library of Congress Cataloging-in-Publication Data

Names: Clise, Jennifer, 1992- author.
Title: The complete guide to yoga props / Jenny Clise.
Description: First edition. | Champaign, IL : Human Kinetics, Inc., [2025]
  | Includes bibliographical references.
Identifiers: LCCN 2024024038 (print) | LCCN 2024024039 (ebook) | ISBN
  9781718223608 (print) | ISBN 9781718223615 (epub) | ISBN 9781718223622
  (pdf)
Subjects: LCSH: Yoga. | BISAC: HEALTH & FITNESS / Yoga | SPORTS &
  RECREATION / Training
Classification: LCC RA781.67 .C55 2025 (print) | LCC RA781.67 (ebook) |
  DDC 613.7/046--dc23/eng/20240621
LC record available at https://lccn.loc.gov/2024024038

ISBN: 978-1-7182-2360-8 (print)

The web addresses cited in this text were current as of March 2024, unless otherwise noted.

Senior Acquisitions Editor: Michelle Earle; **Senior Developmental Editor:** Laura Pulliam; **Managing Editor:** Kevin Matz; **Copyeditor:** Janet Kiefer; **Graphic Designer:** Denise Lowry; **Cover Designer:** Keri Evans; **Cover Design Specialist:** Susan Rothermel Allen; **Photographs (cover and interior):** © Human Kinetics unless otherwise noted; **Photo Production Specialist:** Amy M. Rose; **Photo Production Manager:** Jason Allen; **Printer:** Versa Press

We thank Studio 313 in Emeryville, CA, for assistance in providing the location for the photo shoot for this book.

Human Kinetics
1607 N. Market Street
Champaign, IL 61820
USA

United States and International
Website: **US.HumanKinetics.com**
Email: info@hkusa.com
Phone: 1-800-747-4457

Canada
Website: **Canada.HumanKinetics.com**
Email: info@hkcanada.com

E9222

I lovingly dedicate this book to every soul who has ever graced a yoga mat and to those who are yet to embark on this journey. I extend this embrace to those who are open minded and curious—to the seekers and the sages.

Like life itself, this book is an invitation—a gateway to new realms of understanding and exploration. It is a tribute to the countless mentors who have illuminated my path throughout the tapestry of my existence.

To the yoga instructors who have imparted wisdom in classrooms and teacher trainings and who have shared insights and fostered an environment of endless discovery—this dedication is for you.

Thank you for never claiming exclusivity to your methods, for nurturing a spirit of continuous learning, and for instilling in me the importance of embracing diverse perspectives and philosophies. Your guidance has been the cornerstone of my ever-evolving and infinitely expanding practice.

Contents

Part I   Recognizing the Value of Props

Part II   Integrating Props Into Practice

Pose Finder

Foreword

If yoga is 5,000 years old, then teaching yoga has been going on for at least 4,999 years. Without transmission, yoga would have no more longevity than a mosquito bite. The joy and general good feeling that come with yoga have moved generous practitioners over the centuries to pass along this practice. With teaching come the artifacts of teaching: for learning a foreign language, the artifacts are vocabulary lists; in yoga, there are texts and props. Just as teleprompts are extraneous to a speaker's message, but helpful in its delivery, yoga props may be extraneous to the pose itself, but necessary for even some long-term practitioners to attain them.

For most of its history, the transmission of yoga has been one individual passing down knowledge to one individual. Yet despite the incredible diversity in the educations, cultural heritages, and religious, social, and political environments of yogis living in various eras and locales, and the limited communication between the yogis, yoga has remained an impressively unified activity. We can attribute this unity to two things: Patanjali's *The Yoga Sutras* has remained yoga's single definitive source, and there is a single goal shared by most who seek out yoga: self-improvement, particularly spiritual improvement.

It's only in the last hundred years or so that Europeans and Americans have realized that we humans were not created quite perfect. We may be equal in our rights, but not in our imperfections. So although the texts are unequivocal and single-pointed, and the paraphernalia today is almost universally shared, the application of props harkens back to the one-to-one transmission common to the yoga teachers of old.

This is why a book of the scope and specificity of the present volume is significant. To see how to do a pose, you can look it up in an encyclopedia and in countless places online. But how can you find a reference that will tell you how to adapt an asana to a given individual? As Margaret Mead once observed, "Always remember that you are absolutely unique. Just like everyone else." That is the reason for using props. On one hand, if you just stick to the basic text, what you know about your pupil and their specific strengths and weaknesses will not come into play. On the other hand, if you focus on the idiosyncrasies of any particular student, then everything you have learned of the dynamics of yoga and about precautions to take will get set aside. Therefore, you need a working understanding of the pupil, the pose, and what you can use to bridge the gap between the practice and the pupil. That's where props come in.

I was taught by Mr. B.K.S. Iyengar and have taught his method for more than half my life. I believe he honed his poses so that the closer you come to his ideal, the more beneficial and the safer the poses become. For him, props were a way of attaining what he worked so hard to create: a pose that is a valuable attainment. He, like many other yogis, used props to initiate the novice, to accommodate physiological and anatomical departures from the norm, and for therapeutic purposes.

I once asked him "How do you know when a pose you're creating is complete?" He gestured to the flute in my hand and answered with a question: "How do you know when a song is complete?" The prop is a fine place for art and science, knowledge and intuition, resourcefulness and caution all to meet: In this book they have an intimate and satisfying rendezvous.

Loren M. Fishman, MD, B.Phil. (Oxon)
Columbia University Medical School

Preface

Understanding means throwing away your knowledge.

Thich Nhat Hanh

I am a student *and* teacher of yoga, and I can say with confidence that this book is for both kinds of readers. Yoga is as unique as the individual practicing it, so wherever you might be in your own journey, this is something you can keep coming back to.

My practice has taken many forms and meanings over the years. Coming from a dance background, I lived for the praise and validation that I was doing a good job. So, early in my yoga practice, I didn't want anyone to think I needed a prop because props seemed to be cued primarily as a tool for modification or injury. I thought that if I used a prop, I was self-identifying as a *less advanced* yogi. And while I had an incredible experience in my initial yoga teacher training, instruction in how to use props was not a priority when trying to cram 200 hours of knowledge into our heads. In fact, in my over 1,000 hours of training, I have learned that yoga props are often something that we have to get curious about on our own. My first book on how to use yoga blocks was written mainly out of independent study and things I had picked up over the years from my teachers.

Not all of us are immediately confident or self-assured with teaching or even practicing with props right out of the gates. Heck, when I first started teaching, I called it a win if I even remembered my whole sequence! The lack of confidence from a teacher, though, can perpetuate the reputation that props are for beginners. This is because we often offer them on an as-needed basis. Vocabulary such as "grab a block if you need it" and "use a strap if you have to modify" in a room full of other students who aren't using them can scare students away from them.

> *Mantra: I welcome the boundless power of learning, as I open my mind to endless possibilities and new discoveries.*

The way to remove the mental obstacle for students is to make props a part of the class and to integrate them into your cues more regularly. Let's upgrade props from the question-able side dish to part of the main meal! In my mission to normalize props, I have come to require them in classes for certain poses or exercises (such as chaturanga alignment drills, shoulder mobility exercises, or restorative postures, to name a few). By removing their adjunct title and making them essential to something we are working on, I am giving my students an opportunity to adapt and give them newer meanings.

I want you as readers—whether you are students, experienced teachers, or teachers in training—to feel confident and assured when it comes to integrating props into class. *The Complete Guide to Yoga Props* offers dozens of variations of yoga asanas that can be modified, progressed, or otherwise changed by using a tool such as a block, blanket, strap, bolster, wall, or chair. In this book, you will learn how and where to position the prop, and you will see the benefit of using it to enhance your yoga practice. *An important message of this book is that props can and should be used by everyone, not just beginners.* Props can be used for multiple purposes: to make a pose more challenging, more comfortable, more accessible, or just different than the traditional pose. Using props provides the yogi with unending possibilities for making their yoga practice truly personal for their body and needs.

The first part of this book will offer an introduction to the props we will be using in the book, as well as do-it-yourself substitutes when needed. Along with this, I will provide general safety tips. Some of the props may be used with specific class formats, populations, or one-on-one clients, but you can use them when and where you see fit.

The second part of this book will be chapters of asanas (postures) categorized into groups such as standing or supine. This will be based on the traditional (or nonprop) version of the pose, because we know that once we add props, we may change orientation a little. Within each chapter, the main pose name will be given (both common name and Sanskrit name), then the variations for that pose will be shown with a photo. For each variation, you will learn the instruction and the benefits of using the props for that pose. While this book is comprehensive, it is just the beginning. There will always be endless "prop-abilities," and this book is a good start to encouraging your creativity in making poses work for any body.

In this book, I aim to avoid cues that dictate a specific form of alignment, encouraging you to approach my offerings with a sense of curiosity. My intention is to word the cues in a way that is inclusive of our differences. However, if you ever feel restricted by any instructions in this book, I invite you to experiment and explore, seeking possibilities that better suit your unique needs.

Please remember that this book is not an all-encompassing guide but rather a spark that ignites potential within you. The possibilities I've learned or explored are meant to inspire you to discover your own. It's perfectly fine to resonate with certain content today, recognizing that it might not hold true for you tomorrow. Embrace the mindfulness of being aware and attentive to what truly benefits your well-being in each moment. In both yoga and life, flexibility and adaptability are vital traits to cultivate. Embrace the myriad perspectives of these poses and allow your practice to flow with curiosity and a spirit of exploration!

This practice goes beyond the tangible attributes of this book; it delves into an even deeper layer of mindful awareness. While I may not always provide step-by-step cues on how to get into each pose, I will focus on how to integrate props and harness their purpose to enhance your practice. Alignment cues will center more around the prop's role than the general pose itself since countless cues can be given outside of the prop.

Due to the inherent nature of yoga poses often overlapping and fitting into multiple category types, I've done my best to select the most suitable classification for each pose. However, if you're searching for a specific posture, the index can always come in handy. For instance, you might find the pigeon pose appearing in various sections, depending on its orientation or variation. Additionally, certain arm balances could also be considered inversions and may be included in only one of the sections. Lastly, some poses might seem a bit unconventional in their placement, like side plank, which has a different orientation than plank. Nonetheless, it harmonizes well in the same section as plank.

Because I understand that yoga looks different in different bodies, you will see many practitioners of all ages, bodies, and backgrounds demonstrating the poses in this book. My intention is so that you can see yourself in the pages and know that yoga is for everyone. You can read through this book, page by page, or use it like an encyclopedia, flipping to the posture you want to learn about. I hope that it becomes a valuable resource that you keep coming back to.

Together, let's embark on this journey of discovery, celebrating our individuality and uncovering the profound beauty of our ever-evolving practices.

Acknowledgments

Thank you to all my teachers throughout the years who imparted upon me the virtue of curiosity, the art of questioning everything, and the beauty of learning from the unknown; I offer my deepest gratitude.

To my students, whose relentless pursuit of knowledge challenged me to become a better teacher and whose patience illuminated the path as I sought answers beyond my reach: thank you for your unwavering support and trust.

Thank you to my acquisitions editor, **Michelle Earle**; your role in the genesis of this book is nothing short of serendipitous. Just as I ventured into the realm of traditional publishing, your timely outreach breathed life into my aspirations. It's as if the universe conspired to make our collaboration a reality, and for that, I am profoundly grateful. It was a synchronicity that affirmed my belief in the coincidental nature of life's twists and turns.

To my developmental editor, **Laura Pulliam**: your presence in this journey has been nothing short of a blessing. Your laughter, dedication, and unwavering kindness have been the guiding lights throughout this journey. Your meticulous attention to detail, coupled with your genuine care for both the work and the people involved, has left an indelible mark on this project. Working with you has been a privilege and a joy.

To the teachers and students who make up the pages of this book: thank you! Your diverse backgrounds and educational lineages in yoga enrich the tapestry of this work, embodying the inclusive spirit of yoga and its transformative power. Each of you brings a unique perspective and lived experience to the practice, embodying the human diversity that defines the yoga community. I want to express my heartfelt gratitude to all these incredible individuals and friends! Special thanks to (including page numbers where they first appear): **Brittany Anderson** (33), **Corey Laplante** (30), **Dani Anderlini** (59), **Irene Hodge** (26), **Juan Ayala** (56), **Kiana Charles** (32), **Laureise Livingston Ruef** (88), **Mark Rudy** (53), **Matthew Steinbock** (28), **Milan Sundaresan** (85), **Nikita Mehta** (40), **Reza Ebrahimi** (61), **Sarah Koh** (86), **Taylor Chang** (35), and **Axel Watts** (65). Each of you brings something special to the pages of this book, enriching its content and making it a truly collaborative effort. Your dedication to the practice of yoga and your willingness to demonstrate poses in this book's photos mean the world to me.

Thank you to the photographer, **Mariya Stangl**, whose artistic vision and unwavering commitment to excellence were instrumental in bringing the poses to life. Her talent behind the lens captured the essence of each subject with unparalleled depth and sensitivity, infusing the pages with a palpable sense of authenticity and vitality. The days spent pouring our energy and sweat into this endeavor were far from easy, but facing them together, we emerged with such a beautiful outcome. Looking back, I'll always cherish those moments, recalling them with a fond "Remember when?"

Also, I'd like to extend a heartfelt thank you to **Jess Lynn Goss**, our lighting tech and photo assistant, whose dedication behind the scenes ensured that every image captured the essence of our vision. And thank you to **Haley Housel**, whose unwavering support and infectious positivity brought light to even the toughest moments, particularly on that challenging first day of shooting. Their contributions went far beyond their roles, and I am deeply grateful for their support throughout this journey.

A heartfelt gratitude to **b, halfmoon**, who generously provided the blocks, bolsters, blankets, straps, and mats featured in this book. Reflecting nature's wisdom, the company's commitment to sustainability and planetary harmony resonates throughout all of their offerings. I am thrilled to showcase a brand that not only has incredible products but also prioritizes ethical sourcing and sustainability. I'm grateful for their support and partnership as we journey toward collective well-being and connection.

Thank you to my friend and colleague **Dana Slamp** and Prema Yoga Institute, who provided me with not only a platform for learning but also a community of like-minded individuals dedicated to the therapeutic potential of yoga. The support and guidance empowered me to explore new avenues of practice and study, enriching my understanding of yoga's profound impact on both the body and the mind.

Special thanks to **Loren Fishman, MD**, who stands as a luminary in the field of yoga therapy and whose pioneering work has inspired countless individuals, including myself. His mentorship during my clinical practicum with Prema Yoga Institute opened my eyes to the power of yoga as a therapeutic modality, fueling my passion for further exploration and study in this domain.

To my friend and colleague, **Renee Marie Schettler**: your thought-provoking inquiries and boundless curiosity have challenged me to explore new realms of thought. Our conversations, both profound and playful, have shaped my perspective on yoga and life itself. Our conversations, ranging from the philosophical to the practical, have provided fertile ground for exploration and growth, challenging me to venture beyond the confines of conventional wisdom.

To **Irene Hodge**, whose friendship has brought immeasurable joy and comfort to my life, thank you for your unwavering support and laughter. Your presence, both in moments of triumph and in times of challenge, has been a constant source of strength and inspiration, infusing the pages of this book with a spirit of camaraderie and connection.

And to **my parents**, whose love and guidance have been the bedrock upon which my journey has been built, I owe an immeasurable debt of gratitude. My mom is the epitome of strength and compassion. Despite facing her own challenges, she always finds a way to navigate them with grace and resilience. She has taught me so much about love, empathy, and where to channel my energy, whether I'm having a great day or struggling through tough times. Her lessons have shown me the importance of appreciating the support of others and finding happiness in every aspect of life. My dad has always encouraged me to embrace life's twists and turns. He's the one who taught me to question the status quo and to never be afraid of the unknown. Even though we both have our stubborn moments, he has shown me how to see what I don't know as an opportunity for growth, often asking me, "Well, what are you going to do about it?" His attitude of embracing all the possibilities life has to offer resonates deeply with me and aligns with the spirit of this book—highlighting the ingenuity we all possess when we look beyond ourselves.

But what stands out the most about my parents is their unwavering support for me to be true to myself. They have taught me that it's okay to change my mind and explore new avenues, and they have always encouraged me to follow my heart, even if it leads me down a different path than their own. Together, they represent the myriad threads that have woven themselves into the fabric of my life and work. Their influence and support have been instrumental in shaping the person I am today, and for that, I am deeply thankful.

Introduction

A Brief History of Yoga Props

For me, [a] prop is not only for the asana. It should contribute to the position of the body which in turn can let the mind be calm and state of "chitta vritti nirodha" be experienced. [The body] is my first prop. The body is a prop to the soul.

B.K.S. Iyengar

Within the vast expanse of modern yoga, an ever-growing assortment of types, applications, and functions of props has emerged. Ranging from inventive do-it-yourself contrivances that kindle our ingenuity and adaptability to the contemporary commercially manufactured tools, the realm of yoga props is teeming with possibilities. Yet, to truly grasp the essence and purpose behind these props, we must journey back in time to explore their historical origins. By delving into the intricate tapestry of yoga's past, we unlock the door to understanding where we stand today, firmly grounded in the heritage that has shaped the evolution of yoga props.

Evolution of Yoga: Navigating the Rich Tapestry of Ancient Wisdom and Modern Understanding

Throughout its long history, yoga has evolved and adapted, blending ancient wisdom with modern understanding, making it accessible to people worldwide and continuing to inspire personal transformation and spiritual growth. As we delve into the intricate time line of yoga's history, we'll examine some of the key time periods, pivotal moments, and the significant advancements that have etched an indelible mark on its enduring legacy here.

Yoga's antiquity leads to multiple estimations regarding its inception and historical time line. Considering the diverse accounts of its origins and the evolving nature of historical insights, it's prudent to regard this time line as a rough approximation rather than absolute.

Mantra: The past is my teacher, guiding me wisely in the present moment.

Pre-Classical Yoga

- Despite differing views on the exact beginning, the majority of sources suggest that the origins of yoga trace back well over 5,000 years. Koletsou (2020) asserts that the pre-classical period of yoga commenced circa 4500 BC, and served as the transition from the shamanic era to the era of classical yoga.

- According to Koletsou (2020), the earliest documented mention of yoga dates back to the Indus-Sarasvati civilization. This reference is evidenced by the Pashupati seals, depicting individuals in postures resembling yoga poses such as baddha konasana and mulabandhasana.

- In the pre-classical period, four ancient text collections known as the Vedas were authored, providing practical advice for metaphysical endeavors (Koletsou 2020). The term *yoga* made its initial appearance in the Rig Veda (India's oldest spiritual text), denoting the notion of discipline (Lacerda 2015). Atharva Veda Samhita, which is part of the fourth Vedic text collection, specifically references the term *asana* and recounts myths of ascetics engaging in yoga while seated in lotus posture, or padmasana (Koletsou 2020).

- Following the Vedas were the emergence of the Upanishads, comprising over 200 scriptures dedicated to the exploration of ultimate truth and methods for attaining liberation from suffering (Koletsou 2020). Lacerda (2015) notes that during the Upanishadic Age, the Upanishads introduced a systematic method for achieving enlightenment within Hinduism. They delineated two primary paths of yoga: karma yoga, which underscores selfless service, and jnana yoga, which centers on the study and contemplation of spiritual texts, as noted by Koletsou (2020). This methodical approach entailed a period of learning under the tutelage of a teacher and a lifelong commitment to the practice of yoga (Lacerda 2015).

- One of the significant texts following the Upanishads was the Mahabharata. According to Koletsou (2020), the Mahabharata stands out as a prominent Sanskrit epic, alongside the Ramayana, acknowledged as the longest poem ever crafted. Within the Mahabharata, the Bhagavad Gita holds significant familiarity, presenting a profound dialogue between Krishna and the warrior-prince Arjuna before a crucial battle. Lacerda (2015) mentions that the Bhagavad Gita outlines three methods of devotion: karma yoga, jnana yoga, and bhakti yoga.

Classical Yoga

- According to Koletsou (2020), a significant cornerstone of the classical yoga era was around 200 BC, when Patanjali authored *The Yoga Sutras*, presenting an eightfold path to yoga.

- The eight limbs include yamas, focusing on moral discipline; niyamas, emphasizing observances and personal disciplines; and asanas, encompassing physical postures for strength and flexibility. Pranayama, the fourth limb, involves breathing techniques; pratyahara, the fifth limb, centers around withdrawing senses from distractions; and dharana, the sixth limb, involves concentration practices. Dhyana, the seventh limb, refers to a state of absorption or meditation, leading to samadhi—the eighth limb and ultimate goal of yoga—representing enlightenment and union with the divine, according to Koletsou (2020).

Post-Classical Yoga

- Koletsou (2020) suggests that the post-classical era of yoga history commenced approximately around 500 AD, although alternative sources place it around 800 AD.
- In this period, Swami Swatmarama authored *Hatha Yoga Pradipika*, placing a primary emphasis on the practice of physical asanas (Koletsou 2020). This significant text provided comprehensive descriptions of the various yoga asanas.

Modern Yoga

- Koletsou (2020) defines the modern era of yoga as spanning from around 1700 AD to the present, marking a contemporary phase in yoga's evolution.
- A pivotal moment in this era was Swami Vivekananda's influential 1893 speech at the Parliament of Religions in Chicago, in which he introduced yoga to the United States and emphasized the universality of world religions (Koletsou 2020).
- Lacerda (2015) notes that the 20th century saw the rise of yoga's popularity in Western Europe and America, with figures such as Swami Sivananda Saraswati and the historic event of Swami Satchidananda's speech at Woodstock in 1969 playing crucial roles in spreading yoga's principles.
- Tirumalai Krishnamacharya, often regarded as the father of modern yoga, made significant contributions to the resurgence of hatha yoga in the 20th century, shaping the contemporary yoga landscape. Notable disciples of Krishnamacharya, such as Indra Devi, K. Pattabhi Jois, B.K.S. Iyengar, and T.K.V. Desikachar, played key roles in popularizing and developing different styles of yoga, such as ashtanga yoga, Iyengar yoga, and viniyoga, a more therapeutic approach to yoga (Koletsou 2020).

Diversity of Modern Yoga

Modern yoga has evolved into diverse forms and lineages, each offering a unique approach and focus: vinyasa yoga, hatha yoga, chair yoga, gentle yoga, slow flow yoga, hot yoga, power yoga, jivamukti yoga, yoga therapy, restorative yoga, ashtanga yoga, kundalini yoga, prenatal yoga, aerial yoga, anusara yoga, Sivananda yoga, bhakti yoga, acro yoga, rocket yoga, Baptiste yoga, Forrest yoga, and many more. These expressions demonstrate the flexibility and adaptability of yoga to meet the diverse needs and preferences of individuals, acknowledging roots in other traditions, such as the influence of Chinese medicine on yin yoga. Regardless of the specific form, all branches share a common thread—the pursuit of physical and mental well-being, spiritual growth, and the connection between mind, body, and breath. These diverse lineages contribute to the tapestry of modern yoga, showcasing its ability to adapt and evolve while preserving its core essence, honoring the rich heritage of yoga's historical origins.

Unveiling the Historical Tapestry of Yoga Props

The integration of yoga props into the practice raises the question of their origin and significance within the broader context of yoga. While many credit Iyengar for the modern-day invention of yoga props (more on this later), it is important to acknowledge that these supportive tools have a long-standing history predating contemporary yoga. While Mr.

Iyengar certainly played a significant role in promoting and refining the use of props, evidence suggests that their roots extend far back in the yoga tradition.

An intriguing aspect of modern yoga is its unexpected connection to ancient Indian yoga and asceticism through the utilization of physical props to enhance yogic and meditative practices (Powell 2018). Surprisingly, the practice of using a cloth yoga strap or belt to align the body in specific postures dates back at least 2,000 years, demonstrating a remarkable continuity between past and present traditions. In Sanskrit literature, this ancient prop was known as the yogapaṭṭa and has been defined as, "the cloth thrown over the back and knees of a devotee during meditation" (Monier-Williams 2005, 857) or a "band used by the ascetics to keep their limbs in a position of rigidity" and the related term yogapaṭṭaka as "a garment worn during contemplation" (Sircar 1966, 386). Powell states some of the earliest sculptural depictions of the yogapaṭṭa can be found at the Great Stupa of Sanchi, an ancient Buddhist site in Madhya Pradesh (c. 50 BCE-50 CE). Additionally, ancient writings like the *Yoga Sutras* of Patanjali, believed to have been composed between 200 and 400 CE, refer to the use of aids like blankets and cushions to offer solace and assistance during meditation. These aids were likely used during yoga postures as well, providing support and diminishing the chances of sustaining injuries.

In more recent times, the incorporation of chairs and various props has become prevalent in certain branches of modern yoga practiced for physical fitness (Mehta et al. 1990). The modern introduction of props originated from the innovative approach of B.K.S. Iyengar, a renowned yoga teacher, author, and creator of Iyengar yoga, which aimed to assist students, whether beginners or advanced practitioners, in maintaining proper alignment during different asanas by providing appropriate support. According to Iyengar (2013), ancient yogis utilized natural materials like wood, stones, and ropes to aid their practice of asanas effectively. Building upon this concept, Iyengar introduced props that enable practitioners to hold asanas with ease and for extended durations without strain. Iyengar emphasized that practicing yoga requires both mental and physical fitness. While teaching yoga over the years, he observed that even individuals in good shape sometimes struggle to sustain certain poses for the required length of time. Additionally, certain asanas involve complex movements that may be challenging for even the healthiest students without assistance. Hence, he developed the use of props in yoga to address these challenges. By incorporating props such as walls, chairs, blocks, bolsters, and belts, Iyengar made the practice of asanas more accessible, more enjoyable, and less tiring for practitioners of all abilities, ages, and conditions. He discovered that props not only supported the body but also facilitated key movements and subtle adjustments while improving blood circulation and breathing capacity. These experiences motivated Iyengar to design props that could be tailored to meet the specific needs of individuals, including those affected by illness or injury.

A significant contribution to the history of props was also made by Iyengar through the development of restorative yoga. This innovative approach allows students to find deep relaxation and support while assuming yoga poses. Restorative yoga became a valuable tool for Iyengar's students who were experiencing fatigue, anxiety, muscle weakness, injuries, or the effects of disease and medical treatments. Building upon Iyengar's teachings, his student Judith Hanson Lasater further popularized and refined restorative yoga until it became the form it is known as today.

As you can see, the use of props in yoga evolved over time (Moosbrugger 2015). Initially, blankets and belts were commonly utilized, but in the 1970s, the wooden block became a popular prop. However, these homemade blocks were often uneven in size and difficult to transport. Notably, Iyengar faced this challenge as he traveled between Bombay and his teaching destinations. Some teachers sought more creative solutions to this problem. Dharma Mittra, the founder of Dharma yoga, improvised by using a large telephone book covered with foam and cloth as a block.

Alongside the development of blocks, the use of pillows for pranayama, meditation, and relaxation predates the introduction of yoga in America. However, during the 1960s and 1970s, teachers began to explore different approaches. Meditation played a significant role in yoga classes, and instructors aimed to find effective ways to guide students into a state of relaxation after asana practice. In 1976, after experimenting with various options, Iyengar designed a firm bolster that offered substantial support to both novice and experienced yogis. This bolster became a valuable prop for practitioners during their yoga sessions.

Overall, the evolution of yoga props saw the emergence of wooden blocks, improvised alternatives, and the development of supportive bolsters. All of these contributed to enhancing the yoga practice and supporting practitioners in their journey.

In 1982, Lakshmi Voelker-Binder, who was bestowed her first name by Swami Muktananda, the founder of siddha yoga, introduced a unique method known as chair yoga. This innovative approach was born out of her observation of a young student in her 30s who faced challenges with floor poses due to arthritis. Recognizing the need for an alternative, Voelker-Binder developed a practice that could be performed while sitting on a chair or utilizing a chair for support while standing. This adaptation allowed individuals with physical limitations to participate in yoga and experience its benefits (About Lakshmi Voelker 2021).

Additionally, in 1979, Alice Christensen, the creator of Easy Does It Yoga, introduced this yoga method through the American Yoga Association. This approach incorporates a range of exercises utilizing various props, such as chairs, floor mats, and even beds. In later editions, the practice expanded to include exercises in swimming pools. By incorporating different settings and props, Easy Does It Yoga offers accessible options for individuals to engage in yoga and adapt the practice to their needs and circumstances. It is important to emphasize that chair yoga, although often categorized as accessible or adaptive yoga, can also be a valuable resource for able-bodied practitioners. In this book, you will discover how chair yoga can present both challenges and creative opportunities for individuals seeking to enhance their yoga practice, regardless of their physical abilities.

In summary, throughout the history of yoga, the use of props has played a significant role in enhancing the practice and supporting practitioners in achieving optimal alignment, comfort, and accessibility. From ancient times, yogis employed logs, stones, and ropes to assist them in their asana practice. Over the years, this concept evolved, and in the 20th century, renowned yoga teacher B.K.S. Iyengar pioneered the use of modern props in yoga, revolutionizing the way practitioners approach their practice. Today, a wide range of props such as blocks, straps, bolsters, blankets, and chairs are commonly used to modify and deepen poses, accommodate physical limitations, and facilitate safe and effective practice. Understanding the significance of yoga props and their transformative impact, this book, *The Complete Guide to Yoga Props*, provides comprehensive insights, practical guidance, and a wealth of knowledge to help practitioners harness the power of props to enhance their yoga journey. From understanding the purpose of each prop to learning how to integrate them seamlessly into various asanas, this book serves as a valuable resource for practitioners of all levels, empowering them to explore the limitless possibilities of their practice with the aid of props.

Paying Tribute to Yoga's Historical Roots: Exploring the Sanskrit Origins

Sanskrit, an ancient Indo-Aryan language, holds the distinction of being one of the oldest languages still in use today (Wile 2012). It carries immense historical and cultural significance as one of the languages associated with Hinduism and Buddhism, as well as being one of 23 official languages of India. Various Indian scripts, such as Devanagari, are used to write Sanskrit. To accurately represent Sanskrit sounds using the Latin alphabet, scholars have established a widely accepted system of romanization. Since the late 1800s, Sanskrit has been transliterated using the Latin alphabet, with the IAST (International Alphabet of Sanskrit Transliteration) emerging as the prevailing academic standard since 1912.

Inclusion of a pose transliteration and Sanskrit guide in the appendix of this book serves multiple purposes. It allows us to honor the lineage and origins of the yoga practice by preserving the authenticity of the posture names in their original Sanskrit form. By providing the posture names in IAST transliterations with correct diacritics, we ensure accurate pronunciation and a deeper connection to the ancient language. This guide enables practitioners to explore the richness and beauty of the original terminology. Additionally, the English translations provide understanding for those who are less familiar with Sanskrit. Overall, the guide enhances the educational and cultural value of the book, fostering a deeper appreciation for the historical and traditional roots of yoga.

Part I

Recognizing the Value of Props

Chapter 1

Overview of Props

*For things to reveal themselves to us, we need to be ready
to abandon our views about them.*

Thich Nhat Hanh

In the realm of modern yoga, a multitude of yoga props has emerged, with an ever-expanding array of types, uses, and functions. From the ingenious do-it-yourself (DIY) creations that ignite our creativity and resourcefulness to modern commercially crafted tools such as handstand blocks, yoga stools, yoga wheels, meditation bolsters, and yoga trapezes, the variety seems endless. However, this book focuses on the most common and accessible original yoga props. For example, while the possibilities with an Iyengar wall, which is a rope wall used in some forms of yoga, may be vast, I have deliberately chosen to explore variations that do not require this level of setup, acknowledging that not all practitioners or readers have access to such specialized equipment. Rest assured, dear reader, this book presents an abundance of variations that will keep you engaged, offering a diverse range of options to cater to your needs and desires along your yoga journey.

> Mantra: I possess the tools to meet my
> needs, empowering myself with strength
> and adaptability.

Prop Creativity

This book is a treasure trove of possibilities, designed to ignite your imagination and inspire you to explore new ways of approaching yoga with props. Picture this: You're all set to teach a class, only to discover that the studio lacks the very props you intended to use—perhaps two blocks or a bolster. It's in these moments that creativity comes into play. How can you adapt and still meet the needs of your practice or teaching?

You might find yourself folding an extra mat to provide cushioning, using a bolster horizontally to mimic the height of two blocks, or substituting a wall for a chair (assuming you're not already teaching or practicing chair yoga, where chairs are expected). But what

3

if you're working in a one-on-one setting, such as a home, where you have limited prop options? How can you adapt in those scenarios? These questions have spurred much of the innovation and invention surrounding yoga props. It all boils down to problem-solving.

Imagine if MacGyver himself were teaching or practicing yoga—the TV character known for finding ways to make do with the things at hand—would find a way to innovate, right? Well, the same applies here. There's no rule book dictating how props should be used in one specific way. This book isn't about that. It's about me sharing what I've learned and devised, with the hope that it serves as a comprehensive starting point for you to uncover your own innovations in your personal practice or classes. It's a catalyst for your mind to think differently and serves as a guide to fill in the gaps where you need it most.

This book primarily focuses on the yoga aspect but let me share a little secret: I've found practical uses for props beyond the mat. I have transformed blocks into a nightstand, a strap around my back and shins into a makeshift fold-out chair for sitting on the ground, and even a bolster serving as a cozy sleeping pillow. Yoga props originated from our everyday devices, adapted and refined to meet the specific needs of yoga. Conversely, they can effortlessly revert back to their prop ancestors—common household tools such as bedding, ropes, stairs, and furniture. In addition, sandbags can be wonderful additions for yin or restorative practices, while using props like eye pillows can enhance a meditative experience. Embracing various props can introduce new dimensions of comfort and depth to the practice, allowing practitioners to delve deeper into each posture and find greater relaxation and alignment.

While the assigned functions of items are clear, try to explore using them in unconventional ways. During the COVID-19 pandemic, for instance, when many lacked a proper home prop setup, I discovered that Clorox wipes containers were approximately the same height as blocks!

In essence, all props, whether explicitly labeled for yoga or not, began as DIY inventions. They are born out of a desire to adapt and make the most of what's available. So feel free to experiment. Let your creativity soar as you explore the endless possibilities of props, both within and beyond the realms of yoga.

As you delve deeper into the mechanisms of props, you'll gain a greater understanding of their nature, and with that understanding comes the ability to generate your own ideas that cater specifically to your practice or classes. Enjoy the process as you learn how to harness the power of props and unlock your creative potential.

Variety of Props

There are many props out there, but in this book, we will mostly be discussing how to use yoga blocks, straps, bolsters, blankets, chairs, and walls. There are many different shapes and dimensions of each of these props, but I will keep things uniform by using as close to a standard size as I can in the posture chapters. I do not claim that one size fits all when it comes to this practice, but table 1.1 will help you understand the different options out there and adapt the suggestions in the text to the props you have or the props that work best for you. Let's dive into the different options!

Yoga Blocks

Yoga blocks are also known as bricks in some forms of yoga, such as Iyengar yoga, which I briefly touched on in the introduction. This brick, originally crafted from wood, has evolved to include alternative materials like foam and cork. The most common rectangular size measures four inches by six inches by nine inches (10 cm × 15 cm × 23 cm), which will be used for demonstration in this book, but there are larger and smaller blocks available. Some blocks even have a curved or rounded shape.

The selection of block material depends on practical considerations such as weight, sweat absorption, firmness, and cost. It may also hinge on the specific yoga class or personal preference. Wooden blocks offer excellent durability and can last indefinitely with proper care. They are robust and heavy, making them ideal for supporting postures that require a stable base. However, they are heavy to carry around, and they are the most expensive option. Moreover, their hardness might make certain practices, like restorative yoga, less comfortable without additional padding. Wooden blocks also tend to be the most slippery.

Cork blocks, as shown in figure 1.1, are a favored choice due to their balanced attributes—reasonable price, moderate weight, comfort, and durability. They weigh less and cost less than wooden blocks but still maintain a long life span if they are well maintained. The drawback is that cork blocks can gradually absorb sweat and develop difficult-to-remove odors. Nevertheless, they are sturdier than foam blocks.

Foam blocks are the most budget-friendly option but require more frequent replacements due to wear and tear. They are also more susceptible to getting dirty, although cleaning them is easy. Foam blocks are lightweight and highly portable, making them ideal for on-the-go use. They excel in classes where you relax into the block, such as restorative yoga, and are easier to lift for poses that require holding them up such as overhead, between your hands, or when you wedge a block between your body and a wall. However, they may lack stability in certain poses that demand reinforcement, such as balancing postures resting your hands or feet on the block. Additionally, foam blocks tend to be less eco-friendly than wood and cork options, although some brands now use recycled foam materials.

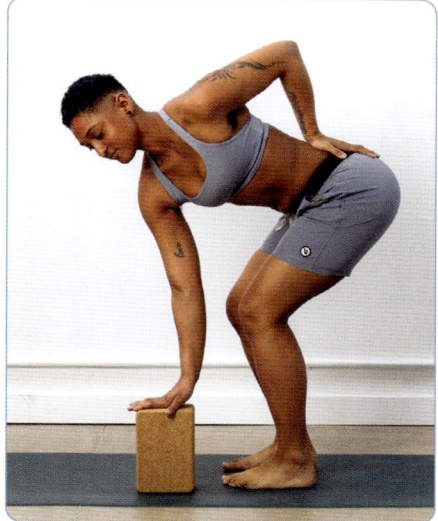

Figure 1.1   Natural cork block that is four inches by six inches by nine inches (10 cm × 15 cm × 23 cm).

Chairs

When it comes to incorporating chairs into your yoga practice, the options are abundant! From a regular chair you have at home to a specialized inversion chair designed for going upside down, the choices are limitless. While nearly any chair can be used to support yoga practice, this book will focus on making use of a folding chair for several compelling reasons.

First and foremost, folding chairs are commonly used in group chair yoga classes, so becoming familiar with this type of chair is advantageous. Additionally, for those who bring their own chair from home when they practice in a studio, a folding chair is the most convenient option, because it is easy to transport and store. To ensure stability and durability, we recommend you select chairs made from robust materials like reinforced metal or steel, especially if you plan to perform weight-bearing variations that involve flipping the chair upside down.

For enhanced flexibility in posture variations, look for foldable chairs that are backless, allowing you to slide parts of your body through the back of the chair (see figure 1.2). Another useful feature to seek is a bar or rung positioned between the legs of the chair. Many chairs come with a bar between the back legs (see figure 1.2*a*), but those with bars between both the front and back legs offer more options (see figure 1.2*b*), reinforcing stability and enabling certain posture variations, such as tucking the feet on the bar itself.

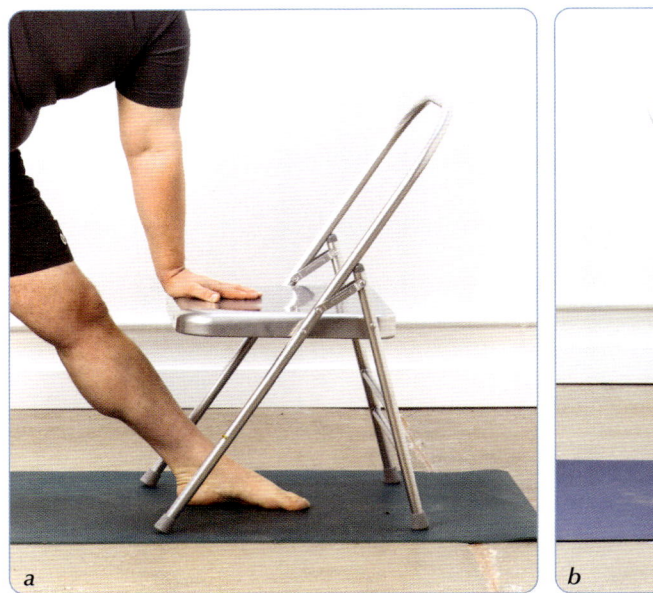 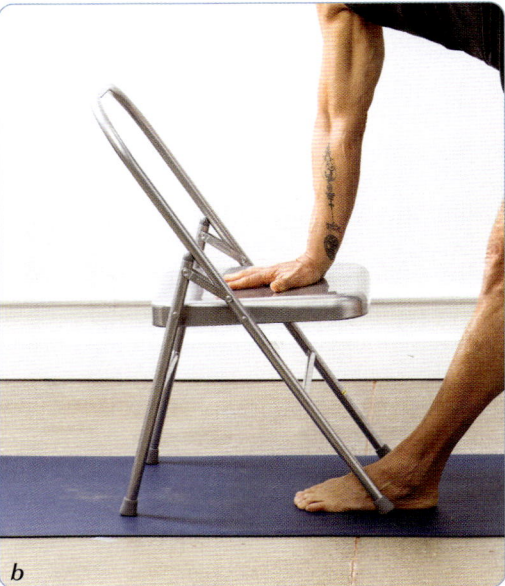

Figure 1.2   Backless and foldable steel chairs with an overall height of 31.9 inches (81 cm) and a seat height of 16.9 inches (43 cm), one with a bar between the back legs (*a*) and one with a bar between the front and back legs (*b*).

Even if your chair lacks a front rung, you can easily create one by looping a strap around the legs of the chair. Yoga chairs come in various dimensions, but a standard foldable yoga chair is typically about 32 inches (81 cm) in height when unfolded. However, you can find chairs that are shorter or taller to better suit your individual needs and preferences.

Straps or Belts

Yoga straps, also known as belts, come in a variety of lengths and materials. Over time, different strap variants have emerged, including elastic options and alternative shapes like infinity bands. However, in this book, we will focus on the more traditional yoga strap, which is a long cotton or polyester strap with a metal ring for fastening (see figure 1.3). These classic straps are incredibly versatile.

The standard sizes for these straps are 6 feet (1.8 m), 8 feet (2.4 m), and 10 feet (3 m). If you're unsure about the length to choose, it's best to opt for the longer version. This way, you'll have enough length to adapt the strap to your specific needs and body requirements. Remember that you can always shorten the strap, but you cannot lengthen it.

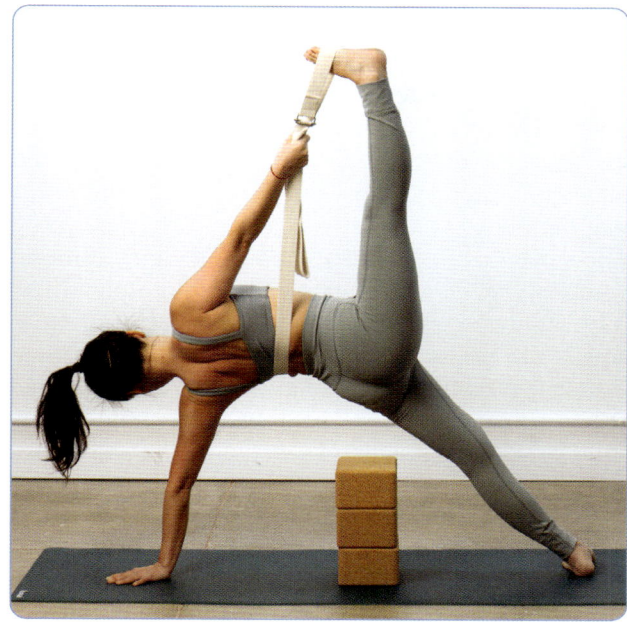

Figure 1.3   A six-foot (1.8 m) organic cotton loop strap.

Various materials and shapes are available for fastening rings. The most commonly known is the *D*-shaped metal ring, which is effective enough. However, my personal preference is the singular rectangular buckle-shaped metal loop that features an adjustable middle bar. This type of fastening provides a more secure hold, ensuring the strap does not slip or slide when looped, offering better stability.

Blankets

A high-quality yoga blanket is characterized by its firmness and is typically crafted from woven wool, cotton, or a blend of materials (see figure 1.4). While there are specialized blankets designed explicitly for yoga, you can also find vibrant Mexican blankets (*sarapes*) at a relatively reasonable price that offer the desired length and firmness.

The key difference between a yoga blanket and an everyday blanket lies in its firmness when folded or rolled. Household blankets might be plush and cozy, but they do not always provide the necessary support for your yoga practice. If you intend to use the blanket to support bony areas of the body, enhance stretches, or raise the height from the ground, you need a blanket that maintains its shape and height even when pressure is applied.

An ideal yoga blanket should stay firmly folded or rolled, offering the required support and stability. By investing in a blanket with these qualities, you can enhance your yoga experience and enjoy the additional benefits of proper support for various postures and exercises.

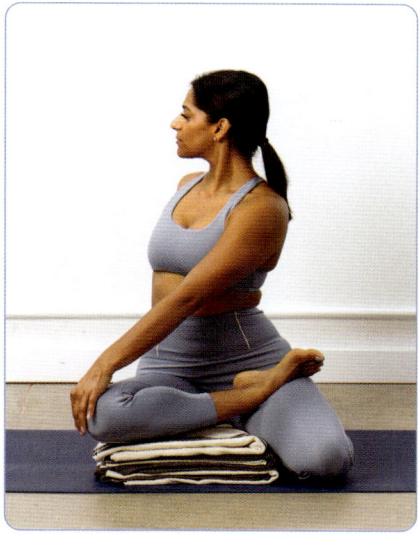

Figure 1.4   A cotton blanket that is 60 inches by 80 inches (152 cm × 203 cm).

Bolsters

Bolsters, like other yoga props, are available in various shapes and sizes. In this book, we will mainly focus on using a rectangular yoga bolster, which is one of the most versatile options (see figure 1.5a). These bolsters are wide, providing a stable and supportive surface for different postures. This book will also show the use of a cylindrical shaped bolster (see figure 1.5b), which offers a nice alternative in instances where one might want to support the natural curves, angles, and arches of the body.

When selecting the best bolster, firmness plays a crucial role for me. Softer and cushiony bolsters have their place in specific postures, but I find that many poses require a firmer backing for optimal support. Less firm bolsters often need reinforcement with additional props or stacking multiple bolsters, which can be inconvenient. Therefore, opting for a firmer bolster from the start prevents issues like flattening or collapsing during practice.

The material inside the bolster is a significant factor influencing its feel. Common fillings include polyester, foam, cotton, wool, and buckwheat hull. However, you don't know how a bolster will feel until you try it. I recommend visiting local studios that provide bolsters to test out different options before making a purchase, especially considering that bolsters can be a substantial financial investment.

Having your own bolster rather than using regular pillows is highly recommended, because bolsters can significantly enhance your yoga practice. They offer greater support and stability. Many bolsters come with removable covers that can be easily washed for convenience and hygiene. Moreover, a bolster for home use can be a fun addition to your yoga space. There is a wide variety of styles, colors, and materials to choose from, allowing you to find a bolster that complements your decor or reflects your favorite color. A good quality bolster can prove to be long lasting, making its purchase a worthwhile investment in your yoga practice.

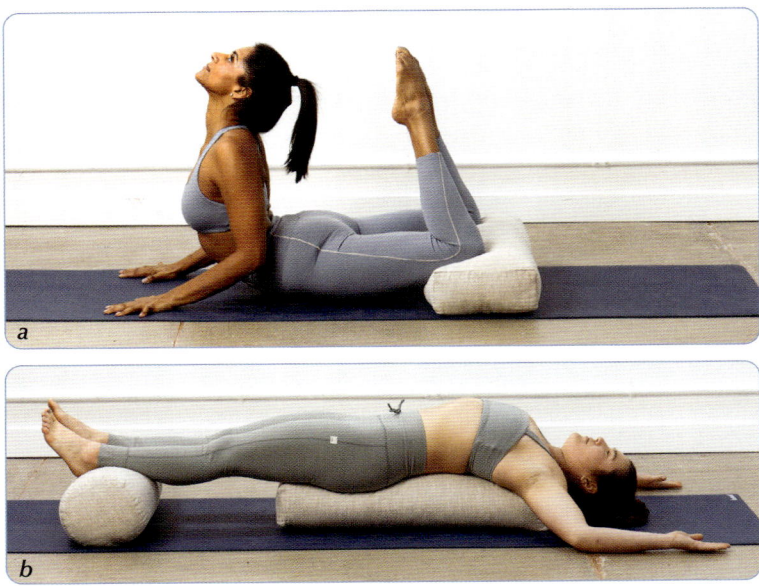

Figure 1.5   Natural linen bolsters: (a) rectangular bolster measuring 5 inches by 10 inches by 28 inches (13 cm × 25 cm × 71 cm) with a cotton fill and (b) cylindrical bolster measuring 8 inches by 8 inches by 24 inches (20 cm × 20 cm × 61 cm) with a cotton fill.

Walls

Walls are one of the simplest props to describe, although not always the easiest to find in a yoga-friendly setup, especially if you have a penchant for home decor. To incorporate wall support into your yoga practice, you require a flat, bare wall that is free from windows and decorations. The most ideal wall space would match the length of your body with arms stretched overhead as well as to the sides.

Many homes lack this kind of dedicated wall space. Sometimes, achieving the perfect wall setup requires creative solutions such as moving furniture. However, the good news is that many yoga studios provide the ample wall space needed for various poses. So, it's worth checking out nearby studios for your practice.

If you are committed to practicing at home and space is limited, fear not! With a little determination and some feng shui magic, you can transform your living area into a yoga sanctuary. Consider rearranging your furniture or temporarily removing artwork to create the necessary wall space. By making small adjustments and being resourceful, you can turn your living space into a yoga shala (a Sanskrit word meaning *home*) in no time. All it takes is a little gusto!

Table 1.1 provides a summary of the yoga props used in this book, along with ideas for DIY alternatives. As discussed in the sidebar at the beginning of the chapter, I always encourage practitioners to explore their creativity and use additional props beyond those listed if they feel inspired to do so.

Table 1.1   Props Used in This Book and DIY Options

Prop	Description of prop	DIY alternatives
Block	In this book, we are using a natural cork block that is 4 inches by 6 inches by 9 inches (10 cm × 15cm × 23 cm), but they come in a variety of dimensions as well as in other materials such as wood or recycled foam.	Stacks of books tied together with a strap, a reinforced box
Chair	In this book, we are using two foldable steel chairs with an overall height of 31.9 inches (81 cm) and a seat height of 16.9 inches (43 cm). One chair will include a front bar between the legs; the other will not. Some Iyengar chairs come with optional attachments such as a back bender for the front of the chair or have special features such as a cushioned seat. You may also see a size range to accommodate height. You may also see chairs with a filled-in back rest. Many products specifically geared toward assisting inversions have more of a stool quality.	A sturdy household chair, a foldable chair without rollers or casters, a stool, a couch, or a bed
Strap/belt	In this book we will be using organic cotton loop straps that are six feet (1.8 m) or eight feet (2.4 m). Our strap comes with a fixed loop on one end to save some time, but any adjustable yoga strap will do for the postures in this book. There is a wide range of yoga straps on the market, differing in material, length, and function. Some attach via two metal D rings on one end or with a singular rectangular shape with a metal bar in the middle such as the one we have in the book. Some straps even have a buckle for ease of use. Some shapes, such as an infinity loop, are made for a particular function, but we will not be using this in the book.	A bathrobe tie, neckties, a mat carrier strap, a dog leash, an exercise band, flat rope

(continued)

Table 1.1   *(continued)*

Prop	Description of prop	DIY alternatives
Blanket	In this book, we will be using cotton blankets that are 60 inches by 80 inches (152 cm × 203 cm), but you can find a variety of options on the market such as wool, recycled blends, or Mexican blankets, which work great and are usually a blend including acrylic and polyester. They come in varied thickness and sizes, but a good rule of thumb is finding one that can cover your full body in savasana.	Thick bath towels, quilts, a rolled or folded yoga mat, pillows
Bolster	In this book, we will be using two kinds of bolsters. The first is a natural linen cylindrical bolster measuring 8 inches by 8 inches by 24 inches (20 cm × 20 cm × 61 cm) with a cotton fill. The second is a natural linen rectangular bolster measuring 5 inches by 10 inches by 28 inches (13 cm × 25 cm × 71 cm) with a cotton fill. There are many bolsters and meditation cushions on the market, all with different dimensions and materials. Some are denser than others, depending on the material, so I suggest trying out a few to find your desired firmness before buying.	Blankets, couch cushions, pillows, meditation cushions
Wall	In this book, we will be using just a plain old wall! That sounds simple enough, but sometimes windows, shelving, wall decorations, or even trimming can get in the way. In some yoga lineages, a wall is specifically designed to support your practice such as an Iyengar rope wall. This book will be catered to those who do not have one of those.	Any clear, flat, solid, sturdy surface

Props and Your Unique Needs

Props can differ significantly even within their own respective categories, and understanding these nuances within the various categories of yoga props can significantly affect your practice. For example, I once had a client practicing bridge pose (setu bandha sarvangasana), with a cork block between her thighs. She immediately communicated to me that the corners of the block were causing discomfort as she squeezed the block because of the denser material. Switching to a softer foam block immediately eased her experience. On the other hand, some of my students find it challenging to maintain balance on foam blocks, because they feel less stable than cork or wooden blocks. For instance, in poses such as half moon pose (ardha chandrasana), where using a block under the hand raises the height of the floor, stability becomes paramount. In this case, the foam material presents a greater risk of wobbling or toppling over, unlike cork or wooden blocks, which provide a firmer and more secure foundation.

Additionally, when using props like blocks for downward-facing dog (adho mukha shvanasana) to reduce wrist and shoulder strain, opting for the least slippery material, such as cork, can enhance the practice. It's essential to consider the specific needs of each pose and choose props accordingly.

Similarly, choosing the right blanket is crucial. While an everyday plush blanket can be a quick substitution for corpse pose (shavasana), certain practices require a firm, rolled blanket. For instance, in thunderbolt pose (vajrasana), using a firm, rolled blanket between the thighs and calves can provide a beneficial massage to the deep tissue of the calf muscles. Attempting the same with a plush throw blanket, however, will likely result in compression or collapse under the weight, because the density of your muscles exceeds that of the blanket.

These same concepts apply to all props, such as the firmness of your bolsters, the length and flexibility of straps, and the availability of walls in your practice space. These are all factors to consider before investing in props. Clarity about your intentions and needs will help you choose the most versatile options for your individual practice. If you work with clients one-on-one, consider having options for them as well since they will have a set of unique needs, goals, and desires different from your own. It may take a few sessions to uncover what works best for them, and they may eventually decide to invest in their props.

If you are taking one-on-one classes, it might be prudent to wait a few sessions before purchasing your props. Your teacher can offer valuable suggestions and guide you in choosing from the options available on the market. Remember that investing in suitable props can significantly enhance your yoga practice and overall experience. We'll learn more about using props for your needs and your body in chapter 2.

Care of Props

Let's now shift our focus to the vital topic of prop care. Once you have acquired or started using props at your favorite yoga spot, it becomes essential to treat them with care, just like any other valuable possession. Even if you're borrowing props, it's crucial to show respect so that others can enjoy their benefits in the same way you do, while also maintaining a sense of reverence for the practice space.

First things first: Let's talk about saucha, a concept rooted in the niyamas of yoga, which are the positive duties or observances spelled out in Patanjali's *Yoga Sutras*. The term *saucha* refers to purity, cleanliness, and clearness. Essentially, this refers to keeping things clean and tidy—yes, I'm talking about cleaning your props!

You'll find plenty of information out there on proper prop-cleaning techniques, but my recommendation is to opt for environmentally friendly cleaning solutions. This helps protect our precious planet, and it also safeguards your well-being. When we practice yoga, we get up close and intimate with our props. Think about it: When you regularly practice with props, they come into close contact with your body. You wouldn't want your skin contacting harsh chemicals, nor would you want to inhale them during a deep breath regulation (pranayama) practice. After all, we're practicing yoga to cleanse and heal our bodies and minds. Thankfully, you can make homemade cleaning solutions or find bio-friendly options on the market to wipe down your mat, blocks, chair, and the like or to wash your straps, blankets, and bolster covers.

Another important consideration is coming into the practice with cleanliness. Yes, you might sweat during your practice (and you should let that sweat flow!), but if you're practicing against a clean wall with dirty feet, you're going to leave your mark.

Now, let's talk about creating a dedicated space. In our practice, we honor the space we practice in. We strive to clear out distractions and clutter, allowing us to delve deeper into clearing our minds and bodies. Of course, life happens, and in this modern era of office yoga, online yoga, and our ever-present technological devices, it can be challenging to create a truly dedicated yoga space. However, we should do our best. If props are an integral part of your practice, it's important to designate a specific space to store them as well. Whether it's in your yoga shala, studio, room, or any other suitable location, find a clean, well-ventilated area to keep your props. This ensures that they are easily accessible and maintained in good condition, enhancing your overall yoga experience.

Finally, proper care of your props supports their longevity. While some props naturally outlast others based on their materials, the overall life span largely depends on how well you take care of them. I'll admit that I'm not a shining example of prop care, but I can certainly share some cautionary tales. For instance, my yoga blocks doubled as my puppy's favorite chew toy! And don't get me started on the fur—my bolster requires daily defurring because I have a pet that sheds . . . a lot. But what if I have a client who needs to use my bolster and is allergic to pet dander? These are the considerations I keep in mind when caring for my props.

Ask yourself how long you have had your current yoga mat (or the one before that). With proper care, a good quality mat should last you well over a year. It is the same with your props. While it may be tempting to use your beloved yoga blanket as a beach towel or picnic blanket, it's important to consider that doing so may shorten its life span. However, you have options! You can easily find high-quality blankets at reasonable prices. My suggestion is to invest in a separate blanket specifically designated for sandy adventures and keep your beloved yoga blanket solely for your yoga practice. Alternatively, instead of purchasing two new blankets, you can repurpose your old yoga blanket as your new beach blanket. This aligns with my earlier point about using props at home and in yoga. If you're going to repurpose your props for everyday activities, consider using the older or more worn-out ones. This approach not only promotes environmental friendliness but also allows you to breathe new life into your props. Let's make sustainable choices while still enjoying the versatility of our props!

Props in Various Yoga Formats

As yoga has evolved over time, various practices have been developed to suit different formats and purposes, and some of them work best with the use of props. Within the realm of niche yoga styles, revolving around the creative use of props, you can find formats such as chair yoga, aerial yoga, prenatal yoga, and even acroyoga, which uses another human body as a structural support for your practice! In the case of chair yoga, having a yoga chair in class is essential, because it serves as the primary tool alongside your own body. Chair yoga is particularly beneficial for individuals who find it challenging to get up and down from the ground, struggle with balance, or rely on modified practices. However, this doesn't mean that chair yoga is limited to specific individuals; it can cater to practitioners of all levels and body types. For example, chair yoga can be a great option for those who can't spare the time for a full yoga class in their day but still want tools to stretch, release stress, and move their muscles at their office desk throughout the day. Moreover, chair yoga has the potential to be both challenging and intricate, making it suitable for a wide range of practitioners.

Certain yoga practices, such as restorative yoga, therapeutic yoga, or Iyengar yoga, heavily rely on the use of props to provide support for the body. In restorative yoga, the focus is on fully releasing into each asana, and props such as bolsters, blankets, and straps play a vital role in allowing the release of tension in the body by allowing the bones to feel heavy and the muscles to soften, as well as reducing stress on specific joints and connective tissue. This setup also facilitates a deeper meditative state and initiates the process of calming the nervous system.

While props may be used in similar ways in yin yoga, the intention behind the practice differs significantly. Some practitioners view props as a form of cheating, associating them with restorative yoga and believing they are unnecessary for achieving the aesthetic aspects of postures in yin. However, Bernie Clark (2015), an influential teacher in yin yoga, counters this perspective, highlighting the multiple benefits of props in yin yoga. They can help adjust stress levels in specific areas, create length and space, make challenging positions achievable, provide support for muscles to release, and increase overall comfort, enabling postures to be sustained for longer durations.

In yin yoga, the focus is on intentionally stressing the connective tissue, which leads to a deeper inner experience and exploration of our neuroanatomy during meditation. As the mind encounters stillness and occasional discomfort, props become essential for safely and effectively applying prolonged stress to the connective tissue. They offer support for joints on hard surfaces and prevent muscles from being overstretched, reducing the risk of harm or injury. Embracing props in yin yoga allows practitioners to delve into their inner experiences and navigate the journey with mindfulness and awareness.

For those seeking a more profound meditation or pranayama practice, incorporating props like a chair, a wall, or meditation bolsters can be highly beneficial during long periods of stillness while sitting or lying down. These props help alleviate any discomfort that may distract the mind and hinder the practice. Moreover, specific props can be employed to enhance the awareness of breath, like breathing into the belly while resting on the floor or using a weighted blanket to feel the release of the diaphragm muscle during each breath. Additionally, looping a strap around the ribs can accentuate the expansion of the rib cage with every breath, further deepening the connection with the breath during the practice. By using these props strategically, practitioners can cultivate a more profound and focused meditation or pranayama experience.

In some yoga practices, the use of props varies depending on the teacher's approach. Personally, I incorporate yoga props into nearly all my classes as they serve specific functions within each session. As explained in the preface of this book, my intention is to empower students to use props effectively rather than simply having them nearby without much guidance. Often, students might feel hesitant or intimidated to use props when given the option to use them if they think they need them. This could be because they are unsure how to use the props correctly or they may not want to be perceived as needing additional support, because props are commonly associated with modifications or injury. I believe that some of the misconceptions surrounding props in more rigorous practices, such as vinyasa classes, might be due to a lack of resources or training for teachers on how to incorporate props effectively. By not intentionally guiding students on how to use props in class, we may unintentionally convey the message that props are only meant for modification until someone is capable enough to practice without them.

However, this does not have to be the case! Props can be incredibly versatile tools that can elevate the challenge of various postures and drills. Using props in this intentional manner not only enhances the overall yoga experience but also allows students to adapt and align to new meanings and perspectives. When props are essential to a particular aspect of our practice, they provide valuable opportunities for growth and exploration. Ultimately, using props strategically can enrich our yoga journey, and they should be seen as valuable allies in our practice rather than just aids for modification.

By now, you've likely grasped that yoga props can serve a multitude of purposes, such as strengthening, assisting, softening, elevating, challenging, providing rest, fostering progression, and even invoking curiosity and play. A better understanding of *how* to use props expands our perspective on *when* to incorporate them into our practice. My aspiration is that you'll gain clarity about the type of practice you need or are offering on any given day and find prop variations in this book that align with your intentions. For instance, if you're practicing hatha yoga and focusing on bridge pose (setu bandha sarvangasana), you can turn to that page in this book and discover options to strengthen and refine the pose's alignment, such as placing a block between your thighs. The very next day, if you wish to practice restorative yoga, you could flip to the same page and find restorative variations, like using a bolster under your sacrum and extending your legs.

Moreover, different yoga styles may employ diverse names and descriptions for poses and the props used. For instance, in Iyengar yoga, you may be asked to grab a *brick* and a *belt*, while in another class, a *strap* and a *block* might be referred to, even though they serve the same purpose. Similarly, a posture may be called pigeon pose in vinyasa and swan pose in yin, yet it remains the same posture. The methodologies across various yoga lineages will also differ, so you might be asked to engage with poses in different ways when transitioning between different teachers.

No matter which style of yoga you prefer, or even if you haven't settled on a specific one, this book aims to be inclusive and adaptable to various styles and teachings of yoga, rather than fitting into a single checkbox or limited to one approach. It offers infinite possibilities and can be tailored to your desired style while inspiring an open mind and encouraging exploration in your practice. This book welcomes all practitioners and facilitators to explore and find value in its contents

Chapter 2

Evidence for
the Use of Props

*Taking an intelligent approach means working toward your goal
step by step.*

T.K.V. Desikachar

In this chapter, we explore the multifaceted nature of props, emphasizing their diverse intentions and reminding ourselves that props serve more than one purpose. They arise when individuals or specific populations have distinct needs, and it is through the ingenuity and inventiveness of countless individuals throughout history that we have discovered multiple ways props can enhance the yoga experience. As we trace the evolution of yoga props over time, we recognize their role in addressing accessibility, amplifying spiritual practices, providing support, and fostering personal growth.

> *Mantra: I recognize that what has aided others can also guide me toward my own healing and growth.*

Understanding the Importance and Impact of Props

Before delving into the nuances and objectives of each prop, it is essential to recognize why props hold such significance and how they have positively influenced practitioners of all abilities and backgrounds. Props offer invaluable support, stability, and accessibility, enabling individuals to reap the benefits of yoga irrespective of age, flexibility, or physical limitations. Moreover, props possess the remarkable ability to adapt a pose or exercise, making it more challenging, comfortable or accessible, or even introducing a unique variation that deviates from the traditional form. Their versatility empowers practitioners to explore and personalize their practice, accommodating individual needs and expanding the possibilities within each pose, and offering adaptability and modification to suit the style or format of the yoga you are practicing. The use of props ensures that each pose can be modified to suit your unique body as these needs shift from one day to another. This fosters inclusivity and bodily awareness, and it encourages the development of a personal practice that meets individual needs. Ultimately, they help create an experience tailored to meet the requirements of our present life journey.

Let's explore some examples of how yoga props enhance our practice. Imagine you have been practicing yoga regularly, and one day, you decide to try a challenging sequence that involves deep hip opening postures like pigeon pose (eka pada rajakapotasana) and monkey pose (hanumanasana). You know that these poses can be demanding on your hips, especially if you've been experiencing tightness or discomfort in that area. You decide to incorporate yoga props to support your practice. Before attempting the sequence, you grab a couple of yoga blocks and a bolster. During pigeon pose, you place a block under your front hip to elevate it slightly, reducing strain on your hip joint and making the pose easier. As you later transition to monkey pose, you slide the bolster under your hips to ground into and to support and cushion the stretch. With the bolster providing gentle elevation, you can focus on the alignment and sensation of the posture without straining your muscles. By utilizing these simple, yet effective tools, you can fully engage in the sequence and explore the postures with a sense of stability and comfort.

Another example of how yoga props can refine and enhance our practice is when working on four-limbed staff pose (chaturanga dandasana). Chaturanga is a challenging and vital pose in many yoga styles, but it can place significant strain on the shoulders and wrists if not performed with proper alignment. To address this, you decide to incorporate yoga blocks to support your four-limbed staff pose alignment. As you enter a plank position, you slide two blocks under your shoulders, placing them at a height that aligns with your elbows. With the blocks providing support, you can now lower yourself into four-limbed staff pose with greater control and ease. The blocks help you maintain a more neutral position for your shoulders and prevent them from dipping too low or collapsing inward, reducing the risk of shoulder injuries. As you engage your core and lower yourself, you find that the blocks guide you to a safe and proper alignment, with your elbows bent at a 90-degree angle and aligned with your wrists. Over time, this focused practice with props helps you progress toward a more sustainable and aligned four-limbed staff pose, enhancing the overall quality of your yoga practice.

Both examples help you maintain proper alignment, deepen stretches, build strength, and protect yourself from injury. These examples highlight how yoga props adapt to our individual needs, empowering us to explore and progress in our practice safely and mindfully. With the support of props, we can approach challenging postures with confidence, and at the same time, nurture our bodies to grow and evolve in our yoga journey.

Contraindications in Yoga

The information provided in this sidebar highlights common contraindications in yoga. However, it is essential to consult with your primary care physician or medical specialist, as these guidelines are not intended to replace medical advice. The best advice I could ever impart on you with yoga though is this: If it hurts, don't do it.

Sciatica

Sciatica can be caused by pinching of the sciatic nerve due to factors such as piriformis syndrome or disc herniation. In the instance of herniation specifically, forward bends can exacerbate the cause of the pain. Instead, try modifying your practice to prevent rounding of the spine, using props, or practice certain hamstring stretches on your back to maintain a long spine.

Sacroiliac Joint Derangement

Sacroiliac joint derangement is another common form of back pain. Postures that include deep forward bends especially with open hips such as a wide-legged forward fold, or asymmetrical hip movement such as postures like half moon pose, can further displace or strain the SI joint. If you are practicing twists, you can also modify them by allowing the hips to move with the spine, such as allowing one knee to come forward in front of the other in a twisted chair pose.

Osteoporosis

Osteoporosis is also something to consider. Yoga has shown to be a great tool in increasing bone density, but it also must be practiced mindfully to mitigate the risk of injury or fracture. One of the biggest things to avoid is flexion of the spine (rounding) as it can increase the risk of fracture.

Pregnancy

Yoga during pregnancy depends on the individual and the trimester they are in. What is recommended is going to vary depending on the type of yoga and how much yoga a person was practicing prior to pregnancy. I recommend working with a prenatal yoga teacher for a tailored approach to the practice, but some general guidelines are avoiding deep twists or belly-down positions that can put pressure on the abdomen. You can also adopt certain forward folds to be wide legged to make room for the belly. Other things to consider are avoiding breath techniques that involve breath retention.

Knee Pain or Injury

The knees are a very common source of pain and injury in yoga. Whether it is due to an underlying injury or inflammation such as arthritis, we want to be mindful of this joint. The knee joint is designed to extend and flex, and it has very little range outside of this, unlike the neighboring ankle and hip joints which provide a much greater range of movement. When dealing with pain or injury, I recommend working "uptown" or "downtown" from the knee joint, working on overall stability and range of motion of these joints to prevent the knees from taking the stress from a pose. Avoid weight-bearing on the knees, locking out the knees, extreme flexion, or extension if you are dealing with pain. Also, some twists where the knee is bent, such as in half lord of the fishes pose, can cause undue stress to the joint. If you choose to stray from these guidelines, please consider the supervision of a qualified physician or instructor who understands the when, why, and how behind stressing connective tissue. Remember, not everyone agrees on these issues! One example of this occurring, in yoga, is within the constructs of a yin yoga class, where certain joint-stressing techniques may be appropriate. When in doubt, remember: Your knees are highly delicate mechanisms that have steep replacement and repair costs financially, physically, and emotionally.

General Joint Pain or Injury in Shoulders, Hips, Wrists, and Ankles

General joint pain should not be ignored. Sometimes the solution is resting the area of pain or injury and then working on strengthening and stretching once it is healed. This book offers many ways to adopt a pose to accommodate pain in these areas, but as always consult with your physician. For example, stretching an injured rotator cuff could be quite painful and worsen symptoms. On the other hand, gently stretching a frozen shoulder might not feel so amazing but can actually be quite helpful.

Certain Diseases or Illnesses

What someone with heart disease practices is going to be something different than someone with cancer or multiple sclerosis. Yoga therapy is a great way to address individual needs in yoga and tailor the practice to help alleviate symptoms of the underlying illness or disease. I recommend consulting with your allopathic care physician in conjunction with a certified yoga therapist to come up with a plan that works for you.

The Evidence Behind Props

As yoga continues to evolve and adapt to the needs of diverse practitioners, the integration of props has become increasingly prevalent. While yoga has stood the test of time, we are now witnessing an increasing amount of research uncovering its benefits. One recurring theme in this research is the incorporation of props, which not only encourage but also maximize the benefits of the practice. Here, we will explore evidence that confirms the efficacy of incorporating props into a yoga practice. From their importance and impact across all bodies and populations to their role in injury recovery and prevention, growth, and enhancing various aspects of well-being, the evidence highlights the invaluable benefits of incorporating props into our practice.

Support for Diverse Bodies

The use of props is supported by evidence and extends to various populations, demonstrating their adaptability and effectiveness for diverse body types. Props can be beneficial for larger-bodied practitioners, pre- and postnatal individuals, older adults, and those with specific health needs resulting from illness, injury, or congenital disorders. However, it is important to emphasize that props are not limited to these populations alone; they are suitable for everyone, regardless of their level of practice or physical ability. While props serve niche populations in unique ways, they can also challenge, support, and deepen the practice of advanced practitioners and individuals who identify as able bodied at any age. The key is to recognize and appreciate the diverse and nuanced ways in which props can enhance the practice beyond accommodating the common needs of individuals.

Now, let's explore some specific examples that highlight how props can effectively support diverse populations in their yoga practice. By delving deeper into these examples, we can gain a better understanding of the valuable role props play in accommodating and enhancing the experiences of individuals with varying needs and abilities.

Timothy McCall, in collaboration with consulting yoga teachers and yoga therapists, writes about clinical geriatric insights in the book *The Principles and Practice of Yoga in Healthcare*, emphasizing the importance of using props to adapt yoga practices for older individuals (Singh Khalsa et al. 2016). Aging brings various challenges such as decreased balance, muscle strength, coordination, and body awareness, as well as conditions like osteoporosis and osteoarthritis, so props play a vital role in making yoga accessible and safe. They aid in maintaining joint mobility, reducing degeneration, improving posture, and enhancing joint and muscle function. Props provide support and stability in standing poses, aid relaxation in seated or lying-down postures, and assist in fall prevention. Overall, props serve as valuable tools in adapting yoga practices for older individuals, promoting physical, emotional, and spiritual well-being.

Yoga practices incorporating props have also been discussed in the context of addressing issues related to race and trauma. In Gail Parker's book *Restorative Yoga for Ethnic and Race-Based Stress and Trauma* (2020), she explains how restorative yoga, a prop-centered practice, is a self-care method for addressing emotional wounds resulting from ongoing stress and trauma related to systemic oppression and racial experiences. Restorative yoga involves practicing receptive forms of yoga that require no physical exertion. It is characterized by stillness and the use of props such as blankets, bolsters, blocks, neck pillows, and eye masks to support the body in different poses for extended periods. The practice focuses on breath, awareness, and attention to stimulate the parasympathetic nervous system, which supports rest and recovery, and it evokes the relaxation response through physiological changes that promote positive health outcomes. Parker goes on to explain that, unlike regular relaxation or sleep, restorative yoga allows individuals to enter a state of deep rest without falling asleep. This enables them to recognize and differentiate between tension and relaxation, even in the presence of chronic stress and anxiety. The practice empowers individuals by helping them shed layers of stress and tension, which they may not have been aware of previously. For people experiencing ongoing, cumulative, and recurrent stress or trauma, restorative yoga is particularly beneficial. By practicing restorative yoga, individuals can identify and release hidden layers of stress and tension, balancing their nervous system and cultivating a sense of safety in stillness. This accessible self-care tool enables people to make deliberate choices, navigate stress with clarity, and foster a sense of belonging.

Improved Physical Function

Props can encourage practitioners to explore deeper expressions of poses, gradually increasing their overall health outcomes, range of motion, and flexibility. One study that was conducted on yoga's effects on physical function and health-related quality of life (HRQoL) in older adults without specific clinical conditions showed that yoga interventions, including prop-based practices like chair yoga, had significant positive effects on physical function (balance, lower body flexibility, lower limb strength) compared to inactive controls (Sivaramakrishnan et al. 2019). Yoga also improved HRQoL outcomes (depression, mental health, physical health, sleep quality, vitality) more than both inactive and active controls. This research supports the inclusion of yoga, including props, as a beneficial activity in physical activity guidelines for older adults, promoting better fitness and mental well-being.

In another example, in a six-week study examining the effects of Iyengar yoga on flexibility, 16 low to moderately active females (aged 52.37 ± 7.79 years) attended one 90-minute session per week. Lumbar and hamstring flexibility were assessed before and after the intervention using a sit and reach test. The results demonstrated a significant increase in flexibility, indicating that a single weekly session of Iyengar yoga for six weeks can effectively improve erector spinae and hamstring flexibility. This suggests that prop-based Iyengar yoga offers a time-efficient approach to enhance flexibility for individuals with limited availability for frequent yoga sessions (Amin and Goodman 2014).

Props offer guidance and support, allowing practitioners to explore and deepen their poses with increased stability and alignment.

Pain Management

Yoga, particularly when employing methods with props, has shown to be a highly effective approach in enhancing the quality of life for individuals coping with chronic pain. A review of 9 out of 13 randomized studies that test yoga's efficacy for persistent pain brought to light the potential role of yoga in pain management for various conditions like chronic low back pain, migraines, chronic pancreatitis, breast cancer, kidney disease, fibromyalgia, osteoarthritis of the hands, and carpal tunnel syndrome (Wren et al. 2011).

These studies predominantly employed hatha and Iyengar yoga practices, with the latter specifically acknowledging the use of props to effectively address chronic pain in yoga practice. The collective findings from these investigations revealed a remarkable reduction in pain and a significant improvement in pain-related symptoms, ultimately enhancing overall quality of life. Among the benefits observed were enhancements in mood, stress, anxiety, depression, pain-related disability, flexibility, decreased reliance on medication, reduced fatigue, improved sleep patterns, diminished joint pain, increased range of motion, strength, and the adoption of various coping strategies.

Injury Recovery and Prevention

The role of props in injury recovery and prevention within yoga is paramount. Props help reduce strain on vulnerable areas, promote proper alignment, and enable practitioners to transition into poses without exacerbating existing injuries or developing new ones. They provide the necessary stability and balance to create a safe and healing environment, allowing individuals to gradually rebuild strength, flexibility, and confidence.

I once found myself driven to perfect the handstand, only to strain my rotator cuff in the process. I turned to the Internet for assistance. It was then that I discovered a remarkable solution through the work of Dr. Loren Fishman, who had studied medicine extensively and practiced under B.K.S. Iyengar. Years later, fate led me to embark on a yoga therapist certification journey, with Dr. Fishman becoming one of my teachers and my eventual mentor.

Dr. Fishman's research on the effects of yoga on osteoporosis deeply resonated with me. I had the privilege of attending his classes with participants in a study examining the impact of selected yoga postures on bone mineral density. This held personal significance, as my mother struggles with osteoporosis, a condition that affects many women and can manifest earlier than in men. I want to emphasize that gender identity and nonbinary experiences were not included in the data or statistics. It highlights the importance of researching yoga's benefits across all populations as we evolve and adapt.

Dr. Fishman's research, a 10-year study involving 741 volunteers recruited online, demonstrated that yoga effectively increased bone mineral density in the spine and femur, offering a safe alternative to Western medical treatments for osteoporosis (Lu et al. 2016). This is remarkable news. Throughout my time studying with Dr. Fishman, props were consistently vital in assisting his students. Chairs, walls, blocks, straps, and other props played a crucial role in creating a safe and supportive environment for everyone working to prevent or reverse this bone disease.

Growth and Empowerment

Beyond injury recovery, props also facilitate growth and progress in yoga practice. Props serve as stepping stones, enabling individuals to access postures that may have seemed unattainable, promoting a sense of accomplishment and motivating further exploration of their potential. The use of props can foster a sense of empowerment for all ages and experience levels, as practitioners experience the stability and support necessary to explore new poses and push beyond their perceived limitations.

The utilization of yoga props extends beyond specific populations, as they can empower individuals of all ages and stages in their practice to progress and reach new levels. Whether it's using blocks to assist in achieving proper alignment, straps to enhance flexibility, or bolsters to provide comfort and relaxation, props serve as valuable tools for personal growth in yoga.

Improved Focus, Relaxation, and Confidence

Props contribute to the enhancement of various aspects of well-being, including focus, relaxation, and confidence. By providing support and comfort, props enable practitioners to release tension, find stability, and deepen relaxation in restorative and meditative poses. They create a nurturing space that allows individuals to direct their attention inward, promoting a heightened sense of mindfulness and self-awareness. Judith Hanson Lasater's book *Relax and Renew* (2011) touches on how prop-supported, restorative yoga can act as an antidote to stress. She explains that restorative yoga poses accompanied by props offer a supportive environment for complete relaxation, counteracting the effects of chronic stress. These poses move the spine in various directions, promoting the wisdom that a healthy spine enhances overall well-being. Inverted poses reverse the impact of gravity, improving blood and lymph fluid circulation, reducing brain arousal, blood pressure, and fluid retention. Restorative yoga also stimulates and soothes the organs, enhancing the exchange of oxygen and waste products within the body. By balancing the masculine (prana) and feminine (apana) energies, restorative yoga ensures practitioners are neither overstimulated nor depleted (Lasater 2011).

This brief overview showed the evidence supporting the use of props in yoga practice is both extensive and compelling! From catering to diverse populations and aiding in injury recovery to fostering personal growth and enhancing overall well-being, props have undoubtedly proven to be invaluable allies. However, it's important to acknowledge that this selection of findings may not encompass all individual needs, as each person's requirements can vary greatly. A vast array of research and resources are out there; they may resonate with you on a personal level, offering tailored support.

This information can help you to broaden your perspective on the significance of props and to encourage you to contemplate how this book can meet your unique intentions and needs. Furthermore, it presents an opportunity for yoga teachers or aspiring teachers to deepen your understanding of your students' distinctive needs, going beyond what is immediately visible in their bodies. By fostering improved communication with your students, you can adapt and tailor their practice to best support them. Remember, there are numerous factors to consider, and it's essential not to make assumptions about the physical, emotional, or mental well-being of your audience. Remain open and adaptable and be prepared to make necessary adjustments. As we progress to the subsequent sections of this book, we will explore specific props and their distinct benefits, empowering practitioners to incorporate these supportive tools into their practice and unlock their full potential.

Part II

Integrating Props Into Practice

Chapter 3

Standing, Kneeling, and Lunging Poses

I am not fully healed, I am not fully wise, I am still on my way.
What matters is that I am moving forward.

Yung Pueblo

In this chapter, we embark on a journey through various yoga postures, exploring the foundational elements of standing, kneeling, and lunging positions along with different ways to adapt them using props. As we delve into these poses, we discover how they serve as a bridge between body and earth, instilling within us a sense of groundedness and balance. They not only enhance physical posture but also foster mental fortitude and willpower, guiding us toward a state of stability and inner strength. Yet, amid the pursuit of these poses, we encounter a valuable lesson—that beauty often emerges from imperfection. The path to mastery is not always graceful; it is a journey marked by twists and turns, demanding patience and compassion. By releasing the weight of expectation, we create space for growth and acceptance, embracing the fluctuating nature of progress. Whether we find ourselves blossoming like a flower or nurturing the bud, each moment within these poses cultivates strength, flexibility, and balance—both in body and mind. In this approach, we utilize props not as a reliance to simply support us, but rather as aids to delve deeper into our potential. At times, these props may propel us forward, while on other occasions, they might guide us toward entirely new paths. Occasionally, they may even provide a nurturing influence, encouraging our growth and exploration. Occasionally, these adaptations may alter the orientation of the posture from its initial standing, kneeling, or lunging form. However, it's important to note that the chapters are structured based on their originally intended forms.

> *Mantra: I stand firm in my unwavering commitment to myself.*

Mountain Pose

Tadasana

ताडासन

Mountain pose is a foundational yoga pose that serves as the cornerstone for many other standing poses. This grounding pose not only improves posture but also works to strengthen the thighs, knees, and ankles, while toning the abdominal muscles. Let's look at a few common variations of mountain pose using props.

Place a block between your feet to activate muscle engagement and inform posture.

Place a block on the lowest height, lengthwise between your feet. Lift through the inner arches of the feet as you squeeze the block, extending the lifting action into the inner thighs. Lengthen your tailbone toward your heels as you lift the pubic bone toward the navel.

Place a block between your thighs to engage your adductors and activate your core stabilizing muscles.

This variation of mountain pose is great if you have a tendency toward bow-leggedness! Place a block between your upper thighs turned to the narrowest width. Squeeze the block up and in toward your pubic bone while engaging the abdomen.

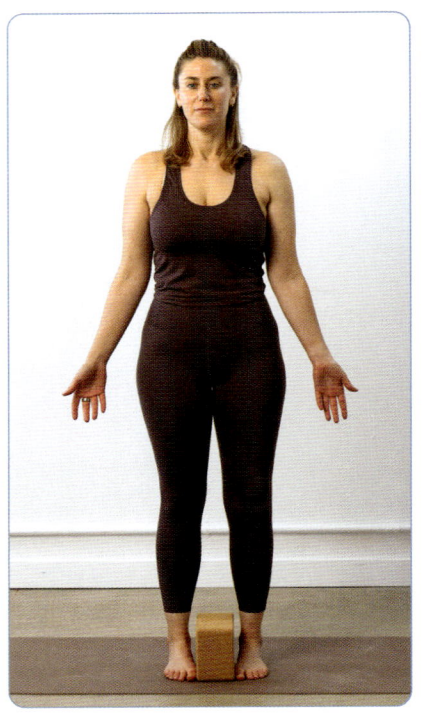

Place a block between your hands to improve overhead range of motion.

Start in mountain pose, then place a block turned to its widest orientation between the palms of the hands. Extend your arms in front of you, squeezing the block while finding a slight external rotation through the upper arms and shoulders. To externally rotate through the shoulders, think about drawing your shoulders down the back and rotating the inner elbows up. Continuing to squeeze the block, raise your arms overhead (or as far as you can). From your natural end range, bend at the elbow, drawing the block toward the upper back. Continue to wrap the elbows toward your midline, externally wrapping the shoulders. Lift up through the top of your sternum without splaying the rib cage open.

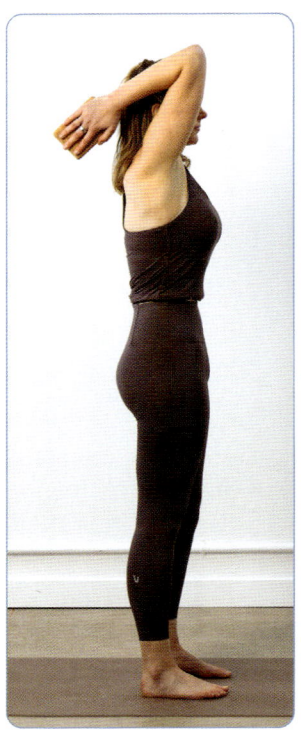

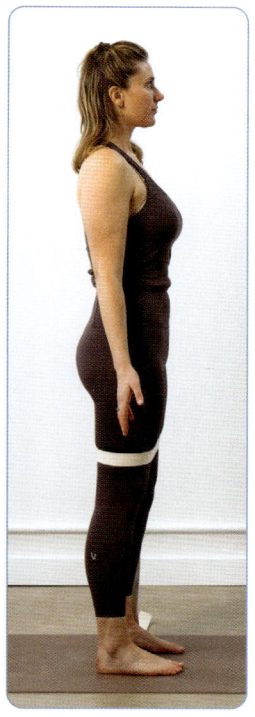

Loop a strap around your thighs to engage the abductor muscles.

This variation of mountain pose is great if you have a tendency toward knock-knees! Standing in mountain pose, loop a strap around your upper thighs and tighten it until it rests comfortably (with no slipping) while standing with the feet hip-width apart. Gently press your thighs into the strap, being careful to not extend this action into the feet by rolling your weight to the outer ankles (referred to as supination). Lengthen your tailbone in the direction of your heels.

Place a block between your sacrum and a wall to lengthen the spine and inform posture.

This is a great variation of mountain pose for monitoring and correcting lordosis, what we commonly refer to as swayback or anterior pelvic tilt. Standing in mountain pose with your back near a wall, wedge a block on its widest side between your sacrum and the wall. The block should rest evenly between you and the wall. This placement encourages a gentle lengthening of the tailbone toward your heels. Be mindful not to overcorrect, though, by overtucking or pressing the hips forward (posterior pelvic tilt). A neutral spine has natural curves; you are simply seeking to align between any extremes and learn more about your natural spinal tendencies.

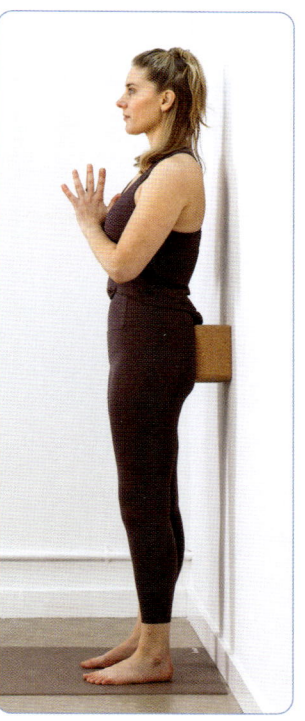

Place your hands on the back of a chair to aid balance.

When working on balance and weight distribution from the feet up, the aid of a chair can help boost confidence! For this variation of mountain pose, perform the pose as you normally would, but with your hands placed on the back rail of a chair. You can always remove your hands when you are feeling ready to, and you can go back to it if needed.

Sit in a chair to inform pelvic and spinal alignment and strengthen postural muscles.

Begin this variation of mountain pose seated on the edge of a chair. If your feet do not comfortably reach the floor, slide blocks or a folded blanket underneath them. Having your sitting bones on the edge of the chair helps to untuck the pelvis, especially if you have tight hip flexors (very common!). Sitting at the back of the chair can sometimes encourage tucking the pelvis, rounding the spine, or relying too heavily on the backrest, all of which deactivate your core muscles. Spread wide through your chest and collar bones and relax your shoulders down your back. Level your chin with the floor and gently retract it until your ears align over your shoulders, stretching through the back of your neck.

One-Legged Mountain Pose

Eka Pada Tadasana   एक पाद ताडासन

One-legged mountain pose is a foundational yoga posture that offers a combination of strength and balance benefits. This pose actively strengthens leg muscles and hips, fostering improved balance and concentration. It also provides a gentle stretch to the hamstrings while strengthening the postural muscles, contributing to overall stability and alignment in your practice. A few ways you can support this pose with props follow.

Practice placing your foot on the seat of a chair for balance and control.

Stepping your foot onto the seat of a chair allows you to practice shifting weight onto one foot without losing your balance. The chair also helps you to stabilize as you build new muscle memory around the posture. Practice hovering your top foot off the chair for a few breaths, then place it back on the chair. Over time, your muscles will strengthen, and you can go for longer holds, or you can ditch the chair completely!

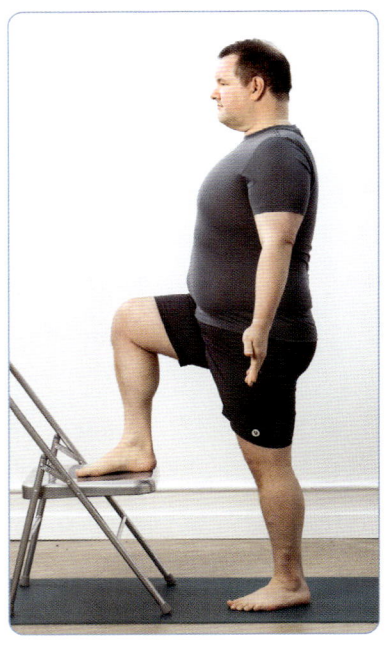

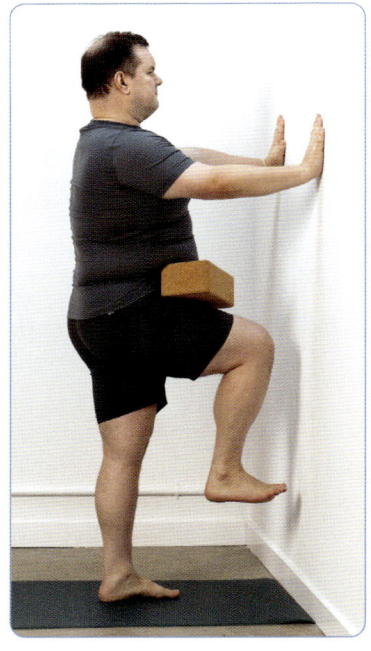

Hug a block between the thigh of your lifted leg and your torso to strengthen hip flexors and improve mobility.

For this variation, you may wish to start with a foam block because it is lighter and softer. You can also begin with a rolled blanket if you want extra cushioning. Using a block will help to strengthen the psoas muscles and deep core muscles. It also helps to increase your active range of motion (using the muscles to produce a desired stretch in opposing muscles). Hugging the block between your thigh and torso lengthens the low back. This helps to correct swayback or arching of the lumbar spine, causing the shoulders to lean back beyond the hips. Engage the thigh of your standing leg and relax the standing foot's toes if they are gripping the mat.

Loop a strap around your lifted thigh and standing foot.

As with the block example, this is an exercise in active mobility. Measure the loop of a strap so that it can comfortably loop around the top of your lifted thigh and bottom of your standing foot. The strap should be taut when the lifted knee is level with the height of the hips. First practice this variation with a bend in your knee. Resisting the force of the strap on both ends, try to lift your leg higher as you press into the other end with your standing foot. You should feel your quadriceps and psoas firing up! To take the challenge up a notch, extend your lifted leg. The strap will naturally want to guide your shoulders back over your hips if you are leaning back, due to the contractions of your core, thighs, and hips. Lengthen the crown of your head away from your standing heel.

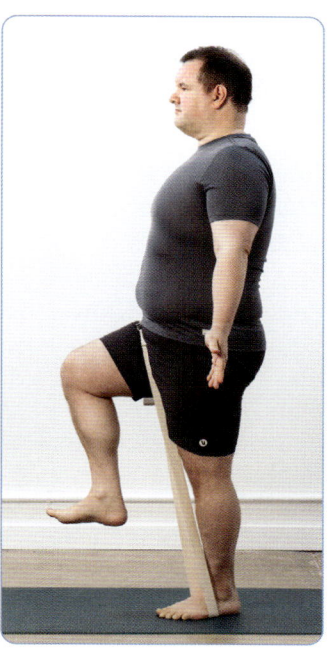

Stand with your back against a wall to strengthen postural muscles and improve alignment.

This variation of one-legged mountain pose requires a lot of muscular activation. Stand with your back against a wall, shift your weight onto one foot, and lift your opposite knee toward your chest. As you enter the posture, you will have to really fire up through your standing leg and core muscles to keep your hips and shoulders against the wall. Imagine lifting through your thigh, as if you were trying to pull your femur bone up into the hip socket. The wall behind you will keep you from shifting your weight back, bringing the shoulders behind the hips (a common occurrence to counterbalance in this pose). If you find this very challenging, you may learn that you tend to sway the shoulders back and press the hips forward when off the wall. Think about lengthening your tailbone in the direction of your standing heel.

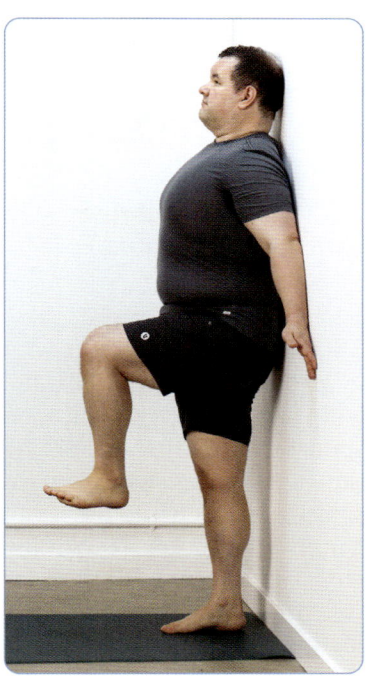

Chair Pose

Utkatasana   उत्कटासन

Chair pose is a dynamic yoga posture that combines strength and balance. This pose effectively strengthens the arches of the feet, ankles, thighs, calves, and spine, while also opening through the shoulders and chest. Let's look at a few common variations of chair pose using props.

Place a block between your thighs to stabilize your pelvis and inform spinal alignment.

Standing with the feet hip-width apart can alleviate certain kinds of lower back pain. Using a block between the thighs can also help to keep the knees and ankles from moving in unplanned directions! Stand and place a block between your thighs turned to the narrowest width as close to the pubic bone as is comfortable. Enter chair pose by sitting your hips down and back, keeping your feet and legs parallel to one another. Squeeze the block between your thighs and work the highest point of the thigh bone toward your heels. Lengthen through your low back and pull your front ribs in toward your spine.

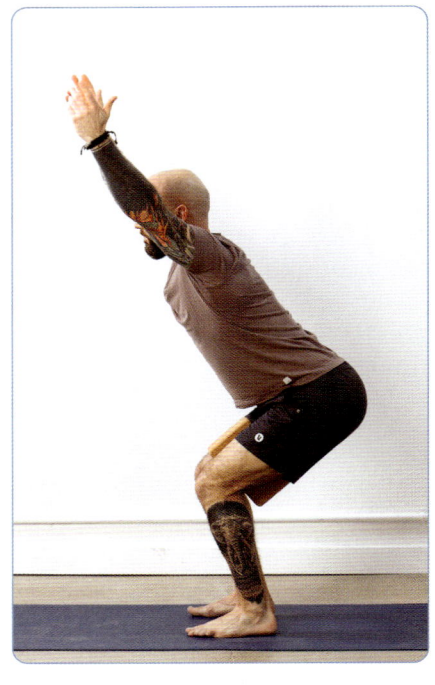

Place a strap around your thighs to stabilize the pelvis and inform spinal alignment.

Just like using the block between your thighs, using a strap around your thighs can help to keep your feet, ankles, and knees aligned while stabilizing the pelvis. In this variation of chair pose, you will loop a strap around your upper thighs so that it is resting comfortably when the feet are hip-width apart. Engage your outer thighs by pressing into the strap. While you are achieving similar goals as with the block, you are engaging a different set of muscles (abductors versus adductors). One may work better for you based on where you need to lengthen versus strengthen. There are many ways to experience one posture, and it cannot always come down to a linear example of certain muscles doing certain jobs.

Sit with your hips against a wall to stabilize the hips.

Begin with your back facing a wall and sit back into chair pose until your sitting bones contact the wall. Adjust the distance between your feet and the wall as needed. The most cued alignment is to stack your knees over your ankles to protect the knee joints. This cue is also beneficial for strengthening the front of the legs. However, if your goal is to increase ankle mobility, working the knees farther forward is OK, especially since the pelvis is stable to support the direction of the knees. It all comes down to intention. You can also experiment with reaching the back and shoulders toward the wall, elongating through your spinal column.

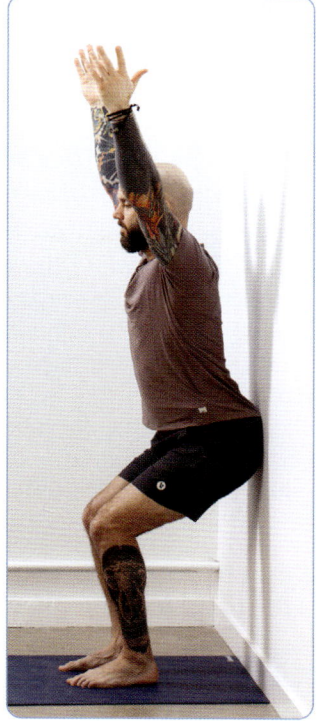

Face a wall with your toes and knees in contact with the wall.

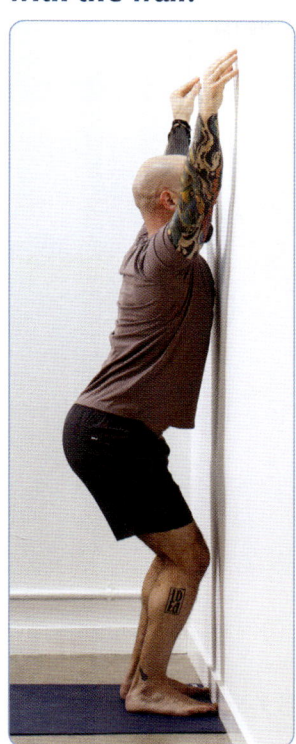

This variation of chair pose supports the cue of drawing the ribs back toward your spine by pressing the fingers into the wall, and it helps to maintain an upright torso—demanding more effort from your core and the lower half of your body. Enter chair pose with your toes and knees in contact with a wall in front of you. From here, slowly start to walk your fingertips up the wall and overhead. When you have walked your fingers as far as you can, press the pads of your fingers into the wall to encourage length in the spine.

Sit in a chair with blocks under your feet and a block between your shoulders and the back of the chair.

Just as in mountain pose, you can practice chair pose in a chair! You will need to use a chair that has a back and not just a rail. For this version, you will need to sit farther back in the chair than you do in mountain pose. Before extending your arms overhead, place a block between your shoulder blades and the back of the chair (for longer torsos, you may need to position the block lower on the back). The moment you feel your posture fading, the block may fall.

Twisted Chair Pose

Parivritta Utkatasana परविृत्त उत्कटासन

Twisted chair pose is a dynamic yoga posture that infuses strength and mobility into the practice. This pose not only encourages rotation of the spine but also provides digestive benefits while strengthening joints, core, back, and leg muscles. Let's look at a few common variations of twisted chair pose using props.

Place a block under your hand to strengthen mobility with support.

By using the block instead of leveraging your elbow into your knee to twist, this variation of twisted chair pose asks for more core engagement, especially the obliques! Place the block to either side and slightly in front of your toes for this variation. As you enter the twist, placing your hand on the block, it is OK to allow one knee to come out slightly in front of the other. Since the lumbar spine and sacroiliac (SI) joint are not designed well for spinal twists when the hips are destabilized, allowing the hips to follow in the twisting motion is often a safer bet.

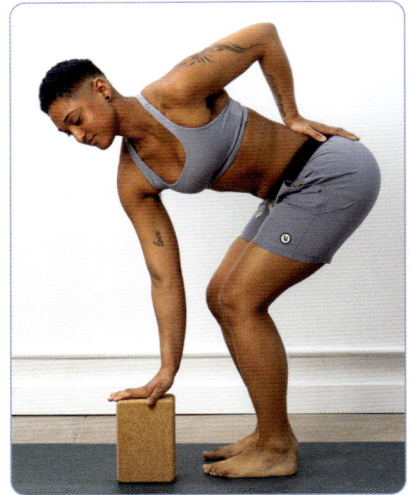

Sit with your hips against a wall to support the sacroiliac joint.

As explained in the previous variation, squared-off knees do not work for every body. By setting your hips against a wall in this variation of twisted chair pose, you are practicing from a more stable pelvis and SI joint. In this version, you can keep the knees aligned with more assurance that your low back will not take the brunt of the twist.

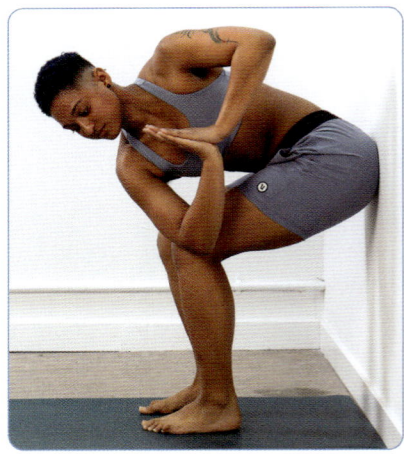

Sit in a chair using the back of the chair for support.

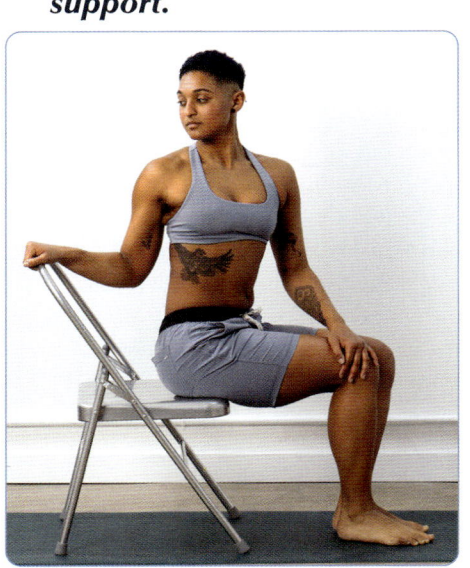

Practice sitting in a chair, using the back of the chair to gently guide you into the twist. This version of twisted chair pose works further into your passive range of motion since you have the leverage of the chair (like the leverage of hooking your elbow outside of your knee in a chair twist). A suggestion here is to sit toward the edge of the chair seat to correct any pelvic tucking and instill a longer spine (axial spinal extension). When the thoracic (middle) spine is rounded, the degree of rotation decreases.

Low Lunge Pose

Anjaneyasana

अञ्जनेयासन

Low lunge pose is a grounding yoga posture that combines strength and flexibility. This pose actively strengthens the quadriceps and gluteal muscles, while simultaneously offering a deep stretch to the psoas and hips. Additionally, low lunge expands the chest, lungs, and shoulders. Let's look at a few common variations of low lunge pose using props.

Place your hands on blocks for stability and alignment.

Blocks not only offer stability in low lunge, but they can help to align. In the version with the back knee grounded (see photo a), blocks can help guide your shoulders over your hips. In this version, think about lifting your pubic bone toward your navel to deepen the stretch in your psoas. Also in this version, you may have to stack blocks if the tallest height of the block is not enough to bring the floor to you. In the runner's lunge variation (see photo b), blocks can assist in lifting your torso off your front thigh by raising the height of the floor. This aids in spinal extension, taking the rounding or slouching out of the upper back.

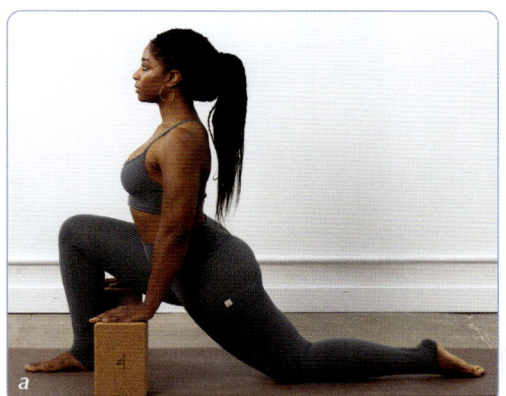 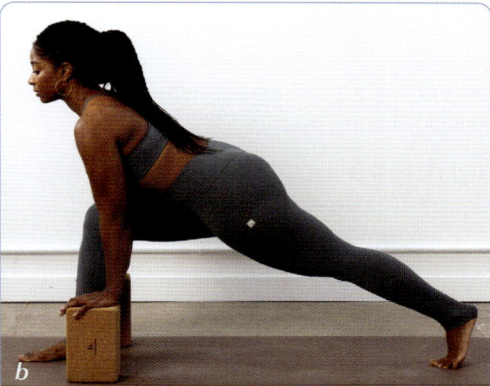

Place your front foot on a block to deepen the stretch.

If you are looking to add a little more intensity to the stretch, place a block under your front foot. You will feel this especially in your psoas, hamstrings, and quadriceps. When deepening into poses, your breath can act as a dial, reminding you when to add or reduce the effort. If you tighten up or shorten your breath here, try returning to the original shape and work your way into this variation of low lunge pose over time. There is no rush in yoga.

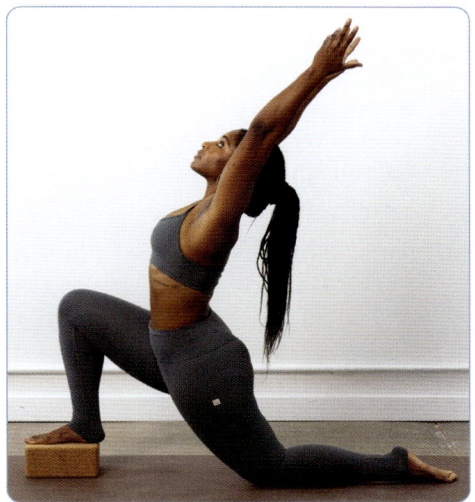

Wedge a block under your front thigh to support extension of the spine.

This variation of low lunge pose is a wonderful reinforcer for both axial extension (lengthening) and extension (backward bending) of the spine. The block provides a platform for your front thigh to engage with, so you can lift out of the sinking sensation in your hips (this one is for

Low Lunge Pose *(continued)*

hyperflexible folks who like to sink into their joints—save all that yummy relaxing into shapes for your yin practice). The block helps you to extend the spine, creating more space in the lower back, and it helps you to engage the muscles that support this movement, mitigating the risk of injury.

Place a blanket under your knee to support the joint.

Any practitioner, regard-less of how long they have been practicing, can bene-fit from adding a softer cushion, such as a folded blanket under the knees. Knees, for how much we demand of them, are not the greatest design in our anatomy, nor do they come with a warranty. A sensitive hinge joint resting between the robust range of motion in our hips and ankles is enough to worry about . . . why not give your knees a little TLC when you can?

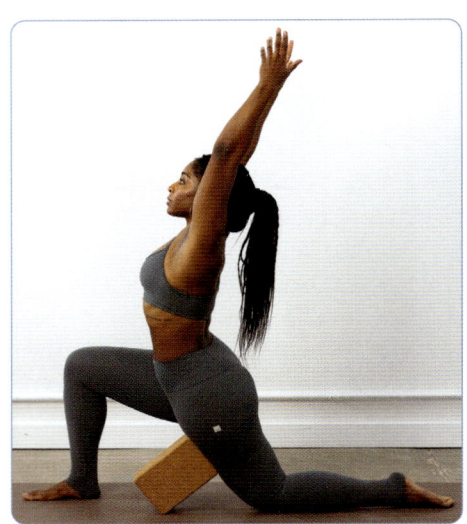

Loop a strap around your front hip and the ball of your flexed back foot.

This variation of low lunge pose is great for deepening the hip stretch by activating your back leg muscles, guiding your front hip back toward and aligning it with the back. I hesitate to say square hips, but it refers to the action of working in a certain direction. The key to this is to first find the size of the loop that best suits you. I find that it is easiest to draw the strap around your back foot, holding both ends in your hands, then loop it from there. Note how it is looped over just the front thigh in the photo. Once the loop feels taut in your lunge, activate through your back heel as you lunge deeper. The strap will naturally guide your front hip back and encourage you to elongate through your spine.

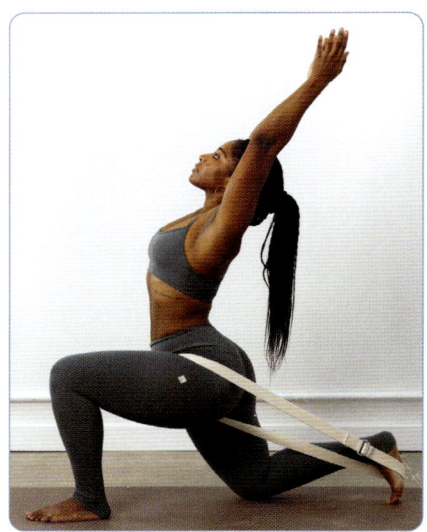

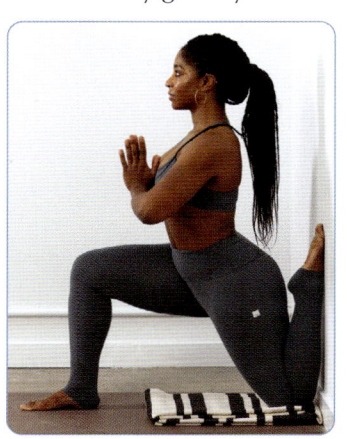

Place a blanket under your knee and your back shin against a wall for a King Arthur variation.

For this variation of low lunge pose, the blanket is vital to protecting your knee joint. Start in a lunge with your back facing a wall. Keep your hands grounded as you walk your back knee and shin to the wall (you can also use a corner to stabilize your shin). From here, walk your hands onto your top thigh or blocks or extend your hands overhead. As you enter your lunge, lift upward through the front of your pelvis. To intensify the quadriceps stretch, work your hips back toward your heel as you continue to lengthen your tailbone toward the back knee.

Lizard Pose

Utthan Prishthasana

उत्थान पृष्ठासन

Lizard pose offers a deep stretch to the psoas, inner thighs, hamstrings, and quadriceps, and it releases tension in the shoulders, chest, and neck. Simultaneously, lizard pose can work to strengthen leg muscles, in some variations, creating a balanced experience. Let's look at a few common variations of lizard pose using props.

Place your forearms on blocks.

Blocks are a great way to bridge the distance between you and the floor so you can relax and breathe deeper. This variation of lizard pose also helps you progress to getting all the way down onto your forearms on the floor. If needed, you can also place a folded blanket under your back knee. As mentioned previously, any practitioner can benefit from adding a softer cushion for the knee.

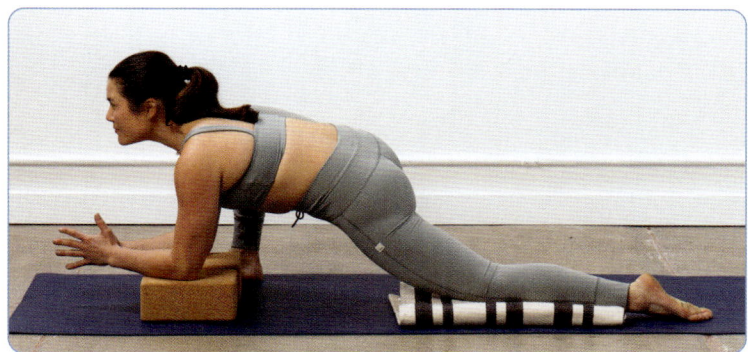

Wedge a block under your back thigh to deepen the stretch in a relaxed way.

This is a little cheat to get an active lizard pose shape, in a more passive form. The block allows the back knee to remain lifted, yet since it is supported, the back thigh can relax. The block can be flush to the floor or tilted at an angle to match the slope of the back thigh. The block may be lower or higher on your thigh as needed.

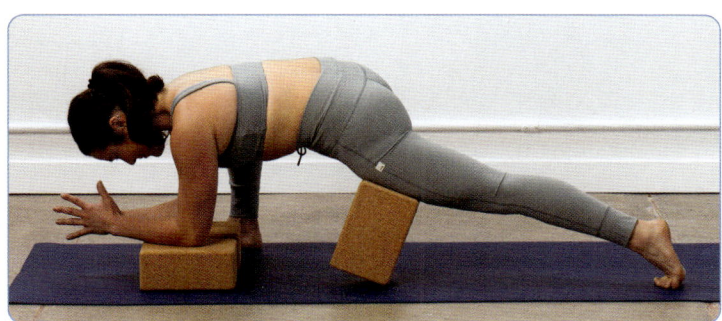

Lizard Pose *(continued)*

Place your foot on the seat of a chair.

Step your front foot onto the seat of a chair with your hands or forearms relaxing down, on the inner side of the front foot. You can control the depth of the stretch in this variation of lizard pose by walking your back leg closer to, or farther from, the chair. Forearms or hands come down on the inner side of the foot on the chair seat. For less of a stretch, place the hands on the back of the chair.

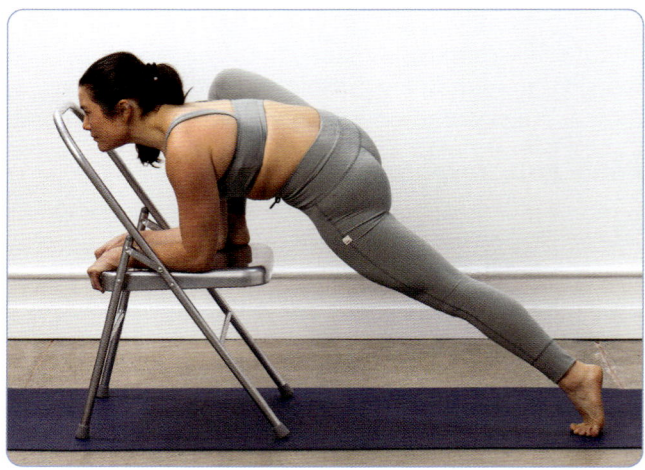

Rest your back thigh on a bolster ramp.

To make lizard pose more accessible for extended periods, particularly during yin yoga practice, you can use a bolster ramp to soften the intensity of the stretch. Adjusting the height of the bolster will help regulate stress levels in your hips, hamstrings, and knees, while also creating more length and space, providing additional support and comfort as you settle into the posture. Lower your back knee into the pose and place a bolster underneath the length of your back thigh. To create the ramp effect, position one or two stacked blocks under the end of the bolster nearest your hip. If you require extra cushioning for your back knee, and depending on your proportions, you have the option of resting your knee directly on the bolster or folding a blanket under the knee behind the bolster.

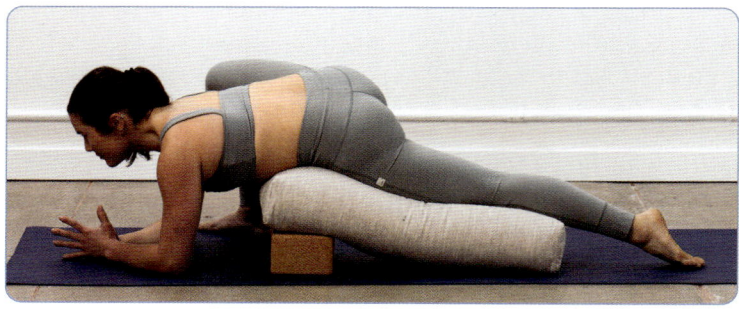

Place a blanket under your knee.

Need I say more? Knee TLC! For this variation of lizard pose, place a folded blanket under your back knee. As mentioned previously, any practitioner can benefit from adding a softer cushion for the knee.

The Complete Guide to Yoga Props

Twisted Lizard Pose

Parivritta Utthan Prishthasana   परिवृत्त उत्थान पृष्ठासन

Twisted lizard pose stretches the psoas, inner thighs, hamstrings, and quadriceps while simultaneously releasing tension in the shoulders, chest, and neck. Twisted lizard pose also strengthens the hamstrings and contributes to the improved rotation of the thoracic spine. Let's look at a few common variations of twisted lizard pose using props.

Wedge a block under your back thigh.

Begin in the block supported lizard outlined under the lizard pose variations. Bend at your back knee, rotating through your spine to reach back for your foot or ankle. This variation of twisted lizard can greatly intensify this stretch so you may decide to add a second block under your front hand to lift the torso a little more. To give lizard pose a twist, move the back shin in both directions: toward your gluteal muscles to deepen the stretch through the front of the leg and hip and away from the gluteal muscles to strengthen those same muscles and deepen the stretch through your shoulders and chest.

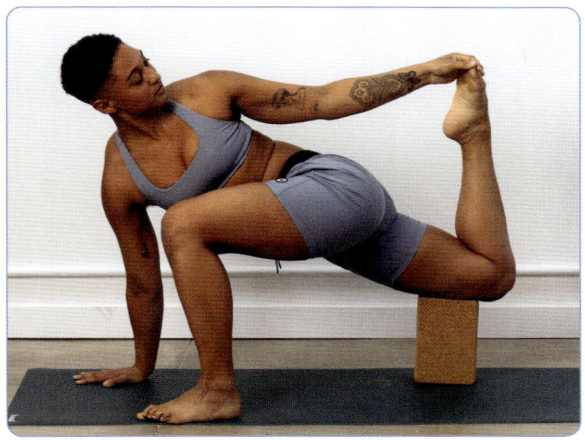

Place a strap around your back foot or ankle.

Straps, just like blocks, are great tools for bridging gaps. The strap acts as a service to you here by bridging the space between your hand and foot. Now you can enjoy the same benefits of twisted lizard pose without pushing yourself too far.

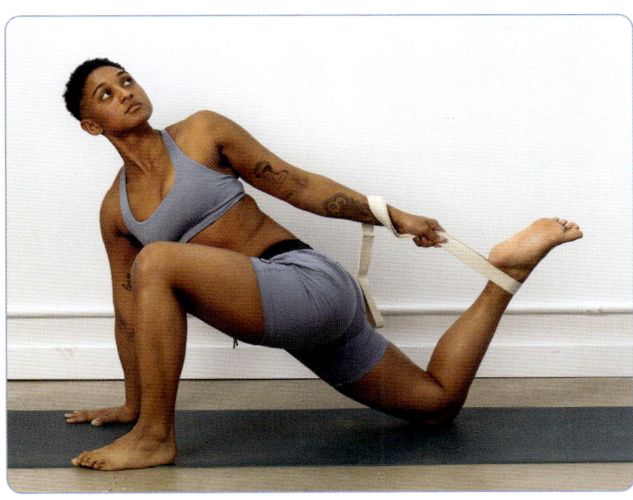

Warrior I Pose

Virabhadrasana I

वीरभद्रासन I

Warrior I pose is a foundational yoga posture that combines strength and flexibility, creating a holistic practice. This pose offers a stretch to the chest, lungs, shoulders, abdomen, and groin, fostering openness and expansion. Warrior I also actively strengthens the shoulders, arms, and back while simultaneously stretching and strengthening the thighs, ankles, and calves. Let's look at a few common variations of warrior I pose using props.

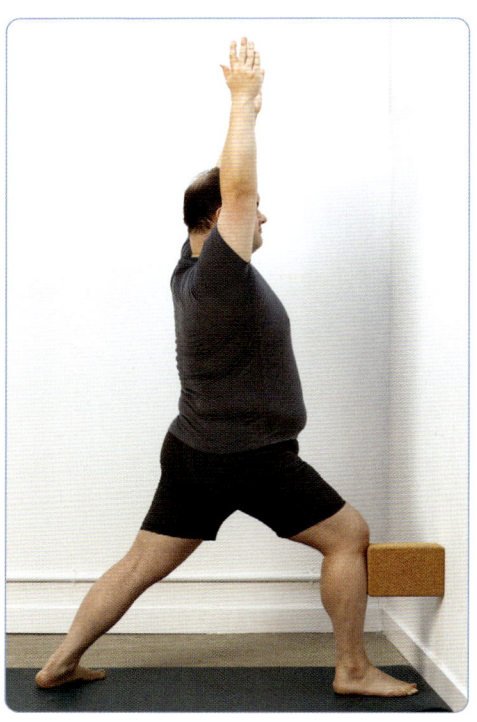

Place a block between your knee or shin and a wall for structural support.

This variation of warrior I pose will allow you to stabilize and align your front knee over your ankle while adjusting the rest of the body. It will also help to alleviate some of the pressure on the front knee. You can pull your front hip back without shifting the direction of the front knee. Think about energetically drawing the inner edge of the front knee toward the block as you draw the outer edge of the front knee away from the block to engage the leg muscles.

Loop a strap around your back foot and front leg hip to engage and align.

Using a looped strap will reinforce the action of pressing into the outer edge of your back foot. This engages the muscles of the back leg, lifting through the arch of your back foot and inner thigh, which also supports the knee. As you press into the strap with your back foot, the front of the loop will gently draw your front hip back, rooting the femur bone into your hip socket. You may need to experiment and play with the size of the loop.

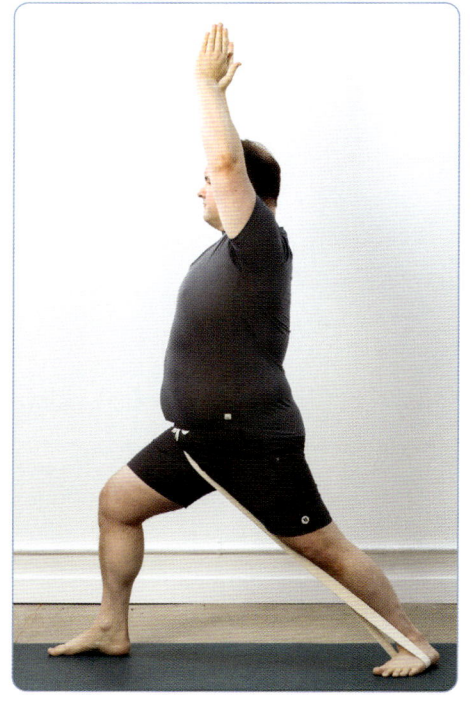

Place a folded or rolled blanket under your back heel.

Grounding your back heel down onto the mat can be challenging and does not always support all bodies. It can add pressure to the back knee or strain in the hips. Placing a rolled or folded blanket under your back heel allows for some grace in warrior I pose for your joints and allows for more comfort and support.

Sit in a chair for stability and balance.

There are a few ways to go about practicing warrior I in a chair; two of them are shown here. Having your sitting bones grounded is great if you need more stability in your hips or are still working on your balance. In photo *a*, the pose is shown with the back leg a little out to the side. Over time, and if there is no other medical contraindication, you can work up the mobility to extend the leg all the way back as shown in photo *b*. If the chair is a little high for you, practice sitting on the corner edge of the chair instead. Practice extending your arms or use the back of the chair for postural support. To begin working into a chair-free warrior I, you can lift the

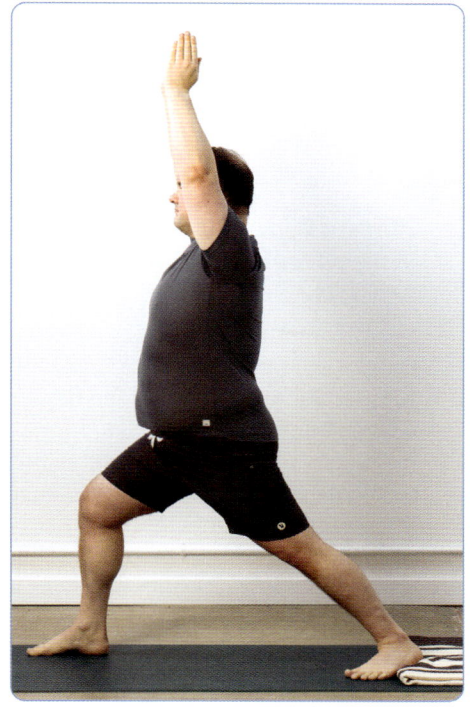

hips slightly to hover over the chair. Hold for a few deep breaths and return to the seat. While the sitting bones are grounded, use this as an opportunity to redirect your focus to the muscle actions of the legs, arms, chest, and shoulders.

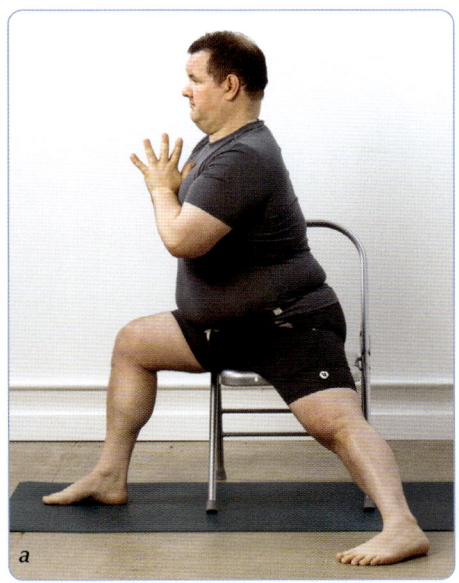

a

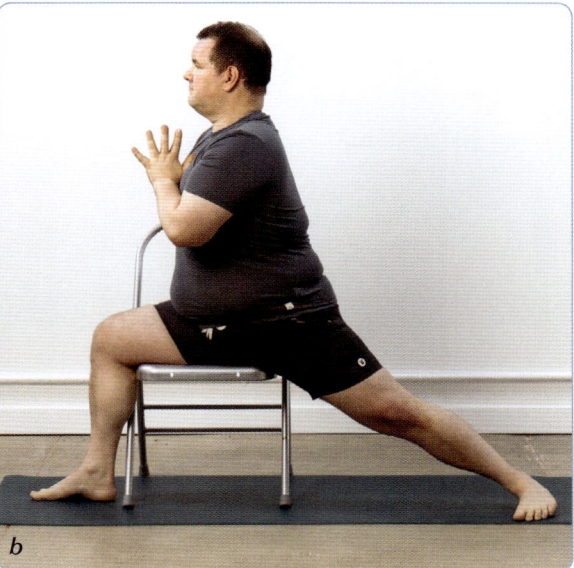

b

Humble Warrior Pose

Baddha Virabhadrasana   बद्ध वीरभद्रासन

Humble warrior pose is a standing forward bend that lives up to its humble name! This pose offers an extensive stretch to the chest, lungs, shoulders, abdomen, and groin, promoting openness and release. Humble warrior actively strengthens the shoulders and arms, while also stretching the muscles along the back of the neck and spine. It also engages and strengthens the thighs, ankles, and calves, contributing to improved balance and stability. Let's look at a few common variations of humble warrior pose using props.

Place a block or stacked blocks underneath your head to release tension.

It can sometimes be difficult to consciously release the head and neck; after all, holding your head up was one of the first things you learned during infancy. The block acts as a reminder and support for releasing through the cervical spine and even softening through the muscles of the face. However, the challenge might be balance! Switching your gaze behind you can be disorienting. Adding stability for your head can be a great way to regain your spatial awareness and direct your focus to the actions of your legs, hips, and shoulders. Stack as many blocks as you need to feel supported in this variation!

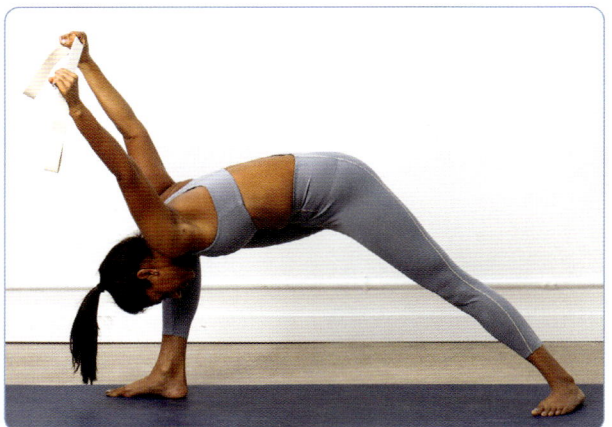

Hold a strap between your hands to create space.

Using a yoga strap is a great tool for bridging the gap if your hands are out of reach from one another. It can also help if the full clasp irritates your shoulders or wrist, alleviating associative pain or strain. A strap may assist in creating enough room in the shoulders to deepen your overhead reach.

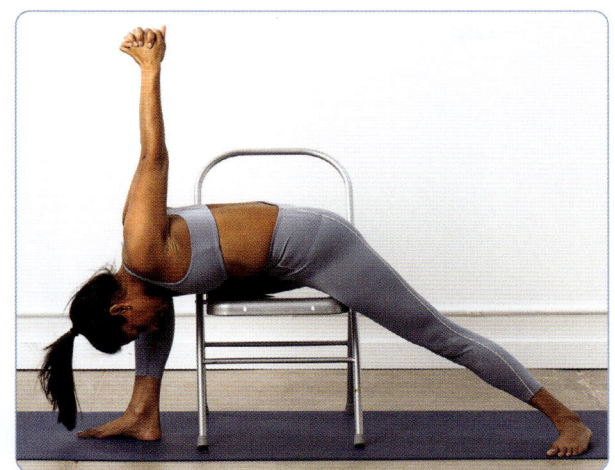

Sit in a chair to assist balance and alignment.

Set up for humble warrior pose by coming into warrior I seated in a chair (shown in the previous pose), then enter humble warrior the same way you would standing—interlacing your hands behind your back, expanding your chest, then folding forward as you exhale. Having the hips grounded on the chair gives you the opportunity to direct your focus on alignment. You should be pulling the front femur bone back and gently adducting the front thigh toward the torso if your shoulder passes your knee. You should also be retracting the shoulders, reaching overhead, and engaging through the back leg. This variation also takes some of the weight off the front leg, making it easier to relax through the head and neck.

Warrior II Pose

Virabhadrasana II   वीरभद्रासन II

Warrior II pose is a foundational yoga posture that brings strength and balance to the practice. This pose actively strengthens the legs and ankles, providing a solid foundation. Additionally, warrior II can help alleviate lower back pain by promoting stability. The pose also gently stretches the chest, shoulders, and groin. Let's look at a few common variations of warrior II pose using props.

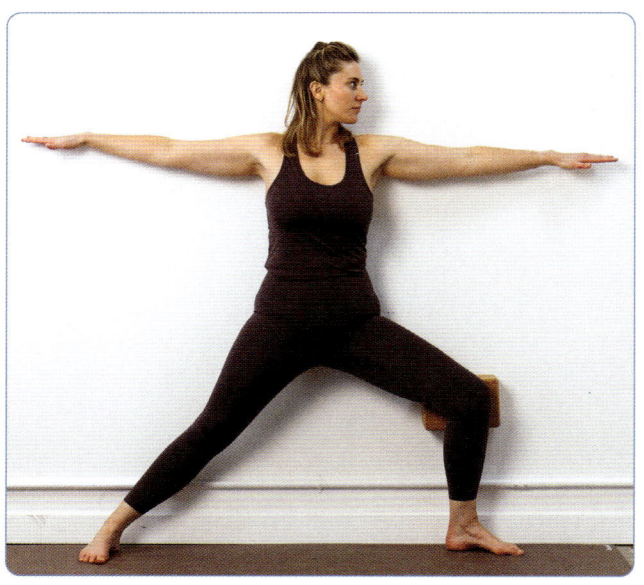

Place a block between the outside of your front knee and a wall to stabilize the knee.

Often in postures such as warrior II or even reverse warrior, the front knee likes to stray away from a right angle to the floor—often toward the big toe. This variation helps to strengthen the muscles along the outer thigh and hips that counteract this stray motion. It also encourages external rotation of the front hip, allowing a more comfortable resting position for the femur bone in the hip socket while strengthening the bones. Enter warrior II with your back facing a wall and wedge a block between the outside of the front knee and the wall, adjusting the distance of the feet from the wall accordingly. Work your front knee toward the pinky toe edge of your foot by pressing into the block and wrap the outer front thigh down.

Place a block between your front hand and a wall.

A common cue for this variation of warrior II pose is to stack your shoulders over your hips. For those with scoliosis, though, this can be quite a challenging task! If your spine curves toward the front knee, try pressing your hand into a block against a wall. This will help to guide the shoulders back and strengthen the muscles on the convex side of the curve and lengthen the tighter muscles on the concave side of the curve.

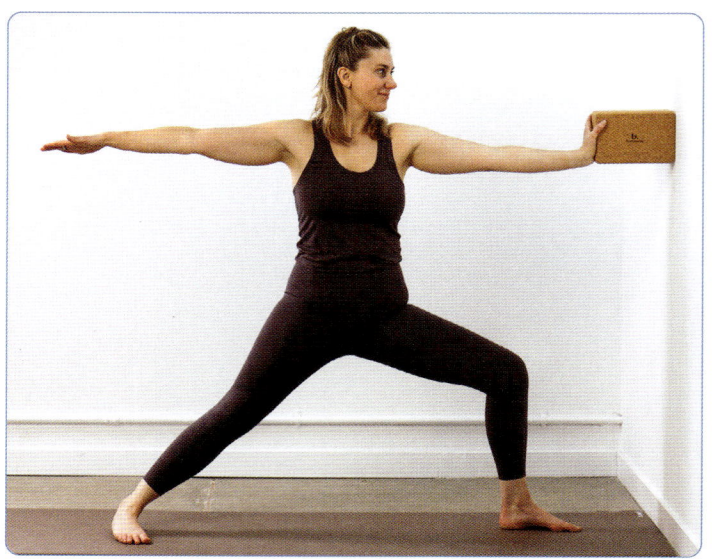

Sit in a chair for stability and balance.

Practicing warrior II in a chair stabilizes the hips and is a great aid if you are working on your balance. While the hips are rooted on the chair, you can focus more easily on the actions of the leg muscles, upper body, breath, and so on—all steps to achieving hovering the hips off the chair for a few breaths and then back down. If the chair is a little high off the floor for you, you can practice sitting on the corner edge of the chair seat instead.

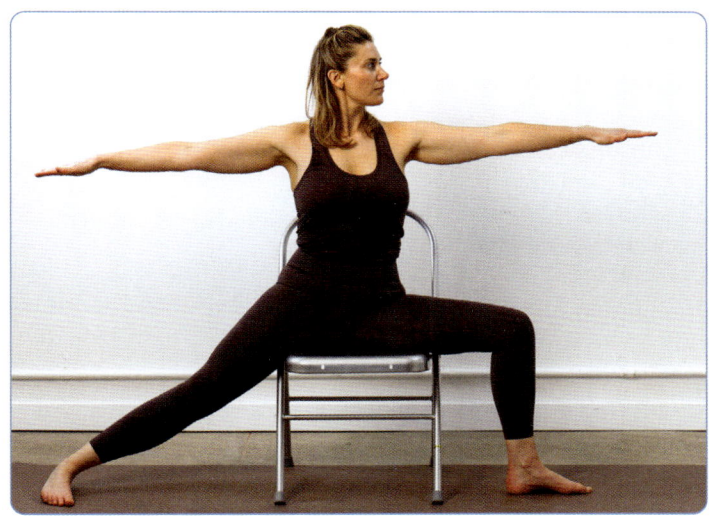

Warrior III Pose

Virabhadrasana III

वीरभद्रासन III

Warrior III pose is a balancing posture that emphasizes strength and concentration. This pose actively strengthens the ankles and legs, establishing a foundation for balance. Simultaneously, it engages the abdomen, shoulders, and back muscles, promoting core stability. To enrich your warrior III experience, let's explore a variety of common variations using props.

Place your hands on blocks or the seat of a chair to support balance and stability.

Blocks or a chair are great tools to help you to find balance while working on the alignment of warrior III. They also help to encourage axial extension of the spine and develop muscle memory for when you are ready to practice hands free. Be sure to have the blocks or chair directly under the shoulders for best support. (See photo a for an example with blocks and photo b for an example with a chair.) If the props are too far forward, this positioning may encourage arching of the spine; if placed too close to your feet, the props' positioning may encourage rounding of the spine and a feeling of less stability. If you are using the chair, you may need to come down onto your forearms or place blocks on the chair to adjust for height.

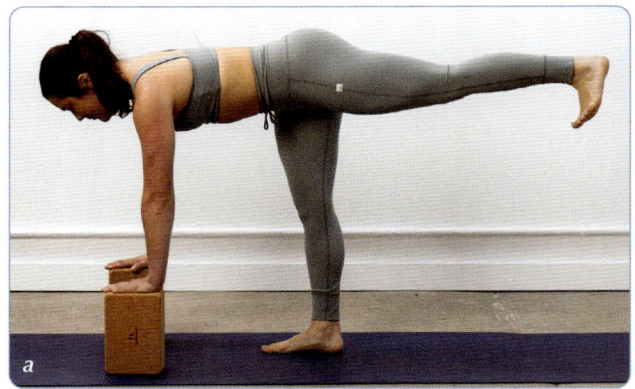

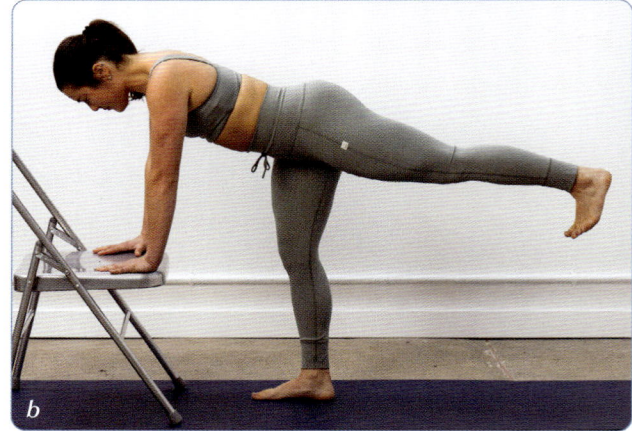

Place a block between your hands with arms extended to engage and energize.

This variation of warrior III is great if you really want to kick this pose up a notch! By squeezing a block between your hands while attempting to raise your biceps toward your ears, you need to really tap into your shoulder mobility and muscles along the back. The block also helps to encourage external rotation of the shoulder; as you squeeze the block, think about wrapping your upper arm bones down and in.

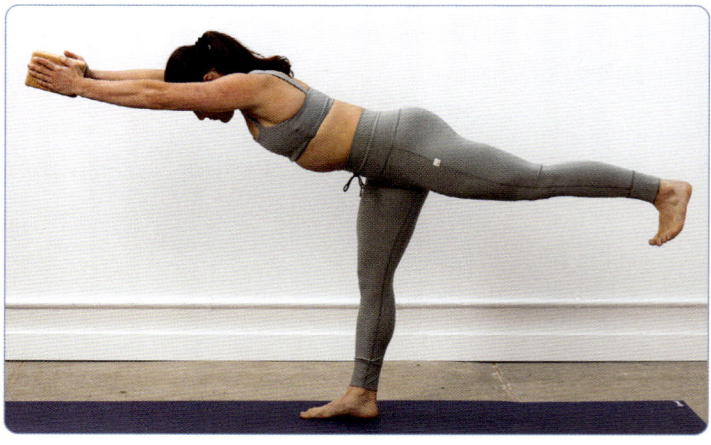

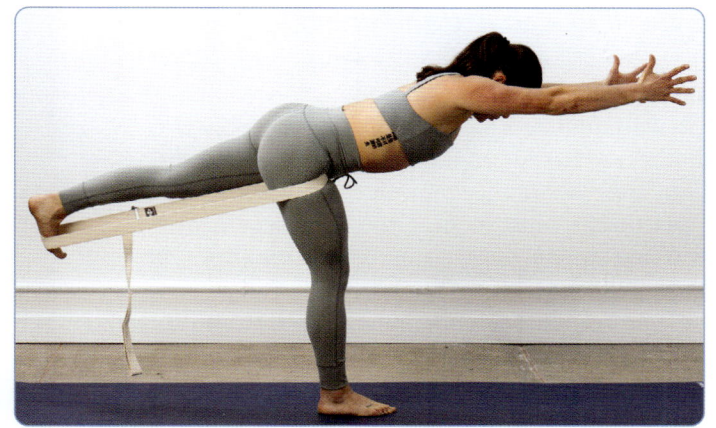

Use a strap to engage and align.

There are a few ways you can adapt warrior III pose using a strap. The first option is by looping a strap around your standing leg thigh and the opposite foot (see the photo). Measure the strap in advance—it is so worth it! The strap simultaneously encourages leveling the hips, anchoring the front thigh back, and engaging through the leg muscles and core stabilizing muscles. By pressing the back foot into the strap, you are also reinforcing a lengthening action in the spine, creating space from your tailbone to the crown of your head. The second option holds many of the same benefits of the previous variation without measuring. Loop the strap around your back foot and hold the ends with your hands. As you hold the strap in your hands, try to keep your arms in line with your torso to inform a neutral spine. This variation also helps to release the shoulder down away from the ears, encouraging length in the cervical spine (neck).

Place your hands on the back of a chair for stability and muscle activation.

In this chair variation of warrior III, your arms will be stretched out in front of you, with your wrists or hands pressing into the back of the chair. Fold a mat or blanket over the back of the chair for more comfort. This variation engages the back muscles, core stabilizing muscles, and the side muscles such as the serratus anterior. The added stability makes it easier to roll the extended leg hip to be level with the other hip—without losing balance as easily.

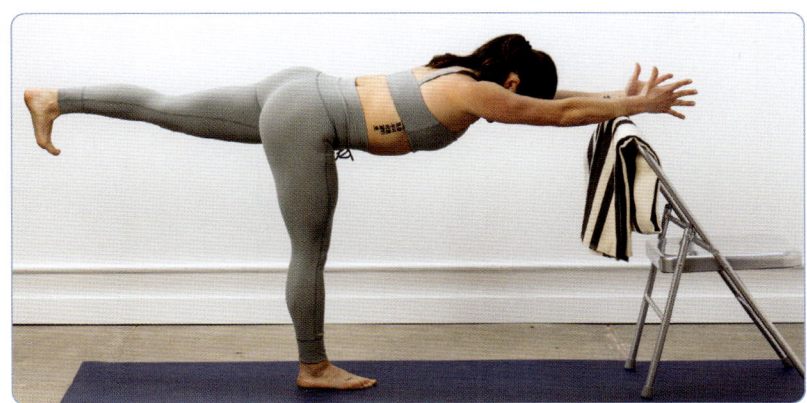

Warrior III Pose *(continued)*

Place your flexed back foot on a wall to stabilize and engage.

This wall variation of warrior III is great for maintaining balance while working on alignment, leveling the hips, and integrating muscle memory for when you are ready to forgo the wall. Place your foot on the wall, level with your hips, and gaze back to ensure all five toes are pointing toward the floor. Actively press your entire foot into the wall to contract the muscles of that leg and hug the front of the standing leg thigh toward the back of the thigh to stabilize the femur bone in the hip socket. Draw your low ribs in toward your spine while simultaneously reaching the rib cage (think thorax region of the upper body) away from your pelvis.

Before you begin, it may help for you to measure your leg distance from the wall by sitting in staff pose (dandasana) with your feet flexed on the wall. The distance from your sitting bones to the wall is the length of your legs. If your back leg doesn't quite reach the wall, or the knee is bent, you can always adjust your distance from the wall!

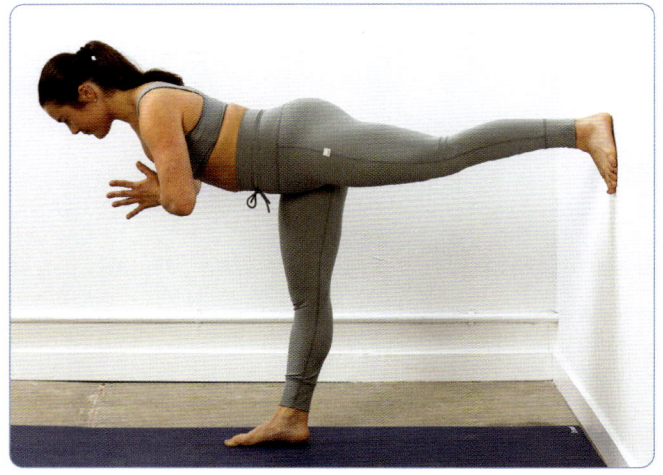

The Complete Guide to Yoga Props

Extended Triangle Pose

Utthita Trikonasana

उत्थिति त्रिकोणासन

Extended triangle pose is a standing posture that not only increases strength and flexibility in the legs, ankles, knees, and hips but also extends a deep stretch to the hips, groin, hamstrings, and calves. Extended triangle pose also opens the shoulders and chest while elongating the spine. Let's explore some ways you can diversify this pose with props.

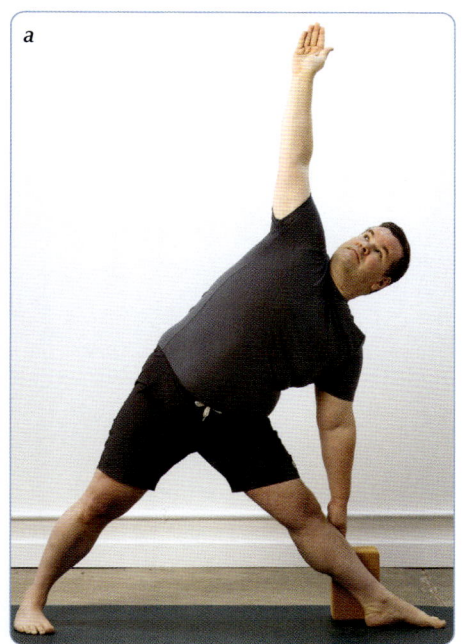

a

Raise the height of the floor with a block or chair.

A block gives you a higher target to reach so you can lengthen the spine and the sides of the body in triangle pose. You can place the block on either side of your front ankle in this posture (see photo a). Placing your hand on a block helps to lengthen the sides of the body by lifting the torso away from the front thigh. Achieving equal length in both sides of the body allows you to breathe more comfortably and makes it easier to roll the chest and shoulders open. If you are looking for even more height, use a chair. Placing your hand or forearm on the seat of a chair can help pave the way to eventually bringing your hand all the way to a block. You can also practice this with the back of the chair framing your front leg and bringing your armpit down to the chair rail to rest as you reach for the chair seat. This helps to encourage stretching through both sides of the waist. See photo b for an example with either the hand or forearm on the chair seat and photo c for an example with the armpit on the back rail of a chair.

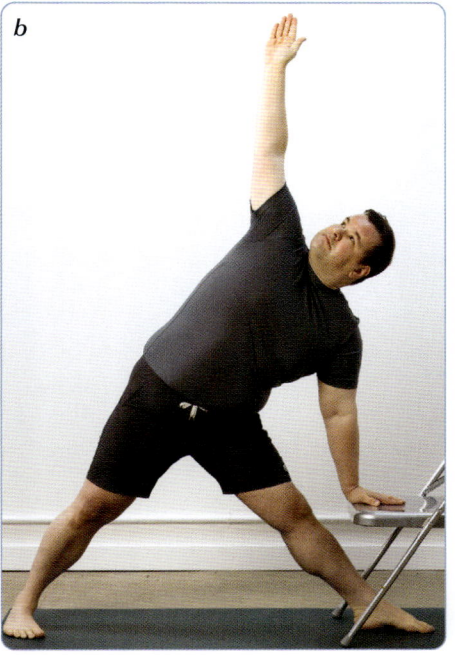

b

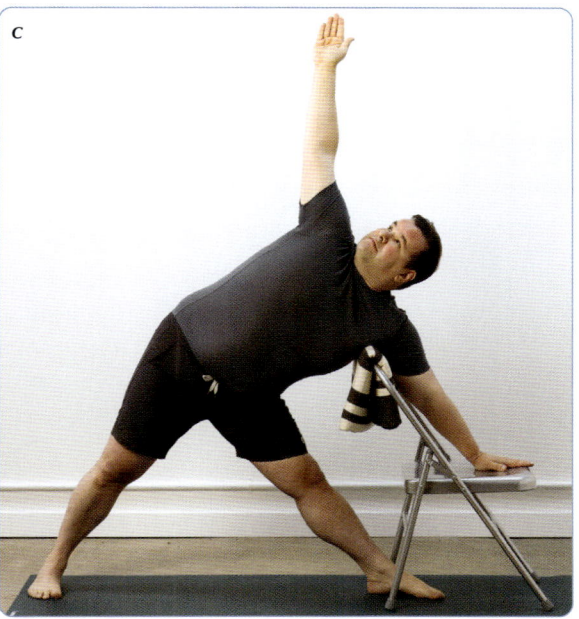

c

Extended Triangle Pose *(continued)*

Place a block between your hands with arms extended to engage your core.

This variation of triangle pose challenges the core, strengthening your obliques, as well as your pectoral muscles, triceps, biceps, serratus anterior muscles, and more. As you hug the block with your hands, try to widen the space between your shoulder blades and draw them down toward your pelvis. Imagine your arms reaching in the same direction as the crown of your head, away from your tailbone.

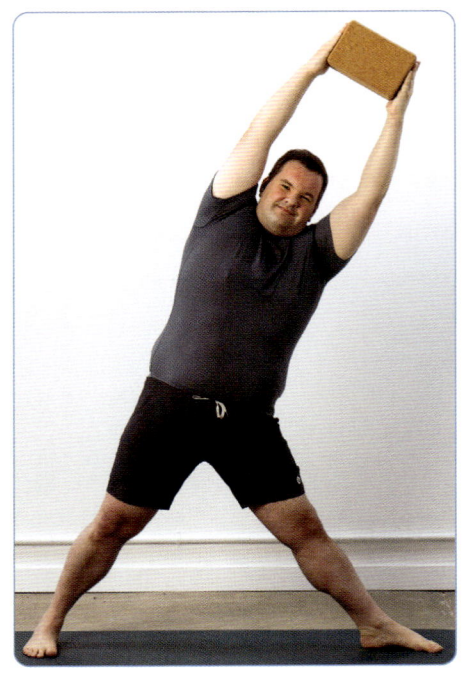

Wedge a block under your front leg calf to counteract hyperextension of the knee.

This variation of triangle pose is a great tool if you tend to hyperextend your legs at the knee joint (when the knees are locked and beyond a normal or safe range). Wedging a block at an angle, under your calf, creates a micro bend in the front knee, helping you to engage the stabilizing muscles surrounding the knee. This means that rather than sinking into bones and joints through your hyperflexibility, the block instead gets you to engage the muscles of the front leg, and it still helps with flexibility! The contraction of the posterior muscles on the front side of the leg helps to lengthen the anterior muscles on the back side of the leg.

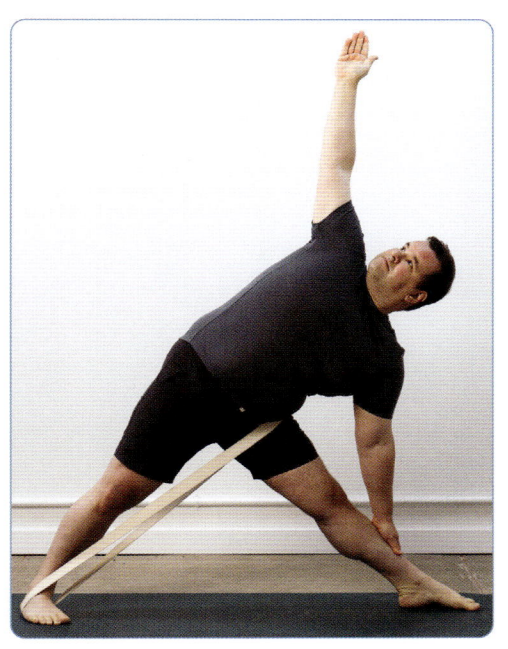

Loop a strap around your front leg hip and back leg foot to self-adjust.

Using a strap in triangle pose helps to pull the femur bone back, freeing up more motion in the hip socket. This helps add length to the side of your waist facing the floor. It also acts as a reminder to engage through the back leg as you push into the strap with your back foot. The back hip should internally rotate some to encourage external rotation of the front thigh. Your front hip will have a bone-on-bone barrier to range of motion if you attempt to externally rotate the back leg; only the front thigh should do this. You may need to play with the size of the loop.

Loop a strap around your back foot and hold it in your back hand.

This is a great variation if you tend to bend from your waist (creating a C shape in the spine), rather than hinging from your hips (creating an I shape in the spine). In triangle pose, imagine two rubber bands, each connecting your low rib bones to your hip points (the anterior superior iliac spine, or ASIS). Strive for equal tension on these two imaginary rubber bands. Hold the strap in your back hand to monitor this. Keep your back arm aligned with the side of your waist and keep tension on the strap. If your spine starts to laterally bend, your back arm and the strap will move away from their previous position. To come back to a long spine, you may have to adjust your bottom hand to a higher position or increase the space between your feet.

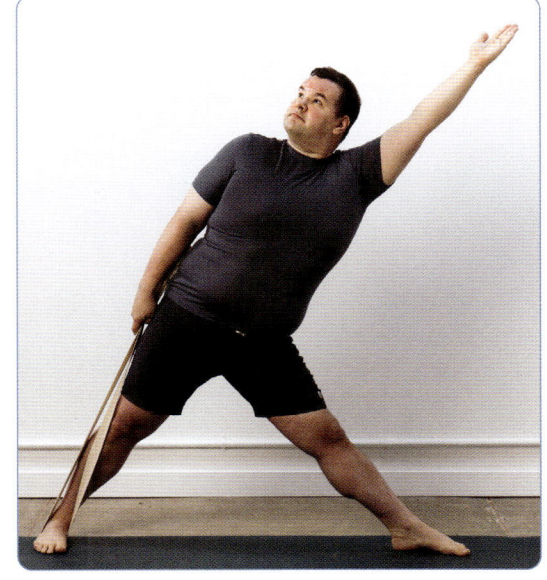

Extended Triangle Pose *(continued)*

Sit in a chair with one leg extended for balance and control.

This modification of triangle pose helps you to stabilize the hips and isolate the movement to the action of the front leg rather than both. Sit on a chair and bring one leg out to the side or at an angle if you can't yet get it all the way out to the side. Enter the pose from there.

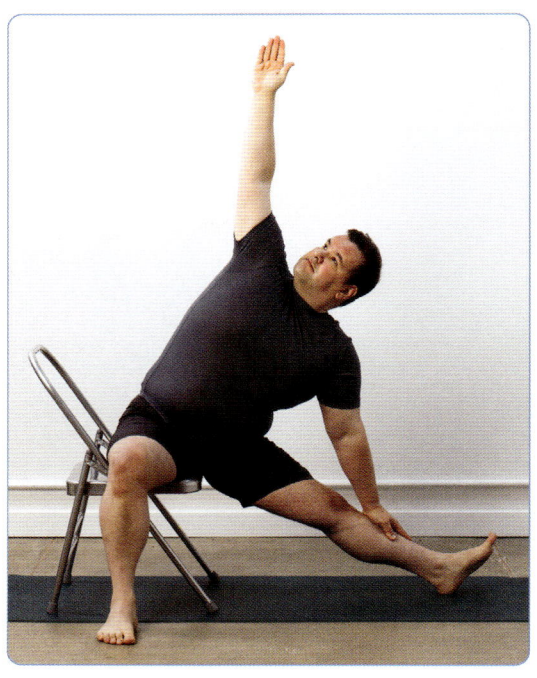

Practice with your back facing a wall to assist in rolling the chest open.

In this variation of the pose, try to align the outer edge of your front foot and your back heel against the wall—adjust though if needed. Enter your triangle pose, paying special attention to the lengthening action of the spine. Start to roll your chest open, steering the backs of your shoulders toward the wall behind you. Instead of the feeling of your top ribs separating from the bottom ribs, imagine your bottom ribs are pushing the top ribs open. Even though the front hip touches the wall, it is OK if the back hip does not; the head of the back femur bone should be internally rotating in the socket. The back toes can be pigeon-toed to assist this.

Intense Side Stretch Pose

Parshvottanasana   पार्श्वोत्तानासन

Intense side stretch pose, most often referred to as pyramid pose, is a forward-bending yoga posture that offers a targeted stretch to the spine, shoulders, hips, and hamstrings. It enhances flexibility and actively strengthens the legs. Moreover, pyramid pose provides a gentle massage to the abdominal organs, contributing to digestive well-being. Let's delve into variations of pyramid pose using props.

Use blocks or a chair under your hands to raise the height of the floor.

Props are a useful tool to bridge the gap between the hands and the mat or floor. They will also assist in finding balance if the floor is out of reach. Try using blocks under your hands to start. If you are working toward a flat back, you can use the blocks to aid in spinal extension as well. You can begin with the blocks right under your shoulders (see photo a), then inhale into a halfway lift, extending through the spine. From here, either fold back into the stretch or walk the blocks forward. Having the blocks farther forward will extend the arms in the direction of the spine, but it is more of a balance challenge! If you are relaxing your spine into the fold, try switching your gaze to the wall behind you to relax the head and neck completely; imagine the brain feeling heavy in the skull. Let the blocks offer support so you can relax deeper into the stretch.

A chair works like blocks under your hands with the key difference being placing your hands on the seat or back of a chair (see photo b). This adds more height than blocks and can be a great step on your way to bringing the hands all the way to the blocks.

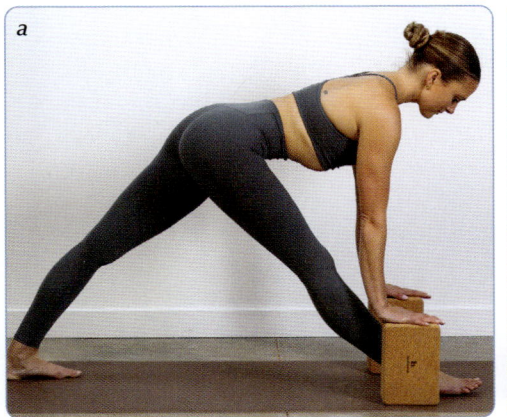

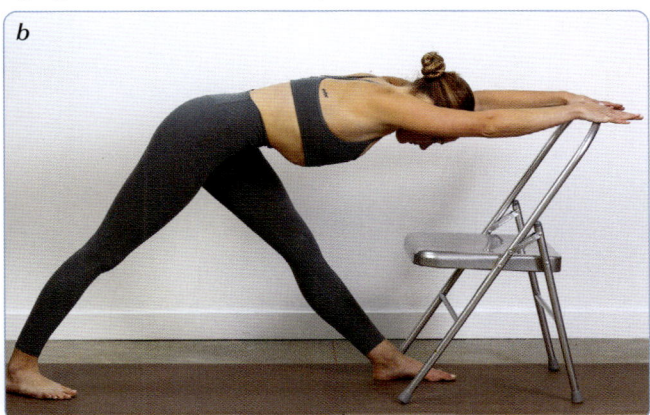

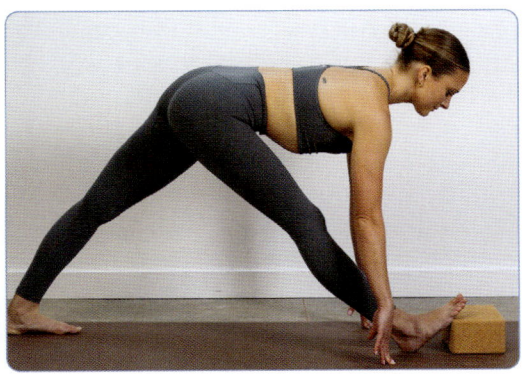

Place a block under your flexed front foot to deepen the stretch.

Using a block in this pose can help to deepen the stretch down the back side of the front leg. Enter your pyramid pose. From here flex through the front foot, reaching the toes back toward the shin and contracting the shin toward the front knee. Turn a block to its lowest height and slide it under the ball of the foot. Inhale, lift halfway, and press through the ball of the foot, contracting the calf. Exhale, fold, and flex the toes toward the shin, releasing the calf muscles.

Wedge a block under your front leg calf to counteract hyperextension of the knee.

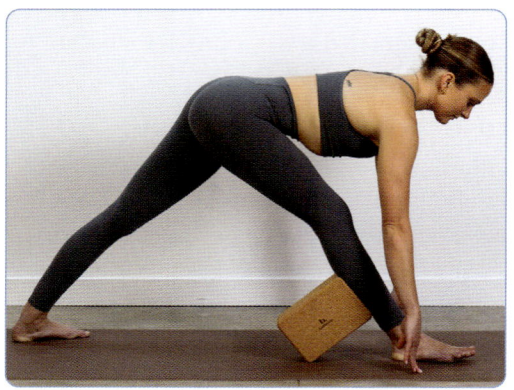

This variation is a great tool if you tend to lock your knees beyond a normal or safe range. A wedged, angled block under your calf creates a small bend in the front knee, helping you to engage the stabilizing muscles surrounding the knee. So rather than sinking into bones and joints through your hyperflexibility, you engage the muscles of the front leg, and it still helps with flexibility! The contraction of the posterior muscles on the front side of the leg helps to stretch the anterior muscles on the back side of the leg.

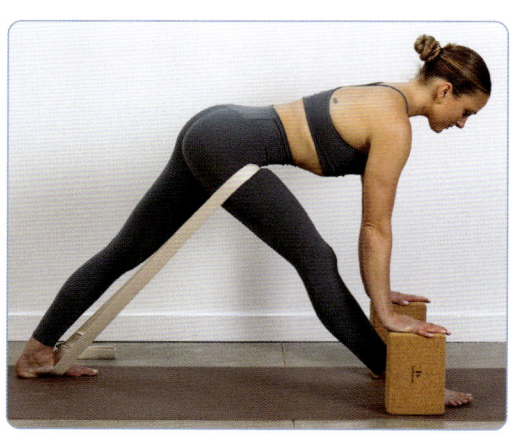

Loop a strap around your back foot and front leg hip to engage and align.

A looped strap in intense side stretch pose reinforces the action of pressing into the outer edge of your back foot. This action engages the muscles of the back leg, lifting through the arch of your back foot and inner thigh, which also supports the knee. As you press into the strap with your back foot, the front of the loop will gently draw your front hip back, rooting the femur bone into your hip socket. You may need to play with the size of the loop to find the best fit.

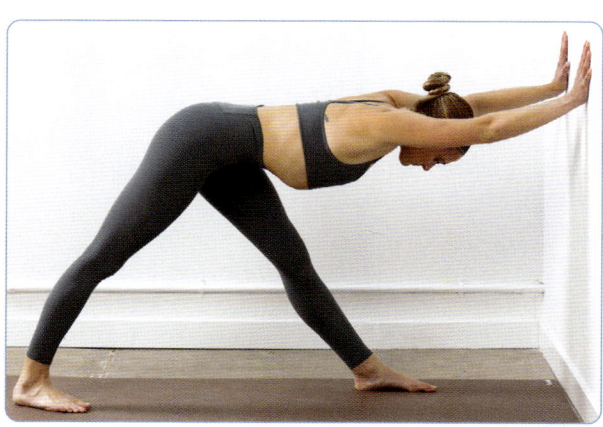

Place your hands on a wall to mindfully uphold the integrity of an extended spine.

If you are working on a fully extended spine in intense side stretch pose, place your hands on a wall in front of you. Start with your hands higher up on the wall, gently pressing into the wall to assist drawing the front hip back and leveling the shoulders. Over time, work the hands farther down the wall, as long as you can still facilitate axial extension in the spine.

Revolved Triangle Pose

Parivritta Trikonasana

परविृत्त त्रकिोणासन

Revolved triangle pose lengthens the gluteal muscles and hamstrings, strengthens the internal and external obliques, opens the chest, and increases twisting mobility in the thoracic spine, providing a comprehensive and revitalizing stretch for the entire body. Explore prop-assisted variations to enhance the benefits of this dynamic yoga posture.

Use a block or a chair to raise the height of the floor.

A block helps reduce the distance between you and the floor, lengthen the spine and through the sides of the body in this posture. You can place your hand on the block on either side of your front ankle to stretch the sides of your body away from the hips and your torso away from the front thigh (see photo *a*). When you achieve equal length in both sides of the waist, it allows you to breathe more comfortably and facilitates the thoracic rotation of the spine. Alternatively, if you require more height, try placing your hand or forearm on the seat or back of a chair (see photo *b*). This works like a block under your bottom hand, but the chair adds more height than a block and can be a great assistance toward eventually bringing the hand all the way to the block.

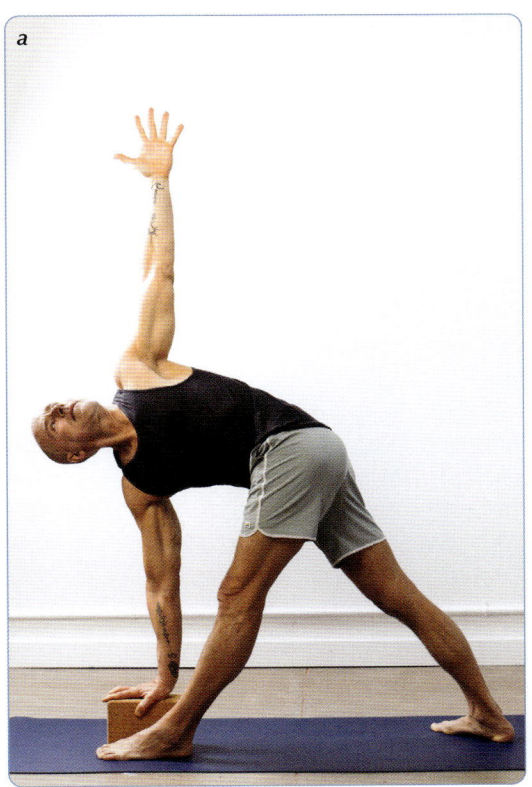

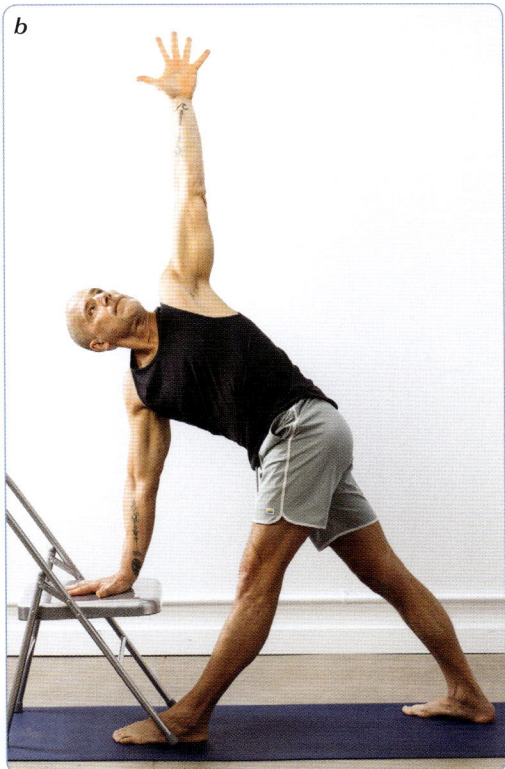

Revolved Triangle Pose (continued)

Loop a strap around your front leg hip and back leg foot to engage and align.

Using a looped strap in this pose reinforces the action of pressing into the outer edge of your back foot and engages the muscles of the back leg, lifting through the arch of your back foot and inner thigh, which also supports the knee. As you press into the strap with your back foot, the front of the loop will gently draw your front hip back, rooting the femur bone into your hip socket. You may need to play with the size of the loop to find the best fit.

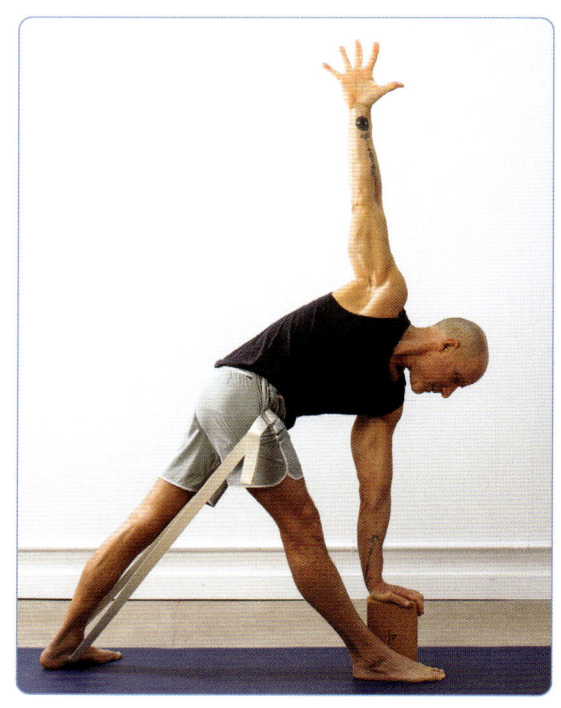

Loop a strap around your rib cage and hold the end of the strap in your top hand to assist thoracic rotation.

Revolved triangle pose requires engaging your internal and external obliques. A strap is a way to self-assist this action! Loop the strap securely around your rib cage to avoid slipping but maintaining breathing comfort. The end of the loop, where the excess strap ends, should be near your bottom ribs (facing the floor as you twist). Hold the excess strap in your top hand, and as you reach your hand toward the sky, the gentle pull on the bottom ribs should encourage the barrel of the rib cage to rotate open—an action generated in the thoracic spine.

The Complete Guide to Yoga Props

Practice against a wall to rotate and align.

You can practice this pose with a wall in a couple of ways on the same side. The first way, with your back facing the wall (see photo a), requires active flexibility known as mobility. The second way, with the belly facing the wall (see photo b), allows you to walk your hand up the wall and use it as leverage, encouraging passive flexibility. Both options help facilitate thoracic rotation of the spine. They also both help you to stabilize the hips, pinning the outer hip to the wall.

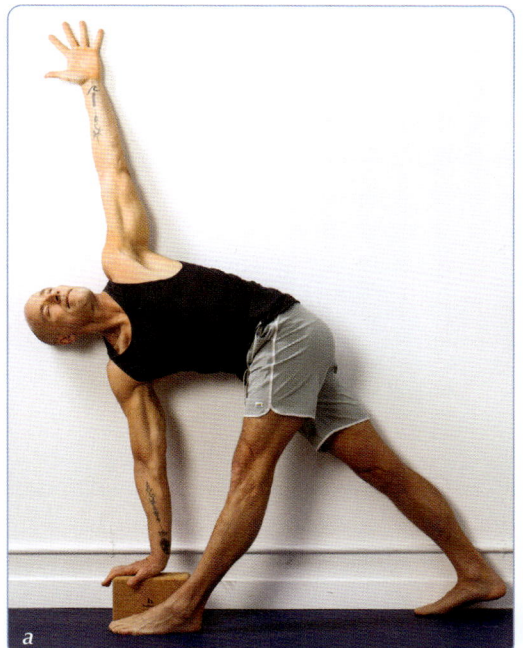
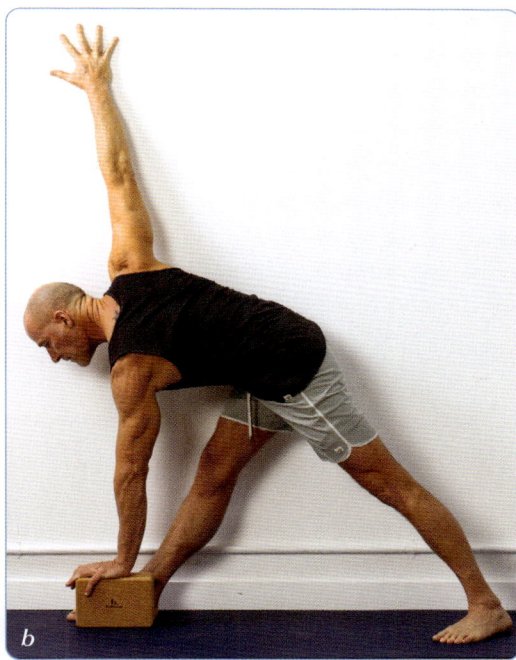

Extended Side Angle Pose

Utthita Parshvakonasana   उत्थति पार्श्वकोणासन

Extended side angle pose strengthens the legs, knees, and ankles, while simultaneously opening the groin, waist, chest, shoulders, and lungs. Additionally, it engages the muscles responsible for spinal extension. Let's explore some prop-supported variations for this pose.

Place your hand on a block to help lengthen and stabilize.

With a block, you can bring the floor to you in extended side angle pose. This variation lengthens the spine as well as the sides of the body. You can place the block on either side of your front ankle in this posture. Placing your hand on a block helps to lengthen the sides of the body away from the hips by lifting the torso away from the front thigh. Achieving equal length in both sides of the body allows you to breathe more comfortably and makes it easier to roll the chest and shoulders open.

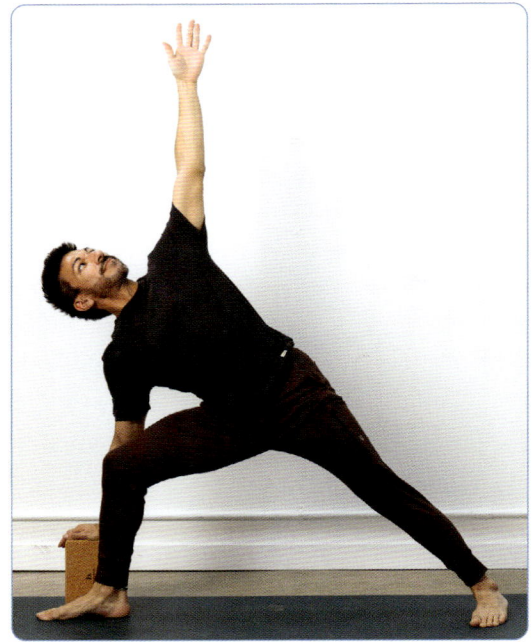

Kneel with a blanket under your knee for joint support.

A great way to modify this posture is by practicing it kneeling. To cushion and protect the knee, you can place a folded blanket underneath.

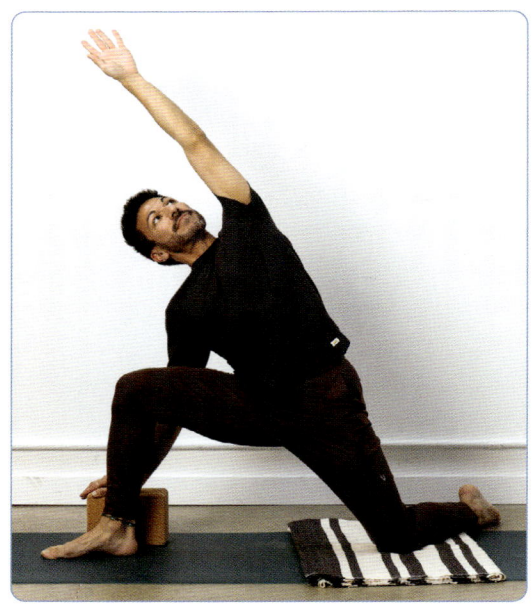

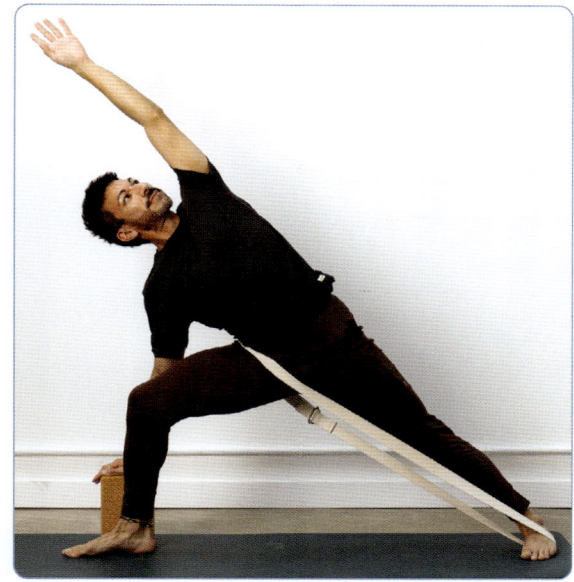

Loop a strap around your front leg hip and back leg foot to self-adjust.

Using a strap here helps to pull the femur bone back, freeing up motion in the hip socket to externally rotate through your front thigh. This helps add length to the side of your waist facing the floor. It also acts as a reminder to engage through the back leg as you push into the strap with your back foot. You may need to play with the size of the loop for proper fit.

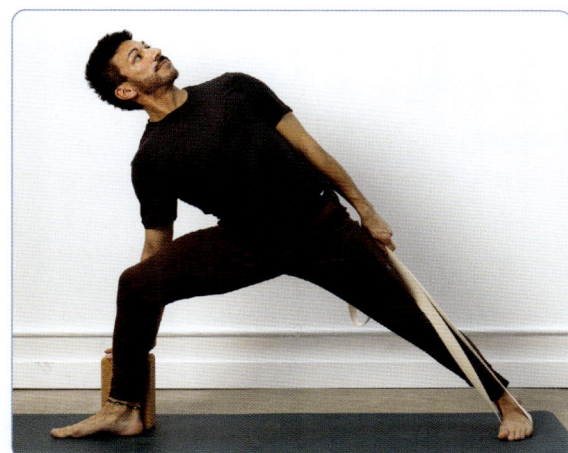

Loop a strap around your back foot and hold in your back hand.

This is a great variation if you tend to bend from your waist (creating a C shape in the spine), rather than hinging from your hips (creating an I shape in the spine). In extended side angle pose, you want to do just that: extend your side angle rather than arch into a lateral bend. Imagine two rubber bands, each connecting your low rib bones to your hip points (the anterior superior iliac spine or ASIS). Work on having equal tension on these two imaginary rubber bands. Hold the strap in your back hand to monitor this. Keep your back arm aligned with the side of your waist and the strap aligned with your back leg. If your spine starts to laterally bend, your back arm and the strap will move away from their previous position. To return to a long spine, you may have to adjust your bottom hand to a higher position or increase the space between your feet.

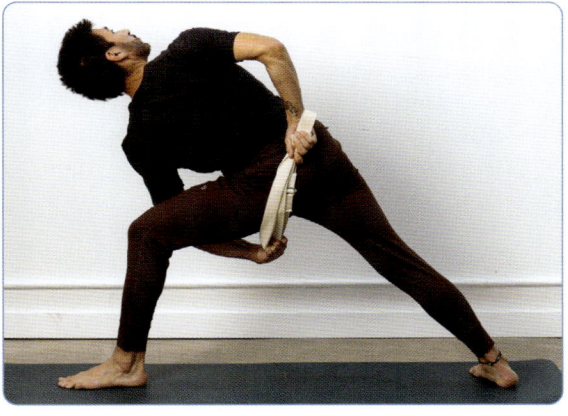

Practice a bind with a strap between your hands to create space.

A strap is a handy tool to free up space in your shoulders in this posture. It can bridge the gap between your hands if they are just out of reach from one another. Even if you can bind your hands, sometimes it is to the sacrifice of your spinal alignment, causing forward hunching, or resting your waist on your thigh via lateral bending of the spine. A strap may come in handy as you maintain length in both sides of the body and gradually work your hands closer together.

Sit in a chair for balance and stability.

When practicing this pose in a chair, the front leg is supported by the chair, which helps you to feel more balanced and aligned. You can even use the back of the chair to practice a half bind by reaching back with your hand for the back railing of the chair, opening across the chest and shoulders.

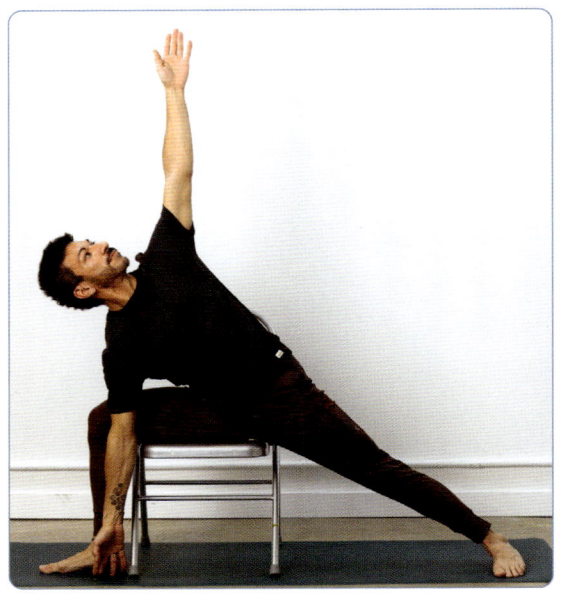

Place your shin against the seat of a chair to align.

Another creative way to use a chair in this posture is to simply inform knee alignment. Place a chair against a wall and bring your knee or shin (depending on height) to the edge of the seat. Your ankle should ideally be directly under the knee with your toes pointing straight at the wall. The contact with the chair seat informs you when your knee strays from the originally-intended position. Reach your top arm to the wall, and if your fingertips reach, gently press them into the wall to strengthen the top side of your waist and lengthen the bottom half.

High Crescent Lunge Pose

Ashta Chandrasana   अष्ट चन्द्रासन

High crescent lunge pose, a dynamic yoga posture, actively opens your groin and hips, tones leg muscles, strengthens the core, increases overhead mobility, and improves balance. Let's look at a few common variations of high lunge pose using props.

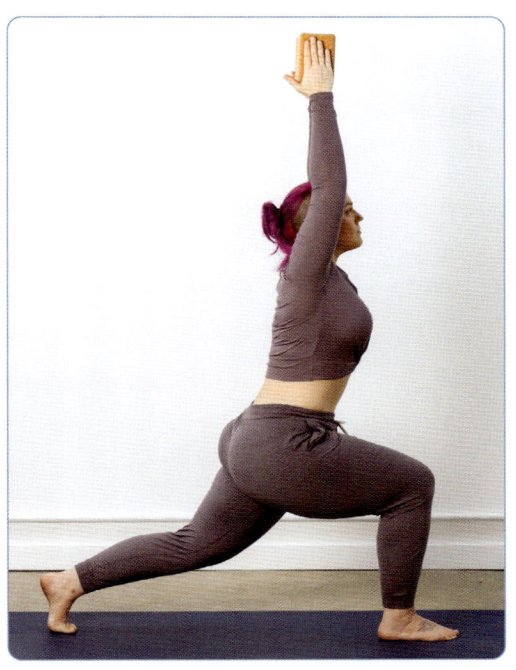

Place a block between your hands.

This variation of high lunge pose lets you really kick this pose up a notch! By squeezing a block between your hands while attempting to raise your biceps to your ears, you need to really tap into your shoulder mobility and muscles along your back. The block also helps to encourage external rotation of the shoulders; as you hold the block between your hands, try to wrap your upper arm bones forward and in.

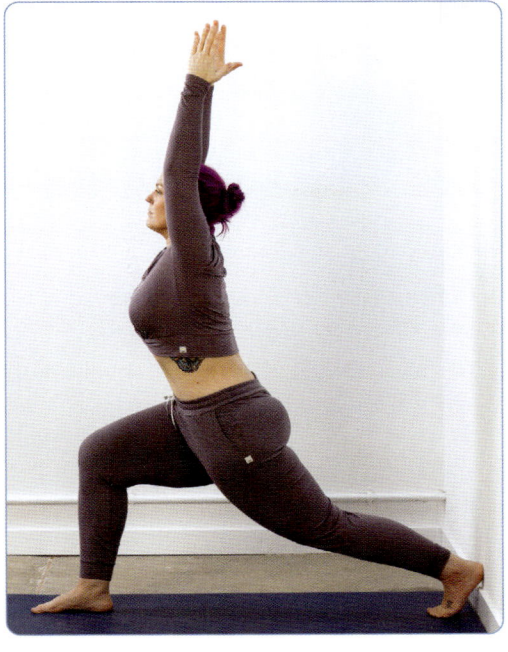

Press your back heel into a wall to stabilize and inform.

Using a wall can inform both alignment and muscle action in high lunge pose. By stabilizing the back heel, you can prevent rolling the ankle to either side. Once the heel is stable you can use the wall to reinforce the actions of your leg muscles so that you are not simply resting in the pose or sinking into your joints. Press your back heel directly back into the wall, firing up through your quadriceps, as if your back knee were lifting toward your hip.

High Crescent Lunge Pose (continued)

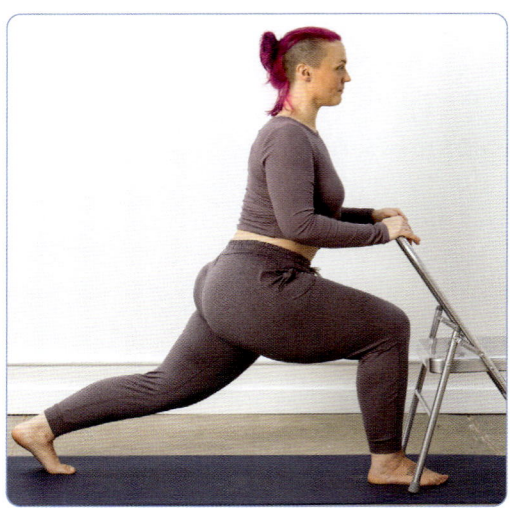

Place your hands on the back of a chair for balance.

Balancing your weight on the sole of the front foot and ball of the back foot in a narrow line can be challenging! To steady your balance, try starting with your hands on the back of a chair. Use the chair to level through your shoulders and practice lifting one hand overhead at a time; eventually progress to lifting both hands, with the chair in place if needed.

Sit in a chair for balance and stability.

When practicing this pose in a chair, the front leg is supported by the chair, which helps you to feel more balanced and aligned. You can hold onto the back of the chair for extra support. If the chair is too high, place blocks under your feet.

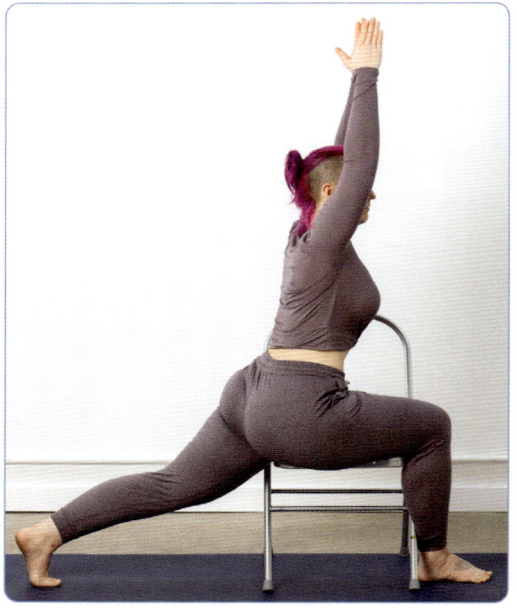

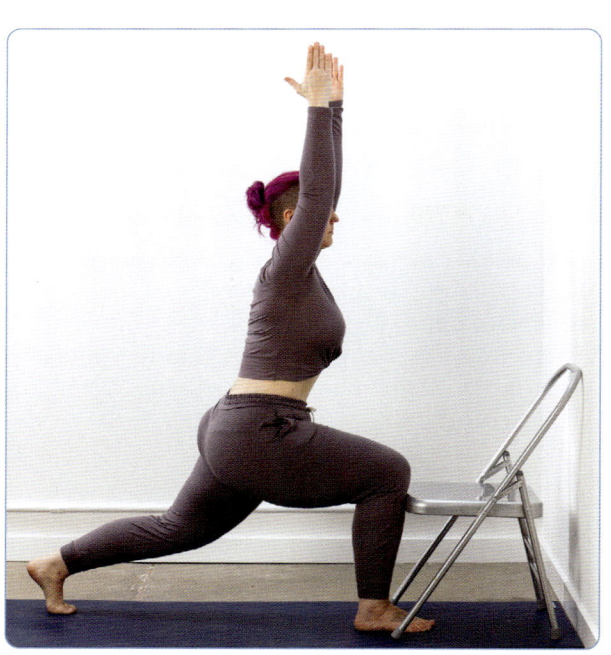

Place your shin against the seat of a chair to align.

This variation supports knee-over-ankle alignment, using the chair seat as reference. Place a chair against a wall and bring your knee to the edge of the seat. Keep your ankle directly under your knee with your toes pointing straight at the wall. The contact with the chair seat informs the placement of the knee so that the knee stays in the right spot.

Revolved Side Angle Pose and Revolved Crescent Lunge Pose

Parivritta Parshvakonasana and Parivritta Anjaneyasana   परिवृत्त पार्श्वकोणासन and परिवृत्त अञ्जनेयासन

These revolved standing postures strengthen the spine, hips, legs, and buttocks. These poses also stimulate and detoxify internal organs and kidneys, contributing to improved digestion. Let's explore a variety of common variations for both poses using props to enhance or access their benefits.

Place your hand on a block to help lengthen and stabilize.

A block helps raise the height of the floor, lengthen the spine, and lengthen through the sides of the body in these postures. Place the block at your preferred height outside your front ankle and then place your hand on the block to help lengthen the side body away from the hips by lifting the torso away from the front thigh (see photo *a* for an example of a revolved side angle pose with a block and photo *b* for an example of revolved crescent lunge pose with a block). Achieving equal length in both sides of the body allows you to breathe more comfortably and makes thoracic rotation of the spine easier.

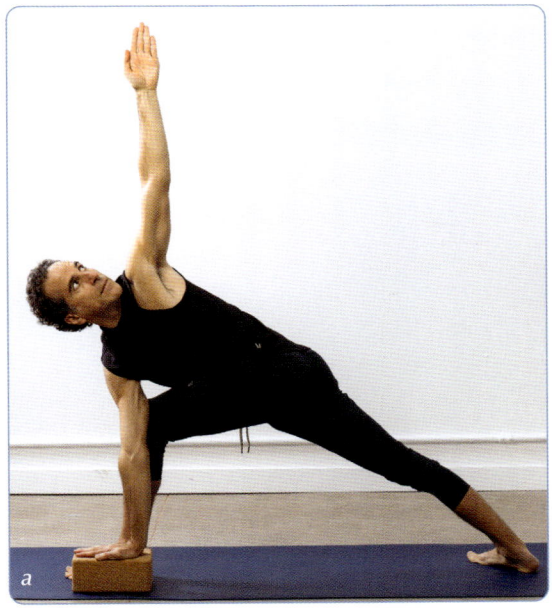
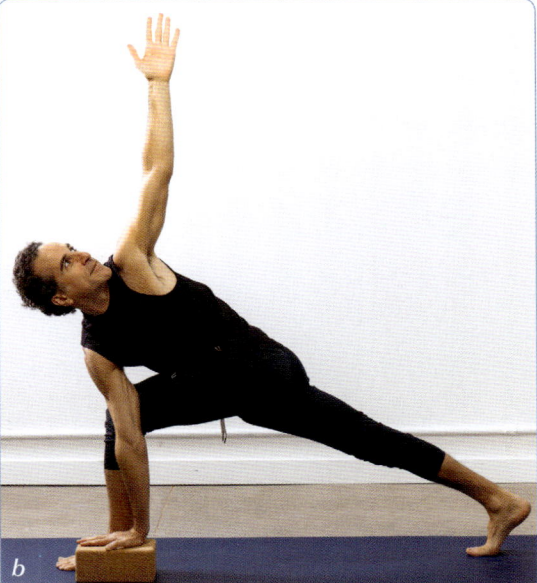

Revolved Side Angle Pose
and Revolved Crescent Lunge Pose (continued)

Kneel with a blanket under your knee to ground and support.

It may prove challenging to balance in revolved crescent lunge with the back knee lifted, so why not ground the back knee to focus your attention on the twist? This provides more stability and support for the sacroiliac joint as you begin your thoracic rotation. Use a blanket under your knee to support your knee.

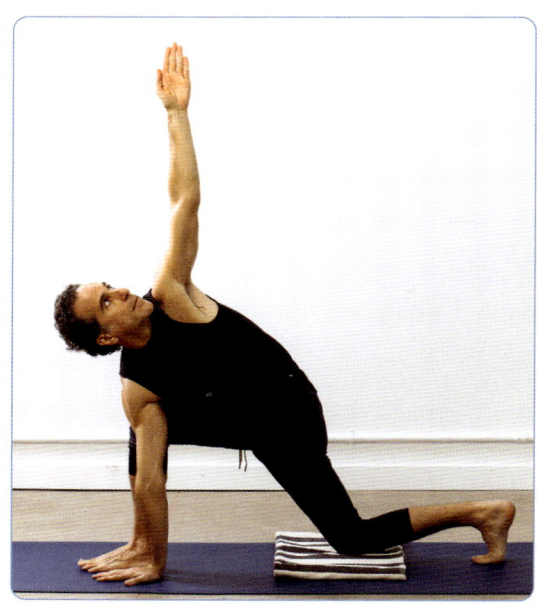

Press your back heel into a wall to stabilize and inform.

Using a wall can inform both alignment and muscle action in revolved crescent lunge. Stabilizing the back heel helps prevent rolling the ankles to either side. It allows you to use the wall to reinforce the actions of your leg muscles so that you are not simply resting in the pose or sinking into your joints. Press your back heel directly back into the wall, engaging the muscles up through your quadriceps, as if your back knee were lifting toward your hip. Continue to press your back heel into the wall and reach your torso forward and away from your hips. This lengthens your spine before you twist.

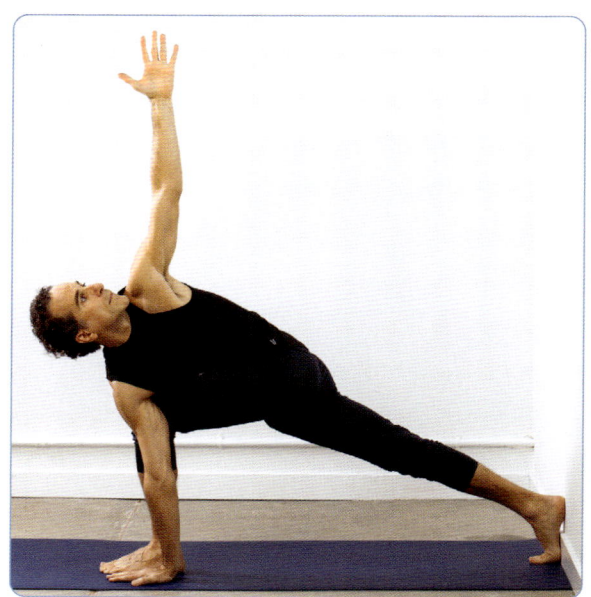

Practice using a wall for support and stability.

This variation of revolved crescent lunge pose can be done standing or kneeling. It offers support for you to deepen into the twist without compromising alignment in the knees or

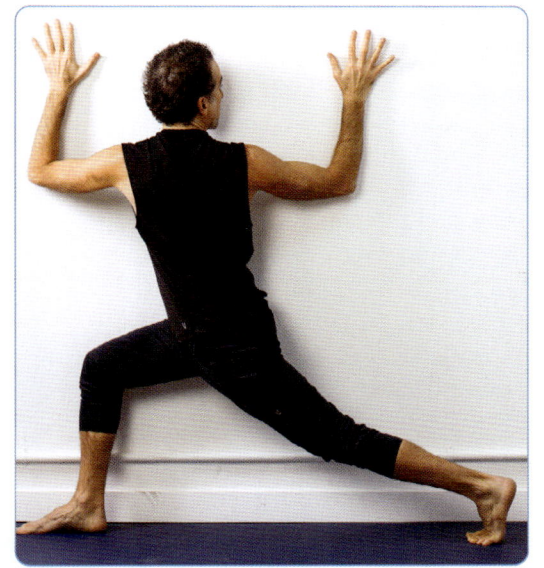

hips. If you experience sacroiliac pain or have a known SI joint derangement, allow the outer hip to roll in slightly rather than trying to have both hips perfectly square. Square hips and twisting are more friendly toward one another when the hips are grounded; otherwise, there is more possibility of straining this joint. In this variation, use the wall to create more space across your chest by raising your arms cactus style and pressing into the wall with the elbow closest to the front leg. The wall also helps to get the shoulders directly over the hips and prevents hunching or rounding the spine.

Sit in a chair.

Here are two ways you can use a chair in revolved side angle and revolved crescent lunge pose. In the first version of this variation, the front leg is supported by the chair seat; the back of the chair is on the side you will be twisting toward. As you twist, you can have both hands on the back of the chair or extend your bottom hand down the leg of the chair or onto a block or the mat (see photo a). In the second version of this variation, you will slide your back leg through the hole in the back of the chair and use the chair seat to support your front leg. Bring your hands to prayer to begin and on an exhale find your twist (see photo b). Reach for the back of the chair with your back hand. If you want to deepen the stretch, you can reach your bottom hand down the leg of the chair closest to your front foot.

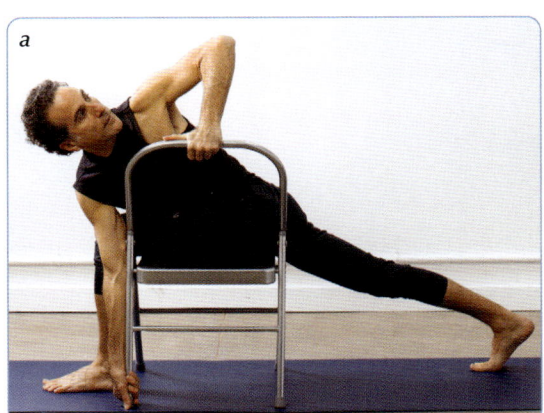

a

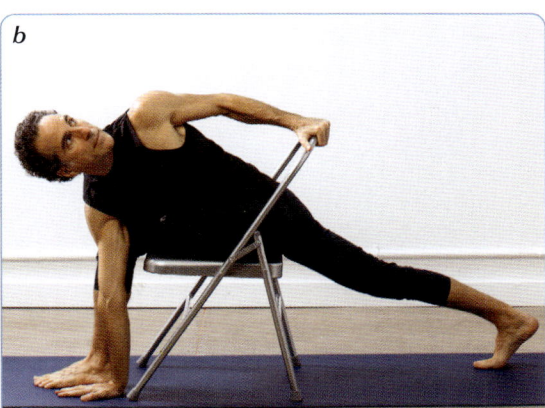

b

Revolved Side Angle Pose
and Revolved Crescent Lunge Pose (continued)

Loop a strap around your rib cage and hold the end of the strap in your top hand to assist thoracic rotation.

In revolved side angle pose, you engage your internal and external obliques. Use a strap to assist this action. Loop the strap securely around your rib cage to avoid slipping but maintaining breathing comfort. The end of the loop, where the excess strap ends, should be near your bottom ribs (facing the floor as you twist). Hold the excess strap in your top hand, and as you reach your hand toward the sky, feel the gentle pull on the bottom ribs that encourages the barrel of the rib cage to rotate open—an action generated in the thoracic spine.

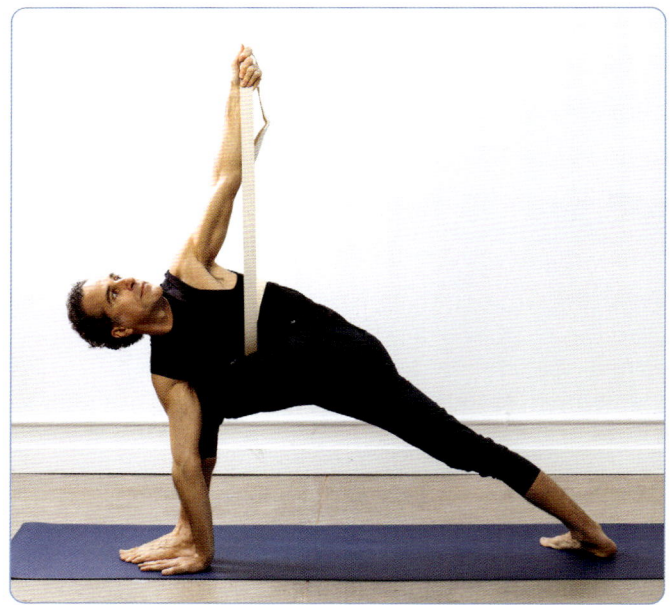

The Complete Guide to Yoga Props

Half Moon Pose

Ardha Chandrasana

अर्ध चन्द्रासन

Half moon pose is a challenging asymmetrical balancing posture that strengthens the spine, hips, ankles, legs, and gluteal muscles. It offers a deep stretch to the shoulders, waist, hamstrings, and calves, contributing to improved flexibility, while enhancing overall balance. Let's review some common prop-supported variations for this pose.

Use a block or a chair to raise the height of the floor.

A block helps reduce the distance between you and the floor, lengthen the spine and through the sides of the body in half moon pose. Place the block in front of your standing foot so that it falls directly below the shoulder of your bottom arm. Placing your hand on a block helps to lengthen the sides of the body and lift your torso closer to level with the height of your hips (see photo a). The block may also provide you with more stability. Alternatively, if you require more height, try placing your hand or forearm on the seat or back of a chair (see photo b). This works like a block under your bottom hand, but the chair is higher than a block and can be a great stepping stone toward bringing the hand all the way to the block one day.

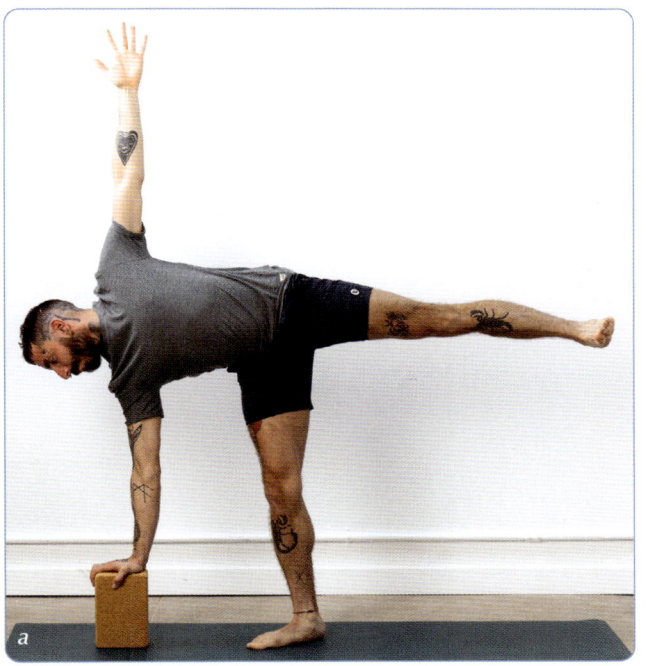

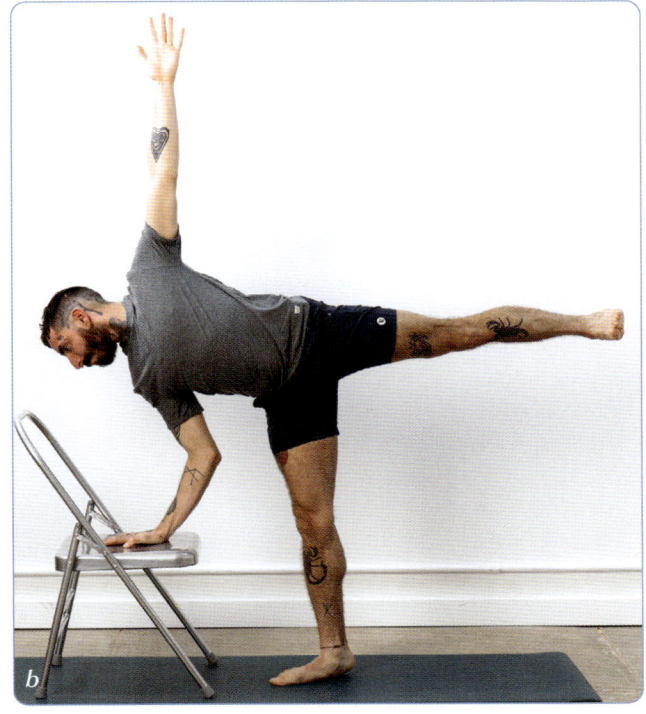

Kneel with a blanket under your knee to ground and support.

This variation allows you to engage your deep core muscles with more stability and provides more surface area to balance on. The bottom hip is not turned out as it is in the standing version, so you're going to feel this in different muscles in the top leg. Instead of the external rotators, you are engaging your leg abductors. You will feel this in the outer hip and glute of the lifted leg especially! Use a blanket under your knee to support your knee.

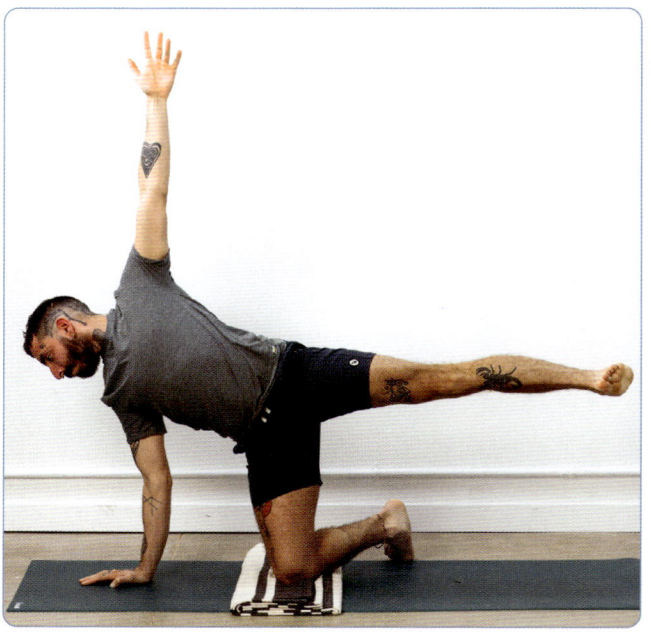

Place your flexed back foot on a wall to stabilize and engage.

This wall variation is great for maintaining balance while working on alignment, leveling the hips, and integrating muscle memory for when you are ready to take the posture off the wall. Place your foot on the wall, level with the height of your hips, and work toward all five toes pointing at a 90-degree angle to the side. Actively press your entire foot into the wall to contract the muscles of that leg and hug the front of your standing-leg thigh toward the back of the thigh to stabilize the femur bone in the hip socket. Draw your low ribs in toward your spine and lengthen through your waist as you roll the shoulder and chest open.

Before you begin, it may help for you to measure your leg distance from the wall by sitting in staff pose (dandasana) with your feet flexed on the wall. The distance from your sitting bones to the wall is the length of your legs. If your back leg doesn't quite reach the wall or the knee is bent, you can adjust your distance from the wall.

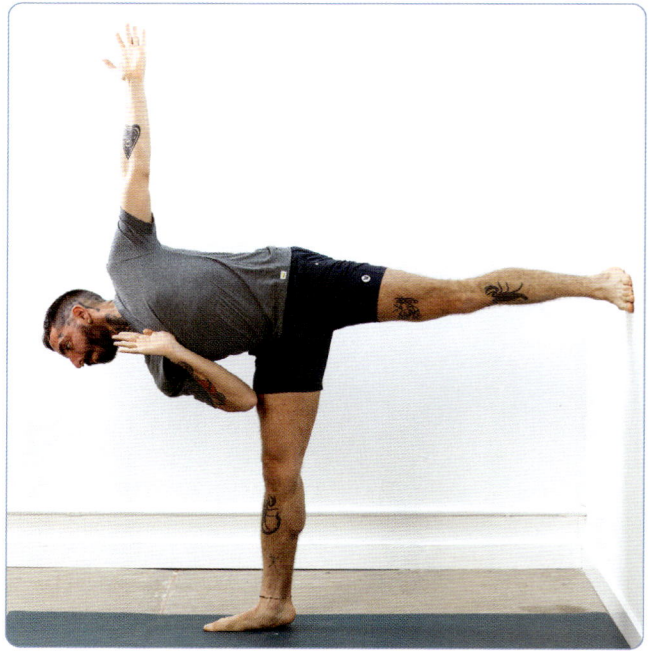

Press your back against a wall to stack the joints.

Using a wall behind you helps you to build muscle memory of where your limbs and joints should be relative to one another. As you enter the half moon pose, feel your top hip and shoulder stacking over the bottom hip and shoulder. Press your back heel into the wall behind you to engage through the leg muscles. Work your top arm in the direction of the wall. Reach the crown of your head away from your tailbone.

Loop a strap around your back foot and hold it in your back hand.

This is a great variation if you tend to hinge at your hips or arch your back in half moon pose. Keep your back arm aligned with the side of your waist and the strap aligned with your back leg. If your spine starts to arch or bend, your back arm and the strap will move away from their previous position. The strap is your alignment guide. Pressing your foot into the back of the strap also helps to create space in the bottom side of the waist, lengthening the spine and lifting your shoulders level with your hips. This is especially helpful if you are working toward lifting your bottom hand off the block or mat. Another option is to hold the strap in your top hand and reach your arm up toward the sky (see the photo). This is especially beneficial if you have thoracic scoliosis. Practice this variation with the convex side of the

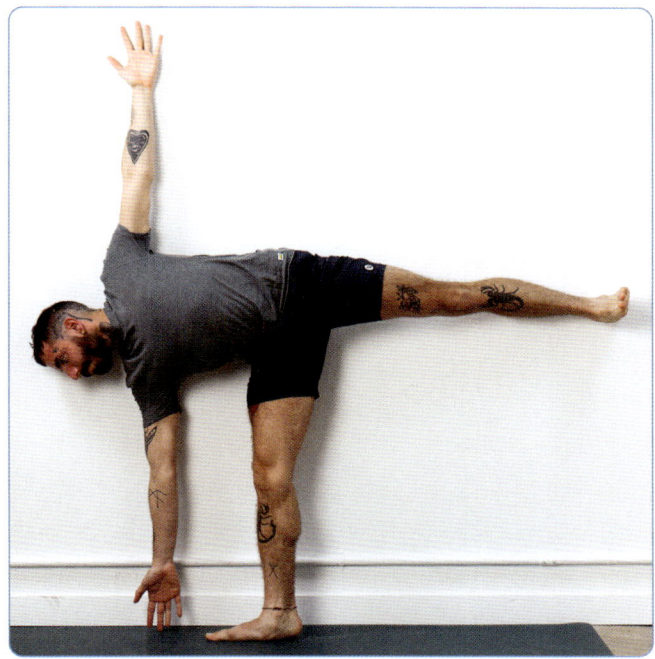

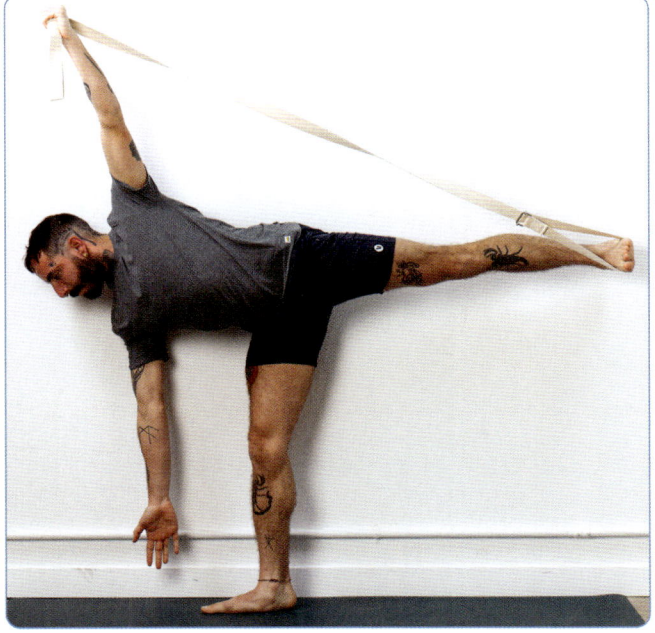

curve facing the floor. You can help to counteract the scoliosis by pulling on the strap, strengthening the thoracic muscles on the lower side.

Half Moon Pose *(continued)*

Practice sugarcane variation with a strap.

Looping a strap around your back ankle is a great way to close the space between your hand and your back foot in sugarcane pose (ardha chandra chapasana). For this variation of half moon pose, you can either loop the strap fully around your ankle and hold the excess in your back hand or have an open loop holding both ends of the strap in your back hand. If you are using the open loop version, flex your back ankle to keep the strap from sliding off. See photo *a* for a version of the pose where your arm is reaching back and you kick your heel away from the gluteal muscles to open the chest and shoulders. See photo *b* for a version of the pose where your arm is reaching overhead and you draw the heel of your foot closer to your head.

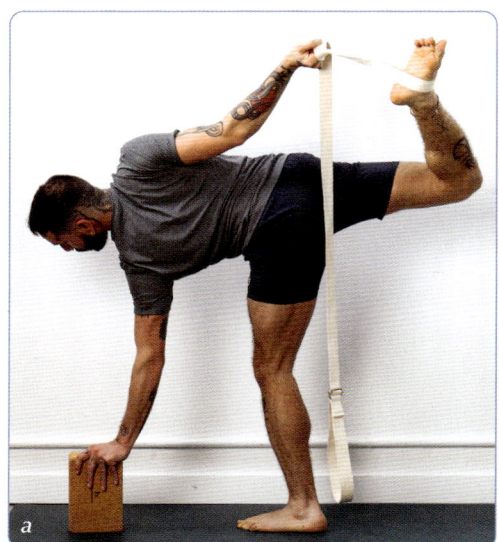 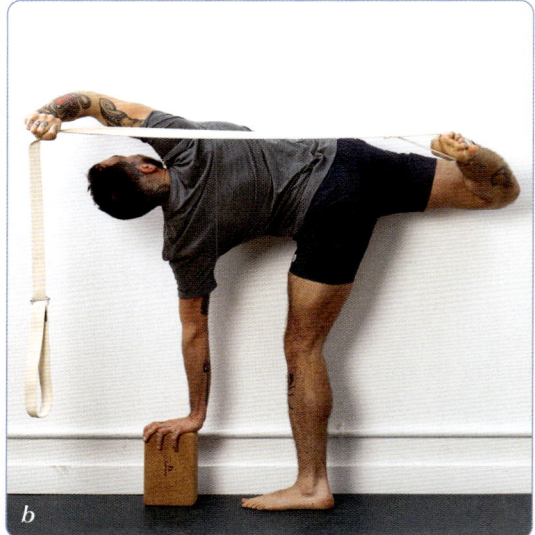

Revolved Half Moon Pose

Parivritta Ardha Chandrasana   परविृत्त अर्ध चंद्रासन

Revolved half moon pose is a challenging posture that not only tests your balance but also enhances mobility through its twisting motion. This pose effectively strengthens leg muscles, engages internal and external obliques, and contributes to overall balance improvement. Let's review some common prop-supported variations for this pose.

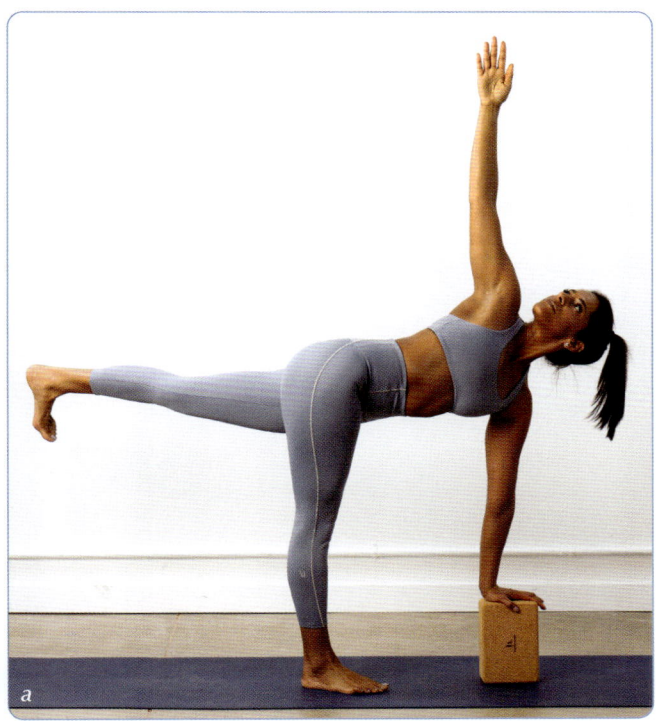

a

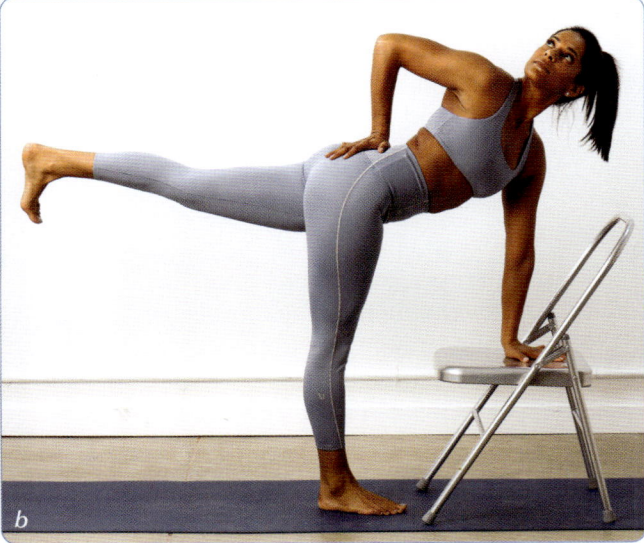

b

Place your hand on a block or chair to raise the height of the floor.

A block helps reduce the distance between you and the floor, lengthen the spine, and lengthen the sides of the body in this posture. You can place the block in front of your standing foot and slightly inside of it, so that it falls directly below the shoulder of your bottom arm. Placing your hand on a block helps to lengthen the sides of the body and lift your torso closer to level with the height of your hips (see photo a). The block may provide you with more stability as well. The added length in the spine will also allow you to breathe more comfortably and makes thoracic rotation easier. Alternatively, if you require more height, try placing your hand or forearm on the seat or back of a chair (see photo b). This works similarly to a block under your bottom hand with the key difference being that the chair is higher than a block and can help you progress to bringing the hand all the way to the block one day.

Revolved Half Moon Pose *(continued)*

Kneel with a blanket under your knee to ground and support.

This variation allows you to engage your deep core muscles with more stability. It may prove challenging to balance in this pose, so an option is to practice kneeling to focus your attention on the twist. Use a blanket under your knee for support. Begin in balancing table pose (dandayamana bharmanasana), extending an opposite leg and arm off the mat from table top position, then roll the chest open, reaching your hand or elbow toward the sky (see photo a). For more stability, you can also ground the back leg (see photo b).

Place your flexed back foot on a wall to stabilize and engage.

This wall variation is great for maintaining balance while working

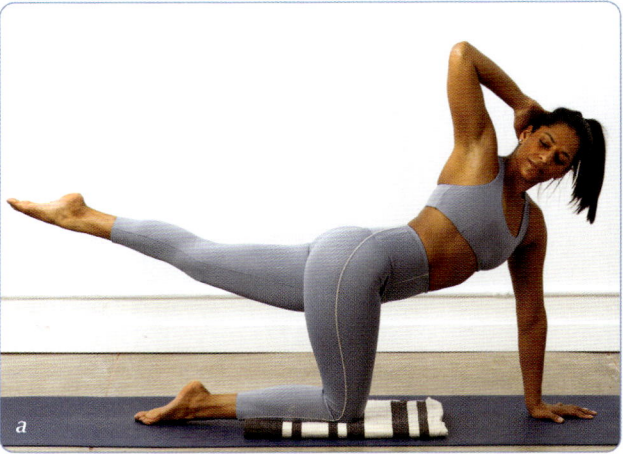

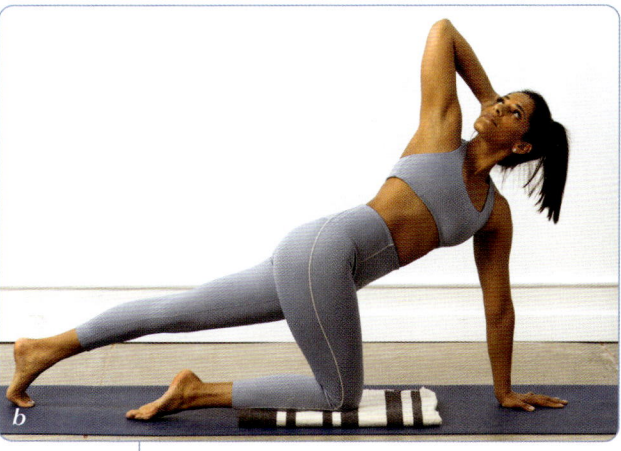

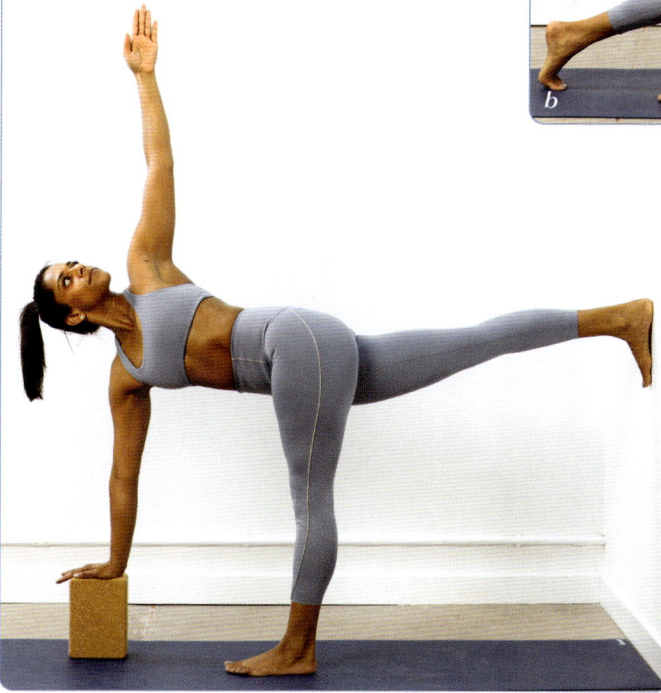

on alignment, leveling the hips, and developing muscle memory for forgoing the wall. Place your foot on the wall, hip high, and gaze back to ensure all five toes are pointing to the floor. Actively press your entire foot into the wall to contract the muscles of that leg and hug the front of the standing-leg thigh toward the back of the thigh to stabilize the femur bone in the hip socket. Draw your low ribs in toward your spine and begin rolling the barrel of the ribs open into your twist.

The Complete Guide to Yoga Props

It may help for you to measure your leg distance from the wall before beginning by sitting in staff pose (dandasana) with your feet flexed on the wall. The distance from your sitting bones to the wall is the length of your legs. If your back leg doesn't quite reach the wall or the knee is bent, you can always adjust your distance from the wall!

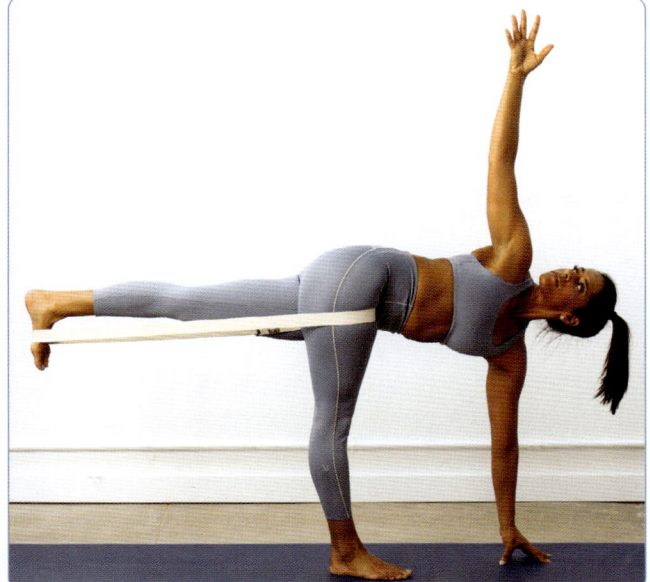

Loop a strap around your front leg hip and back leg foot to engage and align.

Using a looped strap in this pose reinforces the action of pressing into the back foot while squaring the back toes toward the floor. This engages the muscles of the back leg and stretches the torso away from the hips, creating the necessary space for a deeper twist. As you press into the strap with your back foot, the front of the loop will gently draw your front hip back, rooting the femur bone into your hip socket. You may need to experiment with the size of the loop to find the best fit.

Loop a strap around your rib cage and hold the end of the strap in your top hand to assist thoracic rotation.

In this variation, you can ground your back foot against a wall for stability or practice away from the wall as shown. To rotate through the spine, you must engage your internal and external obliques. Use a strap to assist this action. Loop the strap securely around your rib cage to avoid slipping while maintaining breathing comfort. The end of the loop where the excess strap ends should be near your bottom ribs. Hold the excess strap in your top hand, and as you reach your hand to the sky, feel the gentle pull on the bottom ribs. This gentle pull should encourage the barrel of the rib cage to rotate open, an action generated in the thoracic spine.

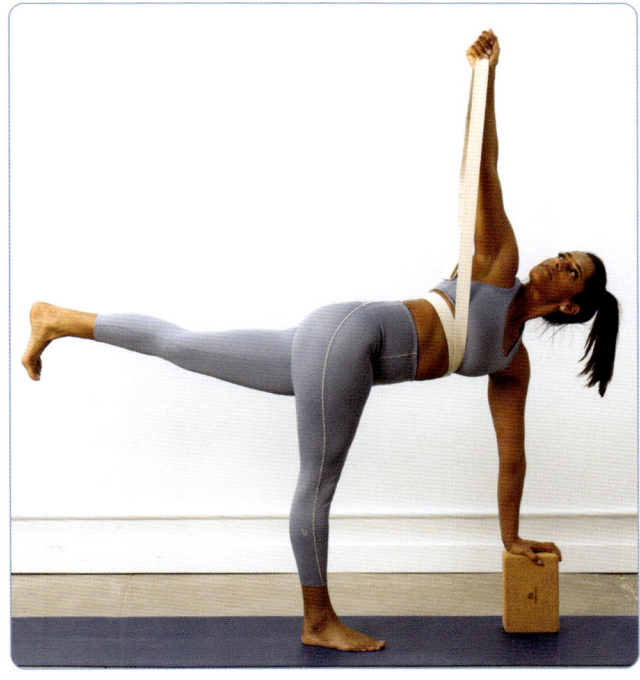

Revolved Half Moon Pose *(continued)*

Practice against a wall to rotate and align.

You can practice this pose with a wall in a couple of ways on the same side. The first way, with your back facing the wall (see photo *a*), requires active flexibility known as mobility. The second way, with the belly facing the wall (see photo *b*), allows you to walk your hand up the wall and use it as leverage, encouraging passive flexibility. Both options help facilitate thoracic rotation of the spine. They also both help you to stabilize the hips, pinning the outer hip to the wall.

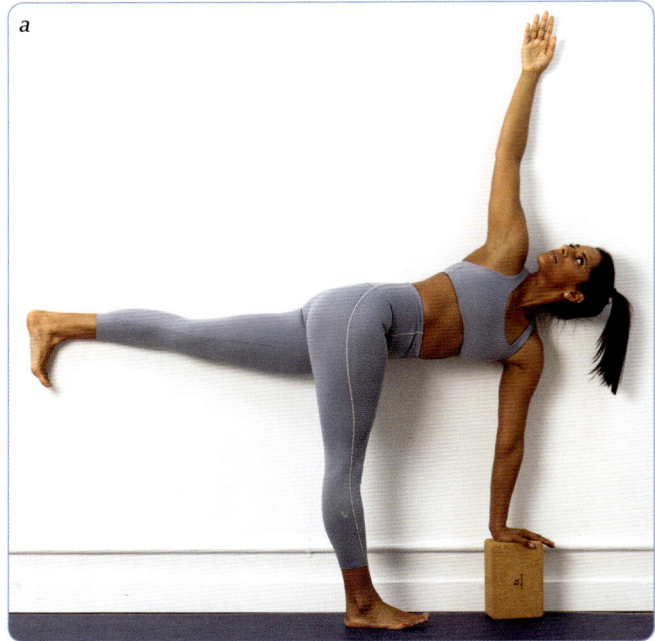

a

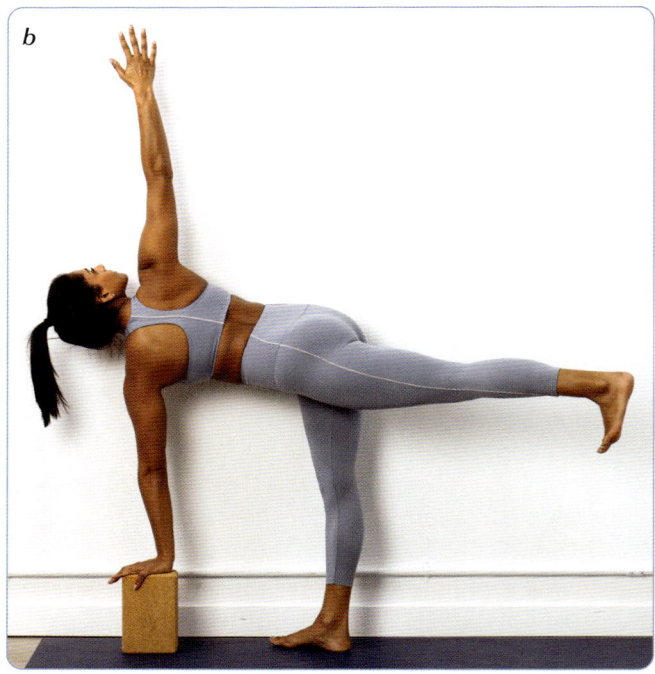

b

The Complete Guide to Yoga Props

Eagle Pose

Garudasana   गरुडासन

Eagle pose is a balancing posture that demands determination and concentration, offering increased circulation to joints and stretching the shoulders and outer hips. Additionally, it strengthens ankles, legs, and the core while potentially benefiting the immune system by stimulating the lymphatic system and aiding in the removal of toxins. Let's explore prop-supported variations to further enrich your experience with this empowering pose.

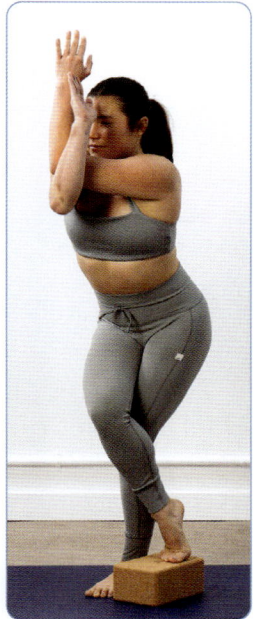

Place a block under your foot to stabilize.

Using a block helps to stabilize eagle pose, improving balance and giving you more control over aligning your elbows and knees. The block stability helps you to sit lower, which may eventually help you wrap your ankle behind the standing leg calf. Begin in chair pose, placing a block on its lowest height outside your left foot. If this is too short, stack two blocks rather than turning the block—it is more stable this way. Wrap the right leg over the left leg and the right arm under the left arm. Rest the foot of the right leg on the block. Repeat on the other side.

Stabilize your hips against a wall.

This is another great variation of eagle pose for finding stability by grounding the hips. Begin with your back facing a wall and sit back into chair pose until your sitting bones contact the wall. You may need to adjust the distance between your feet and the wall. The lower you sit, the easier it will be to wrap the legs. Enter eagle pose from there. There are different takes on how to practice this pose. Some involve forward bending to move lymph. When practicing at the wall, however, try drawing your shoulders back toward the wall, aiming to stack them over your hips. Lift your elbow and reach your hands forward to gently stretch between your shoulder blades.

Sit in a chair to inform pelvic and spinal alignment and strengthen postural muscles.

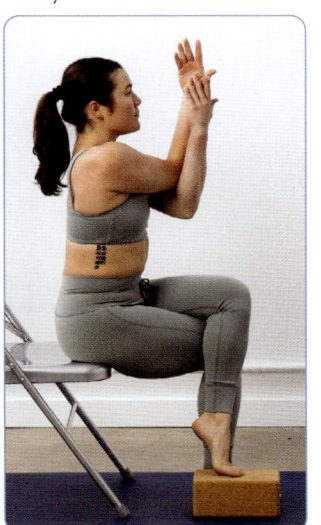

Begin this variation of eagle pose seated on the edge of a chair. If your feet do not comfortably reach the floor, slide blocks or a folded blanket underneath them. Having your sitting bones on the edge of the chair helps to untuck the pelvis, especially if you have tight hip flexors. Sitting at the back of the chair can sometimes encourage tucking the pelvis, rounding the spine, or relying too heavily on the backrest—deactivating your core muscles. Enter eagle pose from here, wrapping one leg over the other and the corresponding arm under the other. Feel the stability in your hips and use it to align through the shoulders and knees.

Tree Pose

Vrikshasana

वृक्षासन

Tree pose is a wonderful introduction to balancing on one leg, providing a foundation for building strength and stability. This pose actively strengthens bones, fosters improved balance, and enhances concentration, making it a beneficial addition to your yoga practice. Let's explore some ways to adapt this pose using props.

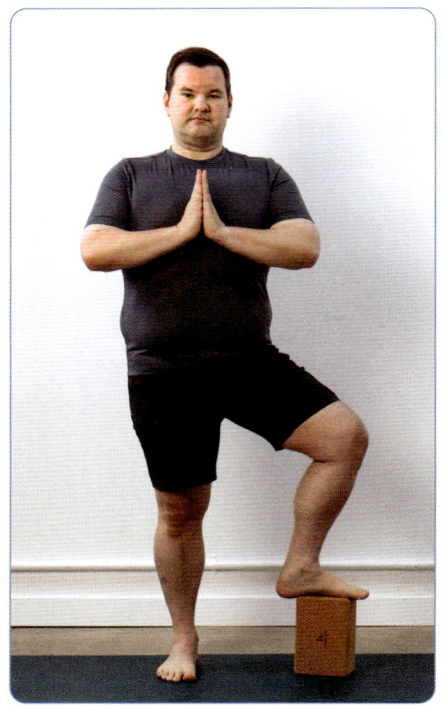

Place a block under your foot to improve balance.

Placing a block or two under your lifted foot is a great way to lift your leg higher without losing the stability of the floor beneath both feet. With both feet grounded, you can fine-tune your postural alignment and work on deepening the external rotation in your lifted leg. You can practice with your full foot on the block and work up to having just the ball of your foot on the block. This is great for those with osteopenia or osteoporosis who are looking to strengthen their bones, with less risk of falling.

Stabilize your hips and shoulders against a wall and a block behind your lifted knee.

This variation requires a lot of muscular activation. Start standing with your back against a wall, turn out one leg and bend at the knee, placing the ball of the foot on the floor, the 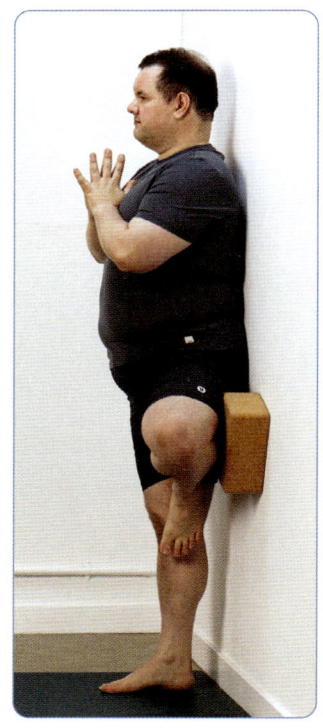 sole of the foot on the calf, or the sole of the foot on the inner thigh (it is often suggested to avoid the opposing knee, but this is still an open topic of conversation). Once you have arrived in the posture, slide a block between your bent knee or thigh and the wall. Work to keep the block from falling while maintaining contact with the hips and shoulders on the wall. As you press into the block, engaging through your outer thigh and hips, think about lengthening your tailbone toward your standing heel. Relax your standing toes if they are gripping. You may want to start with a lighter foam block, then work your way up to a cork block.

Practice with your hands on the back of a chair for stability.

Just as with the block variation, using a chair can help you boost your confidence in this balance. Enter tree pose with your hands on the back of the chair for support. Use this time to breathe and build muscle memory. Over time you can use the chair to empower a hands-free practice. Start by having 10 fingers on the chair, then gradually reduce until you only have 1 finger on each hand on the chair. Then practice lifting both hands from the chair.

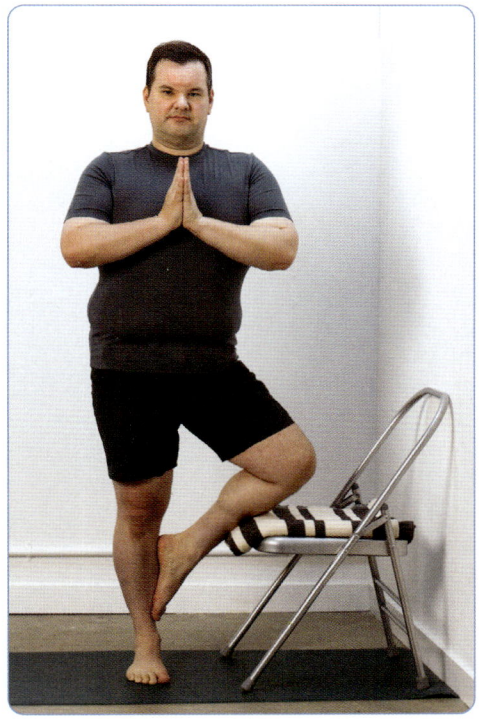

Practice your balance with your shin against the seat of a chair and your foot on your calf.

This tree pose variation decreases the knee flexion for those with knee injuries and supports balance. When practicing, you may decide to fold a blanket or extra mat over the chair seat for comfort. Enter tree pose, placing the sole of your foot inside your standing leg calf. Adjust the height of your foot to accommodate having the shin on the edge of the chair seat, rather than on your knee. With your lifted leg stabilized, root down through your standing leg, while simultaneously lifting through your thigh. Feel the crown of your head rising higher as you release your shoulders down your back.

Lie on your back with a rolled-up blanket under your knee to reduce weight-bearing on the ankles.

Want to practice the structure of tree pose without having to balance on one foot? Take the pose in a supine position, lying on your back. This variation informs good spinal alignment, supports your knees and hips, and reduces strain on the ankle of the straight leg. This reduction in weight-bearing on your feet is great for those with ankle injuries. Lie on your back with a folded blanket within reach. Bend your left knee and place the sole of your foot on your right calf or inner thigh. Slide the blanket under your left knee or thigh to support your hips, especially if you feel your right hip lifting off the mat. Flex through your right foot so that all five toes are pointing to the ceiling. Your palms can come together or you can reach your arms overhead with your arms framing your ears. Press the back of your right leg into the floor as if you were trying to get your shin and thigh bones to touch the mat. Repeat on the other side.

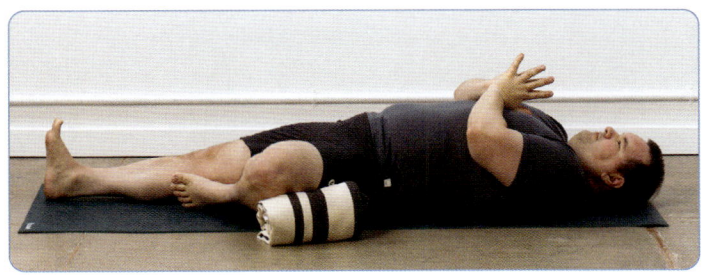

Dancer Pose

Natarajasana   नटराजासन

Dancer pose, sometimes known as lord of the dance pose, demands grace and patience in its execution. This pose not only boosts energy but also enhances balance and concentration while opening the front of the body, including the chest, abdomen, and hip flexors. Let's explore some prop-supported variations to aid in a successful dance!

Practice using a strap to make the pose more accessible.

Using a strap is a great way to start practicing dancer pose with an overhead reach—without torquing the shoulders and hips! Start standing, holding both ends of a strap in one hand. If the strap is in your left hand, shift your weight into your right leg and lift your left heel toward your gluteal muscle, bending at the knee. Loop the strap around the top of your left foot or ankle. Pull both ends of the strap over your shoulder and reach your right hand up and back to grab them as well (both ends should be in both hands). Lift your elbows overhead and kick into the strap with your back foot—working to create a tulip shape in your body. If the flexibility is there, you can walk your hands up the strap, making it shorter. You may need to flex through your toes to keep the strap from sliding off your foot.

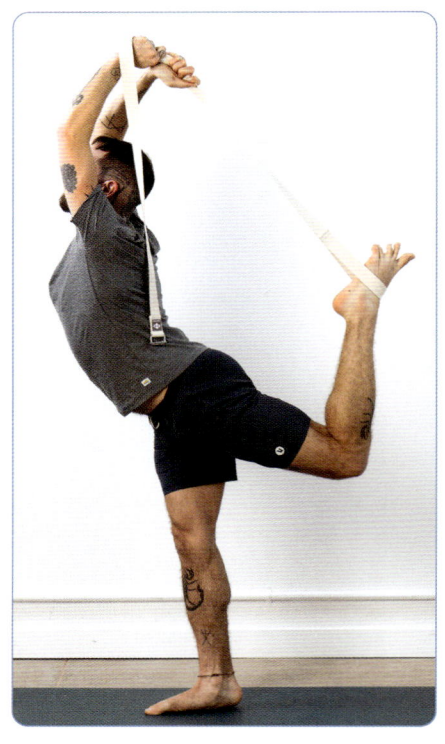

Stabilize your chest and shoulders against a wall.

A great way to stabilize your balance and square through your shoulders and hips is by aligning them with a wall in front of you. The wall also supports lifting the chest, working deeper into your shoulders and upper back, rather than dumping into your lumbar spine. As your chest presses into the wall, use the feedback from the wall to engage the muscles down your back and stretch through the front of your body.

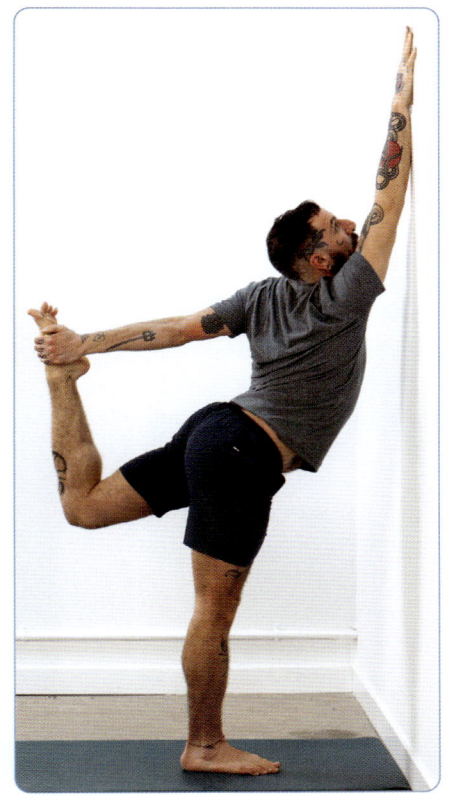

Face a wall and extend your hand up the wall in front of you.

This version of using a wall is a step to finding balance and alignment away from the wall. Rather than having both hands overhead, practice dancer pose with one hand on the wall and the other reaching back for the inside of your foot or ankle. The distance you stand from the wall depends on your mobility, but you can move closer over time. The higher you walk your extended arm up the wall, the more you feel opening across your chest and shoulders. As you kick into your back foot, press your hand into the wall in front of you to stabilize the shoulder of that arm and gently draw the shoulder of your other arm forward to align with it.

Practice with your hips on the back edge of a chair.

Your ability to perform this variation of dancer pose can come down to your height but there are ways to adjust for short stature such as standing on a block or placing blocks under the chair seat. Additionally, you can find a slight bend in the standing leg, as shown in the photo.

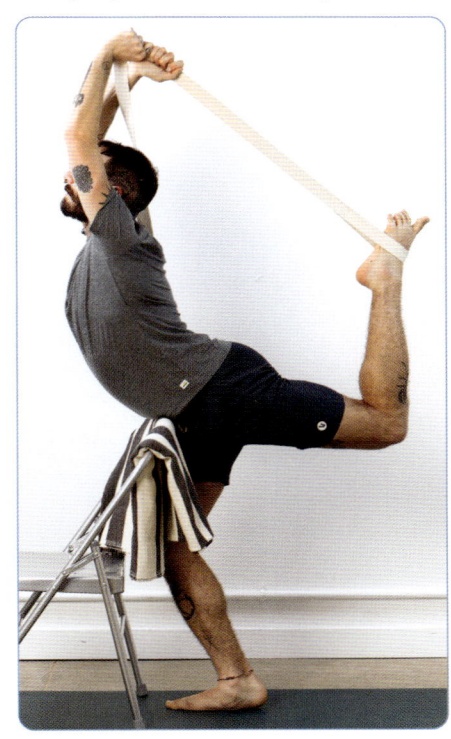

Bring your hips to the edge of the back of the chair, aligning the hip creases with it. Begin coming into the pose, keeping your pelvis secure on the chair. As your hips hinge forward slightly, use the chair as a reference to push the femur bone of your standing leg back. The chair also helps to level the hips by keeping both hip points as points of contact.

Practice with one hand on the back of a chair to aid in balance.

Just as in using the wall, you can use the back of a chair for balance support. Rather than having both hands overhead, practice dancer pose with one hand on the chair and the other reaching back for the inside of your foot or ankle. Use this time to breathe and build muscle memory. Over time you can use the chair to empower a hands-free practice. Start by having five fingers on the chair, then reduce the number of fingers until you only have one finger remaining on the chair. Then you can practice lifting the hand altogether, knowing that the chair is still there for you to come back to at any time.

Extended Hand to Big Toe Pose I and II

Utthita Hasta Padangushthasana I and II

उत्थिति हस्त पादाङ्ग ुष्ठासन I and II

Extended hand to big toe pose I and II are grounding postures that strengthen bones, enhance balance and concentration, and provide a deep stretch to the hamstrings. These poses contribute to the strengthening of ankles, making them a well-rounded and beneficial addition to your yoga practice. Let's look at some common prop-supported variations of these poses.

Practice using a strap to bridge the gap between your hand and foot.

When you can't reach your big toe, usually bending the knee is the next best option. You can avoid this if you have a strap, though. Loop a strap around your foot, holding both ends in the same-side hand as the lifted leg. The strap bridges the gap so you can extend the lifted leg fully. Once the leg is extended, pull your hip and shoulder back so that they are level with the other hip and shoulder. For hand to big toe pose II, bring your leg out to the side, externally rotating through the lifted leg, working your heel toward the sky. See photo *a* for an example of this variation for hand to big toe pose I and photo *b* for hand to big toe pose II.

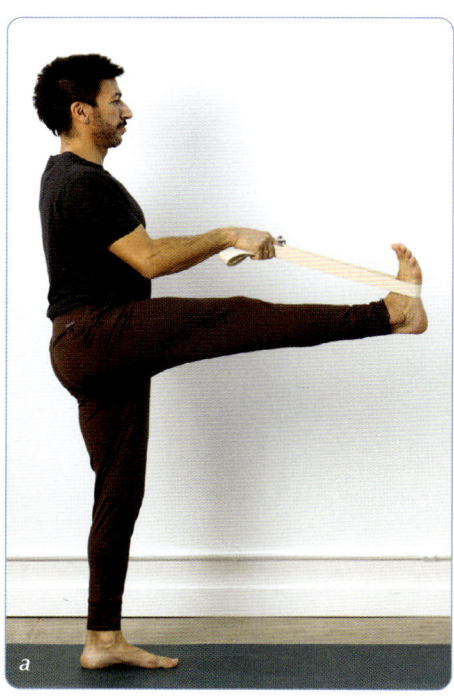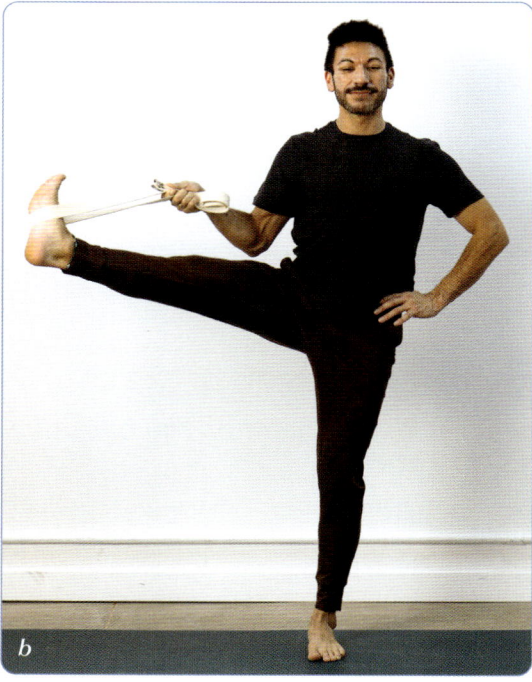

Practice with your back against a wall to stabilize and improve posture.

This variation of hand to big toe pose requires a lot of muscular activation. Start by standing with your back against a wall and shift your weight onto one foot. Reach for your lifted leg just under your knee or grasp your big toe with your hand, or use a strap as shown in the photos. As you enter the posture, you will have to really fire up through your standing leg and core muscles to keep your hips and shoulders against the wall. Think about lifting up through your thigh as if you were trying to pull your femur bone into the hip socket. The wall behind you will keep you from shifting your weight back, bringing the shoulders behind the hips (a common occurrence to counterbalance in this pose). If you find this very challenging, you may learn that you tend to sway the shoulders back and press the hips forward when off the wall. Think about lengthening your tailbone toward your standing heel. If you are practicing hand to big toe pose II, rotate your hip to the side and think about externally rotating through your thigh to level your hips. You will notice if your hip tends to hike upward, or internally rotate, because your back will want to separate from the wall. See photo *a* for an example of this variation for hand to big toe pose I and photo *b* for hand to big toe pose II.

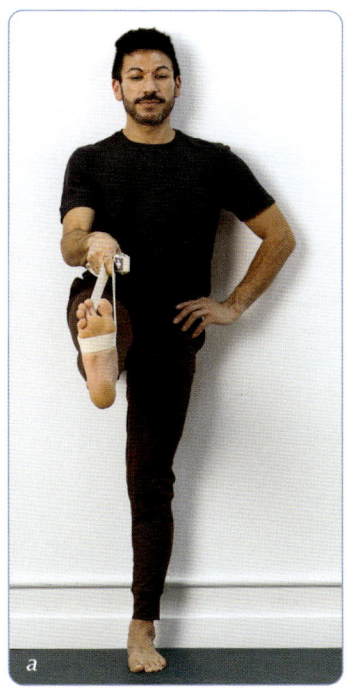 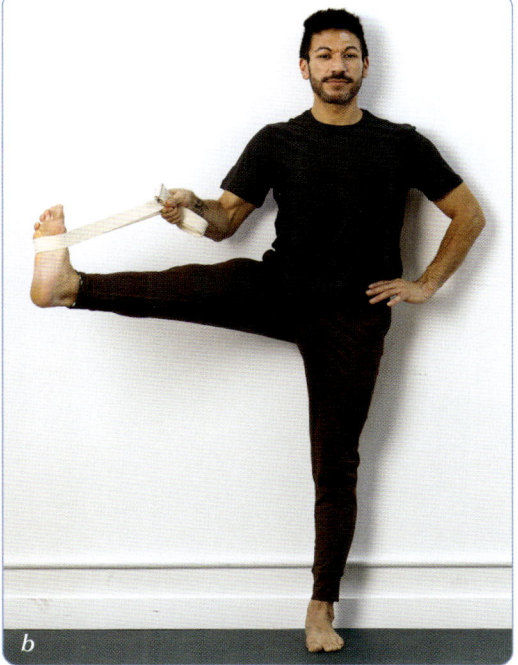

Practice using a strap with your foot pressed against a wall for balance and alignment.

This wall variation of hand to big toe pose I is great for maintaining balance while working on alignment, leveling the hips, and integrating muscle memory for when you take the posture off the wall. Loop a strap around the foot you will be lifting, holding the ends of the strap in one hand. Place the foot on the wall, level with the height of your hips, and ensure all five toes are pointing up. Press your entire foot into the wall to contract the muscles of

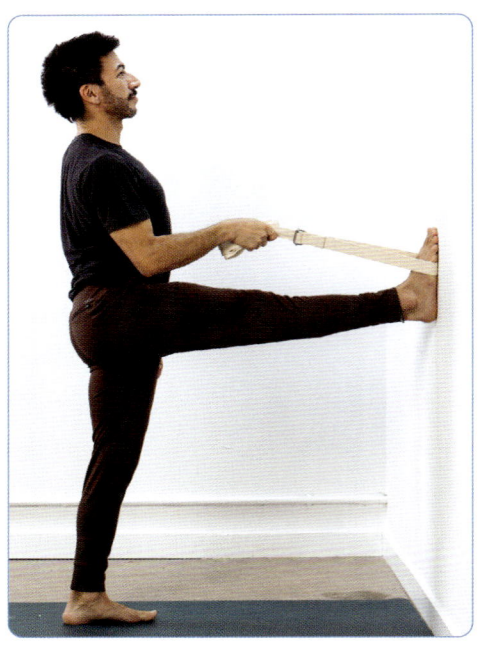

that leg and hug the front of the standing-leg thigh toward the back of the thigh to stabilize the femur bone in the hip socket. Draw your low ribs toward your spine while simultaneously reaching the rib cage (think thorax region of the upper body) away from your pelvis. You want to keep your shoulders over your hips, so over time, if you are working your hand closer to your foot, you will need to place your foot higher up the wall and step in closer.

Before you begin, consider measuring your leg distance from the wall by sitting in staff pose (dandasana) with your feet flexed on the wall. The distance from your sitting bones to the wall is the length of your legs. If your back leg doesn't quite reach the wall or the knee is bent, you can always adjust your distance from the wall!

Practice with a strap, seated in a chair to aid in balance.

The cues for the standing version of extended hand to big toe pose with the strap are the same, but this time you are grounding your hips on the seat of a chair. This offers more stability and control over your postural alignment. If you have osteoporosis or osteopenia, avoid folding forward to loop the strap around your foot. Instead, step on the strap, holding the ends

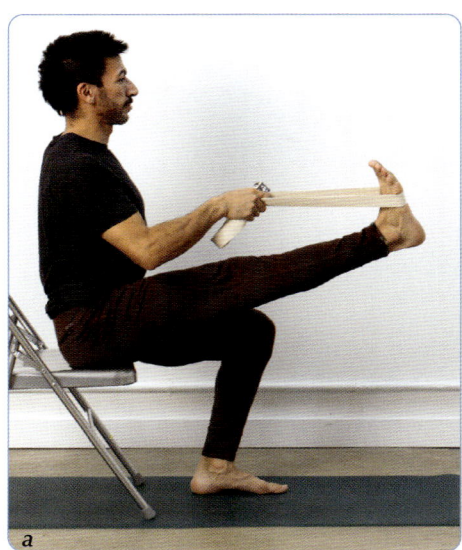

a

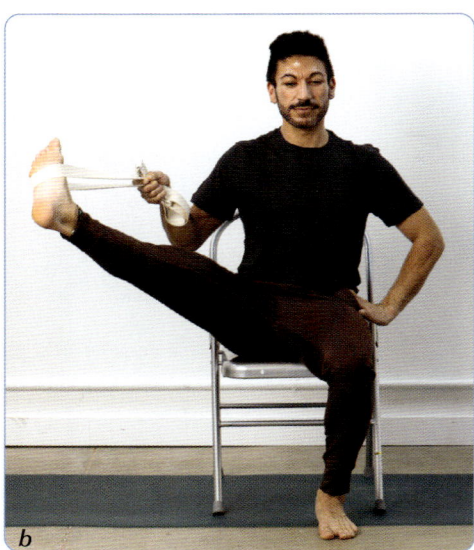

b

prior to sitting down. Forward folding increases the risk of fracture for those with low bone density. For extra support, place the hand that is free on the chair seat and press down to lengthen through your spine. See photo *a* for an example of this variation for hand to big toe pose I and photo *b* for hand to big toe pose II.

Practice with a strap while placing your ankle on the back of a chair with a folded blanket underneath.

Another great example of strap meets prop is using the back of the chair for support. Similar to the wall example, having your lifted leg supported by a structure aids in balance. This version requires a different set of muscles. Rather than pressing your foot *into* the wall, you are pressing the heel or ankle down *onto* the back of a chair. This uses the muscles down the back side of the leg, offering you more stability as you navigate the head of the femur bone into the hip socket. If the back of the chair is too high, start with the chair seat. See photo *a* for an example of this variation for hand to big toe pose I and photo *b* for hand to big toe pose II.

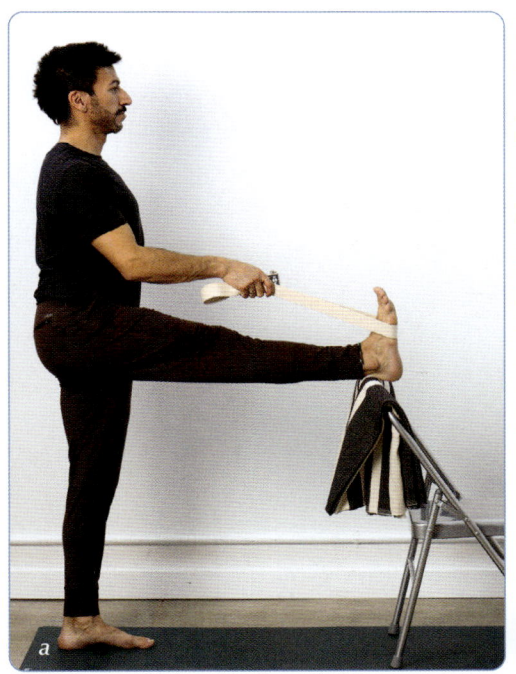 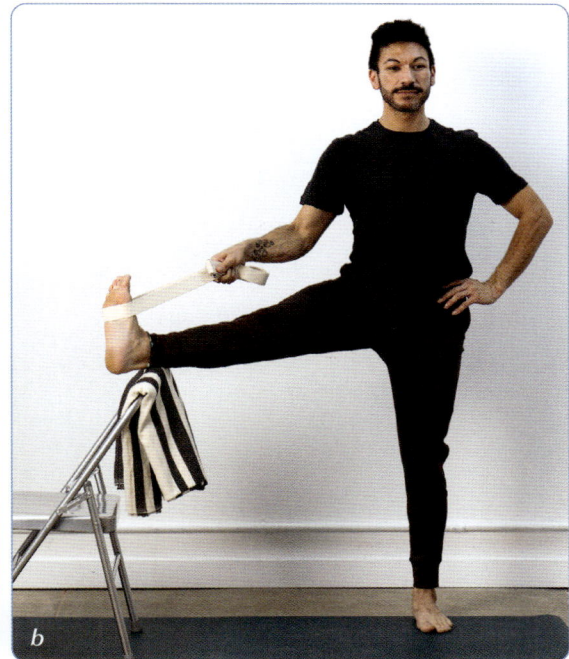

Revolved Hand to Big Toe Pose

Parivritta Hasta Padangushthasana

परविृत्त हस्त पादाङ्ग्ुष्ठासन

Revolved hand to big toe pose, also known as extended hand to big toe pose III or dancing Shiva pose, is a dynamic yoga posture with multiple benefits. This pose enhances thoracic rotation of the spine, promoting improved balance and concentration. Additionally, it aids in detoxification and offers a deep stretch to the hamstrings and outer hips, making it a valuable addition to your practice. Let's look at a few common ways to support this pose with props.

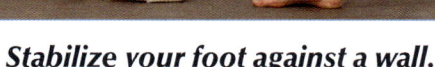

Practice using a strap to bridge the gap between your hand and foot.

When you can't reach your big toe, usually bending the knee is the next best option, but you can avoid this with a strap. Loop a strap around your foot, holding both ends in the hand on the opposite side of the lifted leg. The strap bridges the gap so you can extend the lifted leg fully. Once the leg is extended, lengthen through your spine, and find your thoracic twist.

Stabilize your foot against a wall.

This wall variation of revolved hand to big toe pose is great for maintaining balance while working on alignment, leveling the hips, and integrating muscle memory for when you take the posture off the wall. Practice with your front arms reaching towards or coming in contact with the wall, as shown in the photo, or with the aid of a strap. If using the strap, loop it around the foot you will be lifting, holding the ends of the strap in the opposite hand. Place the foot on the wall, level with your hips, and ensure all five toes are pointing up. Actively press your entire foot into the wall to

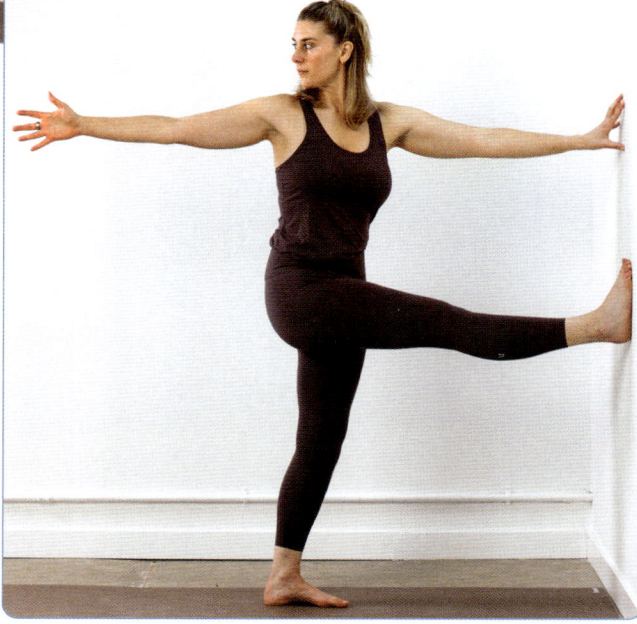

The Complete Guide to Yoga Props

contract the muscles of that leg and hug the front of the standing-leg thigh toward the back of the thigh to stabilize the femur bone in the hip socket. Draw your low ribs in toward your spine, while simultaneously reaching the rib cage (think thorax region of the upper body) away from your pelvis. Try to keep your shoulders over your hips, to facilitate the thoracic rotation of the spine.

Before you begin, it may help for you to measure your leg distance from the wall by sitting in staff pose (dandasana) with your feet flexed on the wall. The distance from your sitting bones to the wall is the length of your legs. If your back leg doesn't quite reach the wall, or the knee is bent, you can always adjust your distance from the wall!

Practice with a strap, seated in a chair to aid in balance.

The cues for the standing version of revolved hand to big toe pose with the strap are the same as the wall variation, but this time you are grounding your hips on the seat of a chair. Another

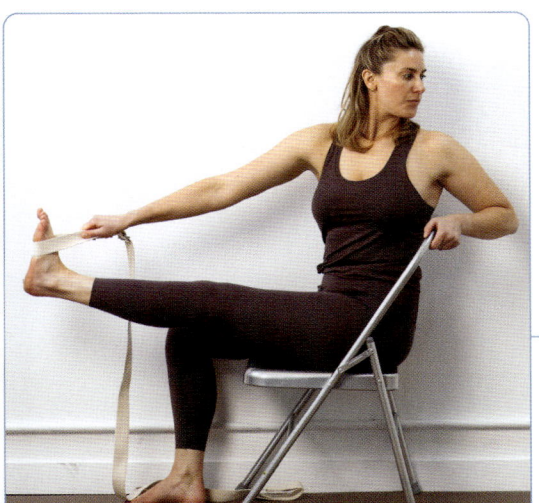

exception to the cues for the wall is that you can use the back of the chair to assist you in your twist, holding on to it with your back hand for more stability and control over your postural alignment. If you have osteoporosis or osteopenia, avoid folding forward to loop the strap around your foot. Instead, step on the strap, holding the ends prior to sitting down. Forward folding increases the risk of fracture for those with low bone density.

Practice with a strap while placing your ankle on the back of a chair with a folded blanket underneath.

Another great example of strap meets prop is using the back of the chair for support. Similar to the wall example, having your lifted leg supported by a structure aids in balance. This version requires a different set of muscles. Rather than pressing your foot *into* the wall, you are

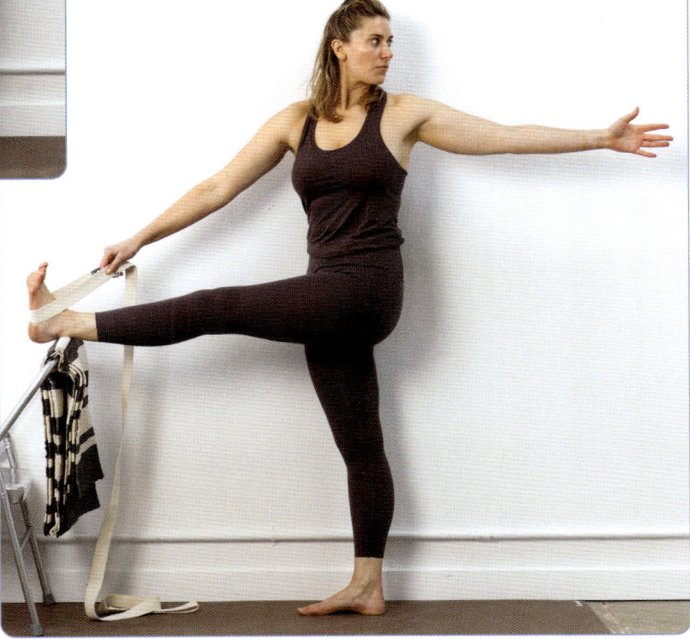

pressing the heel or ankle down *onto* the back of a chair. This uses the muscles down the back side of the leg, offering you more stability as you navigate the head of the femur bone into the hip socket. If the back of the chair is too high, start with the chair seat.

Stabilize your outer hip against a wall to rotate and align.

You can practice with a wall in a couple of ways on the same side. In the first option of this variation, you turn the front of the torso away from the wall in the pose (see photo *a*). This variation requires more mobility. In the second option of this variation, your torso rotates toward the wall, and you use your hand against the wall for leverage, allowing more passive flexibility. Gently press your back hand into the wall to encourage the front shoulder closer (see photo *b*). Both options help facilitate thoracic rotation of the spine. They also both help you to stabilize the hips, pinning the outer hip to the wall.

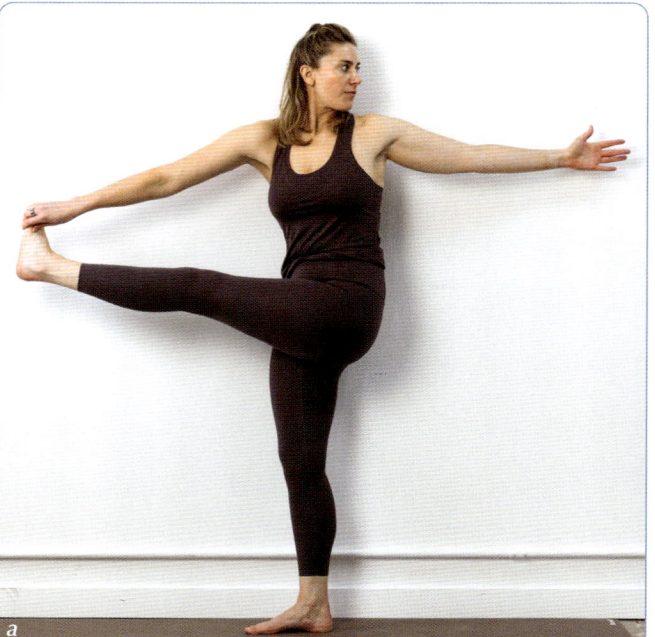

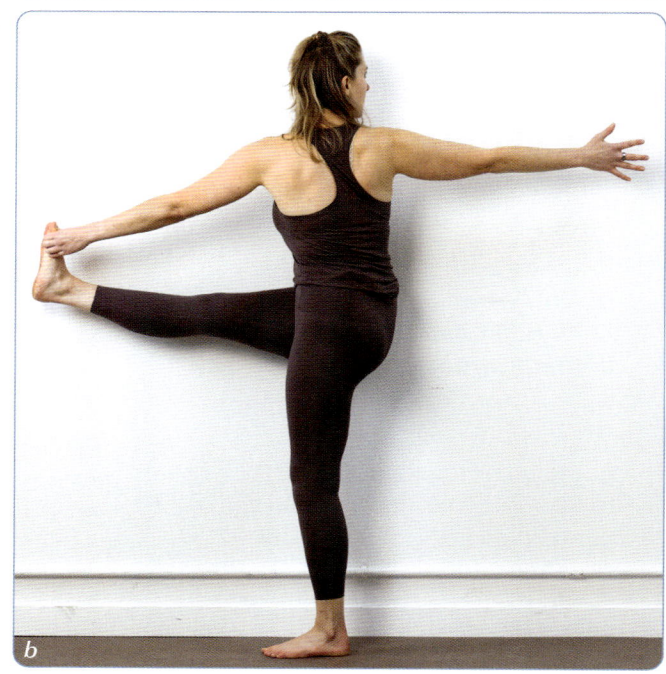

Standing Splits Pose

Urdhva Prasarita Eka Padasana उर्ध्व प्रसारति एक पादासन

Standing splits pose is a dynamic yoga posture that provides a multitude of benefits. This pose actively stretches the hamstrings and hips and strengthens the gluteal muscles, hamstrings, and calves. It enhances balance and concentration, and as an inversion, standing splits improves circulation, adding a revitalizing element to your practice. Here are a few ways you can support this pose with props.

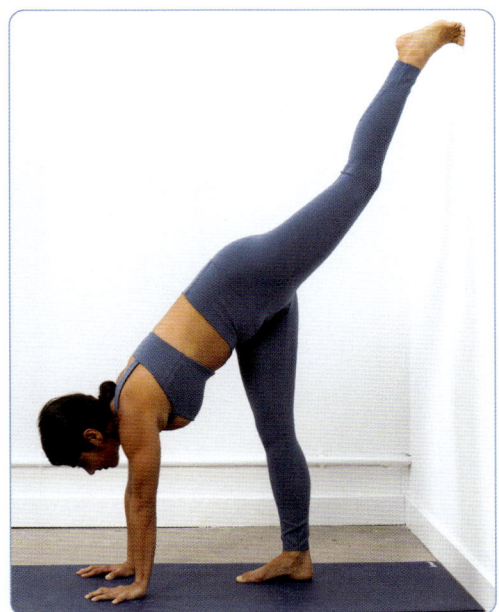

Stabilize the back leg against a wall.

Using a wall under the lifted leg in standing splits increases your passive flexibility. Pressing the back leg into the wall gets the hamstring of the standing leg to lengthen. It also lengthens the psoas of the lifted leg. Another benefit, though, is pelvic alignment. By ensuring the top of the foot is facing the wall, you can better level through your hips. If the foot likes to roll to one side, flex your toes and press them into the wall to ensure the hips are square. Open hips are *fine*, if that is your *intention*. Squared hips target the belly of the hamstrings; open hips move the stretch into the inner thigh.

Place blocks underneath your hands to stabilize.

If the floor feels too far away from your hands, place blocks on the floor to bring it closer to you. The blocks can be turned to three different heights, so you can work your way closer to the floor over time. If you need more stability, try stacking blocks instead.

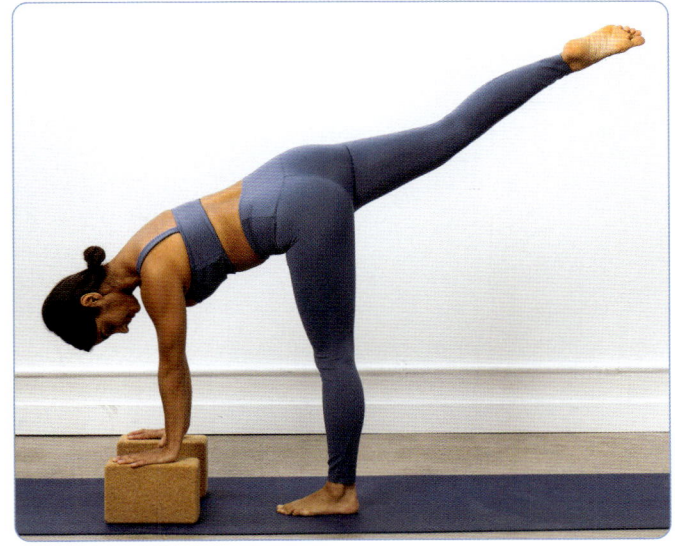

Goddess Pose

Utkata Konasana

उत्कट कोणासन

Goddess pose is a powerful yoga posture that engages the pelvic floor, creating stability and strength. This pose also offers a comprehensive stretch and strengthening effect on the ankles, legs, and hips, while opening the chest and fortifying the back of the body. Incorporating goddess pose into your practice brings a balance of grounding and expansion. Here are a few common ways you can support this pose with props.

Practice with your back against a wall to inform postural alignment.

Practicing with your back against a wall is a great way to check in with your spinal alignment and direct your muscle actions. As you enter the pose, sliding your back down the wall, your feet should be a little bit in front of you and turned out to your natural range of motion (do not force turnout, my ballerinas!). Draw your low ribs into your back, toward the wall. Start to direct your knees back, toward the wall, using your outer thighs and gluteal muscles to commandeer this action. Try lifting all 10 toes off the floor to engage the shin and ankle muscles and distribute weight equally across the feet.

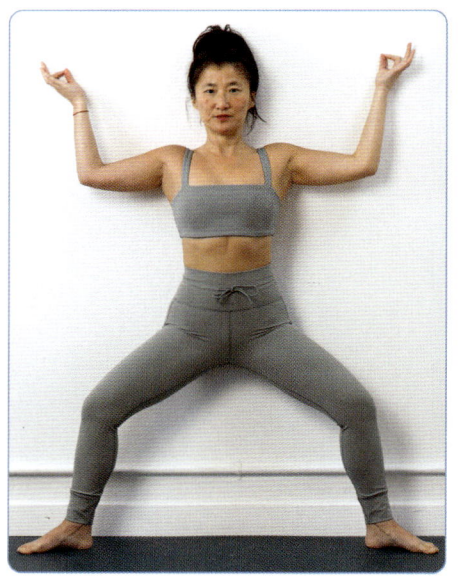

Sit in a chair to stabilize the pelvis.

As you work up the strength and balance to practice this pose standing, try it in a chair. The chair helps to stabilize the pelvis, allowing you to focus on postural alignment and the actions of the legs. While seated, step your feet out to the sides, opening through your hips and inner thighs. You may use sheer muscle strength to do so, or use your hands to guide each leg open, one at a time. With the hips grounded, you may feel more confident playing with new variations, such as adding a side stretch or a forward fold.

The Complete Guide to Yoga Props

Recline with your feet on a wall and bolsters under your thighs or knees.

This is a wonderful restorative take on goddess pose. Begin lying on your back in reclined bound angle pose (supta baddha konasana), with your toes touching the wall. Flex through your feet and begin walking them out to the sides until they are directly in front of the knees. Slide bolsters or folded blankets under your knees and shins for support. The feet should be around the same height as the knees, with the bolsters or blankets taking the strain off the knees. Keep your feet turned out and the soles of the feet against the wall. You may need to adjust the distance between your sacrum and the wall to find the sweet spot.

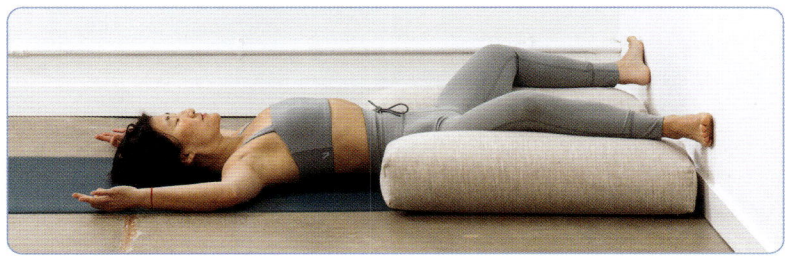

Bird of Paradise Pose

Svarga Dvijasana

स्वर्ग द्वजिासन

Bird of paradise pose is a symbolic and challenging posture that teaches both patience and resiliency as one unfolds into full bloom as does the flower. This pose actively strengthens leg muscles and hips, enhancing balance and concentration. Additionally, it provides a deep stretch to the hamstrings, hips, shoulders, and chest muscles, while also strengthening the postural muscles. The journey into bird of paradise encourages a beautiful blend of strength, flexibility, and mindfulness in your practice that can be supported along the way by some common prop variations below.

Place your foot against a wall for balance and stability.

This pose can offer quite the challenge by asking you to balance on one leg, while finding a deep stretch, practicing a bind, and remembering to breathe! The wall will help you to find your alignment without falling over, aiding in building muscle memory over time. Start by facing a wall and place your foot on the wall, keeping the knee bent. Once the foot is stabilized on the wall, mindfully turn your torso away from the wall and shift your standing foot parallel to the wall. Reach around your lifted leg and behind your back to enter the bind. Press your foot into the wall to engage through the leg muscles and work to externally rotate the thigh into the hip socket. If flexibility permits, you can extend the lifted leg, walking the foot higher up the wall.

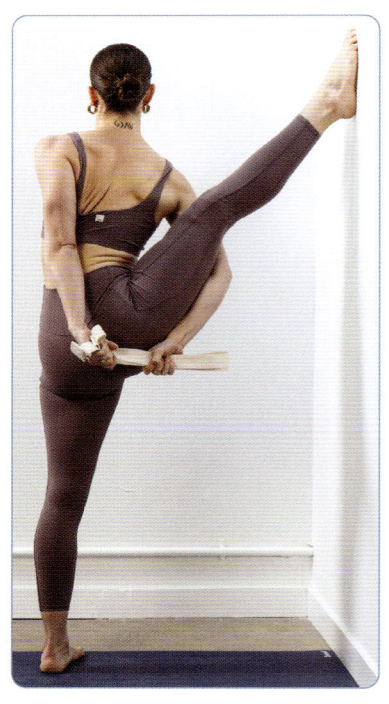

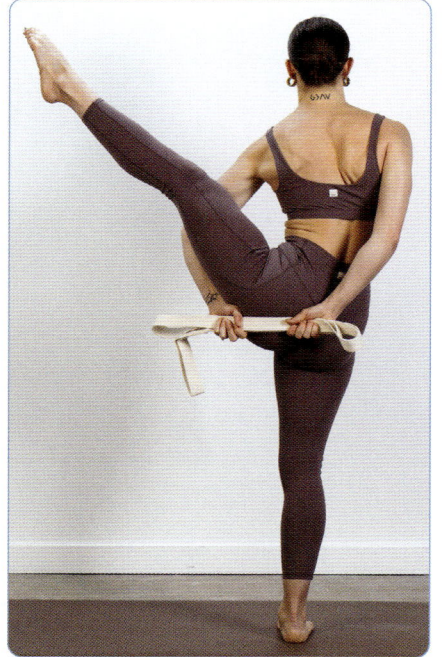

Practice a bind with a strap between your hands to create space.

A strap is a handy tool to free up space in your shoulders in this posture. It can bridge the gap between your hands if they are out of reach. Even if you *can* bind your hands, sometimes it is to the sacrifice of your spinal alignment, causing forward hunching, or internally rotating the thigh, hiking it up. So a strap may come in handy as you maintain length in both sides of the body and work your hands closer together over time from there.

Table Top and Balancing Table Pose

Bharmanasana and Dandayamana Bharmanasana

भरमानासन and दण्डायमान भरमानासन

Table top pose is a foundational yoga posture that offers comprehensive benefits. This pose actively strengthens your abdominal muscles, legs, hips, shoulders, and chest muscles, promoting stability and strength. It also improves balance and concentration while engaging postural muscles. Additionally, incorporating cat or cow movements in table top pose bends and extends the spine, enhancing range of motion and providing a stretch to both the front and back of the torso.

Balancing table pose, commonly referred to as bird dog, is a dynamic yoga posture that provides the same benefits as table top pose. Balancing table pose provides a holistic approach to building strength and enhancing mindfulness in your practice. Let's explore some common prop-supported variations for these poses.

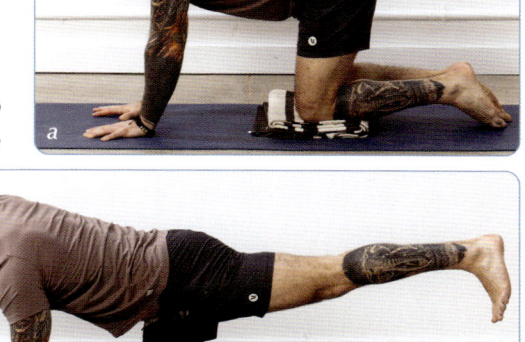

Practice with blocks or a folded blanket under your knee to align.

Using a block or a blanket raises the knee to be level with the heel of your back foot. This can alleviate strain on the knee and ankle by reducing the angle of flexion and returning the angle to 90 degrees. See photo *a* for an example of this variation for table top using the blanket and photo *b* for an example for balancing table pose using the block.

Practice with a block or a blanket under your hands to aid the wrists.

Using a block under one or both of your front hands in these postures can take some of the weight-bearing out of the wrist. You can also roll a blanket and place your hands on it at a slightly downward angle to decrease the angle of flexion in the wrist. This is great for modifying for a wrist injury or for building upper body strength. See photo *a* for an

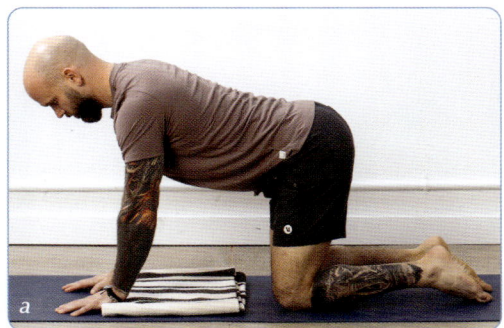

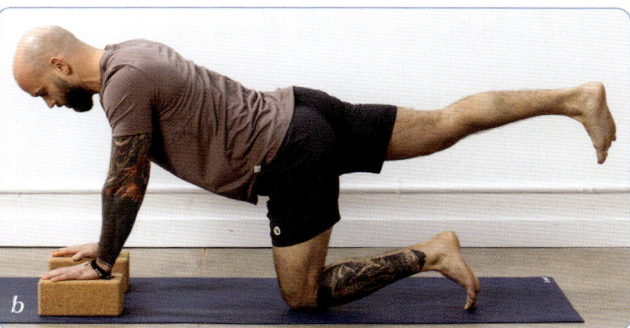

example of this variation for table top with the folded blanket and photo *b* for an example for balancing table with blocks under both hands. From here, you can practice extending the arm opposite your back leg.

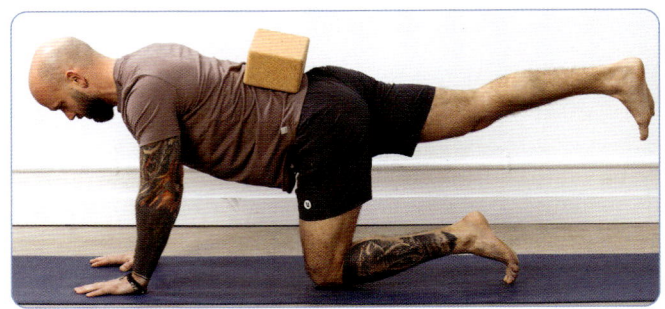

Practice with a block on your low back to level the hips.

For balancing table pose, try placing a yoga block on its lowest height just above your sacrum. Try to maintain a neutral spine and level hips. If the spine collapses or rounds, the block will move. If the hips roll in or out, the block will move. Think of it as sort of a fun game rather than a daunting task!

Practice with a blanket under your knees for support.

A great way to modify these postures is by practicing them kneeling. To cushion and protect the knees, you can place a folded blanket underneath.

Practice with a block between your thighs.

In table top pose, a block helps to keep your knees and thighs parallel, stabilize the deep core and pelvic muscles, and direct orientation of the tailbone. Start by placing a block between your thighs, turned to the narrowest width, high up by the pubic bone and perform cat or cow variations (marjaryasana or bitilasana). Hug the block up toward the pubis, engaging through the inner thighs in cat pose (see photo *a*). Lengthen your tailbone down toward the backs of the knees and draw the navel in toward the spine. Practice in cow pose with that same hugging action, this time lifting through the tailbone and broadening across the chest and collar bones (see photo *b*). You can also try to strengthen your core in table top pose by hovering the knees with a neutral spine (see photo *c*). Continue squeezing the block to stabilize the pelvis. Mentally split the mat in two with your hands to broaden the space between the shoulder blades.

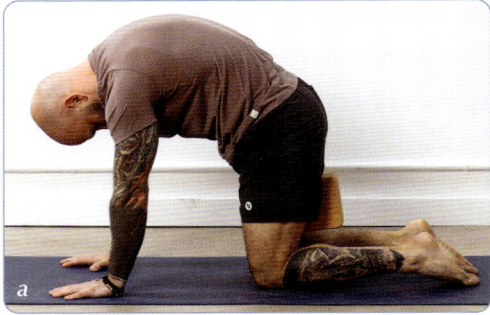
a

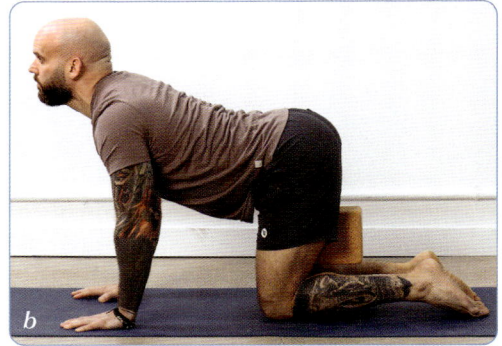
b

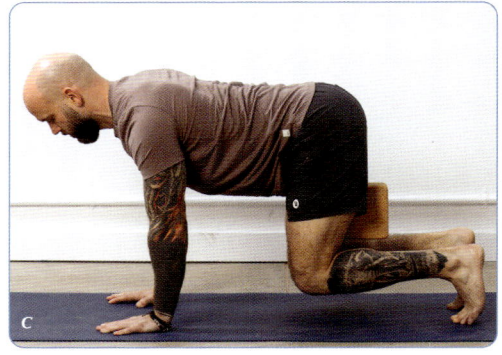
c

Gate Pose

Parighasana   परघिासन

Gate pose is a transformative yoga posture that combines strength and flexibility. This pose actively strengthens and stretches muscles along the back and side of the body. Additionally, gate pose provides a deep stretch to the hamstrings, hips, and ankles, offering a comprehensive release and opening in these areas. Let's dive into a few of the ways you can support this pose with props.

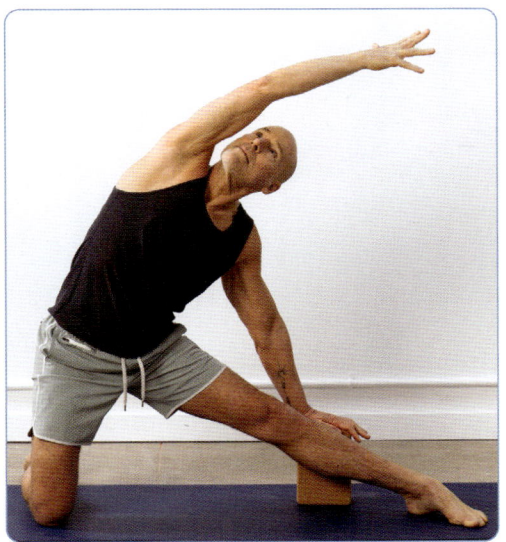

Place a block under your bottom hand.

A block helps raise the height of the floor and lengthen the spine. It also aids in rolling the chest open. Place the block outside your extended leg in gate pose. Placing your hand on a block helps to create more space in the spine to twist and assists those with tight hamstrings.

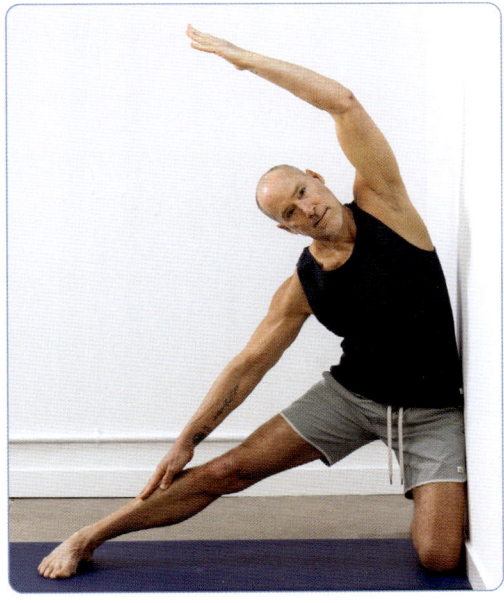

Place your hip against a wall for alignment and reinforcement.

In this variation of gate pose, you will pin the outer edge of your kneeling leg hip to a wall. The wall guides the hip points to be level and stabilizes them as you stretch and rotate through your spine.

Gate Pose (continued)

Place a strap around your foot and hold in your top hand.

A strap is a handy tool to free up space in your shoulders in this pose. It bridges the gap between your hands and your ankle or foot and gives you something to hold while rolling the chest open. The connected grip takes some of the work out of the core muscles in rotating the spine by giving you more leverage. Slide the strap under the foot of the extended leg. You can practice with the foot grounded or flexed to lessen the intensity of the stretch in the hips and ankles. Hold both ends of the strap in your top hand.

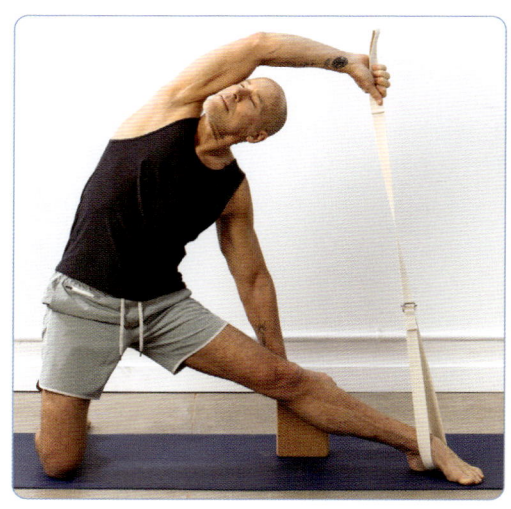

Self-adjust the upper body using a chair.

In this variation of gate pose, the extended leg goes under a chair facing your side. Your bottom arm slides onto the chair seat. You can either keep the arm outstretched or bend at the elbow to bring the palm of your hand to the back of the chair, if your chair has one. Reach your top arm overhead and roll your ribs to face the sky. If you are pressing your bottom hand into the back of the chair, use that as leverage to roll your ribs and sternum open.

Chapter 4

Seated and Squatting Poses

Life will give you whatever experience is most helpful for the
evolution of your consciousness. How do you know this is the
experience you need? Because this is the experience you are
having at the moment.

Ekhart Tolle

In this chapter, we explore a diverse array of seated and squatting yoga postures, exploring various adaptations that use props to enhance our practice. As we ground our sitting bones into the earth, we unlock pathways for deeper connection and growth. Whether we are folding, unfolding, twisting, or simply finding stillness, our bodies become more rooted and responsive to the ebb and flow of our practice. In the embrace of these seated postures, we discover a sanctuary of calm, yet remain fully awakened, striking a delicate balance between focus and relaxation and between effort and ease—much like the preparation for meditation. Seated postures offer a spectrum of experiences, ranging from invigorating to deeply relaxing, meeting our individual needs and states of being. Throughout our exploration, we'll witness how props serve as versatile allies, enriching our poses by providing difficulty, comfort, accessibility, or variability from the traditional forms. It's important to note that the chapters in part II are organized based on each pose's originally intended form, but in some cases the adaptations alter the orientation of the posture from its initial form.

Mantra: In this seated stillness, I find inner
peace and embrace the present moment.

Easy Pose

Sukhasana   सुखासन

Easy pose is a foundational yoga posture known for its simplicity and grounding effects. This pose calms the mind, strengthens the back and postural muscles, and gently stretches the knees, ankles, and hips while you are seated with crossed legs. Explore the variations of easy pose supported by props to deepen your practice and enhance the comfort of this meditative posture.

Place a block, bolster, or blanket under your sitting bones for support.

A little hip elevation can go a long way! Adding height can ease joint tension in a few ways. Having the hips level with or higher than the knees decreases the angle of flexion at the joint, reducing strain. If you have tight psoas (hip flexors), sitting on the edge of a prop slightly tilts the front of your pelvis toward the mat, removing rounding in the low back and bringing the pelvis into a neutral position. A neutral pelvis supports a long and relaxed spine. Once seated, shift your weight back into the sitting bones, distributing the weight evenly between the two. Grow tall through your spine, stacking the shoulders directly over the pelvis. Slightly retract your chin, lengthening the back of the neck, until your ears are above your shoulders.

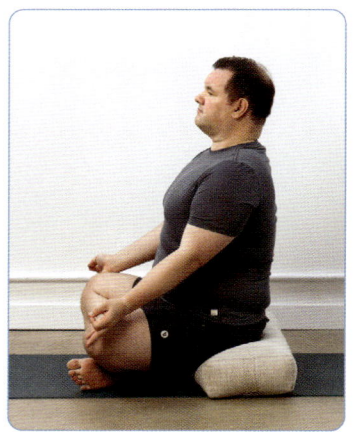

Add a forward fold for a dynamic stretch.

A forward fold brings a nice stretch to this posture. Resting your head on something helps you to fully relax into it. A block can help by bringing the floor closer to you, lessening the intensity of the fold. The block can allow you to rest the muscles of the neck and shoulder and release tension throughout your face. It even extends a sense of deeper relaxation from the top down to your psoas. Start by sitting cross-legged on the mat or the edge of a blanket. Sit tall, lengthening through the spine, then begin to walk your fingertips forward on the mat, extending the torso out and away from the hips. When you can't walk the fingers any farther, allow the spine to round down, lowering the chest toward the mat and softening the belly toward the shins. Rest your forehead on the block at any height. You can massage your forehead muscles by rolling your head side to side on the block.

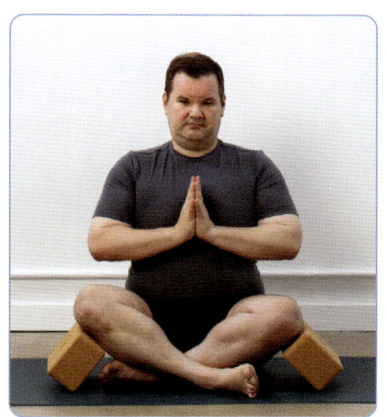

Place blocks under your knees to ease tension or strain.

Blocks slid under your knees are a great way to relieve tension in the knee and hip joints. You can turn the blocks under to any height or even place them at an angle so the slope of the blocks matches the slope of your legs.

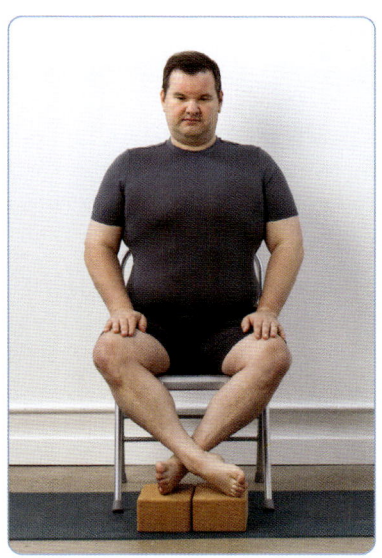

Sit on a chair with blocks under your feet.

Sitting on the edge of a chair adds postural support, like sitting on the edge of a block, blanket, or strap. Having your feet farther away from the hips is a wonderful way to support your knees and work your way up to the ground (a little yoga oxymoron). Once seated, cross your ankles and place them on blocks. Feel free to stack multiple blocks to raise the height of the feet over time!

Staff Pose

Dandasana   दण्डासन

Staff pose is a fundamental seated posture that focuses on building strength in the back and postural muscles while offering a deep stretch to the hamstrings. Simultaneously, it opens the chest and shoulders, promoting improved posture. Delve into various prop-supported variations of staff pose to enhance your practice and experience the full benefits of this foundational yoga pose.

Practice against a wall with blocks under your hands to lengthen and align.

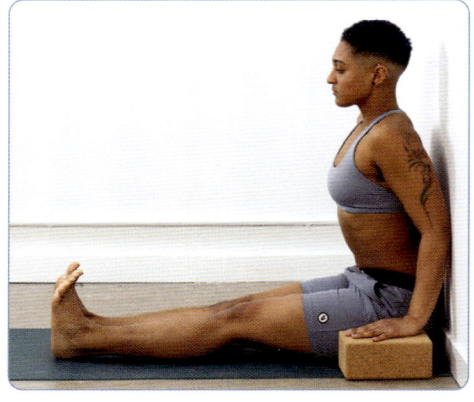

Every body is unique. Not everyone's arms are long enough to reach the floor in staff pose. Even if you can comfortably reach the floor, there are benefits to using blocks. Blocks help to lengthen the torso out and away from the pelvis and aid in neutralizing your pelvis if your hips are feeling tight. If you have wrist pain, slanted blocks help to decrease the angle of flexion on the wrists. Slant blocks against a wall a little wider than the width of your hips. Sit a few inches (several centimeters) in front of the blocks with your legs extended in front of you, parallel to one another. Place your hands on the blocks with your fingers pointing down and press into the blocks, encouraging length through the spine and the top of the sternum. Press into your sitting bones and draw your pubic bone to be level with them. Drive the heels of your feet and the tops of your thighs down toward the floor.

Place a block, bolster, or blanket under your sitting bones to support tight hips.

A little hip elevation can go a long way! If you have tight psoas, sitting on the edge of a prop slightly tilts the front of your pelvis down, removing rounding in the low back and bringing the pelvis into a neutral position. A neutral pelvis supports a long and relaxed spine by making it easier to draw the torso perpendicular to the floor. Once you are seated, shift your weight back into the sitting bones, distributing the weight evenly between the two. Grow tall through your spine, stacking the shoulders directly over the pelvis.

Practice with a block and a wall to improve posture.

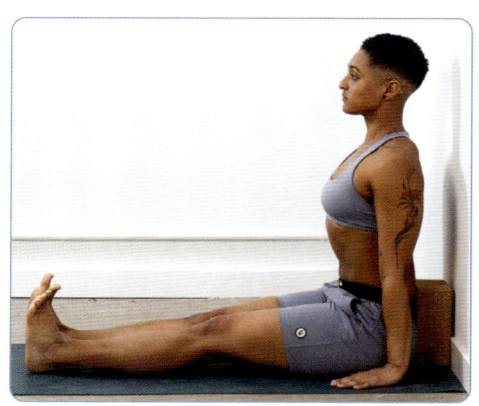

Using a block in staff pose directs the action of the spine from the pelvis upward. Place a block on the tallest orientation between the sacrum and the wall, informing the direction of the pelvis. Try to make contact with the entire block as you align the shoulders to stack over your hips. You can sit on a blanket if you need more space to untuck your hips and extend the spine. Use the space between your torso and the wall for the shoulder blades to draw backward. Try bringing your hands to prayer at the heart center to tone the core muscles and extend through the chest.

Place a rolled-up blanket under your knees to support your hamstrings and hips.

If your hamstrings or hip flexors are feeling tight, rolling a blanket under the knees can help. The slight flexion in the knees shortens the hamstrings and psoas, decreasing the pull you might feel on these muscles. It also directs the sensation (such as pain) away from the attachment points and toward the hamstring muscles.

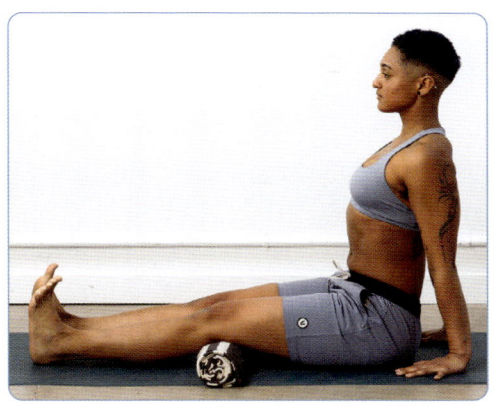

Sit on a chair with your feet against a wall.

To really ease the intensity of the stretch, try staff pose by starting on a chair. Sitting tall at the edge of the seat, extend your legs toward a wall. You may need to measure this distance beforehand to get your feet all the way to the wall. You can also place blocks under your heels if your legs do not comfortably reach the floor or if you are ready to deepen the stretch. Having contact with the wall informs the direction of the legs. The toes should be pointing straight up to avoid any internal or external rotation of the legs.

Big Toe Pose

Ardha Baddha Padma Padangushthasana

अर्ध बद्ध पद्म पादाङ्गुष्ठासन

Big toe pose, occasionally referred to as half lotus tiptoe pose, offers potential relief for joint pain by enhancing circulation. This pose actively strengthens ankles, legs, and core muscles, contributing to improved balance and focus. It may also offer relief from symptoms of sciatica. Explore various prop-supported variations of big toe pose to maximize its benefits and add versatility to your yoga practice.

Use a wall to stabilize your back and to support balance and posture.

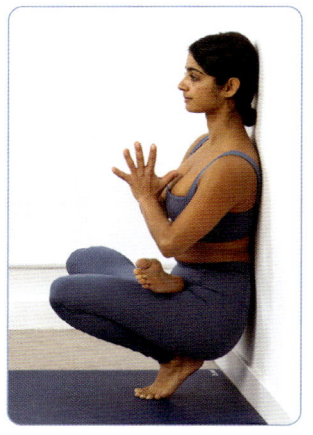

Using a wall will not only inform postural alignment, but it will help you feel more stable and balanced! Start in mountain pose, with your back against a wall. Shift your weight onto one foot, lifting your other leg into either a figure four position (the ankle crossing the thigh above the knee) or a half lotus position (bringing the heel of your foot into your hip crease, pointing the knee of the lifted leg down). Fold forward at the hips (have blocks ready to support you so you don't feel like you are falling forward). Once your hands are on the blocks, bend the knee of the standing leg, drawing your hips down. The weight should be in the ball of the standing foot. Walk your shoulders back to stack over your hips and lean against the wall behind you. With the support of the wall and a newly found tall spine, bring your hands to heart center.

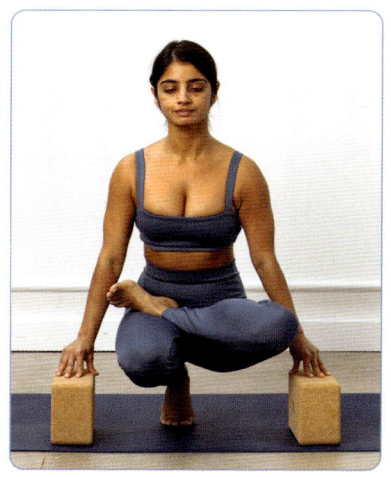

Place blocks under your hands.

Use blocks to bring the floor to your hands. This new point of contact gives you a new sense of balance and control. Once you feel well situated in the posture, practice reaching to your fingertips, then slowly removing fingers from the blocks, one by one, until you can hover your hands over the blocks.

Place blocks under your knees or shins.

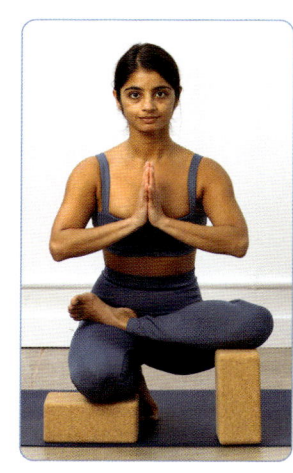

Relying on blocks for support helps your balance and, when you press into the props, relieves pressure on your knees and low back. After coming into this posture, slide a block in its lowest height under your front knee and another block in any position under your other knee. For an extra challenge, press down into the blocks to hover your hips above your heel. Stack your shoulders over your hips and bring your palms to touch at the heart center.

Sit on a chair with your bottom foot on a block to build muscle memory and support.

This is a pretty dynamic pose! Why not take your time with it and work on your flexibility and muscle memory first with the aid of a chair? The chair will take the pressure and weight off your knee and remove the required balancing act. You will still get many of the same benefits. Sit on the edge of a chair and draw one leg into a figure four or half lotus position. Lift your bottom leg and place your foot on a block. Over time, add more blocks to increase the angle of flexion on the knees and hips. You will get the stretch without the force of your body weight and gravity.

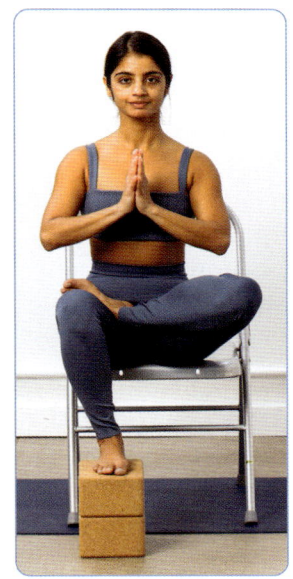

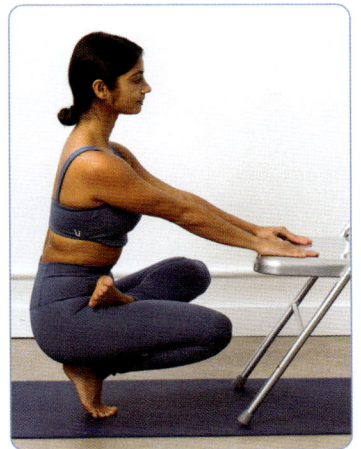

Place your hands on the seat of a chair for support.

This variation works like adding blocks under your hands, only with a little more height! This means you don't have to fold forward as far to reach the desired prop so there is a lesser hamstring stretch. The chair adds a new feeling of balance and control. Have the chair in front of you before your start, so you can reach for it when you begin to find your fold. Once you feel well situated in the posture, you can practice coming to your fingertips, then slowly removing fingers from the chair, one by one, until you can hover your hands over the seat.

Seated Forward Bend

Pashchimottanasana   पश्चिमोत्तानासन

Seated forward bend is a rejuvenating pose that stretches the spine, shoulders, and hamstrings while stimulating the liver and kidneys for detoxification. This posture also calms the nervous system, offering a holistic and grounding experience in your practice. Explore the following prop-supported variations for added depth.

Place a block, bolster, or blanket under your sitting bones to support tight hips.

If you have tight psoas, sitting on the edge of a prop slightly tilts the front of your pelvis toward the mat, removing rounding in the low back and bringing the pelvis into a neutral position. A neutral pelvis supports extension of the spine before you begin to fold forward. The intention is to feel the stretch in your hamstrings more than in your low back, which happens when the psoas are tight and the pelvis tucks under.

Place a rolled-up blanket under your knees to support your hamstrings and hips.

If your hamstrings or hip flexors are feeling tight, rolling a blanket under the knees can help. The slight flexion in the knees shortens the hamstrings and psoas, decreasing the pull you might feel on these muscles. It also directs the sensation (such as pain) away from the attachment points and toward the belly of the hamstring muscles.

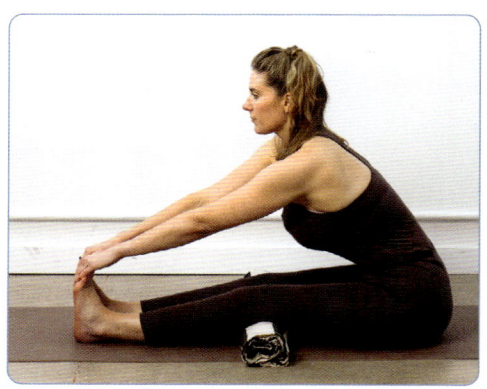

Place a block in front of your feet to deepen the stretch.

Using a block in front of your feet extends the distance beyond your legs, creating a deeper hamstring stretch than reaching for the feet alone. Holding on to the block allows you to use your arm strength to extend your torso farther out and away from the hips, creating more length in the sides of the body and psoas. Place a block on the wide orientation in front of your flexed feet. Extend your torso away from the pelvis and reach the chest toward the block. When you cannot extend the chest any more, start to relax the chest toward the tops of your legs and reach for the outside edges of the block. Gaze toward the block and keep your spine elongated for an active stretch, or round through the upper, middle, and lower back, releasing the chin toward the chest for a restorative quality.

Sit on a chair with a strap.

To really ease the intensity of the stretch, try it by starting the pose on a chair. Sitting tall at the edge of the seat, loop a strap around the front of your feet and extend your legs. Holding the ends of the straps in both hands, begin to hinge at your hips, while maintaining a long spine. Over time, you can walk the hands farther down the strap. The toes should be pointing straight up to avoid any internal or external rotation of the legs. You can also practice this with a wall similar to the example shown in staff pose (dandasana). You may need to measure this distance beforehand to get your feet all the way to the wall. You can also place blocks under your heels if your legs do not comfortably reach the floor or if you are ready to deepen the stretch. Having contact with the wall informs the direction of the legs.

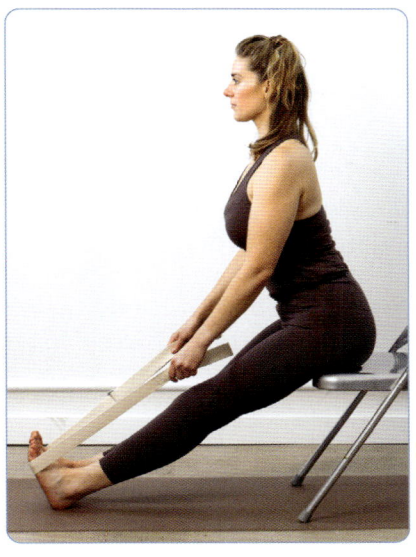

Loop a strap around your feet and hold the ends in your hands.

If your feet are just out of reach, use a strap to bridge the gap! Loop a strap around your feet, holding the ends of the strap in both hands. The strap should give you enough space to extend through the legs fully while still energetically reaching for the feet. You can practice this in a traditional seated position (see photo a), or if you are working on finding a long spine, you can do this on your back (see photo b). Be careful not to overstretch while on your back. Having the hips and spine supported in a neutral position by the floor means you will be facing your hamstring flexibility in its most honest form, where the pelvis and spine are not compensating to achieve the stretch. You can always invite a little bend into the knees if it is too intense.

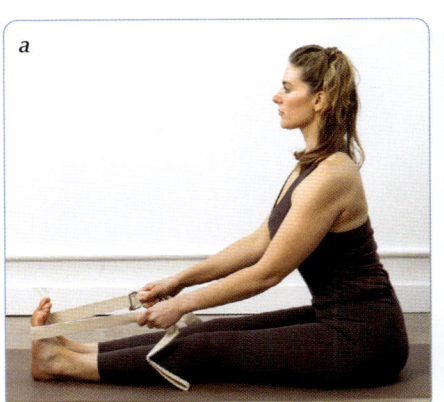

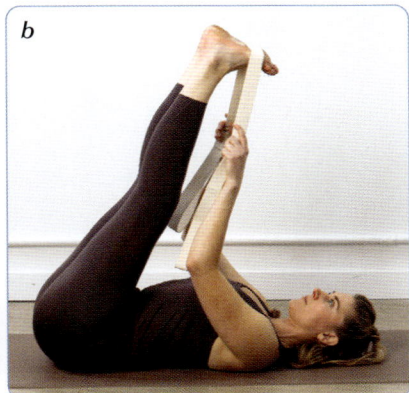

Place a bolster on top of your thighs.

Postures can be practiced in more than one way; it all comes down to intention. If you are looking to release into this pose and have some time on your hands, why not make it more restorative? You control the dial between effort and ease. Slide a bolster on top of your thighs, hugging it in toward your hip creases, and gently

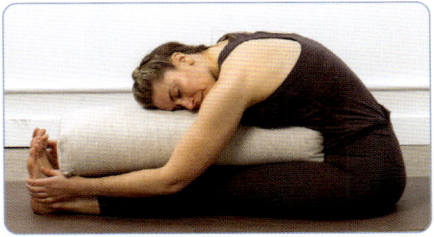

fold over it. You might even get some digestive aid from the belly releasing into the bolster. You can use the bolster as a ramp to add height. To do so, separate your feet slightly and stack blocks under the front end of the bolster. Once you have folded forward, you can use the space under the bolster to wrap your arms through, finding a gentle hug.

Rest or reach using the seat of a chair.

You can also use a chair to release more fully into a posture. Furthermore, you can use the chair to find a more active extension through your spine. To find a more active stretch (see photo *a*), slide both legs under the chair seat and reach for the seat or legs of the chair with your hands, maintaining a long spine. To find a more relaxed and supported version of this posture (see photo *b*), draw the chair close enough to you to release your forehead onto the chair seat, allowing the spine to round. Feel free to place a second mat or blanket on the chair seat for added comfort. In this version, fully release the cervical spine and head, letting tension subside.

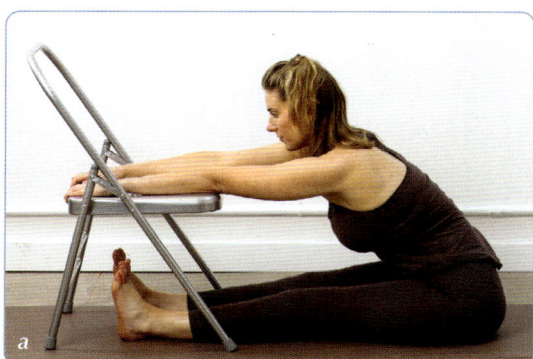 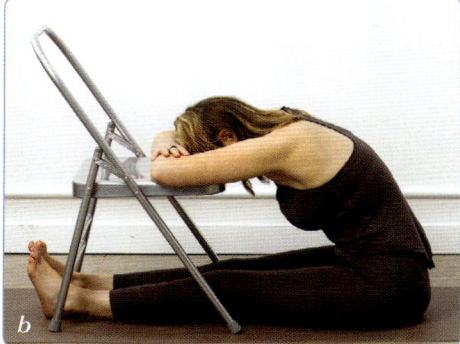

Wide-Angle Seated Forward Bend

Upavishtha Konasana   उपविष्ठ कोणासन

Wide-angle seated forward bend is a beneficial pose that efficiently stretches the insides and backs of the legs. This pose also stimulates abdominal organs, promoting digestive health, and releases tension in the groin area. Explore prop-supported variations to enhance your experience and amplify the benefits of this expansive posture.

Use blocks or a bolster ramp to raise the height of the floor.

Blocks are a great way to bring the floor to you! If you have trouble reaching the floor, placing blocks under your forehead, chest, or forearms can increase relaxation in this stretch and make it easier (see photo a). If the blocks are not high enough, create a bolster ramp! To do so, stack blocks under the front of the bolster and draw the back of the bolster into your hips (see photo b). If your bolster is feeling a little flimsy or is simply too small, stack two bolsters and wrap a blanket over them to prevent sliding. Once you have folded forward, you can use the space under the bolster to wrap your arms through, or wrap around the blocks as shown in the photo.

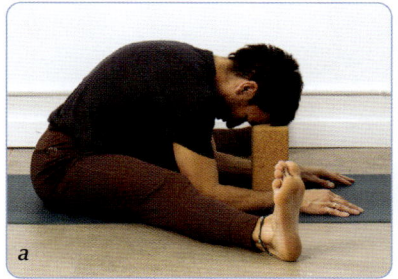
a

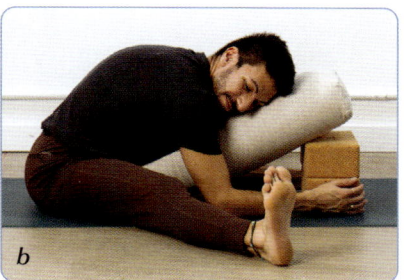
b

Add a leg lift routine over blocks to improve mobility.

Who says props have to be static? Adding some flair to this posture and increasing the mobility of your hips can turn it into a challenging exercise! In this exercise, you use the block to strengthen the psoas muscles and lower abdominal muscles. It also strengthens the muscles on the front side of the thigh (primarily the quadriceps) while lengthening the muscles on the back side of the thigh (primarily the hamstrings). Sit tall in a wide-legged straddle position. Place the block next to the inside edge of one ankle. Frame that leg with your hands and turn the torso toward the leg. Engage through the psoas and core muscles to lift the extended leg to the other side of the block and then back to its starting position. Continue to repeat for 5 to 10 repetitions, then switch sides. Moving slower and with more control makes the exercise more challenging.

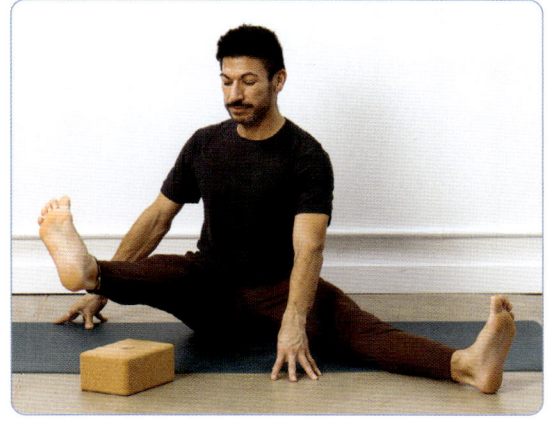

Sit on a bolster or blanket to neutralize tight hips and release your hamstrings.

If you have tight psoas, sitting on the edge of a prop slightly tilts the front of your pelvis down, removing rounding in the low back and bringing the pelvis into a neutral position.

A neutral pelvis supports extension of the spine before you fold forward. The intention is to feel the stretch in your hamstrings more than in your low back (something that happens when the psoas are tight and the pelvis tucks under).

Rest or reach using the seat of a chair.

You can also use a chair to release more fully into a posture. The chair also helps you to find a more active extension through your spine. To find a more active stretch (see photo *a*), have a chair in front of you, equidistant from the feet of the extended legs and within reach. Reach your hands for the seat or legs of the chair; once you contact the chair, work toward maintaining a long spine. Adjust the distance of the chair from you as needed. To find a more relaxed and supported version of this posture (see photo *b*), draw the chair close enough to you to release your forehead onto the chair seat or edge, allowing the spine to round somewhat. Place another mat or blanket on the chair seat for added comfort. In this version, allow the cervical spine and head to release fully, letting tension subside.

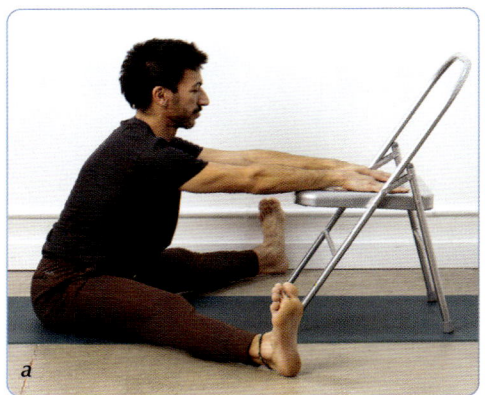
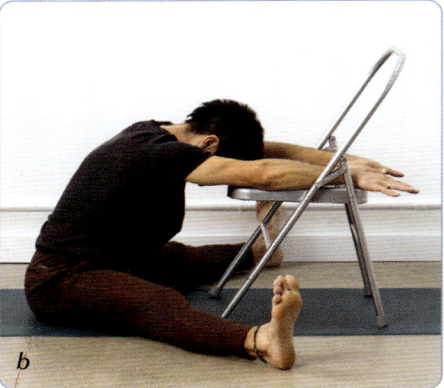

Lie on your back with your legs on a wall to support a long spine.

You can practice this traditional seated position lying down! Gravity gently turns this into a supine legs-up-the-wall position that supports a long spine, stable hips, and an inner thigh stretch. You also get some of the upside-down benefits, including lymphatic drainage, increased blood flow to your head and heart, and downregulation of the nervous system.

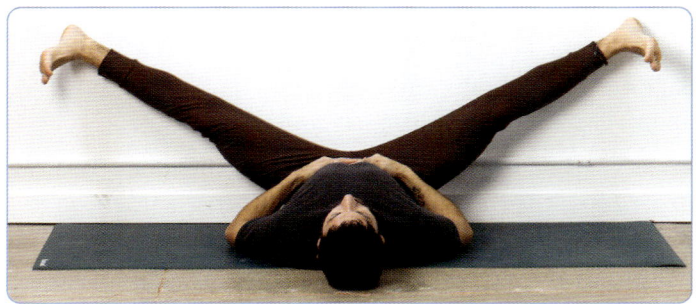

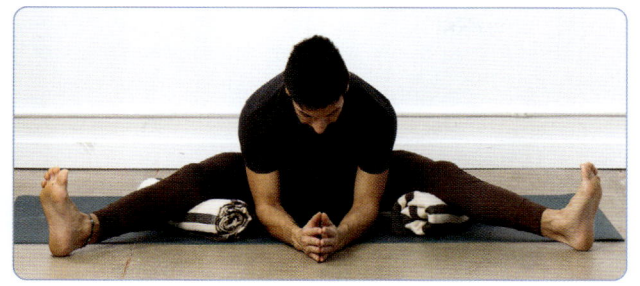

Place a rolled-up blanket under your knees to support tight hamstrings.

If your hamstrings or hip flexors are feeling tight, rolling a blanket under the knees can help by adding a slight flexion in the knees that shortens the hamstrings and psoas, decreasing the pull you might feel on these muscles. It also directs the sensation (such as pain in the backs of the knees) away from the attachment points and toward the belly of the hamstring muscles.

Place straps around feet and hold in your hands.

If your feet are just out of reach, use two straps to bridge the gap! Loop a strap around each foot and hold the end of each strap in the corresponding hand. The straps should give you enough space to extend the legs fully while still energetically reaching for the feet.

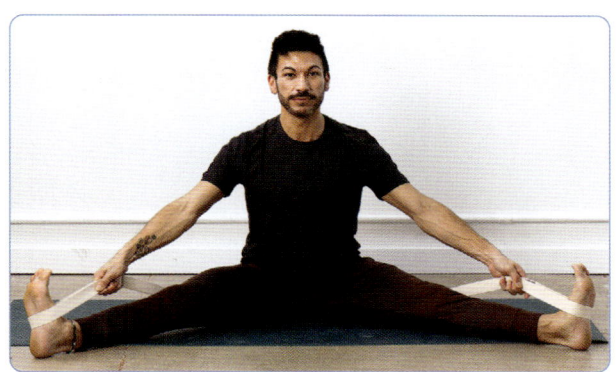

Place blocks or blankets under your heels to deepen the stretch and to prepare for tortoise pose.

If you are working toward tortoise pose, try sliding blocks or blankets under your feet in wide-angle seated forward bend. The additional leg elevation may make sliding your arms under the legs more accessible. If the hamstring stretch still feels too intense, invite a bend into the knees. Over time, practice working your legs closer together to get your legs higher up on your arms.

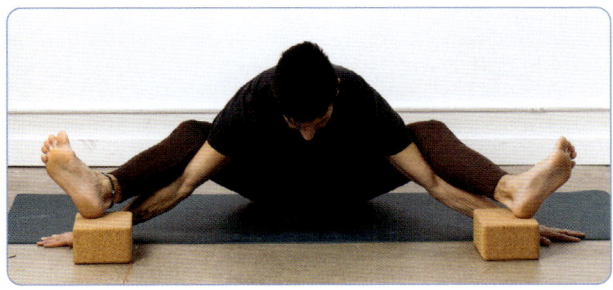

Hero Pose

Virasana

वीरासन

Hero pose is a rejuvenating yoga posture that aids in restoring blood flow to the less vascularized tissues of the knees upon exiting. This pose actively stretches the thighs, knees, and ankles while also strengthening the arches of the feet. Incorporate prop-supported variations to enrich your experience and enhance the benefits of this grounding and therapeutic pose.

Sit on a bolster or place a block between your ankles.

Using a block and bolster in hero pose is a great way to reduce pressure on the knees. It also lessons the intensity through the psoas, thighs, ankles, and shins. Place a block between your ankles turned to its widest orientation (see photo *a*). Stack blocks if needed or place a blanket over the blocks for more comfort. If you are using a bolster, sit on the front edge of it so that your knees can come together, just in front of it (see photo *b*).

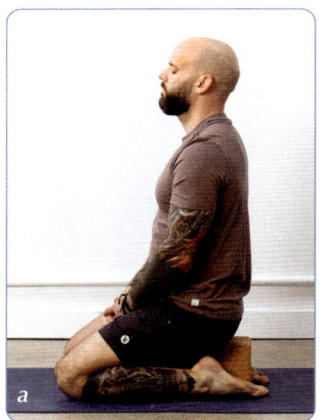 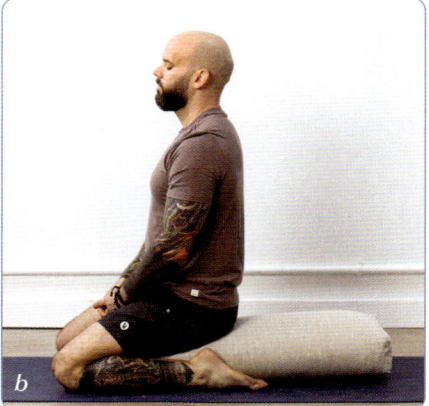

Place a blanket under your knees or ankles to ease joint pain.

You can use one or more folded blankets under the knees and shins to reduce pressure and associated pain in the knees and shins. If you are working your sitting bones all the way to the floor, roll your calves gently out to the sides to make space for the hamstrings as you lower your seat to rest between your ankles.

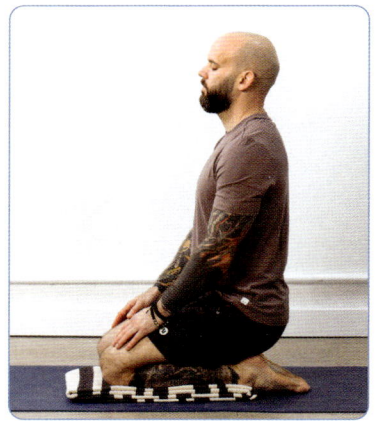

Sit on a chair with a bolster behind the front legs of the chair.

This variation is great for reducing knee strain and is good if you have difficulty getting up from and down on the floor. Slide a bolster behind the front legs of a chair, then sit on the chair. Bend your knees, tucking your feet under the chair and behind the bolster. Allow the front of your feet and ankles to rest on the bolster.

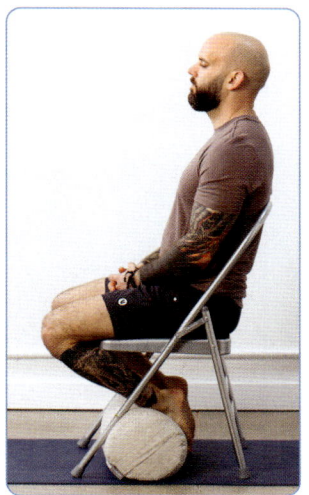

Place a rolled-up blanket behind your knees for a calf stretch.

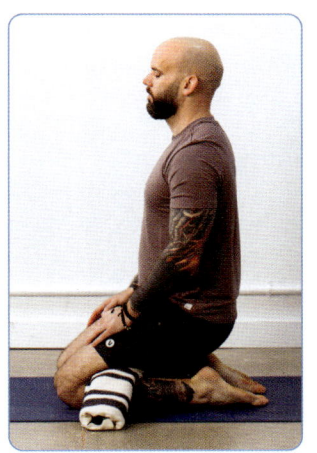

This is one of my favorite deep tissue massage techniques at home! Start by rolling a blanket into a firm cylinder shape. From a kneeling or table top position, slide the blanket behind your knees, then begin to sit back toward your heels. You should feel a deep compression of the tightly rolled blanket into the tops of your calves. If the pressure is too intense, add a bolster or block under your sitting bones. If you would like to target a different portion of the calves, move the blanket farther down. This is also a great home remedy if you suffer from shin splints or charley horses! Because the variation restricts blood flow to a higher degree, be sure to take a down dog position after to bring blood and oxygen back to the knees and ankles. This sudden rush of blood flow is especially healing for the knees because it is less vascularized than other parts of the body.

Support the structure of your legs with a looped strap.

In any variation of this pose, you can use a strap around your thighs to hold the legs and knees together. For the chair variation, the strap will be looped just around the thighs. For all other variations, you can loop the strap all the way around the shins to keep your lower legs from splaying too far and irritating your knees.

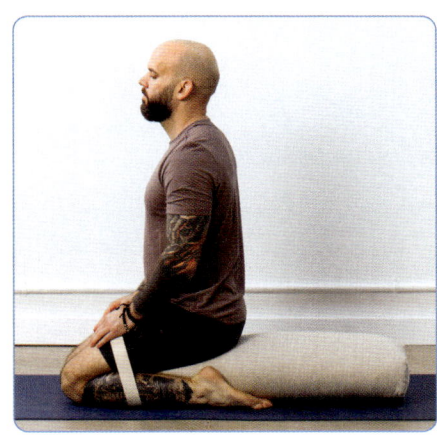

Heron Pose

Kraunchasana

क्रौञ्चासन

Heron pose is a transformative yoga posture that focuses on lengthening the spine and providing a deep stretch to the thighs, hamstrings, knees, and ankles. This pose actively strengthens the arches of the feet. Explore prop-supported variations to enhance your practice and experience the full benefits of this pose.

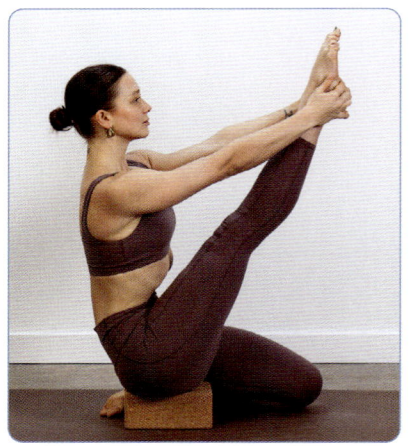

Sit on a block to support your bent knee and hips.

Use a block to add a little height and take pressure out of the knee. Stack blocks if you need more height or place a blanket over the block for more comfort. Start in hero pose sitting on a block, then extend one leg. Bend the knee of the extended leg, planting the foot on the mat in front of you. Reach both hands for the outside of the ankle or around the sole of the front foot and lift the foot off the mat, shifting the weight back onto the sitting bones. Lift your chest toward the sky and start to straighten the front leg. Draw your shoulder blades down the back.

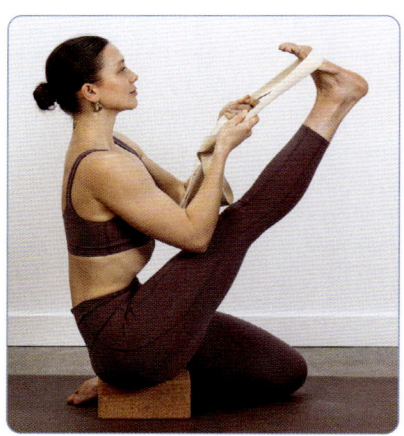

Use a strap to help reach your foot.

Straps are great for bridging the gap between your foot and your hands. They also help you to extend your front leg without sacrificing your spinal posture. Start in hero pose, then extend one leg in front of you. Bend the knee of the extended leg, planting the foot on the mat in front of you. Loop a strap around the ball of your front foot and hold the ends of the strap in both hands. Lift the chest toward the sky and start to lift and straighten the front leg. Over time, walk your hands farther down the strap.

Place your heel on the seat of a chair to stabilize and center yourself.

Using a chair in this pose allows you to relax the lifted leg a little bit and helps you to find your balance. It can feel like there is a lot of weight shifting to one side of the body given the asymmetry of this pose, so the seat gives you more structure and stability. With the foot stabilized, lengthen through your spine. You can achieve this by pressing your heel into the seat to reinforce an opposite lifting-away action of the torso from the front of your extended thigh or by sitting your back against a wall to inform this alignment.

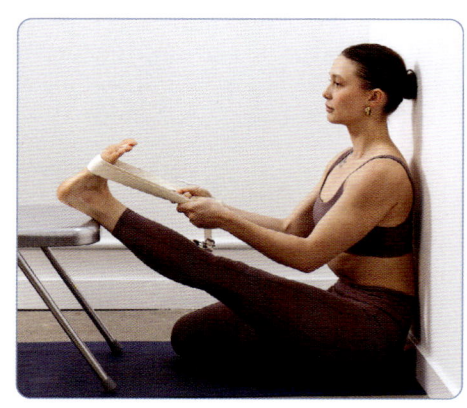

Sit on a chair and use a strap to stabilize and center yourself.

For this variation of the pose, begin seated on a chair with both feet planted on the floor. This offers stability and control over your postural alignment, and it will take some of the pressure off the knees. Draw one knee into your chest and reach for the outside of the ankle or around the sole of the front foot with both hands. Lift the foot off the mat, shifting the weight back onto the sitting bones. Lift the chest toward the sky and start to straighten the front leg (see photo a). Draw your shoulder blades down the back.

You can also bend your bottom knee and place the top of your foot on blocks or on the bar under the chair, or you can use a strap if your foot is just out of reach (see photo b). If you have osteoporosis or osteopenia, avoid the risk of fracture caused by folding forward to loop the strap around your foot. Instead, step on the strap, holding the ends prior to sitting down. For extra support, hold both ends of the strap in one hand and place the free hand on the seat of the chair and press down to lengthen through your spine.

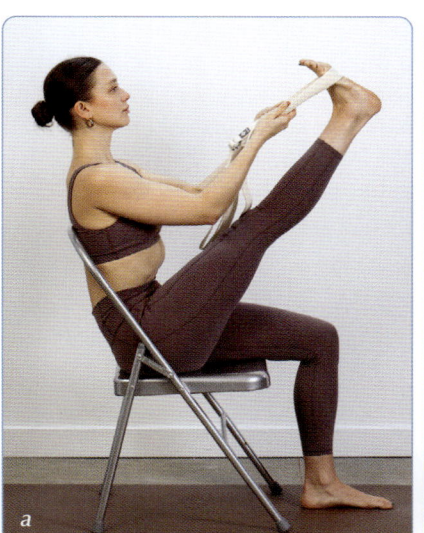
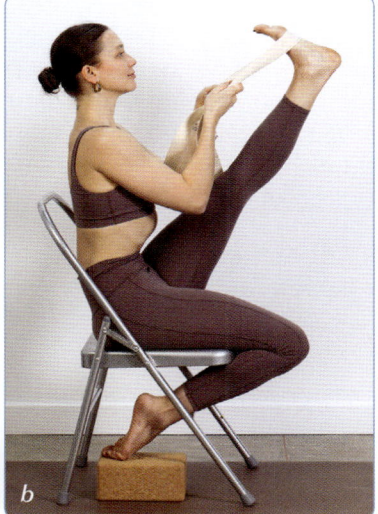

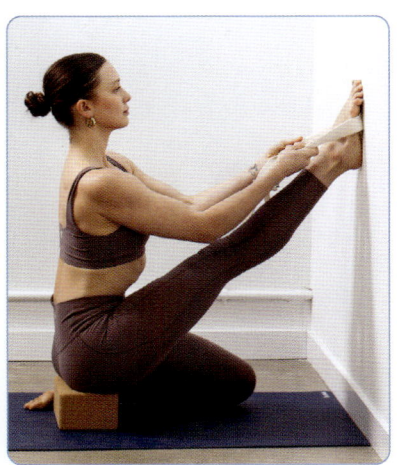

Place your foot on a wall and use a strap to stabilize and center yourself.

This wall variation is great for maintaining balance while working on alignment, leveling the hips, and integrating muscle memory. Loop a strap around the foot you will be lifting, holding the ends of the strap in one hand. Place the foot on the wall, starting with a bent knee. This may be a great place to pause and breathe. If you can maintain length in your spine, inch your front foot a little higher up the wall. If you feel yourself reaching an end range of motion or the spine wants to round, pause and breathe. Over time and with patience, the leg will eventually make its way to fully extend up the wall. You can also adjust the intensity of the stretch by sitting closer to or farther away from the wall. Try your best to keep your shoulders stacked over your hips.

Garland Pose

Malasana   मालासन

Garland pose is a rejuvenating yoga posture with a range of benefits. This pose efficiently stretches the ankles, groin, and back of the torso, fostering flexibility and release. It also tones the abdominal muscles while stimulating digestive organs, promoting a sense of balance and well-being. Explore prop-supported variations to deepen your practice and enhance the therapeutic effects of garland pose.

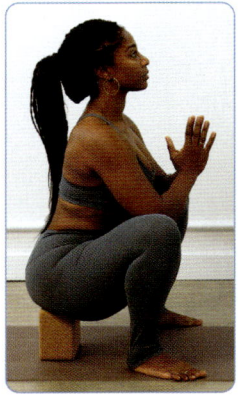

Sit on a block to ground your heels.

Using a block in this pose supports your hips and ankles! The added height from the block allows you to reach your heels to the floor, which stretches the backs of the ankles and calves and strengthens the fronts of the ankles and shins. This variation also decreases the angle of flexion on the knees, lessening tension there, and frees up more space in the spine so you can sit tall. Turn a block to the medium or tallest height under the sitting bones or stack blocks. Bring your hands to the heart center and draw the shoulder blades down and back. Lengthen down through the tailbone as you lift up through the crown of the head. For a deeper stretch, extend the torso forward between the thighs and walk your fingertips out long on the mat, extending through the arms.

Use a block to support leg extension in skandasana (half squat pose).

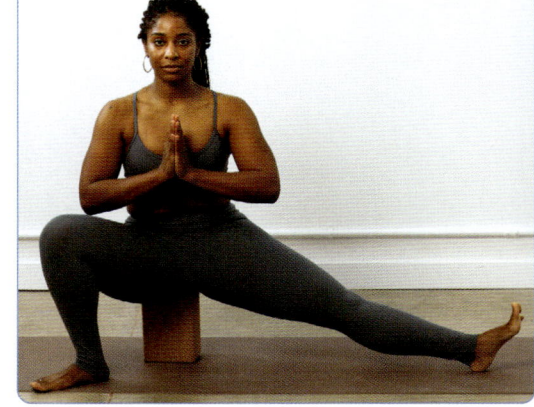

Just as in garland pose, the block supports half squat pose (skandasana), by allowing you to ground the sole of the foot on the bent knee leg without putting too much pressure on the knee. It also makes it easier to lift your shoulders up and back to stack over your pelvis. With the hips grounded, home in on the subtle actions of the legs and upper body. Start in the block-supported garland pose, tracking your knees in the direction of the feet. Extend one leg in the direction of the knee. Bring your hands to the heart center and draw the shoulder blades down and back. Lengthen down through the tailbone as you lift through the crown of the head. Wrap your outer thighs down and back, pointing your kneecaps toward the sky. Press through the heel of the foot of the extended leg. Feel free to take your favorite arm variation such as reaching for your big toe or bind your hands around the bent knee.

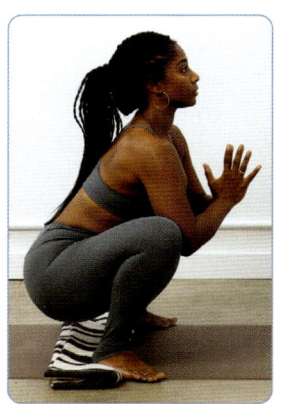

Use a rolled-up blanket to ground your heels.

If your ankles are feeling tight and don't want to flex to the degree this posture demands, slide a folded blanket under your heels. The heels can remain both lifted yet grounded all at once. Being able to ground the heels offers more stability and balance as you focus your powers of concentration on your breath and on the actions of your legs and spine!

Practice a bind with a strap between your hands to create space.

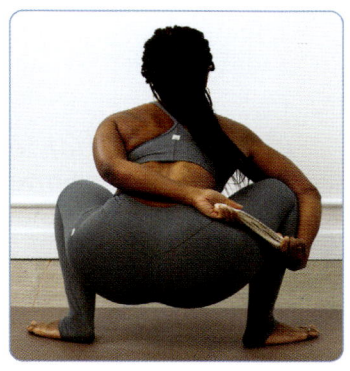

A strap is a handy tool to free up space in your chest and shoulders in this pose. It can bridge the gap between your hands if they are just out of reach from one another. Even if you *can* bind your hands, sometimes it is to the sacrifice of your spinal alignment, causing forward hunching or a wonky positioning in one or both knees (such as the knee caving in toward the direction of your big toe). So a strap may come in handy as you maintain your length in both sides of the body and work your hands closer together over time from there.

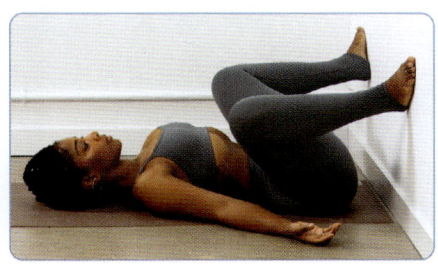

Lie on your back with your feet against a wall to support a long spine and reduce weight on the ankles.

Want to practice the structure of garland pose without compromising posture from the hips up? Take the pose in a supine position. This variation informs good spinal alignment, supports your knees and hips, and reduces strain on the ankles, especially if you have an injury in the foot or ankle that calls for no weight-bearing activities. Place both feet on the wall and begin to bend your knees toward your armpits. I suggest having the feet level with or higher than the knees to protect the knee. You may need to adjust the distance of your sacrum from the wall to find what works best for you. To deepen the stretch, scoot your body closer to the wall; to lessen the stretch, scoot your body farther from the wall.

Loop a strap around your shins and behind your rib cage for alignment.

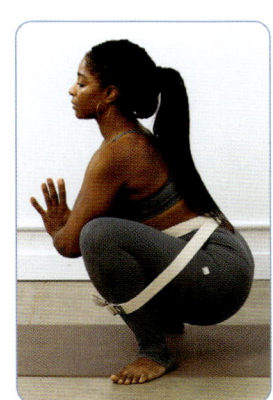

The hardest part about this variation of garland pose is figuring out the strap! Start by folding a strap in half, then enter your squat. Hold the strap behind your back, then loop the folded end of the strap around the top of one shin. Bring the loose ends of the strap around the top of your other shin and close the loop. Shimmy the strap up your back until it is behind the rib cage, then tighten the loop so it is firmly held in place (depending on your unique proportions, you may have the strap a little lower on your back). Start to sit tall through your spine, pressing the back of your ribs into the strap and lengthening your tailbone toward the floor. The action of your spine pressing into the strap should cause your knees to draw back and your hips and inner thighs to open.

Thunderbolt Pose
(Toe Squat Variation)

Vajrasana
वज्रासन

The toe squat variation of thunderbolt pose efficiently opens the fascia on the bottoms of the feet, providing relief and increased flexibility. Simultaneously, it strengthens the ankles and offers a deep stretch to the toes, soles of the feet, and calves. Let's explore some common prop-supported variations to enhance your practice and experience.

Place a block, bolster, or blanket under your knees to reduce intensity.

Using a prop takes the strain off the knees and lessens the intensity of the pose through the soles of your feet, calves, psoas, and thighs. The prop relieves pressure on the feet and ankles, which is more comfortable when you shift the torso back to stack over the hips. Start by kneeling with your feet touching and your toes tucked under your heels. Rock your weight back to lift your knees off the mat and slide one or more blocks, bolsters, or blankets under your knees. Sit tall through your spine. Relax through your shoulders and facial muscles; since this is a deep stretch for the fascia on the bottom of the feet, referred tension can show up in other areas of the body.

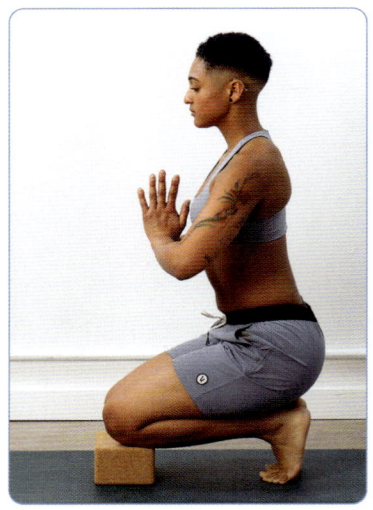

Place a block, bolster, or blanket between your sitting bones and heels to support the knees.

Using one or more props can take pressure out of the knees by reducing the angle of flexion. However, the amount of weight-bearing on the feet may increase some, causing a deeper sensation on the toes, feet, and ankles. Start by kneeling with your feet touching and your toes tucked under your heels. Place a block, bolster, or folded blanket on top of your heels or ankles and sit back.

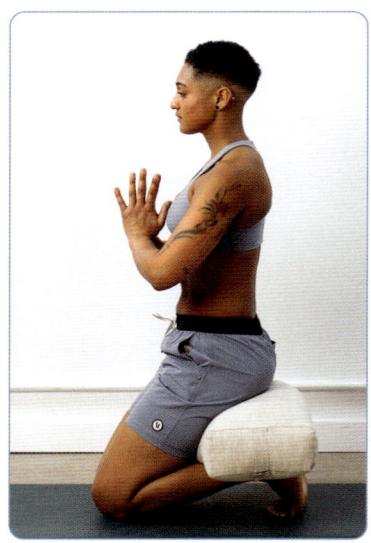

Bound Angle Pose

Baddha Konasana   बद्धकोणासन

Bound angle pose is a restorative yoga posture with multifaceted benefits. This pose effectively stretches the inner thighs, groin, and knees, providing relief and flexibility. It also soothes sciatica and may alleviate menstrual pain, offering therapeutic support. Explore prop-supported variations to enhance your practice and unlock the full potential of this pose.

Sit on a blanket with blocks under your knees to support the knees and hips.

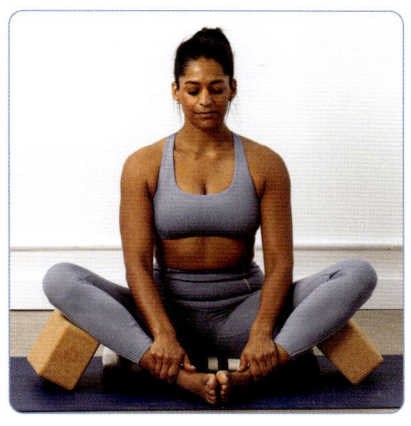

Using blocks in bound angle pose gives the legs something to rest on, relieving tension in the knees and the hips. Sit with the sitting bones pressed into the floor or on a folded blanket to elevate the hips slightly and support a neutral spine. Bring the soles of your feet together and open the knees wide, like opening a book. Draw your heels as close to the pelvis as is comfortable. Place blocks at your preferred height under the knees for support or place them at an angle to match the slope of your thighs. Hold your ankles and sit tall through the spine to start. If you would like to take the posture further, fold forward, bending your elbows out to the sides. Alternatively, slide your feet farther away to create a diamond shape with the legs. This shape generates more decompression and spinal traction as you release tension through the upper and middle back.

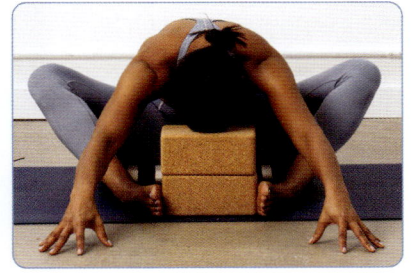

Practice tarasana, star pose variation, with a block between your feet.

Depending on your approach to this posture (whether it be active or passive), you can benefit from both stretching and strengthening your hips and inner thighs. Start seated, then bring the soles of your feet to the outsides of a block and open your knees wide, like opening a book. The orientation of the block is the yogi's choice! Press your feet into the block to activate the stabilizing muscles of your hips and inner thighs or release into a forward bend. If you choose, you can stack blocks and bend forward to benefit from the deeper relaxation that comes with bringing the floor to you. Resting your forehead on stacked blocks allows you to relax your facial muscles and let tension dissolve from the upper body down.

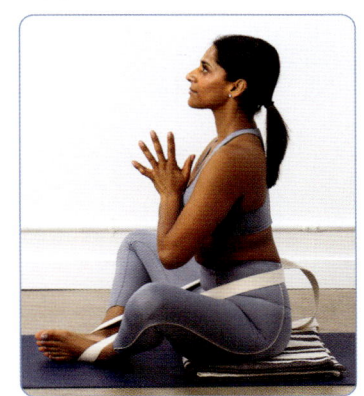

Loop a strap around your lower back and feet.

This variation of the pose is best practiced sitting upright or in a supine position (discussed later). The biggest benefit of using a strap is supporting the natural *S* curve of a neutral spine. Because external rotation of the femur bones in the hip sockets is hard for some people, they might accommodate this movement by curling through the low back or tucking through the pelvis. A strap will help you to gently open the hips while resisting the collapse of your posture. Start in bound angle pose as you normally would with a strap within reach. Create a big loop with your strap, then draw it over your head and torso. Place the back of the loop around the rim of your pelvis and the front of the loop over your ankles and under your feet. The sides of the strap will lie on top of the inner thighs and calves. Begin to tighten the looped strap, pulling your feet closer to your pubic bone—just enough to cause a nice stretch—no strain! The back of the strap will pull forward simultaneously due to the increased tension, helping you to sit up straighter. The gentle resistance you may have for the back of the strap will also reinforce posture.

Wrap a rolled-up blanket around your feet and under your ankles to support the knees.

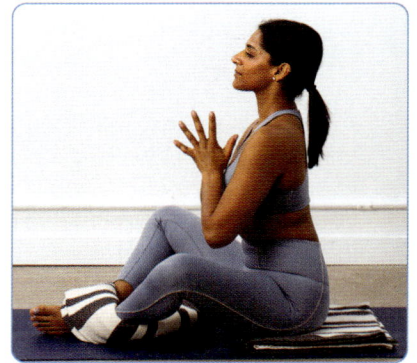

This is my favorite alternative to sliding props under the knees! This variation still supports the knees and hips, but it also gives the ankles more cushion and support, which is especially helpful if a supinated foot position causes you strain! The blanket also holds the feet together in a way that just allows you to release fully without thinking. Roll your blanket to your desired thickness. Place the rolled blanket over the tops of your ankles and wrap it around the sides of the ankles, tucking it under. Depending on the thickness of your roll, the blanket may be under the calves more than the ankles; play around with it and find out where the sweet spot is for you. It can change depending on the day! Release fully through your legs, allowing the blanket to support your weight.

Slide a bolster under your knees for support.

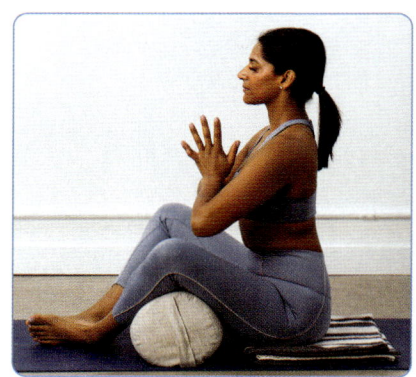

All the same concepts apply in this variation as they do in the first variation with blocks under the knees, with the difference being prop height and texture. A bolster guarantees a softer cushion than blocks with their defined edges.

Lie on your back with your legs on a wall to support a long spine.

You can practice this traditional seated position lying down! Turning this into a supine legs-up-the-wall position supports a long spine, stable hips, and an inner thigh stretch gently directed by gravity. In addition to this, you get some of the upside-down benefits, including lymphatic drainage, increased blood flow toward your head and heart, and downregulation of the nervous system.

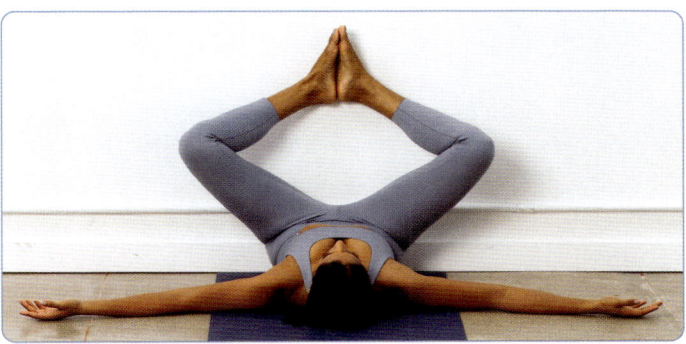

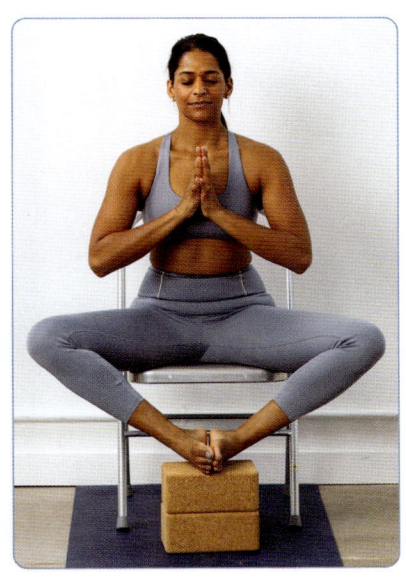

Sit on a chair with your feet on blocks or blankets.

This variation is for those who have difficulty getting up and down from the floor or have knee or hip strain or injury. Sit on the edge of the chair to release tension through the hips and comfortably lengthen the spine. Place the feet on the blocks or blanket then move the knees away from each other to bring the soles of the feet together. To deepen the stretch, over time, stack more blocks or blankets under your feet to bring your heels closer to your pelvis.

Fire Log Pose

Agnistambhasana

अग्निस्तिम्भासन

Fire log pose is a focused yoga posture that targets and stretches the hips, specifically the piriformis, along with the groin and low back, providing targeted relief and flexibility. This pose also strengthens the ankles when the feet are flexed. Delve into various prop-supported variations to enrich your practice and maximize the therapeutic benefits of this pose.

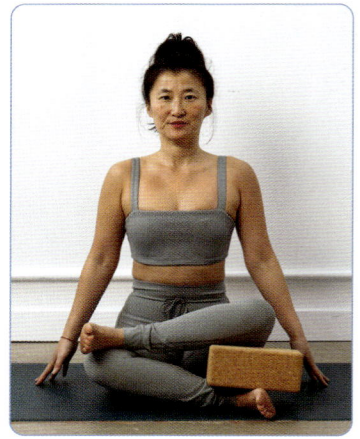

Place a block or rolled blanket between your knee and ankle.

Not everyone's knees and ankles will stack perfectly on top of one another. Blocks or blankets are wonderful tools for bridging the gap between the top knee and bottom ankle. The prop gives the top knee something to rest on to ease strain or discomfort. It also aids in relaxing through the psoas, which you may have been working to stabilize and hold the elevated knee in place. Start in a seated cross-legged position. Bring your bottom heel forward until your bottom shin is parallel to the edge of the mat, then stack your top shin directly over the bottom one. If this is too much, you can start with the top foot folded toward your hip crease, then eventually work the top ankle to stack over the bottom knee so both shins are parallel to the top of the mat. If your top knee is hovering over the bottom ankle, bridge the gap with your block or rolled-up blanket. Flex the feet and toes to shorten the muscles pulling on the knee; to protect the knee. Drive your sitting bones into the mat and sit tall. You can also fold forward for a deeper hip and hamstring stretch.

Place a block or rolled blanket under your bottom knee for support.

Just as in the prior example of your knee hovering over the bottom ankle, the bottom knee may want to hover over the floor. Don't worry if your knee does not initially rest down on the mat. Blocks and blankets are wonderful tools for bridging the gap between the bottom knee and the floor or mat. The prop gives the knee something to rest on to ease strain or discomfort. It also prevents injury that could be caused by the force of the top foot or ankle pressing on an unsupported knee.

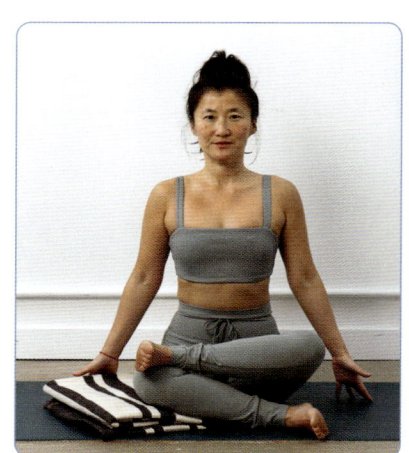

Fire Log Pose (continued)

Place a block or rolled-up blanket under your foot in front of your bottom knee.

This variation of the posture allows for a deeper hip, thigh, hamstring, and groin stretch without putting added stress on the knees. The block decreases the pressure on both knees by taking the force of the top foot off the bottom knee and reducing the angle of flexion in the top knee. For further reduction, use a blanket instead of a block. I love this variation because it gives you the option to work on parallel shins while protecting the health of your knees!

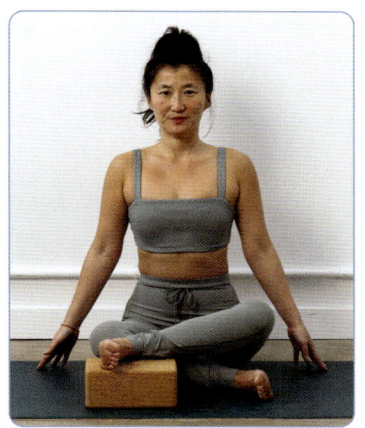

Place a bolster or folded blanket under your sitting bones to support tight hips and a long spine.

A little hip elevation can go a long way! Adding some height can ease joint tension in a few ways. Having the hips level with or higher than the knees decreases the angle of flexion at the joint, reducing strain. If you have tight psoas, sitting on the edge of a prop slightly tilts the front of your pelvis toward the mat, removing rounding in the low back and bringing the pelvis into a neutral position. A neutral pelvis supports a long and relaxed spine. Once seated, shift your weight back into the sitting bones, distributing the weight evenly between them. Sit tall through your spine, stacking the shoulders directly over the pelvis.

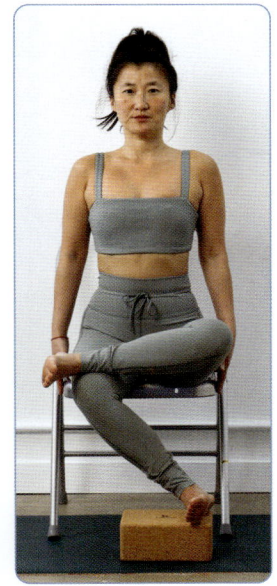

Sit on a chair, with your bottom foot rolled to its outer edge on a block.

If you have difficulty getting up from and down on the floor or have knee or hip strain or injury, this variation is for you! Sit on the edge of the chair to release tension through the hips and comfortably lengthen the spine. Cross one leg over the other knee, coming into a figure four position. If this strains your knee or low back, stack blankets on the seat under your hips to add height. Have your bottom foot on a block or stack of blocks beneath you. The block should be between the front legs of the chair and slightly in front of the chair (the same distance in front of the chair as your knee), but you can deepen or lessen the stretch by sliding the block to the right and left from this baseline point. Begin to roll to the outer edge of the foot that's on the block. You can let the ankle relax fully or support the ankle and knee by actively flexing through the bottom foot—flexing the foot prevents assuming a supinated foot position and shortens the extensor muscles that can pull on the knee when relaxed. You can fold over the legs, resting your hands on the seat with your feet on the blocks below, or you can let them release fully toward the floor. Alternatively, you can grab the back of the chair as you hinge forward at the hips to extend through your spine, flattening your back. To progress over time, stack more blocks under your bottom foot to bring it closer to your top knee.

Monkey Pose

Hanumanasana   हनुमानासन

Monkey pose, also recognized as a lateral split, is a dynamic yoga posture that actively stretches and opens the thighs, hamstrings, and psoas, fostering increased flexibility and release. It also stimulates the abdomen, adding a vitalizing element to this invigorating pose. Explore prop-supported variations to enhance your practice and fully experience the benefits of monkey pose.

Place blocks or chairs under your hands to raise the height of the floor.

Using props that bridge the gap between you and the floor can help you fine-tune alignment and level the pelvis. Having blocks or chairs under your hands helps maintain good spinal alignment by stacking your shoulders over your hips. This spinal alignment supports the pelvis by counteracting the tendency to roll weight into the outer hip of your front leg. When the torso is upright, the front of the pelvis will have to lift upward rather than tilt forward, which deepens the psoas and quad stretch through the back leg. For a half split, start in a low lunge with your hands on blocks or the seats of chairs, framing the hips. Stack your shoulders over your hips and lengthen your tailbone down toward the back of your knee. Straighten through the front leg, walking the heel forward so that your hip aligns over the back knee. You can stop here and bend over the front leg, taking the half split. See photo *a* for an example of half splits with blocks.

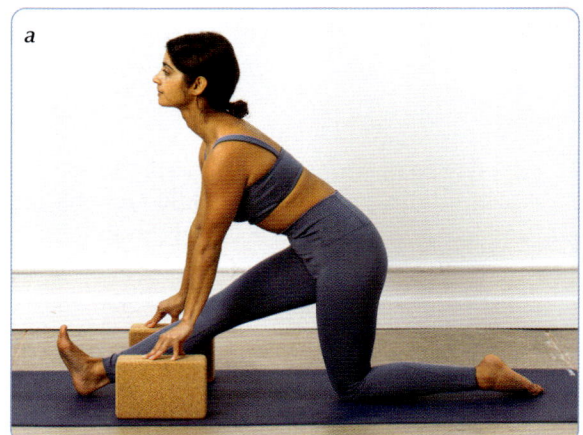

If you are working toward a full split, keep your shoulders stacked over your hips and start to walk the back leg knee back. Keep driving your tailbone down toward the mat and your pubic bone up toward your navel. Only go as far as you can keep your front knee pointing up and your back knee pointing down while maintaining level hip points (anatomically referred to as the anterior superior iliac spine, or ASIS) that are an equal distance from the floor below. Relax your shoulders down and away from your ears as you draw your front ribs in toward your back body. See photo *b* for an example of full splits with chairs.

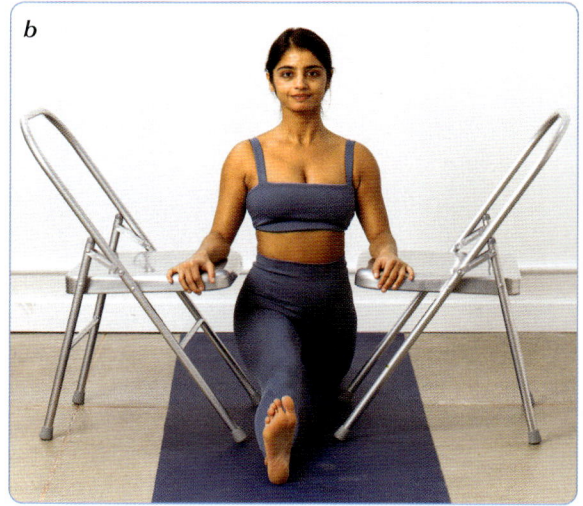

Place a block, bolster, or rolled blanket under the hips.

When there is a gap between your hips and the floor, you may naturally want to resist overstretching by tensing up and straining to fight gravity. Alternatively, you may try a less intense stretch by tilting your torso and pelvis forward. With blocks, bolsters, or blankets

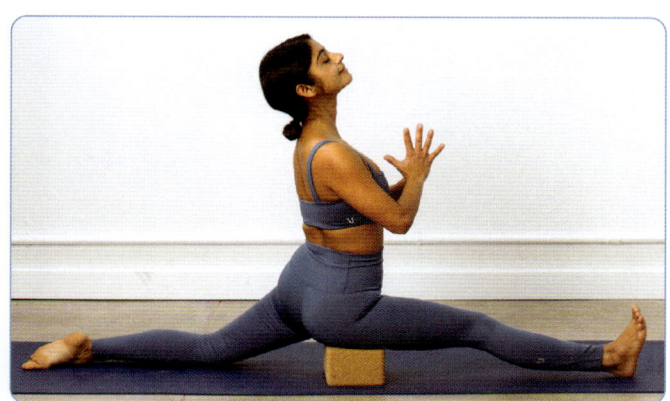

under your pelvis, you can bring the floor to you, providing yourself with the support you need to relax the upper body and level the hips. Slide your prop of choice under the sitting bone and buttock of the extended front leg to bridge the gap between your hips and the mat. Relax your shoulders down and away from the ears as you draw your front ribs in toward your back body.

Use two chairs and a wall for structural support.

This variation may require a little more setup, but it is a great option for tighter muscles and alignment fine-tuning. Line two chairs up in front of a wall, with the backs of the chairs facing the wall. You may have to play with the distance of the chairs from the wall, depending on the length of your legs. Step your back leg through the back of the chair closest to the wall and extend the leg until your back foot is flexed against the wall with

your back toes pressing down into the floor, or for added height, a block as shown in the photo. For extra height or comfort, place a folded mat or blankets on top of the seat. Hold the sides of the chair to lift your front leg onto the chair in front of you (or have someone assist you). Hold the back of the chair in front of you to lift your torso over your pelvis. Press your back foot into the wall behind you to lengthen through your back leg and square through your hips. Over time, you can practice moving your back leg farther up the wall behind you.

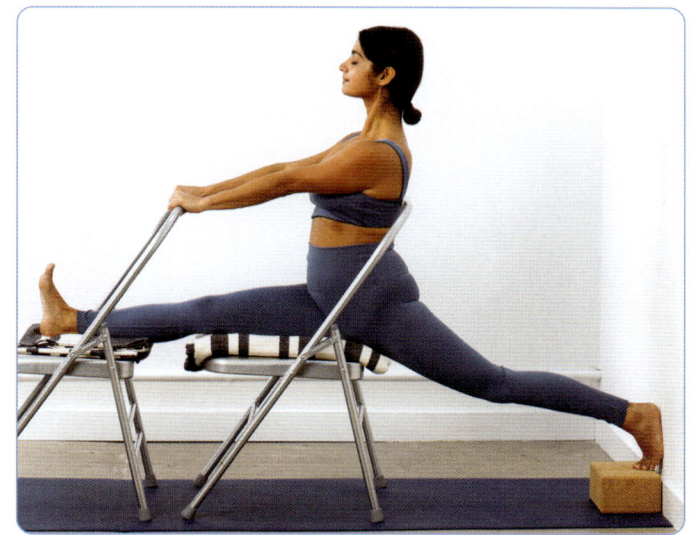

Monkey Pose *(continued)*

Loop a strap around your front hip and the ball of your flexed back foot.

This variation is great for deepening the hip stretch by activating your back leg muscles and guiding your front hip back in to align with the back hip. I hesitate to say "square hips," because all hips are different, but it's the action of working in a certain direction. The tricky part is determining the size of the loop that best suits you. I find that it is easiest to draw

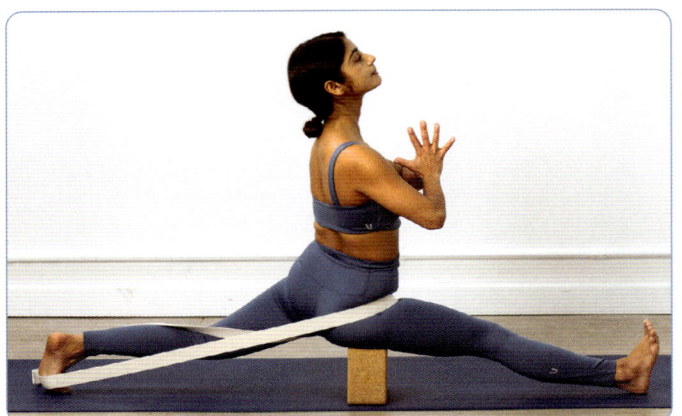

the strap around your back foot, holding both ends in your hands, then loop it from there. Note how it is looped over just the front thigh in the photo. Once the loop feels taut, activate through your back heel, lengthening through your back leg. The strap will naturally guide your front hip back and encourage you to elongate through your spine. If the hips don't reach the mat, slide a prop under.

Cow Face Pose

Gomukhasana   गोमुखासन

Cow face pose is a targeted yoga posture that actively stretches muscles connected to the deep bands of connective tissue down the outer legs, fostering increased flexibility and release. This pose also enhances shoulder range of motion and strengthens multiple muscle groups, including the chest, hips, thighs, triceps, shoulder joints, ankles, and spine. Cow face pose may also provide relief for symptoms of sciatica and assist in resetting the sacroiliac joint if derangement is present. Explore prop-supported variations to enrich your practice and unlock the full therapeutic potential of the pose.

Place a block under your sitting bones to raise the hips.

Having a block under your sitting bones in cow face pose is helpful in a couple of ways. First, it takes some pressure off your low back by releasing some of the tension associated with tight hip flexors. This also helps to neutralize the pelvis if your hip flexors are the cause of pelvic tucking or low back rounding. Second, it will relieve some pressure on the knees by bringing the hips level with or higher than the knees.

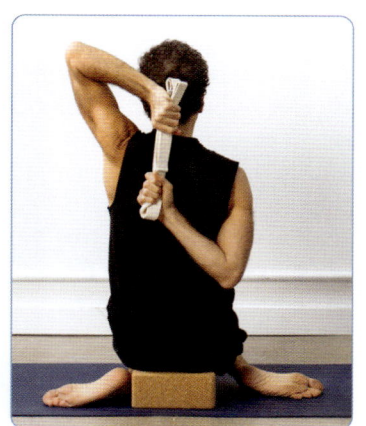

Practice a bind with a strap between your hands to create space.

A strap is a handy tool to free up space in the chest and shoulders in this pose. It can bridge the gap between your hands if they are just out of reach from one another. Even if you *can* bind your hands, sometimes doing so alters your spinal alignment, causing forward hunching of the cervical spine or overarching of the thoracic spine. A strap may come in handy as you maintain axial extension (lengthening) of the spine and work your hands closer together over time.

Turn the bind into a passive stretch by practicing supine with a block or bolster under your hips.

This is one of my favorite restorative or yin-like takes on cow face arms. It makes the bind more accessible and lets you passively rest during the stretch. It also allows you to support a long spine. Start lying on your back with both feet firmly planted on the floor, knees pointing up to the sky. Bring your hands behind your head, setting up for an abdominal crunch. Lengthen your tailbone forward and draw your belly button in toward your spine.

On an exhale, find your crunch, lifting the backs of your shoulders from the mat. Grab one elbow with the opposite hand to assist sliding the other hand between the shoulder blades or as close as you can. Lie back down, resting your upper back or head on your arm—sort of like a pillow! Continue to lengthen your tailbone forward, then press your

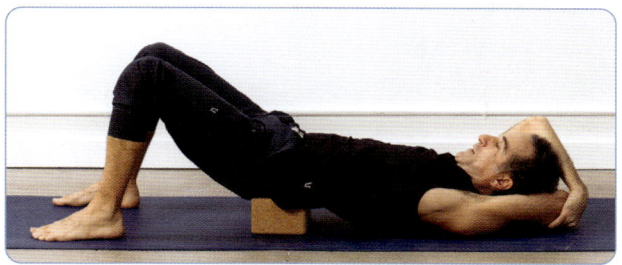

feet down into the mat to lift the hips up toward the sky, coming into bridge pose (setu bandha sarvangasana). Use the hand that was on your bent elbow to slide a block or bolster under your hips, coming into supported bridge pose (salamba setu bandha sarvangasana). This bridge variation will support extra length in the low back and aid in knitting your low ribs in toward your spine.

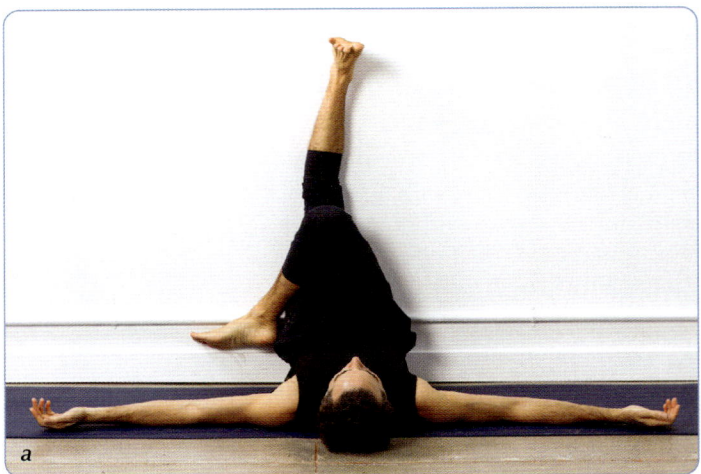

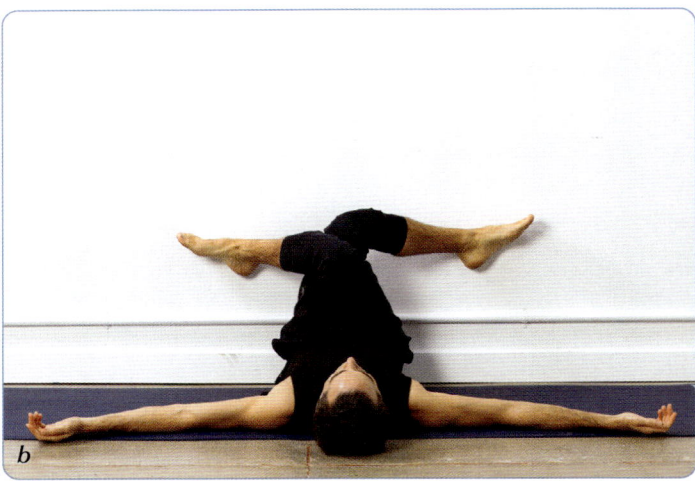

Lie on your back with your legs on a wall to support a long spine.

You can practice this traditional seated position lying down! Turning this into a supine legs-up-the-wall position supports a long spine, stable hips, and an outer thigh stretch gently directed by gravity. You also get some of the upside-down benefits, including lymphatic drainage, increased blood flow back toward your head, and heart and downregulation of the nervous system. Start in legs-up-the-wall pose (viparita karani), then cross one leg over the other, bending the knee of the top leg. The foot of the bent leg should bend toward the outer hip of the extended leg. If this is too intense, move your hips farther away from the wall to lessen the stretch. You can stay here in the half version of the pose (see photo *a*) or proceed to bend the bottom knee into a similar position (see photo *b*).

Head to Knee Pose

Janu Shirshasana · जानुशीर्षासन

Head to knee pose is a focused yoga posture that actively stretches the back of your body, homing in on the quadratus lumborum for increased flexibility and release. This pose provides targeted relief for tightness in the low back, hips, gluteal muscles, and hamstrings. It also stimulates abdominal organs, including the lower intestines, kidneys, and liver. Head to knee pose induces a calming effect, potentially offering support for managing symptoms of depression and anxiety. Explore some common prop-supported variations of this pose as described here to enhance your practice.

Slide a block or rolled blanket under the bent knee to support the knee.

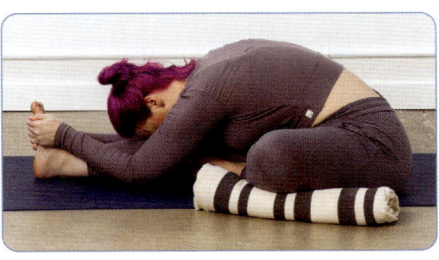

Using a block or blanket gives the leg something to rest on, relieving tension in the knee and the hip. Sit with your legs extended, with both sitting bones anchored into the floor or on a folded blanket to elevate the hips and support a neutral spine. Bring the sole of one foot toward your inner thigh or calf muscle, bending at the knee. Draw your heel as close to the pubic bone as is comfortable. Place a block or rolled blanket at your preferred height under the knee for support. Turn your torso to hover over your extended leg, then fold forward on an exhale.

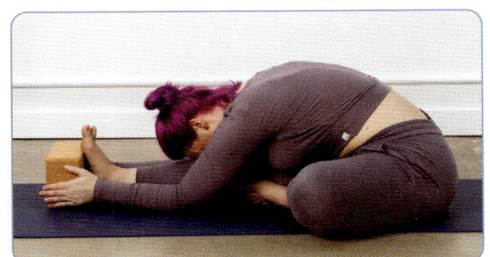

Place a block in front of your foot to deepen the stretch.

If you feel comfortable in this stretch and are looking to deepen your flexibility, you can extend the length of your leg by placing a block in front of your extended leg foot. The block will also prevent your legs from rolling in or out by reminding you to have all five toes and your knee pointing up toward the sky.

Support your arms on blocks or rest on the seat of a chair to relax the upper body.

To access the downregulating (nervous-system pacifying) effects of this pose, release the upper body fully into the pose. If the floor feels too far away, place blocks under your hands or forearms (see photo a) or slide your extended leg under the seat of a chair and rest your arms or head on the chair (see photo b).

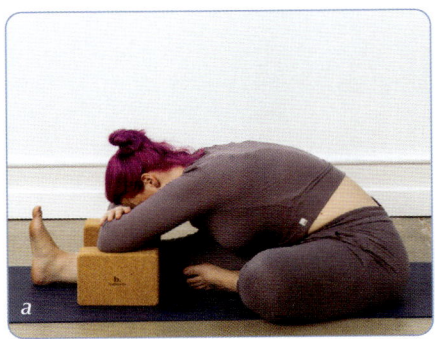
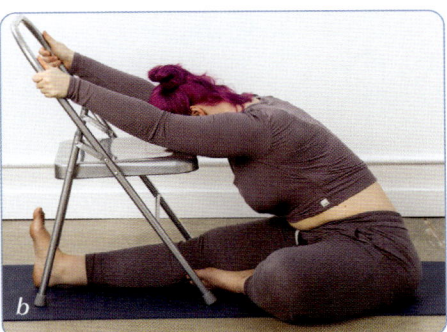

Use a strap to bridge the gap between your hands and the foot of your extended leg.

When you can't reach your foot, you usually bend the knee. But you can bridge the gap by looping a strap around your foot, holding the ends in each of your hands. This allows you to extend the leg fully. Once the leg is extended, gently rotate your shoulders and chest so they are framing the extended leg and, on an exhale, release into the forward bend.

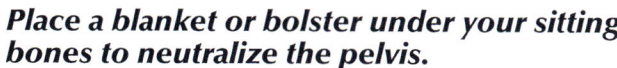

Place a blanket or bolster under your sitting bones to neutralize the pelvis.

A little hip elevation can go a long way! If you have tight psoas, sitting on the edge of a prop slightly tilts the front of your pelvis down, removing rounding in the low back and bringing the pelvis into a neutral position. A neutral pelvis supports a long and relaxed spine by making it easier to draw the torso toward the extended knee.

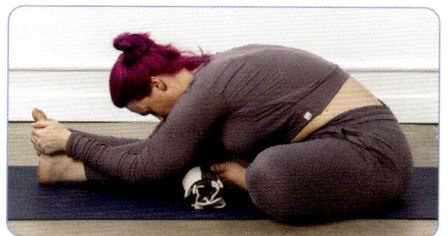

Place a rolled-up blanket under your knee to support tight hamstrings.

You can use a rolled blanket under the knee to lessen the intensity of the hamstring stretch or counteract hyperextension in the knee. A soft bend in the knee will move the stretch into the belly of the hamstring muscles and release tension from the knees and hips.

Lie on your back with your legs on a wall to support a long spine.

You can practice head to knee pose lying down! Turning this into a supine legs-up-the-wall position supports a long spine, stable hips, and an inner thigh stretch gently directed by gravity. You also get some of the upside-down benefits, including lymphatic drainage, increased blood flow back toward your head and heart, and downregulation of the nervous system. Start in legs-up-the-wall pose (viparita karani), then bend one knee out to the side, sliding the sole of the foot down the inside of the extended leg.

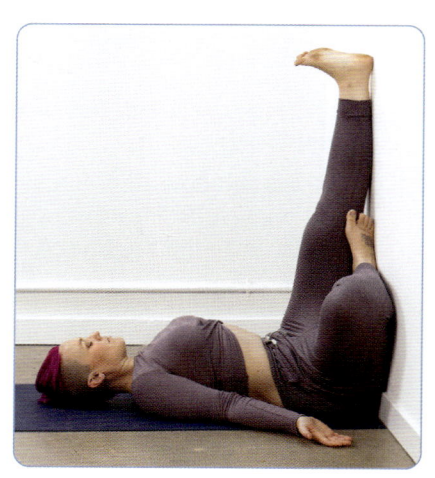

Sit on a chair with one knee bent and the other leg extended.

If you have difficulty getting up from and down on the floor or have tight hamstrings, this variation is for you! Sit on the edge of the chair to release tension through the hips and comfortably lengthen the spine. Step one foot out to the side, keeping the knee bent and leg turned out. Extend the other leg in front of you and begin to fold forward, bending at your hips. As you bend over the leg, rest your hands on the seat, blocks below, or let them release fully toward the floor. You can also loop a strap around your foot and hold it in your hands or grab the back of the chair as you hinge forward at the hips to extend through your spine (think flat back). To progress over time, stack

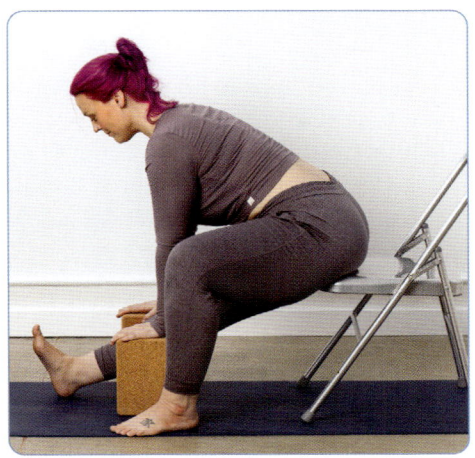

blocks under the heel on the extended leg, bringing your leg closer to you.

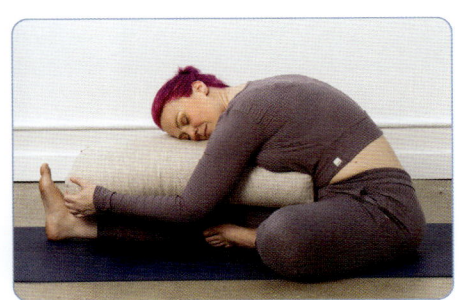

Place a bolster on the top of your thigh for a restorative twist.

Having a bolster on top of your thigh is great for many reasons! It gives you something to relax on, raises the height of your leg, and adds a slight compression to gently massage the abdominal organs. Stack as many bolsters as you like. To prevent sliding, secure them together by folding a blanket over them or looping a strap around them.

Revolved Head to Knee Forward Bend Pose

Parivritta Janu Shirshasana परविृत्त जानु शीर्षासन

Revolved head to knee forward bend pose is a dynamic yoga posture that actively stretches and releases the sides of the body, hips, gluteal muscles, groin, shoulders, and hamstrings. This pose induces a calming effect, opens the chest and ribs, engages core muscles for gentle spinal rotation, and stimulates abdominal organs, promoting overall well-being. Explore some common prop-supported variations of this pose to enhance your practice.

Slide a block or rolled blanket under the bent knee to support the knee.

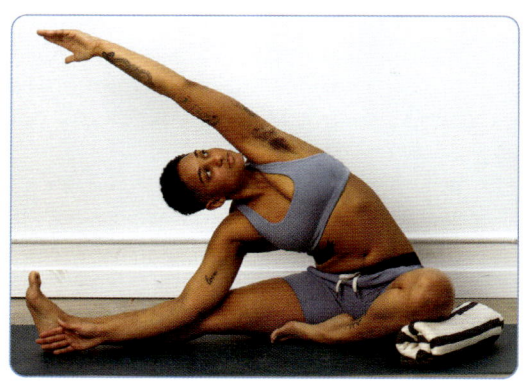

Using a block or blanket gives the leg something to rest on, relieving tension in both the knee and the hip. Start in a wide-legged straddle (wide-angle seated forward bend) with both sitting bones anchored into the floor or on a folded blanket to elevate the hips slightly and support a neutral spine. Bring the sole of one foot toward your inner thigh or calf muscle, bending at the knee. Draw your heel as close to the pubic bone as is comfortable. Place a block or rolled blanket under the knee for support. Extend both arms overhead and begin to find a lateral stretch toward your extended leg. If you can, rest your arm closest to the floor inside your knee and grab your foot with the other hand. On an exhale, begin to rotate your chest toward the sky and your shoulders toward the floor.

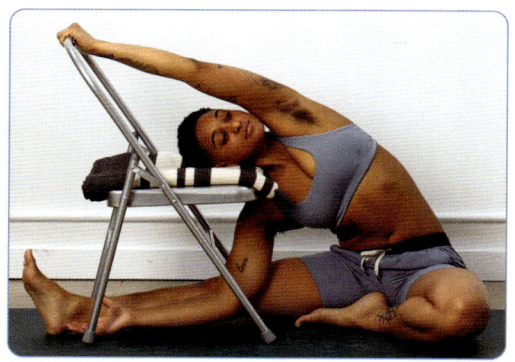

Support your head and neck on the seat of a chair while reaching your top arm to the back of the chair.

This variation allows you to create a platform on which to rest your head and neck and to gain leverage and space in your shoulder. Start in a wide-legged straddle (wide-angle seated forward bend), with one leg extended under the seat of a chair. Bend the other knee, bringing the sole of your foot toward your inner thigh or calf muscle. As you come into the side stretch, reach your top arm for the back railing of the chair and slide the bottom arm under the chair, inside the leg. Rest the side of your head on the chair seat, using a folded blanket or mat for comfort. If you can, grab a leg of the chair with your bottom hand. Use your grip on the back rail of the chair to help you rotate through the spine, spinning your chest up, away from the floor. Depending on how far the spine rotates, you might roll your head, bringing the back of the skull onto the chair instead of the side.

Place a block under your bottom arm to raise the height of the floor.

If the floor is out of reach, stack a block or two under your forearm so you can release further into the stretch with support. The blocks should ideally be inside the leg, but if you need more space, you can start with them outside the leg.

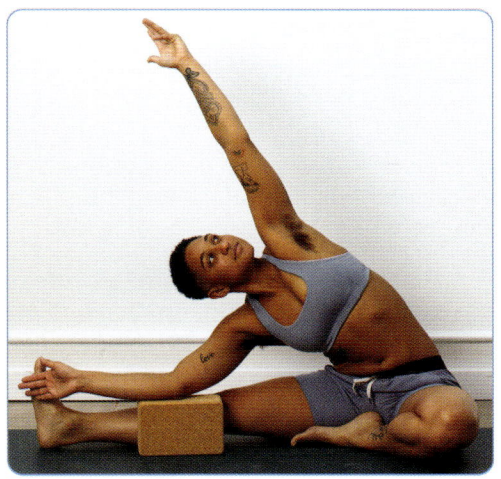

Use a strap to bridge the gap between your hands and the foot of your extended leg.

If you can't reach your foot, you could bend the knee to help, or you could bridge the gap with a strap. Loop a strap around your foot, holding the ends in your bottom hand (see photo a) or your top hand (see photo b). The strap bridges the gap so you can extend the leg fully. Once the leg is extended, gently rotate your shoulders and chest so your back is working toward facing the floor and your heart is turning up. If the strap is in the top hand, you can use it to find more rotation.

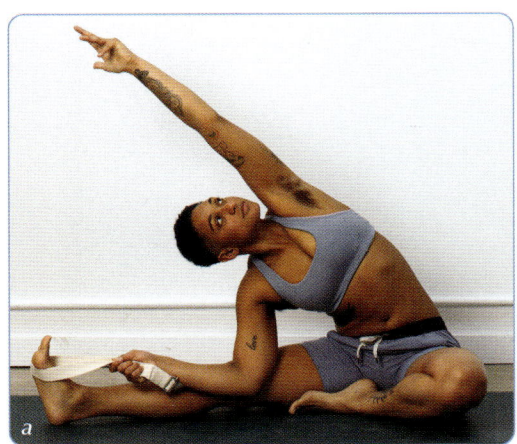 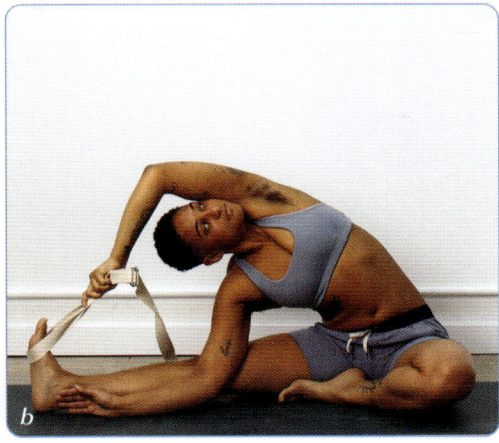

Revolved Head to Knee
Forward Bend Pose *(continued)*

Place a blanket or bolster under your sitting bones to neutralize the pelvis.

A little hip elevation can go a long way! If you have tight psoas, sitting on the edge of a prop slightly tilts the front of your pelvis down, removing rounding in the low back and bringing the pelvis into a neutral position. A neutral pelvis supports a long and relaxed spine by making it easier to draw the torso toward the extended knee. This will come in handy when working into the lateral stretch and thoracic rotation of the spine because rounding can inhibit these actions.

Place a rolled-up blanket under your knee to support tight hamstrings.

You can use a rolled blanket under the knee to lessen the intensity of the hamstring stretch or counteract hyperextension in the knee. A bend in the knee will move the stretch into the belly of the hamstring muscles and take tension away from the knees and hips.

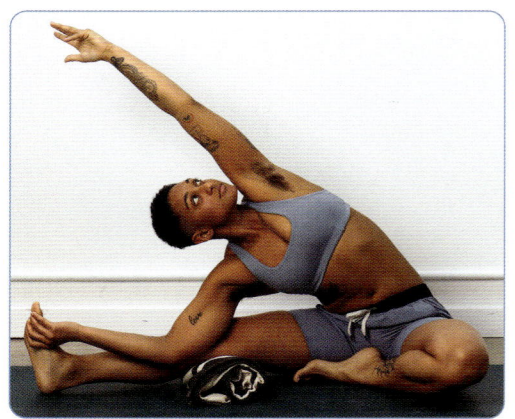

Seated Side Stretch Pose

Parshva Upavishtha Konasana   पार्श्व उपवष्टि कोणासन

Seated side stretch pose is a rejuvenating yoga posture that actively stretches the hips and the back of the body. It lengthens the backs of the legs while contracting the tops of the legs, providing a comprehensive stretch. It strengthens and stretches the waist, promoting flexibility and core engagement. This pose may also have a calming effect on the mind. Explore some common prop-supported variations of this pose to enhance your practice and fully experience its therapeutic benefits.

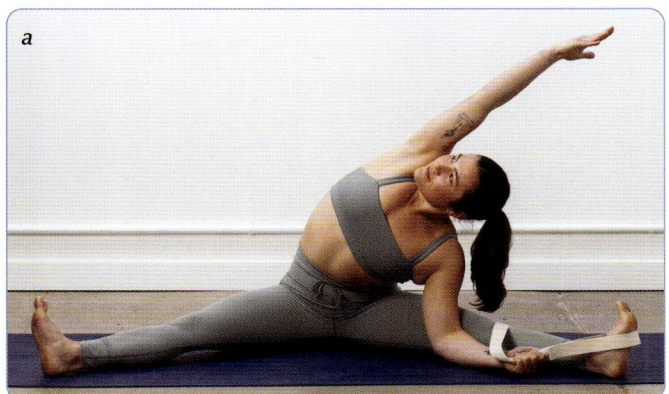

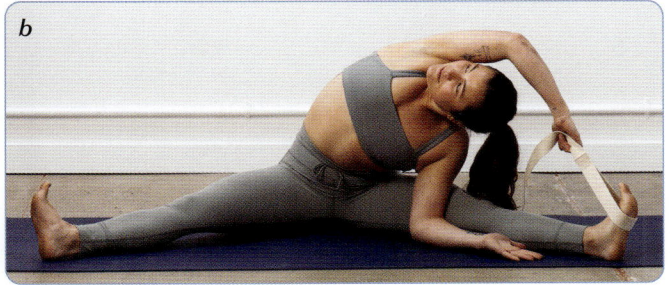

Use a strap to bridge the gap between your hands and foot.

If you can't reach your foot, you could bend your knee, but you can also bridge the gap with a strap. Loop a strap around your foot, holding the ends in either your bottom hand (see photo *a*) or your top hand for a deeper stretch (see photo *b*). The strap bridges the gap so you can extend the leg fully. Once you come into the side body stretch, you can begin to work your hand farther down the strap toward your foot.

Place a blanket or bolster under your sitting bones to neutralize the pelvis.

A little hip elevation can go a long way! If you have tight psoas, sitting on the edge of a prop slightly tilts the front of your pelvis down, removing rounding in the low back and bringing the pelvis into a neutral position. A neutral pelvis supports a long and relaxed spine by making it easier to draw the torso toward the leg. This will come in handy when working on the lateral stretch because rounding in the spine can inhibit this action.

Place a rolled-up blanket under your knees to support tight hamstrings.

You can use a rolled blanket under the knees to lessen the intensity of the hamstring stretch or counteract hyperextension in the knees. A soft bend in the knees will also move the stretch into the belly of the hamstring muscles and take tension away from the knees and hips.

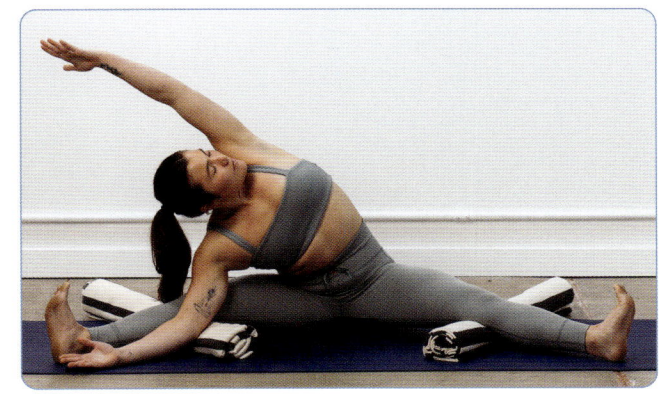

Sit on a chair with legs bent or extended.

If you have difficulty getting up from and down to the floor, or if you have tightness in your low back or hamstrings, this variation is for you! Sit on the edge of the chair to release tension through the hips and comfortably lengthen the spine. Keep the knees bent and turn your legs out to the sides by stepping both feet out or using your arms to move one leg at a time. This should look like a seated goddess pose. Hold one side of the seat and on an inhale, extend your other arm overhead. As you exhale, begin to find a side stretch toward the side of the hand gripping the chair, or you can slide that hand down the leg, reaching for your ankle (see photo *a*). Alternatively, you can practice with extended legs, sitting on the corner edge of the chair (see photo *b*). If you are doing this version, have stacked blocks or another chair nearby to rest your bottom arm on or rest your arm on your leg as shown in the photo.

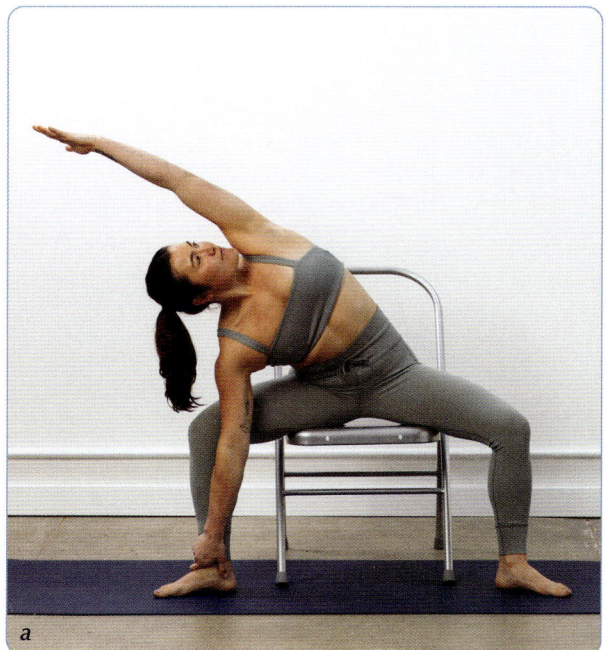
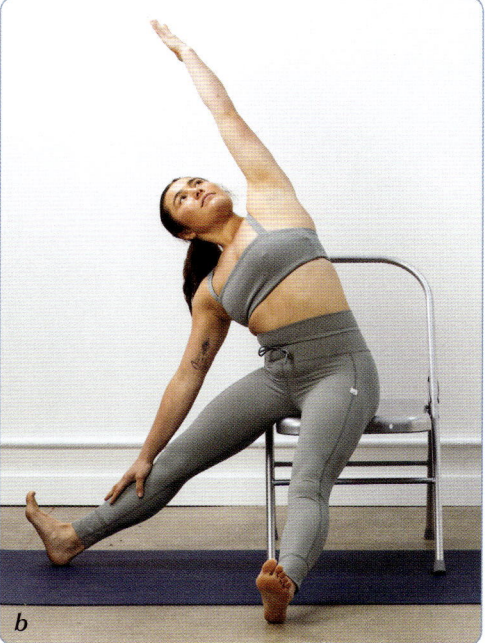

a

b

Lotus Pose

Padmasana   पद्मासन

Lotus pose is a meditative, yet challenging yoga posture that actively opens the hips while lengthening internal rotation muscles and engaging external rotation muscles. This pose benefits those with arthritis or osteoarthritis by lubricating the knees. It also puts pressure on bones, aiding in countering osteoporosis, and it tones the abdominal muscles. Lotus pose also holds the power to focus the mind. Explore some common prop-supported variations of this pose to enhance your practice and fully experience its therapeutic benefits.

While this pose may offer many benefits, I think it is especially important to note that no benefit outweighs a knee injury. If you have a history of knee pain or injury, or feel tremendous force or pressure trying to get into the pose, don't do it. Work on opening the muscles that support this posture in the meantime, and perhaps return at a later time. There is no rush in yoga.

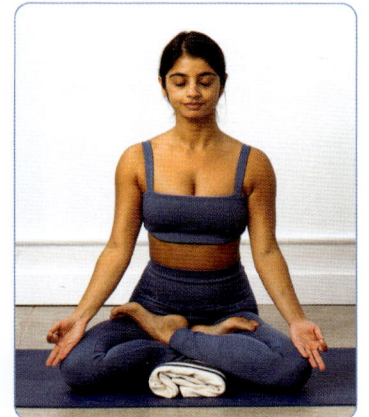

Place a rolled-up blanket under the ankles.

Lotus pose can put a lot of stress on the ankles by forcing them into a supinated position where the toes curve inward and the heels drop back. This position of the ankles can then lead to stress on the knee. To counteract this action, try tolling a blanket and placing it under your bottom ankle. This should help to keep the ankles from rolling until your mobility improves to support this action over time.

Place a blanket under your sitting bones if your hip flexors are tight.

Adding height can ease joint tension. Having the hips as high as or higher than the knees decreases the angle of flexion, reducing strain. If you have tight psoas, sitting on the edge of a prop slightly tilts the front of your pelvis down, removing rounding in the low back and bringing the pelvis into a neutral position. A neutral pelvis supports a long and relaxed spine. Once seated, shift your weight back on the sitting bones, distributing the weight evenly between them. Grow tall through your spine, stacking the shoulders directly over the pelvis.

Place a rolled-up blanket under your top knee to release tension if it is lifting off the floor.

Having a surface to support your knee, such as a blanket, makes the pose easier and releases tension in your hips and inner thigh muscles. Because this pose has a bit of a reputation for stressing the knees, when practiced in a forced manner, it is crucial that you offer yourself support and patience. This is your best route for mitigating risk of harm or injury.

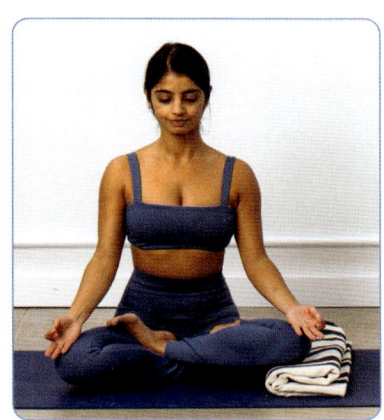

Practice half or full bound lotus with a strap.

Using a strap can be helpful in more ways than one! The strap acts as a bridge in the gap between your hand and your foot. Due to the nature of the bind, the strap also frees up more space in your chest and shoulders, so you do not have to compromise your posture. Loop the strap around your foot and hold the ends in the hand that is bound behind your back. Sit tall through the spine, and over time, work towards bringing your hand further down the strap towards your foot (see photo a). If you are practicing fully bound lotus (see photo b), you will need two straps or one big looped strap that goes behind the back and loops around both feet.

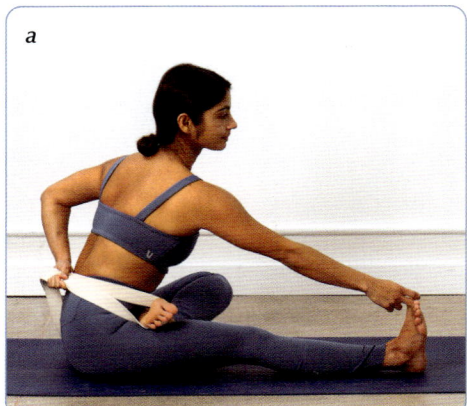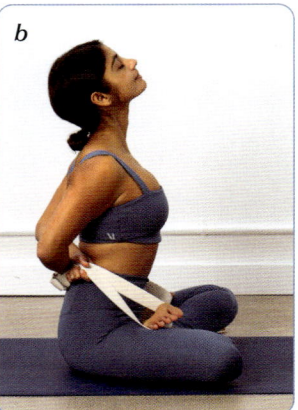

Seated Compass Pose

Parivritta Surya Yantrasana   परविृत्त सूर्य यंत्रासन

Seated compass pose is a dynamic yoga pose that actively strengthens the arms, promoting upper body strength. This pose also increases hip mobility and range of motion while opening the chest and lungs for improved respiratory health. The pose also enhances spinal flexibility and stimulates the digestive and reproductive systems, inspiring confidence. Explore some common prop-supported variations of this pose to enhance your practice.

Place your foot against a wall for balance and stability.

This pose can offer quite the challenge! It will stretch you in more ways than one—getting into your hips, legs, shoulders, waist, chest, rotators, and others, all while remembering to breathe! The wall will help you with your alignment without compromising stability, aiding in building muscle memory over time. Start sitting cross-legged facing a wall and place one foot on the wall in front of you, keeping the knee bent. Once the foot is stabilized on the wall, turn your torso and hips away from the wall, stopping when you start to feel gentle resistance in the hips. Extend through the bent knee, walking your foot up the wall. If this is too intense on the hamstrings, start

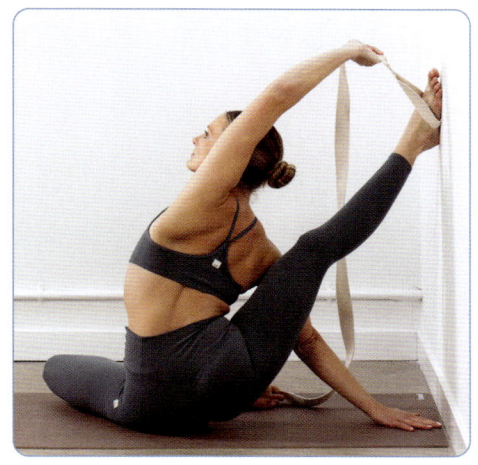

over with your hips farther from the wall. Press your foot into the wall to engage through the leg muscles and externally rotate the thigh into the hip socket. Bring your arm closest to the wall inside the extended leg and your hand down onto the floor just outside the hip. Gently lean your weight into this arm as you reach your other arm behind your head toward your foot, ankle, or calf. If you cannot contact your foot, practice energetically reaching toward your foot or use a strap. If you do make contact, leverage holding the leg to assist you in rolling your chest open, away from the wall.

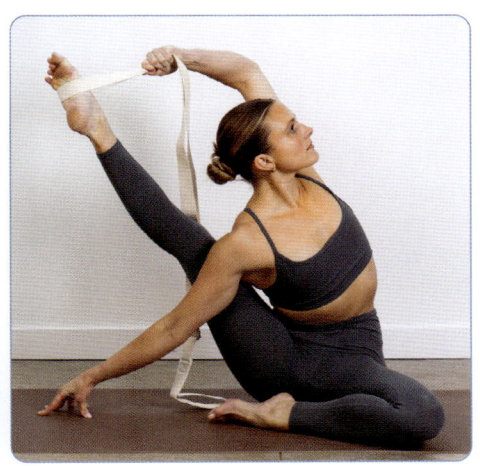

Loop a strap around your foot and hold both ends in your top hand to create space in the shoulders.

Straps are an excellent tool for bridging gaps. In this pose in particular, the strap will allow you to form a connection with your foot while also allowing more space in your chest and shoulders. Rather than grabbing your foot, loop the strap around, holding both ends of the strap in your hand. As you extend through your leg and kick into the strap, you will feel a stretch, opening through the side of your torso that is opposite the extended leg. Gently pull on the ends of the strap to guide your head and chest in front of the overhead arm. Continue to use this leverage to assist you in rolling your chest open, away from the extended leg.

Seated Compass Pose *(continued)*

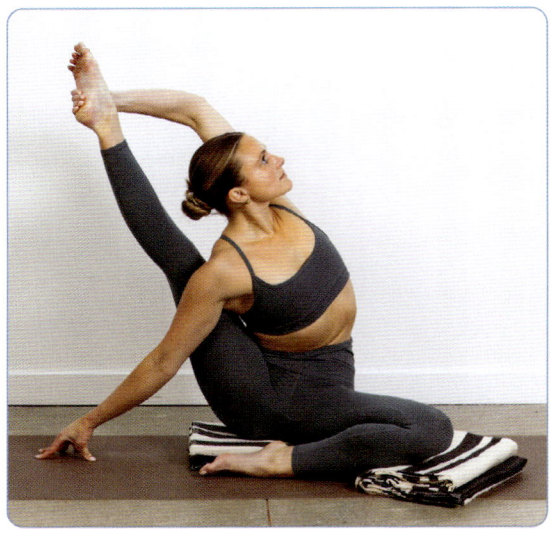

Place a blanket under your sitting bones or a rolled-up blanket under your bent knee to ease knee and hip tension.

Using blankets in this variation gives the grounded leg something to rest on and adds elevation to the pelvis, relieving tension in both the knee and the hip. Start in a cross-legged seat on a folded blanket to elevate the hips slightly and support a neutral spine. If you are extending your right leg, wedge a rolled blanket under the left knee for support. Lift the right leg, cradling your shin in your right elbow crease and left hand, then thread your right arm under the right knee, bringing your right hand to the floor, just in front of and outside the right hip. Move your left hand to grip the pinky toe edge of your right foot. Once you have a firm grasp, begin kicking into your hand. Shift your weight into your right hand and hip as you begin to pull your chest through under your arm. Roll your chest open, away from your right leg. Try to shift some weight back into the left hip, gently pressing the bent leg down into the blanket. Repeat on the other side.

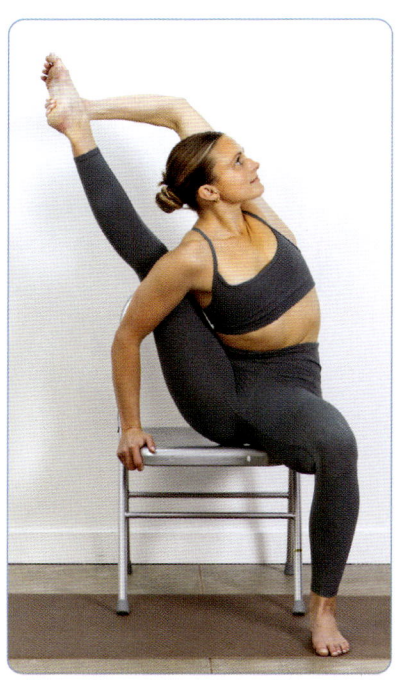

Sit on a chair for stability and support.

This variation is great for reducing knee strain due to less flexion in the grounded leg, and it is good if you have difficulty getting up from and down to the floor. The cues for this pose are like the seated version but with a few minor adjustments. Instead of sitting on the floor, start by grounding your hips on the seat of a chair. Sit near the front edge of the chair to untuck the pelvis if you have tight psoas. This will offer more stability and control over your postural alignment as you practice. Another difference from the seated version is that instead of placing the hand on the floor outside your hip, you grab onto the outer edge of the seat. This should offer you more control and stability as you transition into the pose.

The Complete Guide to Yoga Props

Half Lord of the Fishes Pose

Ardha Matsyendrasana   अर्ध मत्स्येन्द्रासन

Half lord of the fishes pose is a dynamic yoga posture that actively increases spinal mobility, enhancing overall flexibility. This pose tones the abdominal muscles, promotes core strength, and provides a deep stretch to the shoulders, neck, and hips. It also stimulates digestive organs, fostering digestive health. It may also offer relief for symptoms of sciatica by lengthening the piriformis muscle, although it is contradictory if sciatica is due to herniation. Explore some common prop-supported variations of this pose to enhance your practice.

Place a blanket under your sitting bones to ease knee and hip tension.

If you have tight psoas, sitting on the edge of a folded blanket slightly tilts the front of your pelvis down toward the mat, removing rounding in the low back and bringing the pelvis into a neutral position. A neutral pelvis supports extension of the spine before you begin to twist. Bringing the hips a little higher than the knee can also help to reduce knee strain.

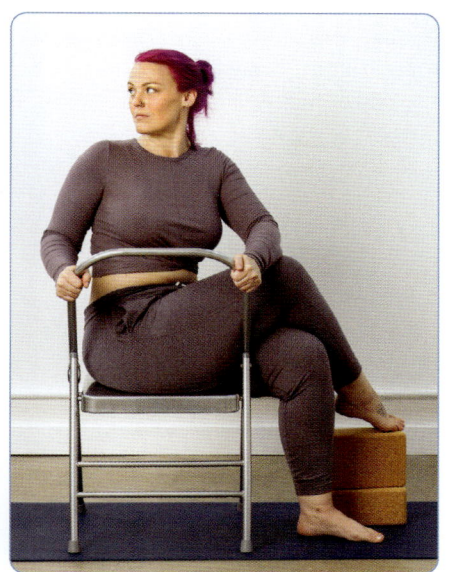

Sit on a chair, with the option to place a block under the foot of the top leg.

Using a chair is a great way to modify this posture. It is also great if you have a desk job and need a quick stretch! This variation also reduces knee and hip strain because external rotation in the bottom hip is not necessary, and the bottom knee has more forgiving flexion than in the seated version. Start by grounding your hips on the seat of a chair, then cross one leg over the other. You can also ground the foot of the top leg by stacking blocks under your foot. As you come into the twist, hold the chair with your back hand or turn the chair sideways so you can hold on with both hands, as shown in the photo. This will offer more stability and control over your postural alignment as you practice.

Twist toward a wall for support and mobility.

This variation offers support for you to deepen into the twist without compromising spinal alignment. Hooking your elbow outside your knee can encourage rounding in the spine, so the wall can help you to find leverage without compromise. In this variation, have your bottom leg fully extended so that you can situate your outer hip flush against a wall. As you come into the

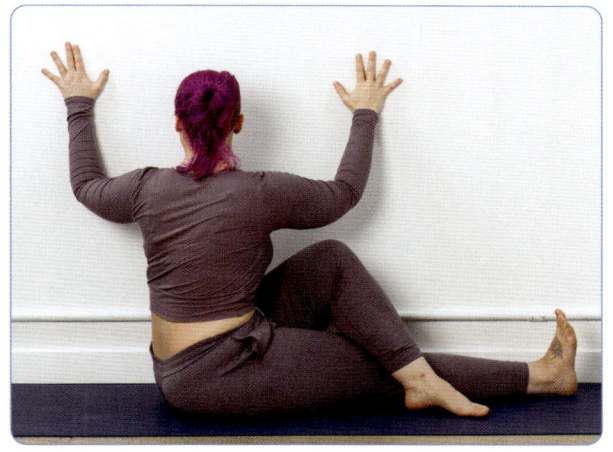

Half Lord of the Fishes Pose *(continued)*

thoracic twist, use the wall to create more space across your chest by raising your arms cactus style and resting your forearms against the wall. Sit tall through your spinal column and press into the wall with the forearm that is farthest back to draw the opposite side of the chest closer to the wall.

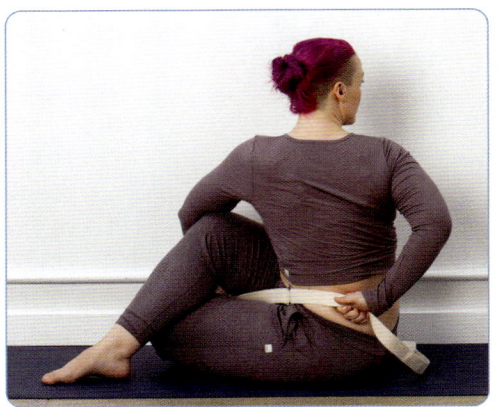

Practice a bind with the help of a strap between your hands to create space.

A strap is a handy tool to free up space in the chest and shoulders. It can bridge the gap between your hands if they are just out of reach from one another. Even if you *can* bind your hands, you might sacrifice your spinal alignment by hunching forward as you twist. So, a strap may come in handy as you maintain your length in both sides of the body and work your hands closer together over time.

Pose Dedicated to the Sage Marichi I, II, III, and IV

Marichyasana I, II, III, and IV   मरीच्यासन I, II, III, and IV

The series of poses dedicated to the sage Marichi (whose name means "ray of light" in Sanskrit) is a set of four postures within the ashtanga primary series. Versions I and II are deep forward folds, stretching your back, shoulders, and legs while extending the spine and providing a cleansing squeeze to your organs. Perform these poses near the end of your practice after warming up your hips, hamstrings, and shoulders to experience the calming and stress-reducing benefits. Versions III and IV are twists and deep shoulder stretches, massaging your abdominal organs and offering detoxifying benefits, especially to the liver and kidneys.

Place a block under your forehead.

When folding forward in the pose dedicated to the sage Marichi I (photo *a*) or II (photo *b*), you can use one or more blocks to raise the height of the floor to your forehead. The structural support of the block will allow you to rest your head and neck, releasing through the cervical spine.

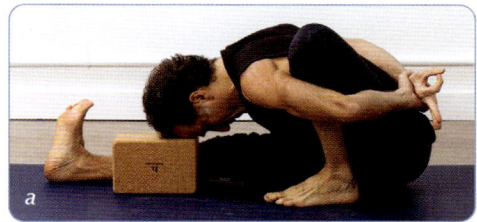
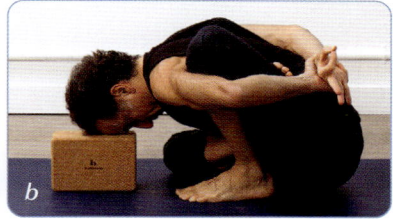

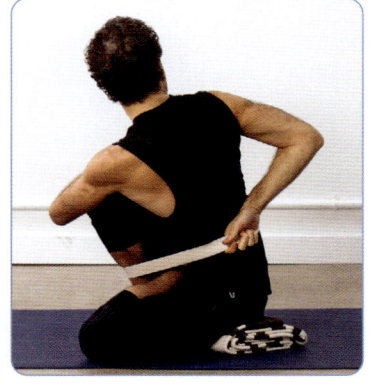

Loop a strap around your front ankle and lower back to assist you in the full bind.

Using a strap in the pose dedicated to the sage Marichi IV will assist you in remaining compact, hugging the bent knee in, and give you something to grab onto as you work toward the full bind. Begin in staff pose (dandasana), bringing your left foot into a half lotus position inside the right hip crease. Bend the right knee, placing the heel of your right foot as close to your sitting bones as is comfortable. Pull a looped strap over your body so that the back of the loop is around your lower back and the front is securely looped around your right shin or ankle. Tighten the strap so that if you let go of your legs, the right knee will not be able to fall to the side. Move the knee across the midline of the body a little as you come into your twist toward the right leg. Your left arm will try to hook outside of the right knee and reach around the front of the right shin, but you can modify as shown in the photo by wrapping the arm from the inside of the knee. Grab the looped strap on the other side. The right arm will be reaching behind your back, also holding the loop. Use the strap as a bridge to work your hands closer together over time. Repeat on the other side.

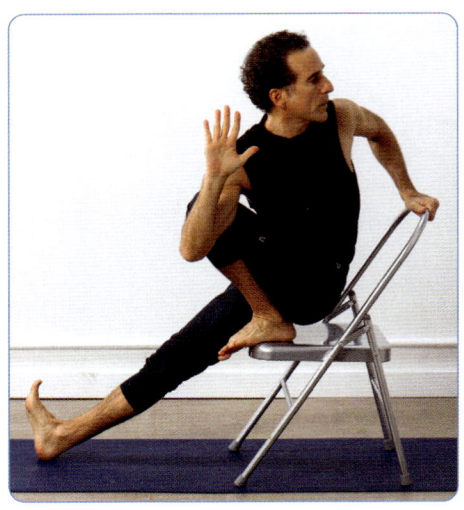

Sit on a chair, with one foot on the chair and one leg extended.

For this variation of the pose dedicated to the sage Marichi III, you can also use blankets on the seat of a chair to raise the height of the hips if you find yourself hovering, as in the photo, and want more support. You also use blocks under your extended leg if the foot does not reach the floor. The chair version supports you when getting up from or down to the floor is challenging. It also makes the twist more accessible and the hamstring stretch less intense. If desiring added height and comfort, start by folding blankets to stack on the back half of the chair seat, leaving room on the front of the seat for your foot. Come to a seated position on the blankets and then begin to engage your abdominal muscles to lift and hug your left knee into your chest. Place the left foot on the chair, just under the bent knee and in front of the blankets. Try to extend the right leg fully, bringing the heel of your right foot onto the floor or stacked blocks for added height. As you come into your twist, use the back of the chair as gentle leverage, holding it with your left hand. Repeat on the other side.

Twist toward a wall for support and mobility.

This variation of the poses dedicated to the sage Marichi III (photo a) and IV (photo b) offers support for you to deepen into the twist without compromising spinal alignment. Hooking your elbow outside your knee can sometimes encourage rounding in the spine, so the wall is a nice alternative for finding leverage without compromise. In this variation, situate your outer hip of the leg you will be twisting flush against a wall. As you come

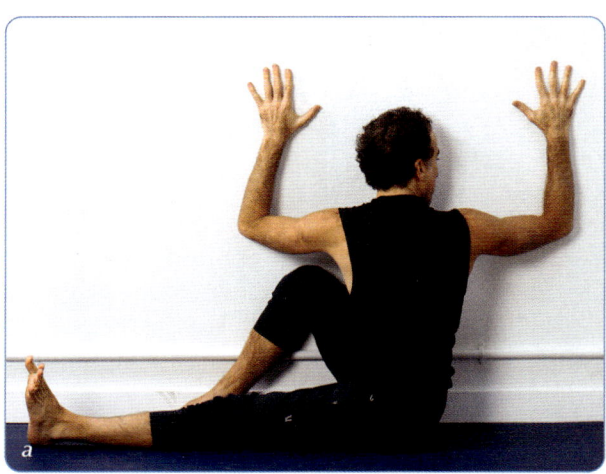

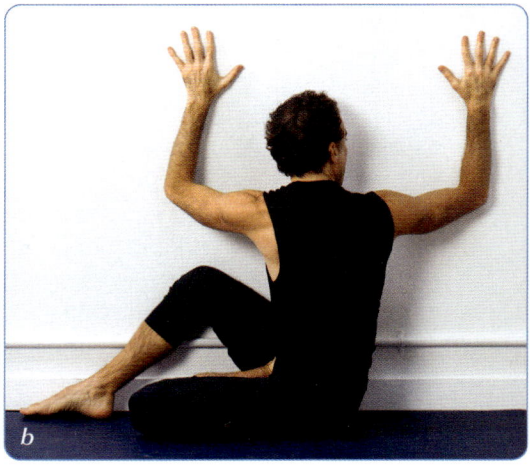

into the twist, use the wall to create more space across your chest by raising your arms cactus style and resting your forearms against the wall. Sitting tall through your spine, press into the wall with the forearm that is farthest back to draw the opposite side of the chest closer to the wall.

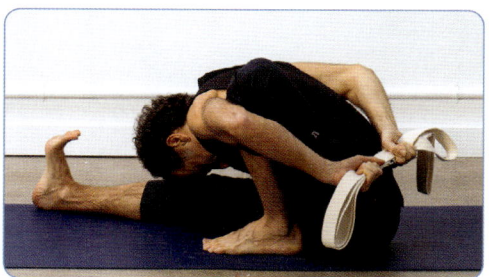

Practice a bind with the help of a strap.

You can use a strap to assist you in binding in all four versions of the pose dedicated to the sage Marichi. To do so, hold one end of a strap in each hand and then walk the hands closer together over time. The photo shows how this is done in the pose dedicated to the sage Marichi I, but it can be applied to any of the versions.

Place a blanket under your sitting bones or roll one under your bent knee to ease knee and hip tension.

A little hip elevation can go a long way in easing joint tension. This can be accomplished in all four variations in a few ways. Having the hips level with or higher than the knees in half lotus in versions II and IV decreases the angle of flexion at the joint, reducing strain. If you have tight psoas, the added height may reduce some of the strain in the hips, too, helping to untuck the pelvis in all four variations. In variations II and IV where both legs are bent, you can also use a blanket under your open hip or your knee for comfort. This is especially helpful if you are working toward the half lotus variation and your front

knee lifts off the floor. Folded blankets under the knee can fill that gap and give something for your leg to rest on, helping you to release tension through the hips. In pose dedicated to the sage Marichi I and III, a rolled blanket under the knee of the extended leg can support tight hamstrings (see photo for example in Marichi I).

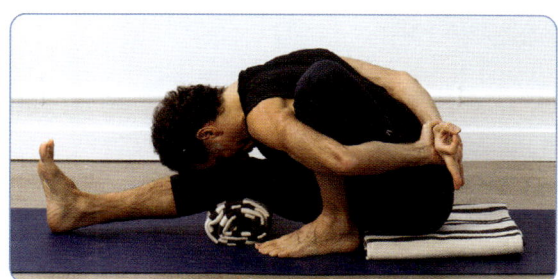

Simple Sitting Twist Pose I and II

Bharadvajasana I and II   भरद्वाजासन I and II

Simple sitting twist poses I and II are versatile yoga postures that offer a myriad of advantages, actively enhancing core strength and fortifying the muscles supporting the spine. These poses foster flexibility in the knees, ankles, and feet, and they also promote mobility in the shoulders and spine. Simultaneously, they provide a rejuvenating massage to abdominal organs, improving digestion, relieving stress, and augmenting spinal and shoulder flexibility. Version II involves half lotus pose, adding an extra layer of depth. Let's explore some common prop-supported variations to enrich your practice.

Practice a bind with the help of a strap.

Using a strap in this pose can help you to deepen into the thoracic twist in simple sitting twist pose I and bridge the gap between your hand and your foot in simple sitting twist pose II. For simple sitting twist pose I, loop a strap around the thigh that you are twisting away from and loop it close to the hip. As you come into the twist, hold the long end of the strap with your back hand and slowly work your hand up the strap closer to your hip (see photo a). Gently pulling on the strap should also assist your back sitting bone to anchor into the floor. For simple sitting twist pose II, have the strap looped around the top of your foot or ankle that is folded into half lotus (see photo b). Gently work your way up the strap toward your toes over time.

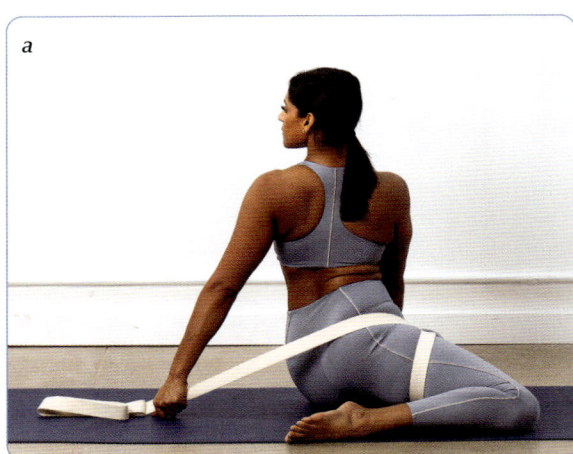
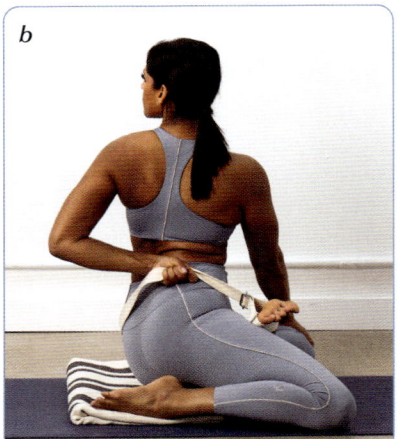

Place a blanket under your sitting bones and knees to ease tension.

A little hip elevation can go a long way in easing joint tension. In both variations, using a blanket to level the hips or position them higher than the knees decreases the angle of flexion at the joint, reducing strain (see photo a for an example in simple sitting twist pose II). If you have tight psoas, the added height may also reduce strain in the hips and make it easier for you to sit tall through your spine. You can also use the blanket under your knees as an extra layer of cushioning. Finally, if you are practicing simple sitting twist pose II and your knee in half lotus lifts off the floor, folded blankets under the knee can fill that gap and give something for your leg to rest on, helping you to release tension through the hips (see photo b).

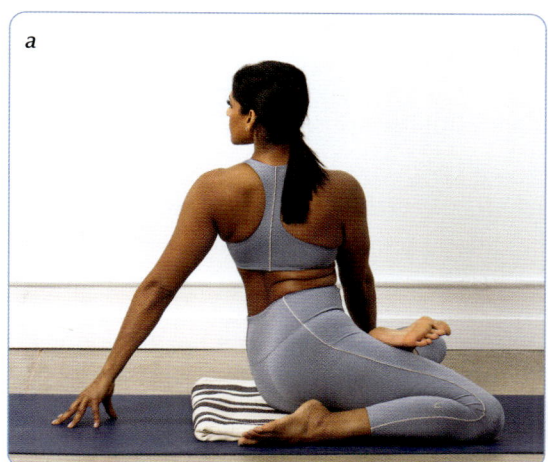 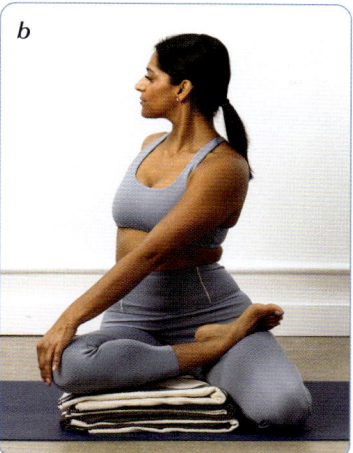

Sit on a chair with your bottom leg folded under and stacked on blocks or the bar between the legs of the chair.

I love this chair variation for both options of the pose because it is helpful in so many ways, especially if you find getting up from and down on the floor challenging! Begin seated on a chair with both legs through the opening in the back of the chair, so that your torso is facing the back of the chair. Lift your left leg and place your foot across your right thigh, coming into a figure four position. If your knee and hip can support the lotus position comfortably, work the top of your left foot up toward your right hip crease and hook the foot around the railing of the back of the chair beside your hip. Bend your right knee, engaging your hamstrings to lift your right heel toward the bottom of the seat, then place the foot on blocks or place it on the rail connecting the legs of the chair if there is one, as shown in the photo. On an inhale, lengthen through your spine, holding the back railing of the chair. As you exhale, use the railing as leverage to find your twist. Over time, work toward a bind, reaching your left hand behind your back for your foot. Repeat on the other side. Simple sitting twist pose II is shown in the photo, but if you prefer to simplify, keep your top foot across your thigh closer to your knee. If this is still too much on the top knee, keep the foot grounded.

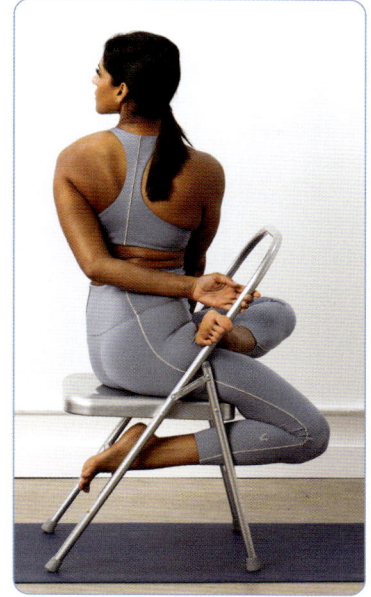

Boat Pose

Navasana

नावासन

Boat pose is a dynamic yoga posture that actively strengthens the abdomen, hip flexors, and spine, providing comprehensive core engagement. This pose also stimulates the kidneys and improves digestion. Now let's explore some common prop-supported variations to enrich your practice and deepen the benefits of boat pose.

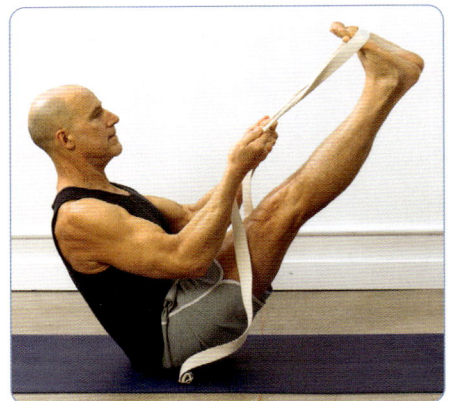

Place a strap around your feet for balance and alignment.

This variation is great if you are working to straighten your legs fully. The strap provides additional support as you build core strength. It will also offer structural support as you try to find your balance on your sitting bones. Start in seated position with your knees bent and your feet planted firmly on the floor. Flex your feet upward to loop a strap around the balls of the feet. Hold the ends of the strap in both hands. Press your feet firmly into the strap as you begin to lift the feet and legs off the floor. Start by trying to bring your shins parallel to the floor, then build up to straightening the legs fully. You can adjust your grip by adding slack to lessen the intensity of the stretch. Gently pull the ends of the strap to straighten through your spine, lift your sternum up toward the sky and draw your shoulder blades down and back.

Loop a strap in front of your feet and behind your upper back for balance and alignment.

Using the strap will reinforce extension through your spine as you extend through your legs. This variation will also help you to more easily find balance and alleviate tension in your lower back. Start in a seated position. Place one end of a looped strap around your upper back, right at your shoulder blades, and place the other end around your feet (you may need to bend your knees to do so), as shown in the photo. You have the option here to place a block between your feet and the strap. The block informs leg and feet alignment by ensuring the feet are parallel, which will

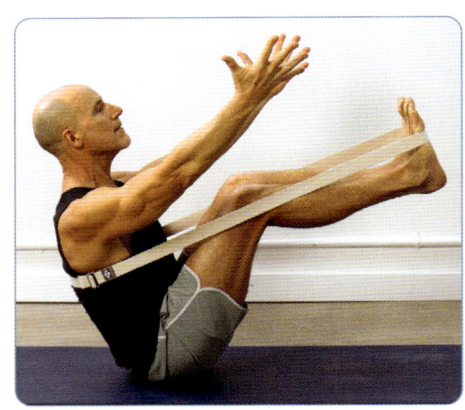

prevent the legs from rotating. Bring your hands to the floor alongside the body and shift your weight onto your sitting bones. Press your feet firmly into the block or strap as you extend your legs out and up. Feel the chest lifting up toward the sky, and your shoulder blades being drawn down and back by the strap as you kick into the loop. With a big enough loop, you can practice with straightening your legs fully or with your knees bent and your shins parallel to the floor. As you continue to build core strength and engage through your abdominal muscles, try lifting your arms parallel to the mat or overhead.

Squeeze a block between your thighs for engagement and pelvic stability.

Using a block helps to stabilize the pelvis and core, firm through the legs and inner thighs, and informs alignment, keeping the knees and thighs parallel to one another. Sit with your feet

The Complete Guide to Yoga Props

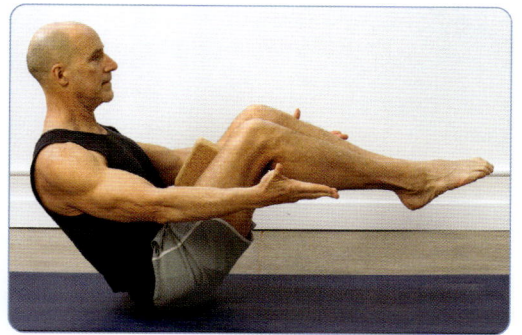

together in front of you, knees pointing up toward the sky. Place a block between your upper thighs turned to the narrowest width. Grab the backs of your thighs and use your biceps strength to pull the top of the sternum up and roll the shoulder blades down the back. Roll your weight forward on the tailbone to try and untuck the pelvis. Without changing the shape of the spine, try to lift the shins parallel to the mat. Squeeze the block in toward your pubic bone as you lengthen up through the spine. Play with extending your arms alongside your shins or straightening your legs. Work the head of the thigh bones toward the mat and lengthen the back of the neck by lifting the chin slightly away from your chest.

Hold a block between your hands to strengthen your core with boat rows.

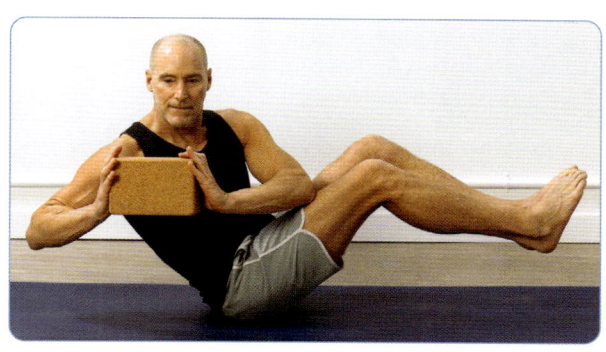

Using a block provides a fun core challenge! Start in boat pose with a block between your hands. Squeeze the block to draw the shoulder blades down and broaden through the chest and collar bones. Twist through the middle of your back so that the right elbow is moving down toward the mat. Try to avoid moving your knees out of their parallel position by isolating the lower body as you find the twist in the middle and upper spine. Return to center and repeat on the opposite side. You should be inhaling through the center and exhaling as you twist. Repeat multiple rounds on each side, adding repetitions over time as your abdominal muscles strengthen!

Sit on a chair holding the seat or back of the chair.

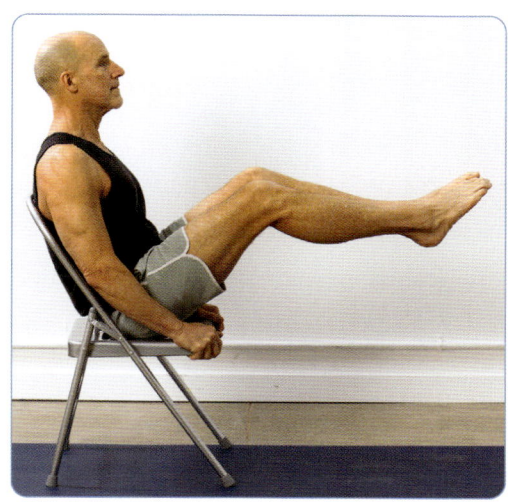

If getting to the floor is difficult for you, boat pose may be practiced on a chair. You can do this with the back of the chair behind you or on either side if you are feeling confident in your core strength. Sit at the edge of the chair, holding the sides of the chair seat for support to start. Begin to lean back, keeping your spine elongated and your lower belly drawing up and in. Come onto your tiptoes, and if you want to progress, lift the feet up off the floor. Eventually work your way up to bringing your knees level with your chest and your shins parallel to the floor or even extending the legs fully. Engage through your inner thighs and the back muscles. You can use your grip on the seat to help you puff up through your chest and lengthen through the spinal column or to test your balance, extending your arms in front of you.

Place your feet on a wall for balance and focus.

Placing your feet against the wall in boat pose can help you maintain a sense of balance so you can turn your attention to your core and pelvic muscles. Start in half boat pose with your feet against a wall and your shins parallel to the floor. You can have your hands grounded beside you, or you can hold the backs of your thighs to help you lengthen through your spine. If you feel comfortable, extend through your legs, walking your feet higher up the wall. Lift your heart up and draw your shoulders down and back. To add a final challenge, lift your hands off the mat with your arms parallel to the floor or overhead.

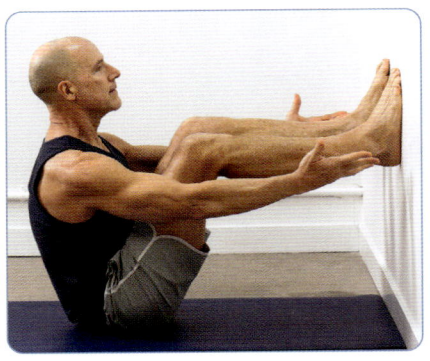

Wedge an angled block under your low back to support posture.

Using a block here is a handy tool to keep the low back from rounding, but it will require you to fire up through your psoas and deep abdominal muscles! Set up for boat pose as

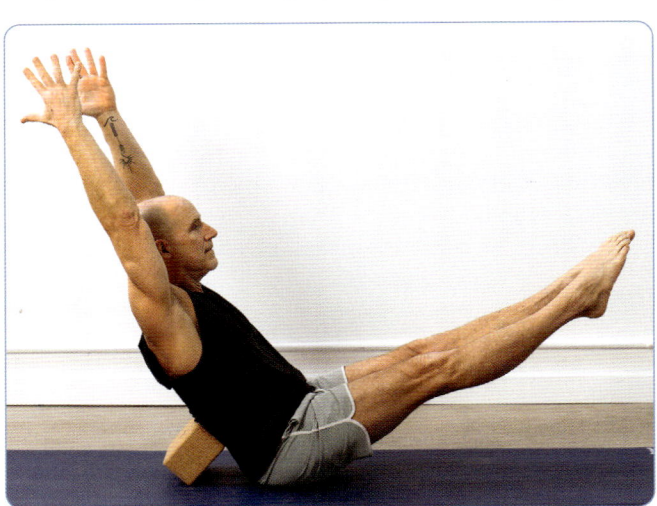

you normally would. Begin to lean back, but before lifting your feet off the mat, wedge a block at an angle on its widest orientation between your lower back and the mat. It is important to practice on a mat or grippy surface so that the block does not slide. Angle the block so that when you lean your torso into it, the block is flush against you. Work toward getting to your tiptoes or lifting the feet fully off the floor. You may find that when the block is there to prevent rounding in the low back, it is more challenging to lift the legs!

Use Props to Improve Posture

Concluding this exploration of seated yoga postures, focus on the practical benefits of incorporating props to enhance postural alignment. Regardless of the pose, strategically using props can have a profound impact on everyday life. Delve into common seated postures, uncovering practical insights that translate seamlessly into improved postural alignment for enhanced comfort and well-being in your day-to-day activities.

Place a block between your shoulders and the back of a chair or wall.

This is a wonderful way to tune up your posture, even outside of your regular yoga practice! When practicing in your chair, you will know just how quickly your postural muscles give up on you by how long it is before your block drops. You will need to practice on a chair that has more than just a back railing for this pose. Sit on a chair, then scoot your sitting bones back enough to wedge a block between your shoulder blades and the back of the chair. If the back of the chair is not high enough, you could turn the chair sideways against a wall to place the block between your shoulder blades and the wall instead. If you feel yourself starting to slouch, the block will move from its intended position.

Sit on a chair and place blocks under your feet.

This block trick is great for more than one reason. The most obvious reason is if your feet do not reach the floor! One of the less obvious reasons is that it will provide relief to your hip flexors and low back by raising the height of your knees to be level with the hips if the feet do not reach the floor. The shortening of the psoas means less strain on them.

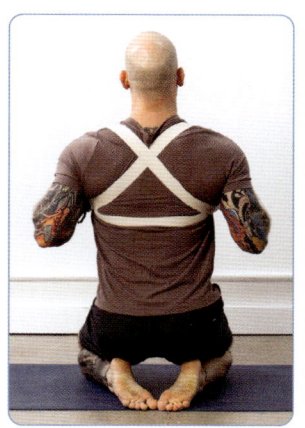

Support your posture with a strap.

This posture trick is something you can use any time of the day to train your body to assume healthier postures by anchoring your shoulders back and down and to open across your chest. Wrap a strap around your back at your shoulder blades and under your armpits. Then loop the ends of the strap forward over the fronts of your shoulders to drape behind you again. Cross the two ends of the strap over your upper back, creating an X. Bring the ends back under your armpits to seal the loop just below your sternum. Have the strap tight enough that you feel your shoulder blades being drawn down and back, resisting any postural urge to slump or hunch!

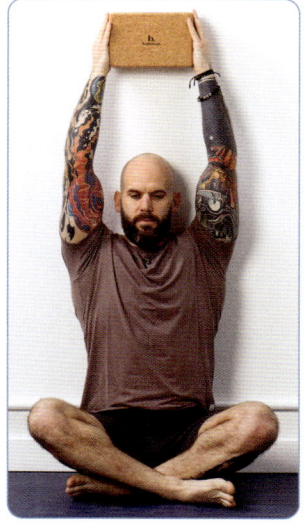

Hold a block between your hands and place your back against a wall to improve overhead mobility.

Start in a seated position with your back against a wall. Place a block turned as wide as possible between your palms. Extend your arms in front of you, squeezing the block while finding a slight external rotation through the upper arms and shoulders. To externally rotate through the shoulders, imagine drawing the shoulders down the back and spinning the inner elbows up toward the sky. Continue to squeeze the block and raise your arms overhead toward the wall as far as you can. Once you have reached the end of your range of motion, draw

(continued)

Use Props to Improve Posture (continued)

your low ribs back and in towards the wall. Continue to wrap the elbows in toward your midline, externally wrapping through the shoulders. The amount of space between your arms and the wall is the gap between your range of motion and full overhead mobility. If you were to bring your arms all the way to the wall, what compromise would your body make? Give it a try as an experiment. This may help you to understand where in your body you may be compensating (such as arching the back or internally rotating your shoulders) to get your arms overhead in other postures such as downward dog or handstand. The more you work on this, the easier the other postures will become over time.

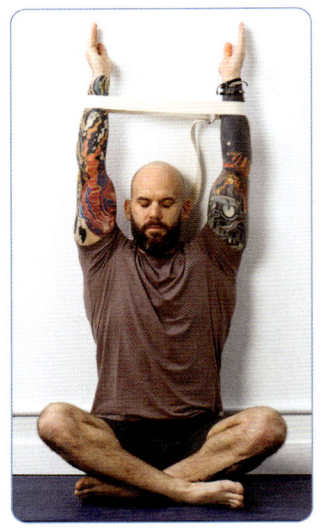

Place a strap around your arms and your back against a wall to improve overhead mobility.

As in the previous example with a block, you can repeat the same exercises with a strap looped around your arms, just above your elbows, leaving room for your head. Press your arms into the strap to wrap your shoulders down and back. Imagine sliding the shoulder blades around the sides of the ribs, away from the spine to create space in the upper back (external rotation). Refer to the previous example with the block for mobility cues.

Seated shoulder flossing with a strap.

This is a great exercise for releasing through your chest and shoulders, improving range of motion, moving synovial fluid in the shoulder joints, and breathing more easily by releasing tension in the diaphragm muscle if it is locked. From a comfortable seat, with a strap between your hands, raise your arms overhead. From here you can explore several movements. One such possibility involves keeping the spine upright and reaching the arms back behind you. The hands can slide farther down the strap to make room in the shoulders for the movement (see photo a). Alternate bringing the strap forward and back with your breath. You can also work to improve your side stretching range of motion by exhaling into a lateral stretch, feeling the opposite side of the body fan open, and alternating sides with your breath (see photo b).

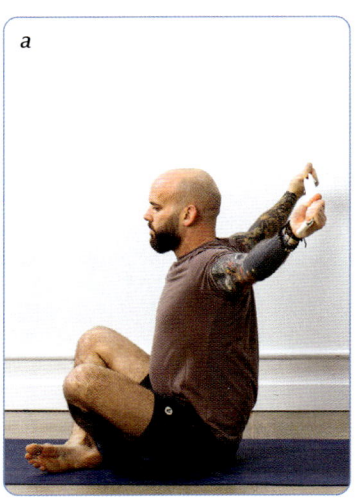

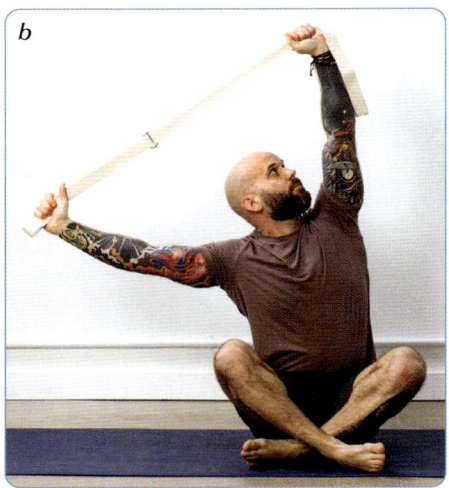

Chapter 5

Backbending and Heart-Opening Poses

Your vision will become clear only when you look into your heart. Who looks outside, dreams. Who looks inside awakens.

Carl Jung

In this chapter, we explore various backbends and heart-opening poses, showcasing diverse adaptations made possible with the use of props. Heart-opening poses provide insights into self-awareness, and nurturing the experience through gentle attention becomes paramount. As we expand through the chest, we expose our hearts to the world, yielding experiences that transcend mere physical benefits. The poses offer an opportunity to connect with our innate kindness and the universal energy surrounding us. Heart opening can elicit a spectrum of emotions, akin to the vulnerability of baring one's heart. While an open heart can foster love, compassion, and openness, it may also evoke fear or a protective instinct. Practicing control over these experiences proves beneficial in safeguarding our vulnerabilities. Backbends are also known for their ability to stimulate the adrenal glands, which regulate essential bodily functions such as metabolism, blood pressure, and stress response. As a result, they have the potential to enhance circulation and elevate heart rate. These backbend postures serve as catalysts for infusing a revitalizing energy into daily activities and promoting cardiovascular well-being. Additionally, heart-opening poses provide relief from weakened back muscles, tension in the chest and shoulders, and postural issues resulting from prolonged hunching. The use of props with these poses facilitates body awareness and fosters a gradual, comfortable progression toward an open heart. In addition to the poses in this chapter, some heart-opening poses are featured in other chapters, strategically placed where they align more seamlessly with the overall flow.

> Mantra: My heart is open, and love flows
> freely within and around me.

Melting Heart Pose

Anahatasana   अनाहतासन

Melting heart pose, also commonly known as extended puppy pose, is a transformative yoga posture with multifaceted benefits. This pose actively opens the chest and back of the arms, and if the chin is on the floor, it also lengthens the front of the neck. Melting heart pose also lengthens the side of the body and stretches the intercostal muscles, preparing you for deeper backbends with arms overhead. Explore some common prop-supported variations to enrich your practice and fully experience the therapeutic benefits of this pose.

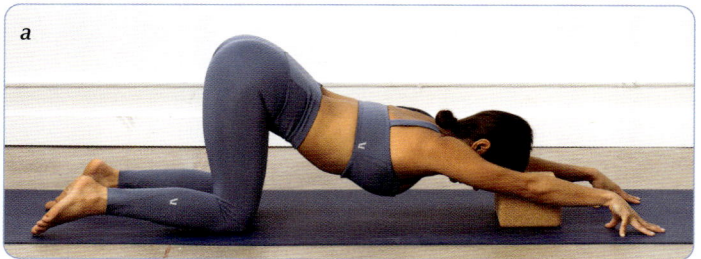

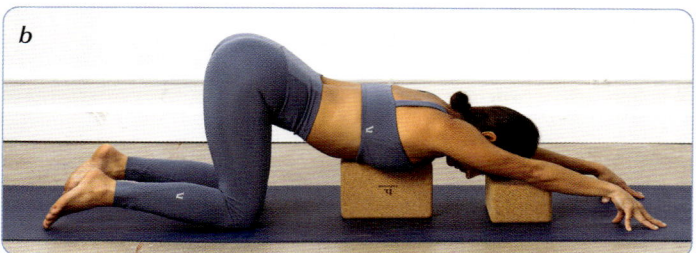

Place a block under your forehead and chest to bring the floor to you.

Not only does this prop-supported position reduce the distance between you and the floor, softening the stretch, but it also allows your head and neck to rest, reducing strain and tension. Start in a table top position. With your hips stacked over your knees, walk your hands forward, extending through your spine. When you reach the point where you cannot walk any farther without shifting your hips in front of your knees, start

to melt the chest toward the mat. As you do so, continue to wrap your upper arms down, creating space in the upper back. Place a block under your forehead, relaxing the neck and face (see photo *a*), or extend the support to your chest by sliding a prop under your sternum as well (see photo *b*). Breathe deep into the belly, inflating it like a balloon as if the belly button were trying to kiss the mat. Let every exhale soften the belly and deepen the stretch through the chest.

Place blocks under your elbows with reverse prayer hands to deepen the stretch.

This block variation offers a deeper chest and heart opener. The blocks also create more space between you and the mat, offering more room for you to work into bringing prayer hands to the back of your heart. Start in a table

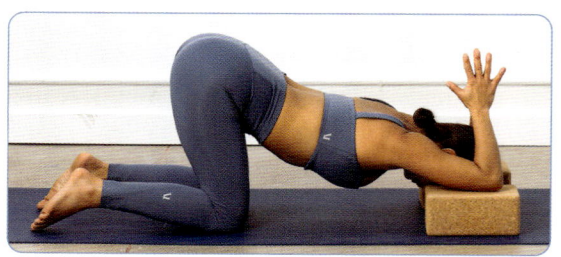

top pose with two blocks in front of your hands, with the long edges of the blocks running parallel to the long edges of the mat. You can place a blanket over blocks for comfort if desired. Bring your elbows onto the blocks and walk your knees back until your hips are directly over your knees. Bring your hands together in prayer and bend at the elbows, working your hands toward the upper back between the shoulder blades. Descend your chest toward the mat. Imagine you are wrapping your shoulders down and back toward the sides of your body to keep the shoulder blades from collapsing inward. Breathe horizontally across the chest and back, stretching through the muscles between your ribs. You can press down through the elbows on the inhale and release on the exhale to deepen the range of motion.

Place blocks under your hands.

This variation creates a deeper stretching sensation and facilitates a wider range of motion. Begin in a table top position, with your hands or fingertips on blocks. Start with the block on the lowest height

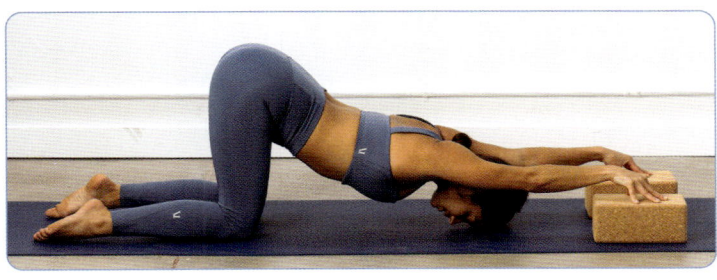

and work your way up to higher block heights. Start to walk your knees back until they stack under the hips, then melt your chest toward the mat. As you do so, continue to wrap your upper arms down, creating space in the upper back. As you inhale, press your hands or the pads of your fingers firmly into the blocks, rotating the armpits toward each other. As you exhale, stop pressing and release the chest deeper toward the mat. Consider lowering the head, neck, and chest below the arm, but don't strain to do so if you are still working up to that!

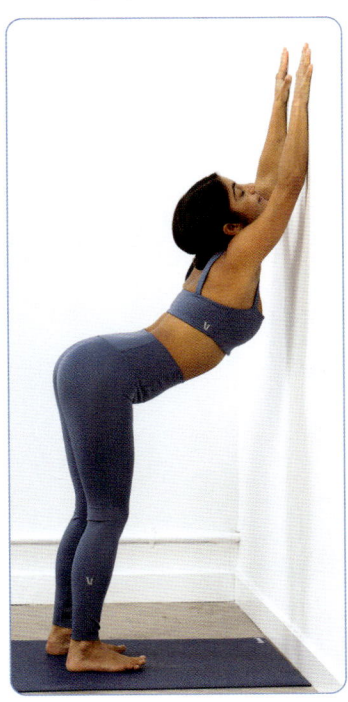

Stand against a wall to support your knees.

If knee flexion or weight-bearing is not an option, you can still benefit from this posture by practicing it standing! Face a wall, standing with your feet about hip-width apart. Place your hands on the wall about shoulder-width apart and step back until your arms are fully extended. Walk your hands up the wall, melting your chest in the direction of the wall. You can adjust your distance from the wall as needed but be sure to keep your hips stacked over your ankles, even if it means your chest is farther from the wall. The goal is to receive the stretch, not to get your chest to the wall. If you hyperextend in your knees, or experience tightness in your low back, softly bend the knees.

Use a chair to reduce knee strain.

These are two great variations for reducing knee strain, and to help if you have difficulty getting up from and down to the floor. In the first chair-supported option, you can practice standing facing the back of a chair. Place your hands on the back of the chair and walk your feet back as you melt through your chest. Be sure to keep your hips stacked over your ankles, adjusting your distance from the back of the chair accordingly (see photo a). The second variation offers more core stability and balance support. It also helps to ensure your hips are in alignment with your knees.

Melting Heart Pose (continued)

Sit on the edge of a chair, facing a wall. You can adjust the distance of the chair from the wall to vary the depth of your stretch in this posture. Place your hands on the wall in front of you, shoulder-width apart, and walk your hands (or fingertips) up the wall. As you do so, melt your chest in the direction of the wall (see photo *b*).

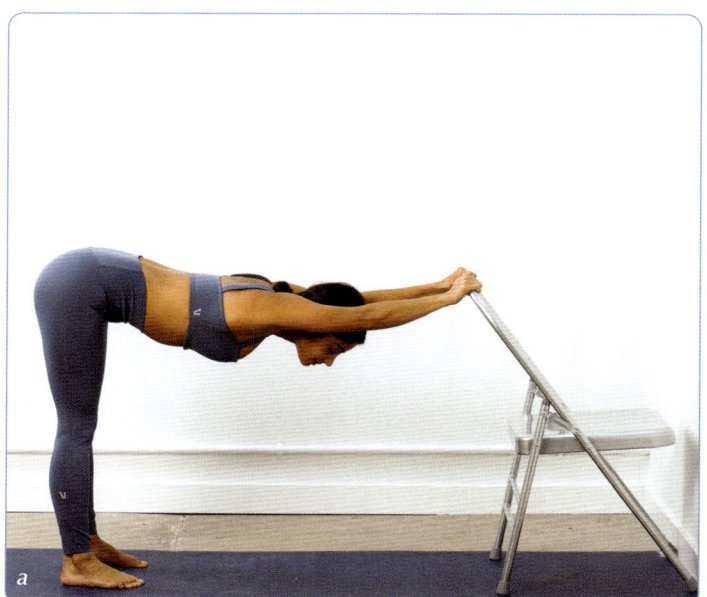
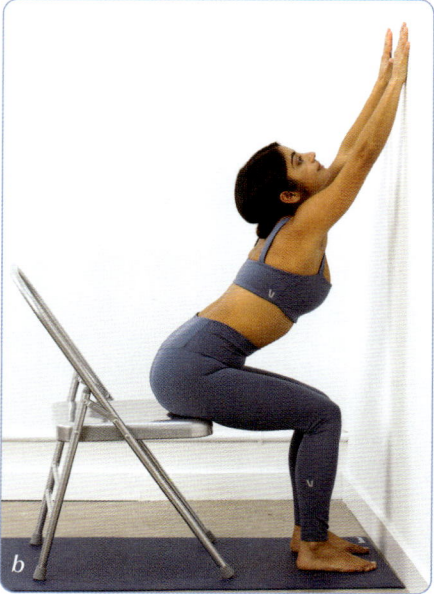

Place a strap around your shins to encourage space in your lower back.

If you notice your feet wanting to come together in this pose, try looping a strap around your shins and pressing into the strap to bring them parallel to each other. This encourages space in the lower back by narrowing your hip points and aids in pelvic stability.

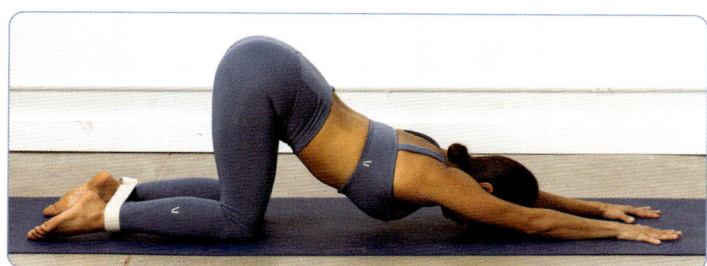

The Complete Guide to Yoga Props

Upward-Facing Dog Pose

Urdhva Mukha Shvanasana ऊर्ध्व मुख श्वानासन

Upward-facing dog pose is a dynamic yoga posture that strengthens and tones the spine, arms, wrists, and thighs, offering comprehensive benefits to your practice. This pose also provides a deep stretch to the chest, lungs, shoulders, and abdominal muscles while firming the buttocks. Explore some common prop-supported variations to enhance your practice and fully experience the transformative benefits of this energizing pose.

Place blocks under your hands to support your wrists and spine.

Using blocks gives the spine more space in the backbend so you are not moving the bend solely into the lower back. The target area for extension is the thoracic spine, which is your middle back. Using the blocks also makes lifting your knees off the mat easier, protecting your lumbar spine (lower back). Start in a downward dog pose with your hands on the blocks, then shift your weight forward into a high plank pose. Start to lower the hips as you lift your chest and gaze to face forward.

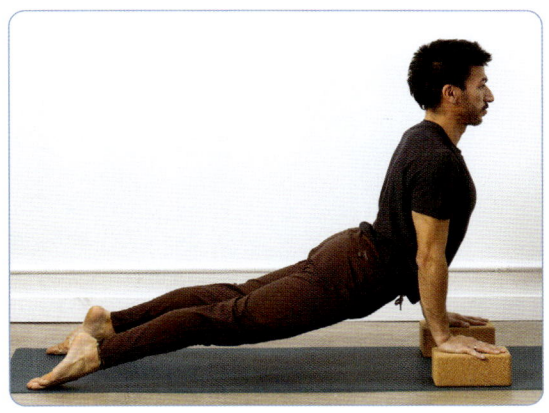

If you can, untuck your toes and come to the tops of the feet. Press down as if your hands were trying to press through the blocks. Broaden across the chest and collar bones. Draw your shoulders down, away from the ears. Hug your front lower ribs in and lengthen the tailbone toward your heels to take pressure out of the low back. Roll up slightly through the inner thighs to narrow the front hip points and create space in the low back. Elevate your knees off the mat by contracting through the front of your thighs.

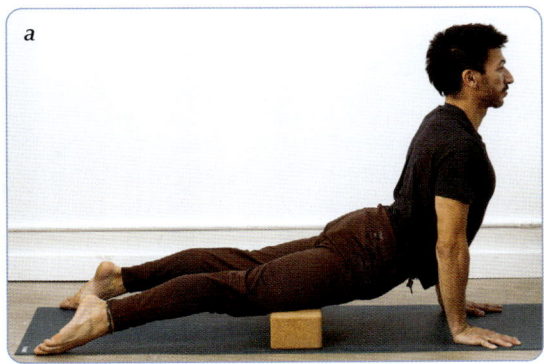

a

Place blocks or a bolster under your thighs to support your lower back.

This is another great way to utilize props to support your spine by lifting your knees off the mat. The props support you as you develop the strength in your thighs and shins to lift your knees on your own and will help you build leg muscle memory for optimal structural support. Lifting the knees off the floor aids the spine by preventing dumping or compression into the lower back. It also engages the muscles supporting the low back and hips. Practice by either placing blocks under your thighs at the low or medium height (see photo *a*) or by sliding a bolster or two under the thighs (see photo *b*).

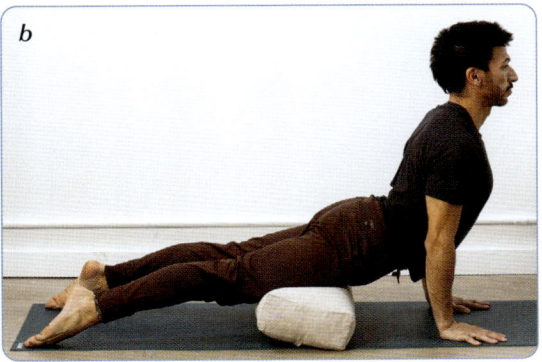

b

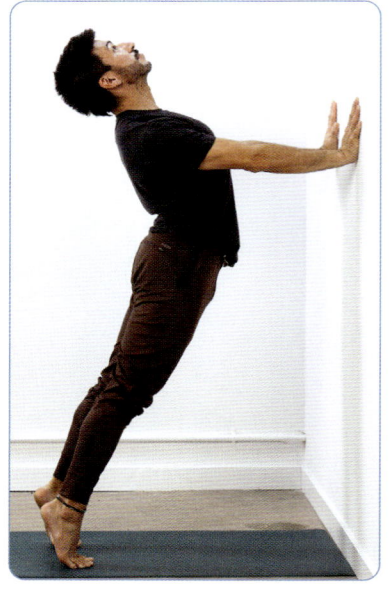

Use a wall to support your back and wrists.

Using a wall is beneficial for building muscle memory, alleviating wrist pressure, improving alignment, and gradually strengthening your back muscles without compromising form. The absence of a floor to press into encourages engagement of postural muscles for support. Stand a foot or two (0.3-0.6 m) from a wall, facing it. Extend your arms and place the palms of your hands on the wall at shoulder height. Your elbows should be slightly bent; if your arms are straight, step closer to the wall. Bring your hands shoulder-distance apart and your feet hip-width apart and parallel to one another. Spread your fingers and make sure your wrist creases are parallel to the bottom edge of the wall (to avoid turning the wrists). Press into your hands and come into a backbend by leaning slightly back with your upper body. You have the option to come onto your fingertips here. Keep your ears in line with your shoulders, so that the natural curve of the spine does not abruptly change at your cervical spine. Lengthen your tailbone toward your heels and lift your pubic bone toward your navel. Broaden through your chest and draw your shoulder blades down. Engage your thighs as if you are lifting your knees toward your chest. Imagine you have a string attached to your sternum, lifting your chest toward the sky. You can step closer to the wall to increase the bend or come onto your tiptoes to practice balance.

Use a chair to lessen intensity.

Using a chair can lessen some of the intensity and strain from this posture. It will also significantly reduce the amount of weight-bearing on your wrists if you are still building strength or recovering from an injury. There are two great variations that use a chair that is leaning against a wall as you lean your weight into it. For the first variation, prop the back of the chair against a wall and place your hands on the seat of the chair. Walk your feet back toward a modified plank position, keeping your wrists stacked under your shoulders. Gently lower through your hips and lift through your chest. Contract through your thighs to support your lower back (see photo *a*). The second option is a bit of a stepping stone from the wall to the seat of a chair. Turn the chair to face the wall and place your hands on the back of the chair. Walk your feet back, bringing your body to a lesser version of the modified plank from earlier in the paragraph and engage your core. Lower the hips slightly and lift through your chest (see photo *b*).

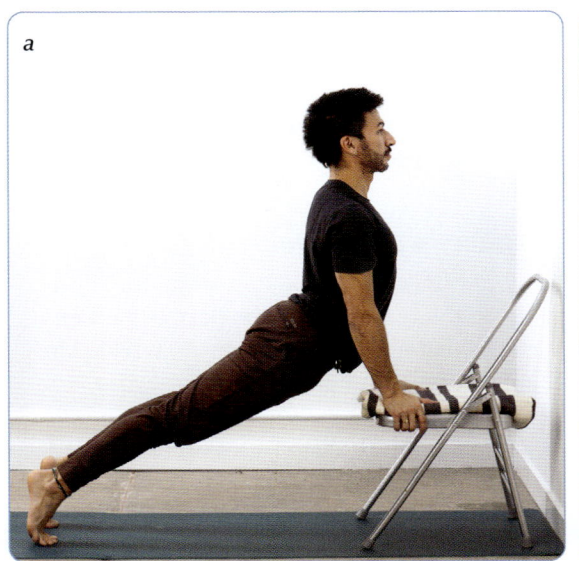

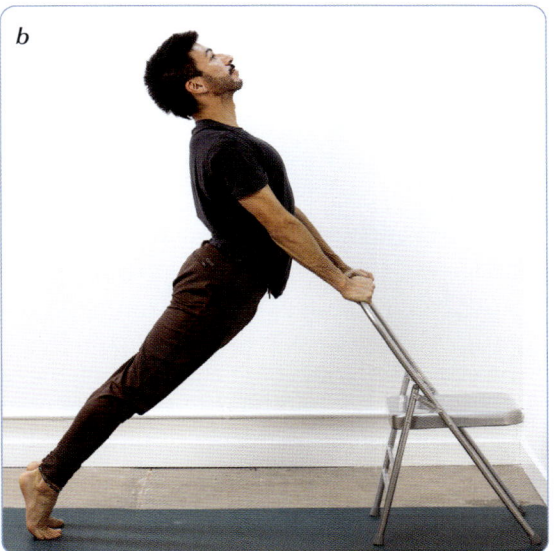

Place a blanket under the hands to alleviate wrist pain.

If full wrist flexion causes you pain or strain, this modification might help! You can use this trick in your plank and downward-facing dog as well. Place the edge of a folded blanket or mat under the heels of your hands. This should elevate the lower half of the hands an inch or so above the top half of the hands and fingers, decreasing the angle of flexion in the wrists.

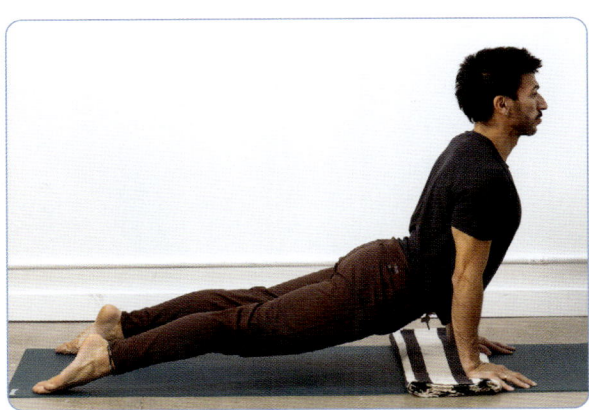

Upward-Facing Bow Pose

Urdhva Dhanurasana   ऊर्ध्व धनुरासन

Upward-facing bow pose, commonly referred to as wheel pose, is a dynamic yoga posture that actively stretches and opens the abdomen, chest, and lungs, providing a profound release. This pose strengthens the arms, wrists, legs, and spine, offering comprehensive toning and support. Upward-facing bow pose also boosts energy by stimulating the thyroid and adrenal glands. Explore some common prop-supported variations to enhance your practice.

Place blocks under your hands to create space in the upper back.

Using blocks can help to create more space in the upper back so you can straighten your arms. You can use two blocks running lengthwise on the mat or you can slant the blocks against a wall to help ease wrist pain by decreasing the angle of flexion of the wrists. Lie on your back with your head between the two blocks. Bend your knees and plant your feet on the mat, hip-width apart, with your heels directly below the knees. Bend your elbows overhead and bring the hands on top of the blocks with your fingers pointing toward the shoulders. Drive your heels into the mat and start to lift the tailbone toward the pubic bone. Try to keep your knees and feet parallel, pressing through the inner arches of the feet. Come to the crown of the head first and check in with the elbows. If they are splaying toward the side of the room, draw them back in so that the elbows point straight up toward the sky. Press more actively through the hands, straightening through the elbows and lifting the head off the mat. Shift your shoulders in the direction of your hands, but don't pass the wrists. If you feel the lower back is crunching, try lifting the heels to create more space. Roll your inner thighs down and soften through your buttocks. Hold and breathe for five deep breaths. To exit the pose, gaze up toward the sky and lower the back of your head, then lower your torso and hips. (See photo *a* for an example with the blocks flat on the floor and photo *b* for an example with the blocks slanted against a wall.)

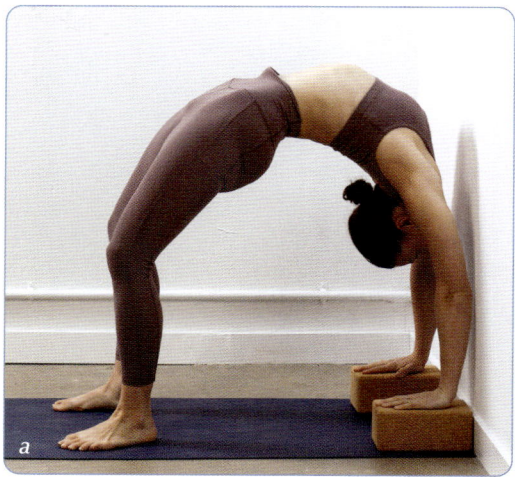 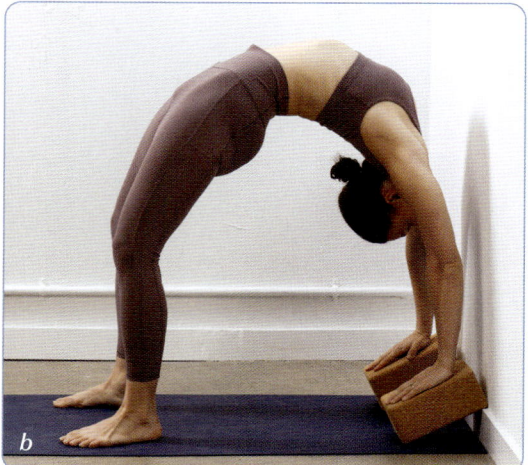

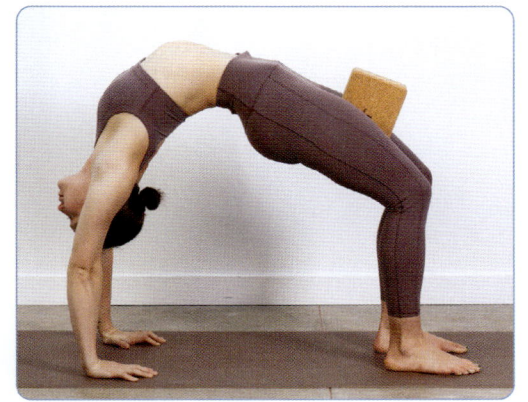

Place a block between your thighs to support your lower back.

Use of the block in this way helps to facilitate more space in the lower back by narrowing the hip points. It informs engagement through the inner thighs and relaxation through the buttocks, reducing strain and tension in the lumbar spine. It also reduces the tendency for leg abduction or external rotation which can strain the lower back. Lie on your back with your feet parallel and your knees up toward the sky. Place a block turned to its narrowest width high up between the inner thighs and walk your heels so they are positioned under the knees. Bend your elbows overhead and bring your hands to the mat with your fingers pointing toward the shoulders. Drive your heels into the mat and lift the tailbone toward the pubic bone. Squeeze the block between the thighs and roll the block down slightly; this will create more space in the low back and allow you to soften your gluteal muscles. Come to the crown of the head and check in to ensure your elbows are as close to perpendicular to the mat as possible. Press more actively through the hands, straightening through your elbows and lifting the head off the mat. Shift your shoulders in the direction of the hands, but don't pass the wrists. Press through the big toe mounds and keep the toes pointing straight forward. Hold and breathe for five deep breaths. To exit the pose, gaze up toward the sky and lower to the back of your head, then lower your torso and hips.

Place a strap around your thighs to support your lower back.

Just as in using the block between your thighs, looping a strap around your thighs can also help to maintain parallel and engaged legs, supporting the lower back and stabilizing through the sacroiliac joint. This informs the muscle actions of the legs differently, though, and may be a better suited variation if you have knock-knees or pigeon toes. This variation works by strengthening the outer thighs and hips without risking turning out the legs. If you tend to roll to the outer edges of your feet, try

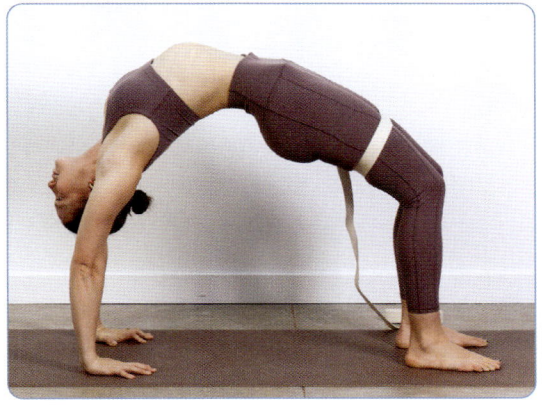

placing the block between the inner thighs first. Loop the strap around your thighs and tighten it enough that the legs, knees, and ankles are parallel and hip-width apart. Once you come into wheel pose, press your outer thighs into the edges of the strap to engage through your legs and create space in the spine.

Place a strap around your upper arms to open through your chest.

Looping a strap around your upper arms in wheel pose can help expansion through your chest without allowing the elbows to splay. Loop the strap around the upper arms, just above the elbows, so that the strap does not get in the way of your head and neck. As you come into wheel pose, press your outer arms into the edges of the strap to inform opening across the chest and shoulders without risking internal rotation or compression in the rotator cuff.

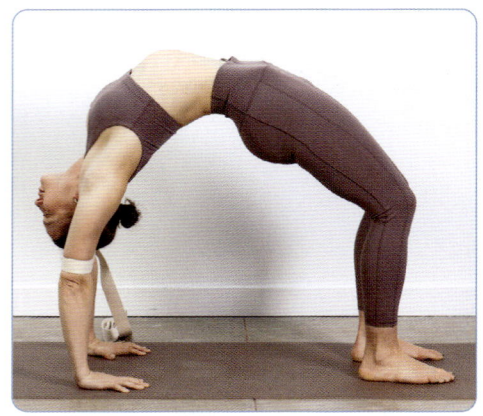

Place blocks under your feet to support your lower back.

Just as blocks under your hands can help create space in the spine for tighter shoulders and chest, blocks under your feet can help to create space for your lower back and hips if they are tighter and mobility is limited. To practice, set up just like you normally would for wheel pose but place two blocks, lengthwise and parallel, directly under your feet before you begin. You can even stack blocks but have a teacher there to ensure they do not slide and to assist you into the posture because it will demand more downward force as you press into the blocks to lift the hips.

Hold the legs of a chair to support your wrists.

This is a great option for those who have wrist pain because it removes the flexion in the wrists. It also helps to create more space in the chest and shoulders by increasing the height of the floor. There are two ways you can do this variation. Both begin with you placing the back of the chair against a wall so that it is stable when you enter the posture. For the first variation, lie down with your head between the legs of the chair, then reach overhead to grab the legs. The palms of your hands should be facing one another and with elbows drawn in, as if they were trying to point up toward the sky. Press into your feet to lift through your hips, then press into the chair to lift through your chest and shoulders (see photo *a*). If you require more space in the shoulders, sit with the back of your shoulders against the front edge of the seat of the chair. Reach your arms overhead and grab on to the side railings of the back of the chair. Lift through your hips and walk your feet forward enough to create ample space in the lower back. Your head and shoulders should be resting on the seat of the chair and your hands are still grabbing the back of the chair overhead. Press into the railing, using your shoulder and arm strength to lift the chest (see photo *b*).

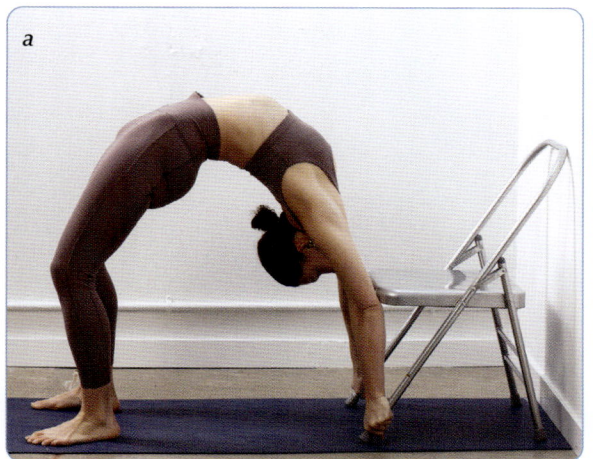

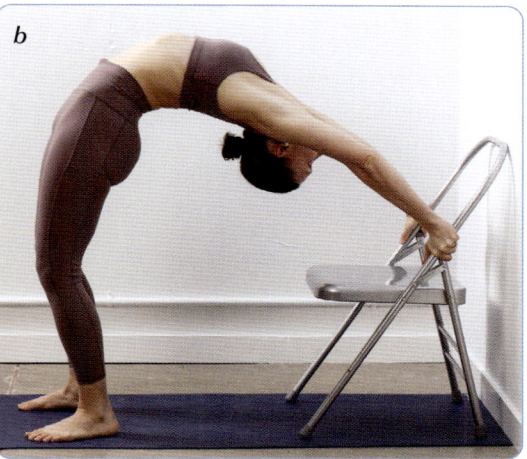

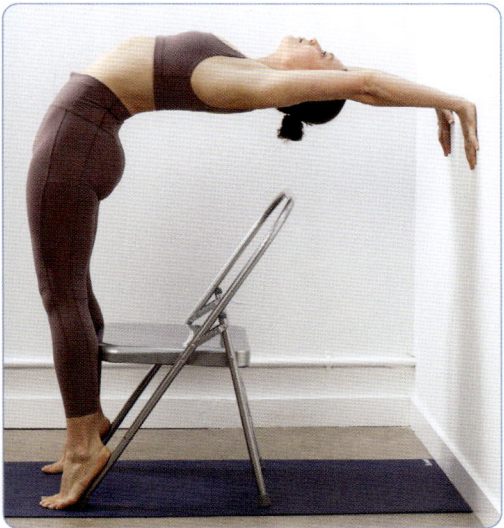

Use a chair and a wall for structural support.

This is another creative and supportive way to utilize a chair in this posture! To ensure the chair does not slide in this variation, make sure it is on a mat with grip. Place the chair near a wall, facing away from the wall. The distance of the chair from the wall will depend on your own mobility and proportions. Sit on the chair and reach your arms up overhead for the wall. If your fingertips contact the wall, you're close enough. While seated, have the heels of your feet on the legs of the chair, as shown in the photo. This will help to create more space in the lumbar spine as you enter the posture. Your upper back will rest on the back of the chair as you come into your overhead extension. Fold a blanket over the top railing of the chair for comfort as needed. Once your arms have contacted the wall behind you, press into your feet to elevate through your hips. You may find that you have room to bring your hands all the way to the wall or even walk your hands down the wall a little! If you are feeling a little intimidated by this, you can ask a teacher to spot you, sitting on the floor behind the chair.

Place your feet on the seat of a chair.

In this chair variation, use the chair to create more room in the lower half of the spine. Lie down with your feet planted firmly on the front edge of the chair seat. Make sure the chair is supported by a sufficiently grippy mat or a wall behind it so that it does not slide. Extend your arms overhead, planting your hands on the floor behind you, with your fingers pointing toward the tops of your shoulders. Press into your feet to elevate your hips off the floor, then press into your hands to lift the shoulders. Since your feet are higher off the floor, you should have more room to shift your chest in the direction of your hands and straighten through your arms.

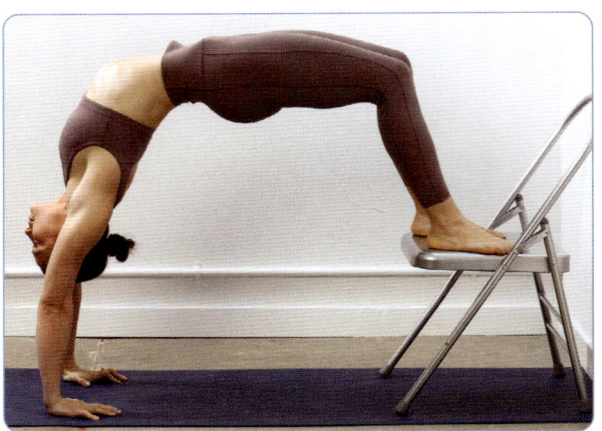

Work your chest toward the wall for a deeper stretch.

If increasing shoulder and chest mobility is your goal, this variation offers a nice challenge! Set up for wheel pose as before. This time, have the heels of your hands against a wall. As you enter the posture, use the wall as a reference point for steering your chest over your wrists. This version will help open your shoulders with reference to the wall, but it is not necessary to extend this far in a traditional wheel. Use caution and curiosity when moving into deeper spinal stretches and listen to your body's subtle cues to tailor your practice.

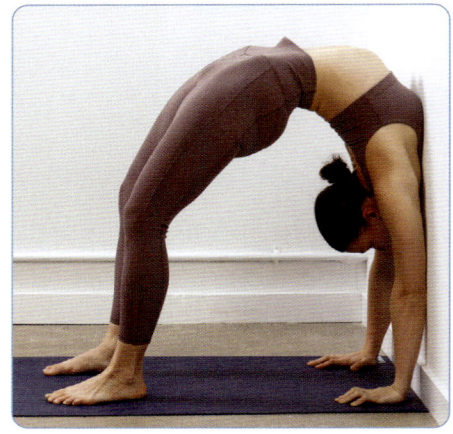

Place your hands on a wall to support your wrists and upper back.

If full weight-bearing on the wrists is not accessible to you, or if you are working up to a more challenging transition such as drop-backs, this option works for both! This is a perfect example of how the same prop can help you to modify and advance your practice! For this version, you may need a teacher to spot you, depending on how far you would like to walk your hands down the wall. Stand with your back to a wall and reach your arms overhead. Gaze up and back toward your fingertips as they contact the wall behind you. For some, having the elbows bent is a fine start! If you feel ready to deepen a bit more, you can walk your feet farther from the wall and extend through your elbows. Be sure your feet are parallel throughout this process to minimize crunching in the lower back. A final option is to begin walking your hands down the wall, which is also a great preparatory strategy for learning drop-backs. A good rule of thumb is to only walk your hands down as far as you have the strength to walk them back up. Practice at a capacity where you can still breathe with ease.

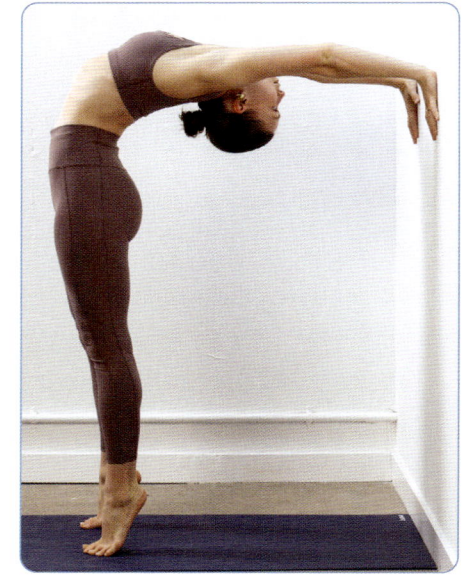

Two-Legged Inverted Staff Pose

Dwi Pada Viparita Dandasana   द्विपाद विपरीत दण्डासन

Two-legged inverted staff pose, commonly referred to as forearm wheel pose, is an invigorating yoga posture that actively strengthens the chest and lungs, providing a deep opening for increased breathing capacity. This pose also increases energy and builds strength in the upper arms, shoulders, and spinal muscles. It enhances shoulder flexibility and dexterity while lengthening the anterior chain muscles and strengthening the posterior chain muscles. Explore some common prop-supported variations to enrich your practice and fully experience the transformative benefits of this dynamic pose.

Place a block under your forearms to create space in the upper back.

Using blocks enhances upper back space in two ways: by raising the height of the floor or by decreasing the amount of spinal extension required by slanting the blocks against a wall. Lie on your back with your head between two blocks lengthwise on the mat and right above the shoulders. If you are using the wall, have the blocks slanted against it. Bend your knees to stack over your ankles as you plant your feet on the mat, hip-width apart. Bend your elbows overhead, bringing the hands on top of the blocks with your fingers pointing toward the shoulders. Drive your heels into the mat and start to lift the tailbone toward the pubic bone. Try to keep your knees and feet parallel, pressing through the arches of the feet. Press more actively through the hands, straightening through the elbows and lifting the head off the mat. If your elbows splay toward the side of the room, bring them back in so that the elbows point straight up toward the sky. Shift your shoulders in the direction of the hands, but don't pass the wrists. Lower your forearms onto the blocks and bring your hands together. You can hold the front edges of the blocks with your fingers if you would like extra support. If you feel the low back is crunching, try lifting your heels. Roll your inner thighs down and soften through your buttocks (see photo *a* for an example with the blocks flat on the floor and photo *b* for an example with the blocks slanted against a wall). Hold and breathe for five deep breaths. To exit the pose, first walk your weight back into your hands, coming back into wheel pose, gaze up toward the sky and lower to the back of your head, then lower your torso and hips.

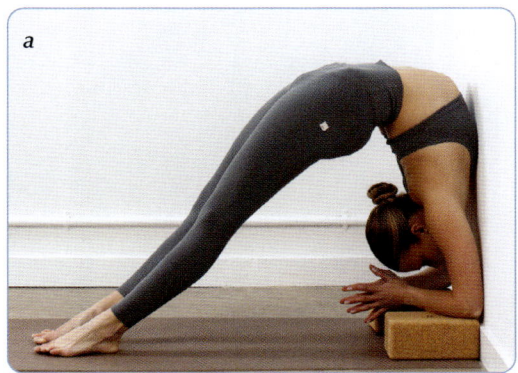 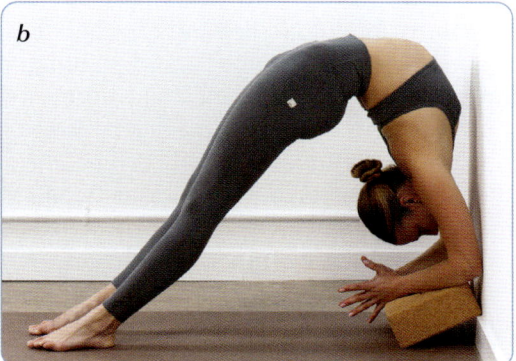

Two-Legged Inverted Staff Pose (continued)

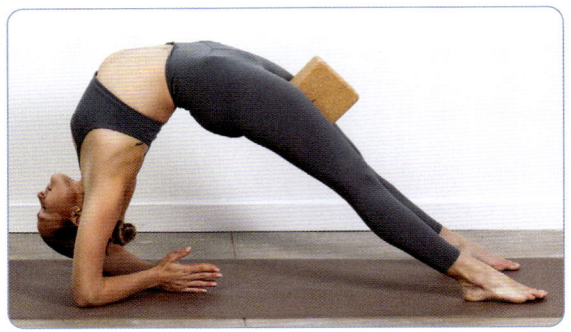

Place a block between your thighs to support your lower back.

Using the block in this way facilitates more space in the lower back by narrowing the hip points. It gets us to engage through the inner thighs and relax through the buttocks, reducing strain and tension in the lumbar spine. It also reduces the tendency for leg abduction or external rotation which can strain the lower back. Lie on your back with your feet parallel and your knees up toward the sky. Turn a block to its narrowest width and place it high up between the inner thighs. Walk your heels as close to your buttocks as is comfortable. Bend your elbows overhead and bring your hands to the mat with your fingers pointing toward the shoulders. Drive your heels into the mat and start to lift your tailbone toward your pubic bone. Squeeze the block between your thighs and roll the block down slightly; this will create more space in the low back and allow you to soften your gluteal muscles. Come to the crown of the head and check in to ensure elbows are as close to perpendicular to the mat as possible. Press more actively through your hands, straightening through your elbows and lifting your head off the mat. Shift your shoulders in the direction of your hands, but don't pass your wrists. Lower onto your forearms, going into the posture. Press the big toe mounds and keep the toes pointing straight forward. Hold and breathe for five deep breaths. To exit the pose, first return your wheel pose, shifting your weight back into your hands, gaze up and lower to the back of your head, then lower your torso and hips.

Place a strap around your thighs to support your lower back.

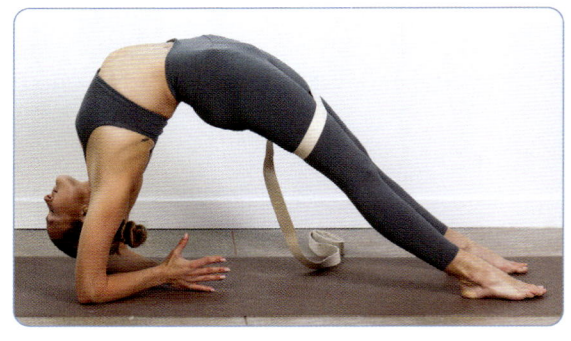

Just as in using the block between your thighs, looping a strap around your thighs can also help to maintain parallel and engaged legs, supporting the lower back and stabilizing through the sacroiliac joint. This informs the muscle actions of the legs in a different way. It may be a more suitable variation if you have knock-knees or pigeon toes. This variation works by strengthening the outer thighs and hips without risking turning out the legs. If you tend to roll to the outer edges of your feet, try placing the block between the inner thighs first. Loop the strap around your thighs and tighten it enough so that the legs, knees, and ankles are parallel and in alignment with your hip points. Once you enter the posture, press your outer thighs into the edges of the strap to engage through your legs and create space in the spine.

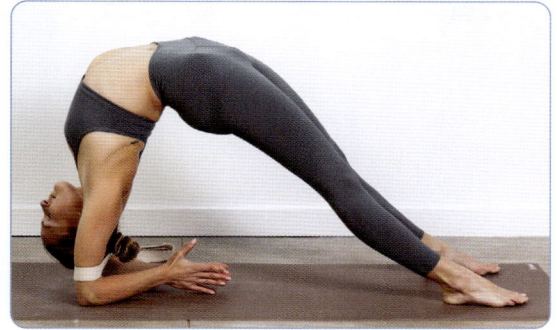

Place a strap around your upper arms to open through your chest.

Looping a strap around your upper arms in forearm wheel pose can facilitate expansion through your chest, without allowing the elbows to splay. Loop the strap around the upper arms, just above the elbows, so that the strap does not get in the way of your head and neck. As you enter the pose, press your outer arms into the edges of the strap to inform opening across the chest and shoulders without risking internal rotation or compression in the rotator cuff.

Place blocks under your feet to support your lower back.

Just as blocks under your forearms can help create space in the spine for tighter shoulders and chest, blocks under your feet can help to create space for your lower back and hips if they are tighter and mobility is limited. Set up just like you normally would for forearm wheel pose but place two blocks, lengthwise and parallel, directly under your feet before you begin. You can even stack blocks. Have

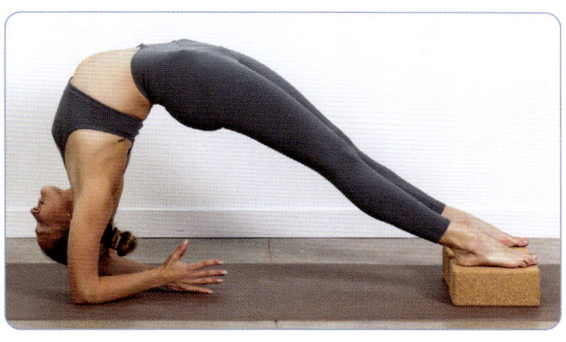

a teacher there to ensure the blocks do not slide and to assist you into the posture, because it will demand more downward force as you press into the blocks to lift the hips.

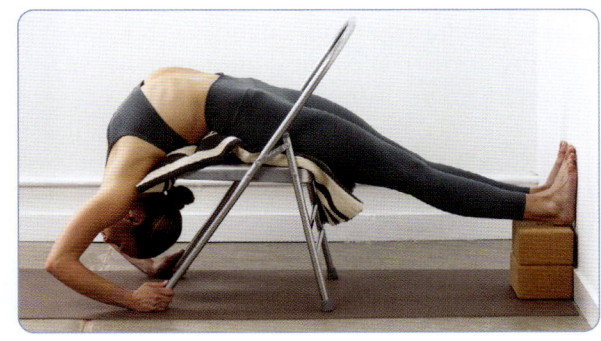

Use a chair for structural support.

This chair variation is a great, safe way to learn this posture. For this variation, you may want to place a folded or rolled mat or blanket on the seat of the chair for extra comfort and support for your spine. Sit on a chair with your legs through the back of the chair and your hands grabbing the back of the chair. Hold the back of the chair as you lower your back toward the seat of the chair. Your head should not touch the seat of the chair. Walk your feet out under your knees or practice extending the legs fully. To take this a step further, reach your arms overhead and try to grab the legs of the chair with your hands as shown in the photo. Hug your elbows in to align with the distance between the wrists. If your feet cannot reach the floor, or you need more space in your lower back, step onto blocks.

Two-Legged Inverted Staff Pose (continued)

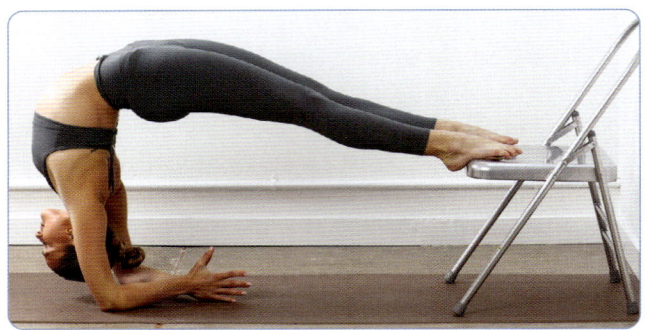

Place your feet on the seat of a chair.

In this variation, use the chair to create more room in the lower half of the spine. Lie down with your feet planted firmly on the front edge of the chair seat. Make sure the chair is supported by a sufficiently grippy mat or a wall behind it so that it does not slide. Extend your arms overhead, planting your hands on the floor behind you, with your fingers pointing toward the tops of your shoulders. Press into your feet to elevate your hips off the floor, then press into your hands to lift the shoulders. From your chair-supported wheel pose, lower to your forearms, one at a time. Since your feet are higher off the floor, you should have more room to shift your chest in the direction of your elbows.

Work your chest toward the wall for a deeper stretch.

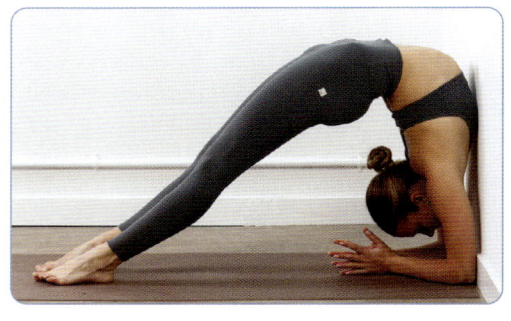

If increasing shoulder and chest mobility is your goal, this variation offers a nice challenge! Set up for a forearm wheel pose, as before, except this time, have the heels of your hands against a wall. As you enter the posture, use the wall as a reference point for steering your chest over your wrists, then lower your elbows to the floor. This version will help to inform how open your shoulders are with reference to the wall, but it is not necessary to extend this far in a traditional forearm wheel. Use caution and curiosity when moving into deeper spinal stretches and listen to the subtle cues of your body to tailor your practice to you.

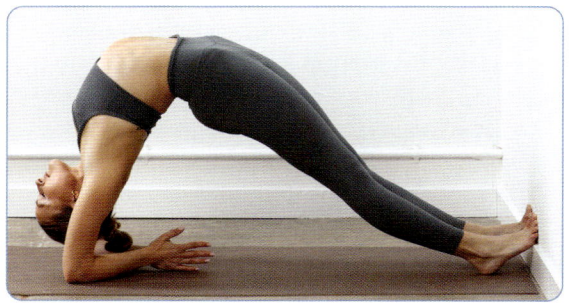

Flex your feet against the wall.

If you are working toward straightening your legs fully in this posture, this version is a great stepping stone! Flexing the feet against the wall informs leg and hip alignment by ensuring all ten toes are pointing up toward the sky, and the flexion shortens the shin muscles, making the stretch less intense. You can even practice this variation in the chair-supported version shown before!

Step both feet onto a wall.

You can practice this in two ways. The first variation is supported by the chair. Sit on a chair with the back of the chair facing a wall and your legs extended through the back of the chair. When you extend your legs, your flexed feet should reach the wall. Hold the back of the chair as you lower your back toward the seat of the chair. Your head should be released from the seat of the chair. Walk your feet out extending the legs fully and place your flexed feet on the wall. To take this a step further, reach your arms overhead and try to grab the legs of the chair or, depending on your distance from the wall, you can work your forearms all the way down to the mat (see photo a). Hug your elbows in to align with the distance between the wrists. This variation will allow more space in your back as you build your way up to extending your legs fully with your feet planted firmly on the floor. The second variation involves walking your feet up the wall from the bent-knee version of forearm wheel pose and pressing into the wall to straighten through your legs and open through your chest (see photo b). While this variation offers more space in the lower back to work toward leg extension, it is a much more challenging version that involves firing up your deep core and hamstring muscles. It is recommended that you have a teacher spot you.

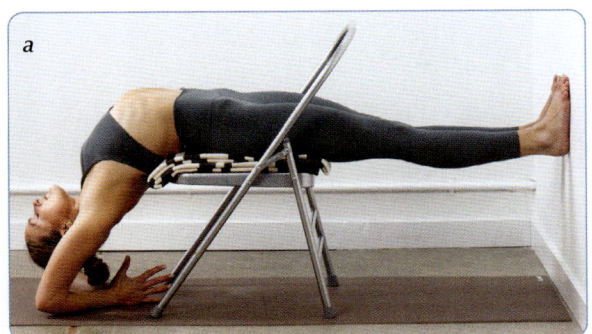
a

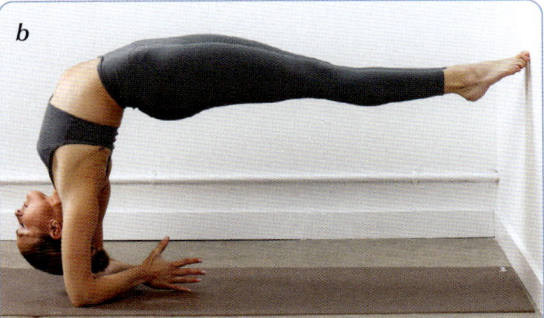
b

Bridge Pose

Setu Bandha Sarvangasana   सेतुबन्ध सर्वाङ्गासन

Bridge pose is a versatile yoga posture that actively stretches and opens the chest, neck, and spine, fostering flexibility and release. This foundational pose further stimulates the thyroid, aiding in energy balance and lowering blood pressure. Bridge pose also engages and strengthens the legs, providing comprehensive support to the lower body. Let's explore some common variations of this pose that props can enhance.

Place a block, bolster, or blanket under your sacrum for restorative effect.

A restorative take on this posture allows you to release through your hip flexors and low back, to support extension of the spine, and to encourage downregulation by promoting a parasympathetic nervous system response. Lie on your back with your feet on the floor and knees up toward the sky. Your feet and knees should be

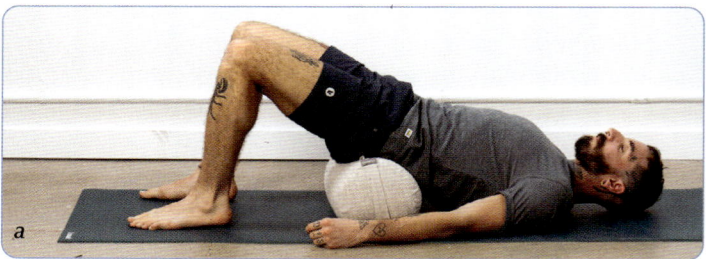

a

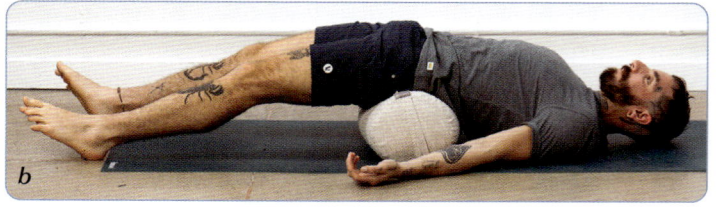

b

parallel to one another. Press through the inner edges of the feet to raise the hips. Place a bolster, folded blanket, or a block on your preferred height under the sacrum. Roll your inner thighs down and relax through your gluteal muscles. Lift your chin away from the chest slightly and soften through the muscles of the neck and throat (see photo a for an example using a bolster). Gently stretch through your belly by breathing deeply. Explore extending your legs fully to deepen the stretch through your psoas and hips (see photo b for an example using a bolster).

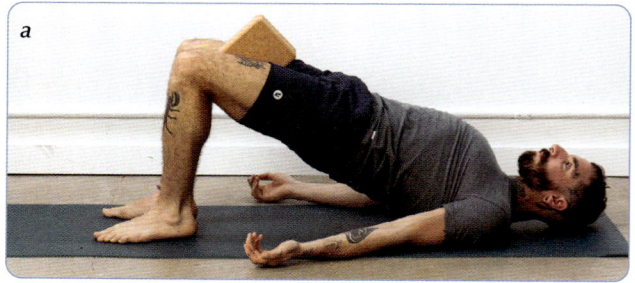

a

Squeeze a block between your thighs.

This variation stabilizes the pelvis and helps to create more space in the lower back by keeping the legs parallel and engaged. Lie on your back with your feet on the floor and knees up toward the sky. Your feet and knees should be parallel to one another. Place a block on the narrowest width between the thighs, as close to the pubis as is comfortable. Drive the heels of the feet

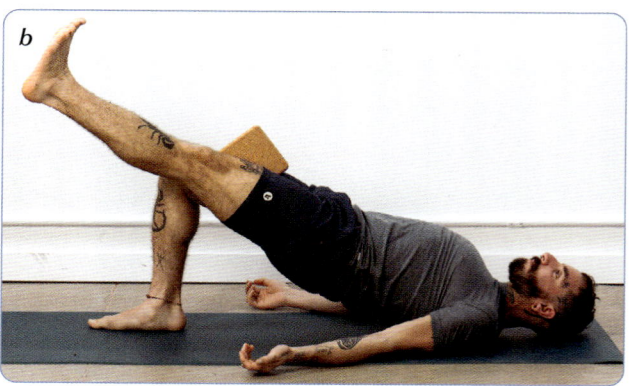

b

into the mat to lengthen the tailbone toward your feet, with the lower belly scooped in and the lower back against the mat. Squeeze the block between your thighs as you raise the hips. Roll your inner thighs down and lengthen the tailbone toward the backs of your knees. Reach your knees forward, contracting the thighs and softening the gluteal muscles a little. Draw your heels back simultaneously, engaging the hamstrings. You can flex your toes toward your shins while keeping the soles of your feet grounded to contract your shins up toward your kneecaps. You can grab the outside edges of the mat for support, have your hands on the mat, or interlace your fingers under the low back, creating a shoulder shelf for the heart and chest to rest on (see photo *a*). To add a little challenge to the legs, hips, and back muscles, try extending one leg forward, reaching through the heel of the foot. Squeeze the block to keep your knees and thighs parallel (see photo *b*).

Loop a strap around your thighs.

Just as with using the block between your thighs, looping a strap around your thighs can also help to maintain parallel and engaged legs, supporting the lower back and stabilizing through the sacroiliac joint. This variation works by strengthening the outer thighs and hips without risking turning out the legs. If you tend to roll to the outer edges of your feet, try the block 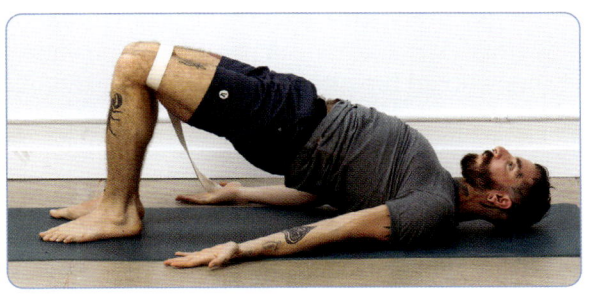 between the inner thighs first. For this variation, loop the strap around your thighs and tighten it enough so that the legs, knees, and ankles are hip-width apart. Once you enter the posture, press your outer thighs into the edges of the strap to engage through your legs and create space in the spine.

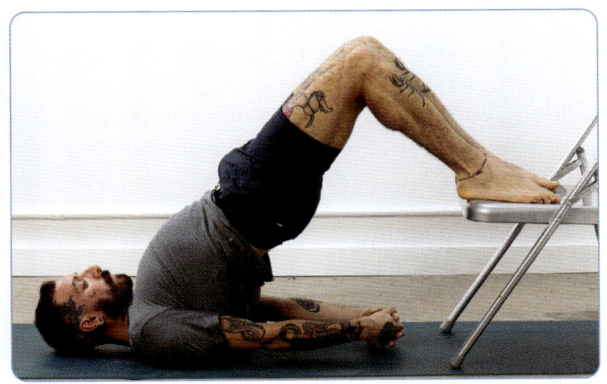

Place your feet on the seat of a chair.

In this variation, you use the chair to create more room in the lower half of the spine. Your chair should be on a sufficiently grippy mat or against a wall for stability and to ensure it will not slide away from you as you enter the pose. Lie down with your feet planted on the seat of a chair (or the edge of the seat if that is more accessible). Have your arms by your sides or hold the outer edges of your mat for extra support before going into the pose. Press into your feet to elevate your hips off the floor while squeezing through your shoulders to open across your chest. Since your feet are higher off the floor, you should have more room to shift your chest in the direction of your chin and possibly clasp your hands under you. Aim to keep your neck in a neutral position, gently lifting the chin away from the chest, if needed, to breathe comfortably.

Bridge Pose (continued)

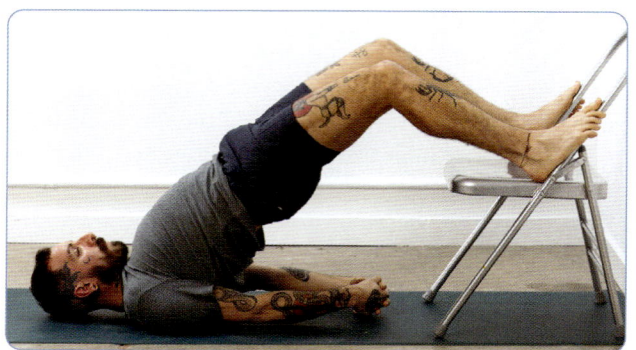

Place your feet on the back of a chair.

In this variation, you use the chair to create more room in the lower half of the spine. Lie down in legs-up-the-chair pose with your calves on the seat of a chair and your feet on the back of the chair. Press into your feet to elevate your hips off the floor while squeezing through your shoulders to open across your chest. Since your feet are higher off the floor, you should have more room to shift your chest in the direction of your chin. Aim to keep your neck in a neutral position, gently lifting the chin away from the chest, if needed, to breathe comfortably. You can utilize the legs of the chair for support if they're within reach, or alternatively, you can press your arms down onto the mat or bind them, as shown in the photo.

Hold straps or the outer edges of your yoga mat.

There are two great ways to modify bridge pose while working to open the shoulders and chest. The first variation involves holding the outer edges of the mat to create more leverage and stability as you elevate through your hips. As you grip the

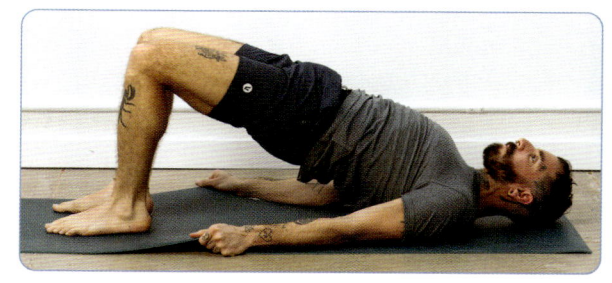

mat, imagine pulling your arms away from one another to draw the shoulder blades closer together (see photo). The second variation is a great stepping stone to clasping your hands together under your back. As you set up for bridge pose, have a strap lying flat on your mat beneath you and hold the edges of the strap in both hands. As you lift your hips, gently pull the ends of the strap away from one another to open across your chest. If you can, walk your hands closer together on the strap as you draw your shoulders closer together under your back. Continue to press your arms into the floor as you do so.

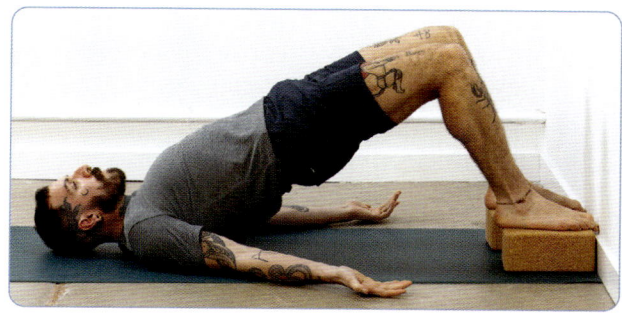

Place your feet on blocks against a wall.

Utilizing blocks under your feet can help to create more room in your lower back and hips if they are tighter and mobility is limited. To practice, set up just like you normally would for bridge pose, but place two blocks, lengthwise and parallel, directly under your feet. To keep the blocks from sliding, place them flush against a wall to ensure stability. If more room is required, stack blocks to add more height.

Fish Pose

Matsyasana

मत्स्यासन

Fish pose is an enriching yoga posture that actively stretches the throat, chest, and abdomen, promoting flexibility and release in these areas. This pose also strengthens the upper back as it stretches and stimulates the organs of the belly and throat. It also provides a targeted stretch to the psoas. Explore prop-supported variations to enrich your practice and experience the benefits of fish pose.

Place blocks under your shoulders and head.

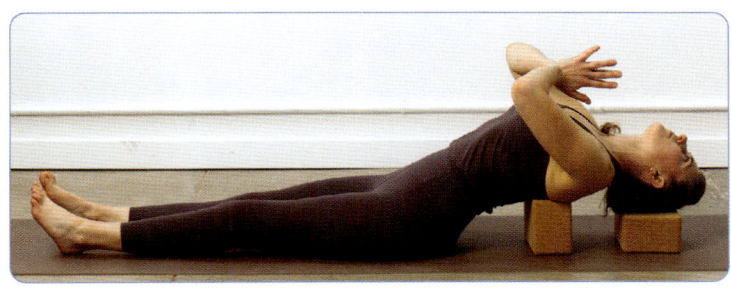

Using blocks will allow you to receive the support you need to find deeper relaxation in the stretch. It can also aid in allowing more extension throughout the thoracic spine and opening through the pectoral muscles, creating space for deeper breathing. Sit with your knees bent and the soles of your feet on the mat in front of you. Place a block behind you turned to low or medium height with the long edge running parallel to the top of the mat. Walk your hands and forearms back until the shoulder blades are resting on top of the block; adjust the block as needed for comfort. Walk the hips forward a little if there is too much pressure in your lower back. Relax the crown of the head back toward the mat, opening through the chest, rib cage, and throat. You have the option to extend the legs for a deeper stretch through the torso and hip flexors. Your arms can rest comfortably by your sides or in your favorite arm variation. Take deep breaths into the entire upper body, softening through the muscles with every exhale.

You can also place a second block under the head to further support to the head and neck, lessening the extension of the cervical spine. By reducing the amount of extension, you are also supporting ease of breath because it offers more opening in the airway. This second block is placed on its lowest height (or the same height), several inches behind the block that goes under the shoulders. Relax the head back on the block, slightly tilting the chin up and away from the chest, opening through the chest, rib cage, and throat.

Use a bolster to practice a restorative version.

This variation is good if you have tight shoulders or if the traditional version of fish pose is too intense. Place a bolster lengthwise on the mat and sit in front of it. Lie back on the bolster with your head and shoulders supported. Relax your arms by your side or extend your arms overhead and relax.

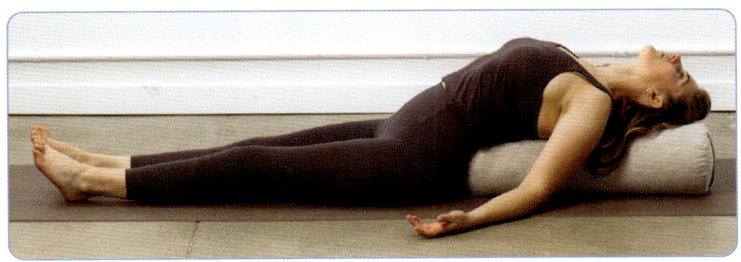

Fish Pose *(continued)*

Place a rolled blanket under your shoulders.

This is another great restorative offering if you have tightness in your chest and shoulders and you wish to find more ease and comfort in the pose. Place a folded or rolled blanket under your upper back, supporting the shoulder blades. The blanket will provide support and allow you to relax into the pose.

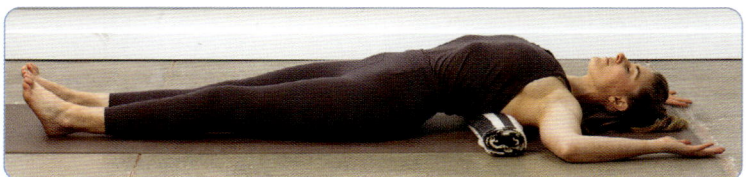

Align your legs with a strap.

Using a strap to bundle the legs together maintains a supportive hip and leg alignment, keeping the legs parallel. It will allow you to relax through your leg muscles without risking external rotation and potential tightening in the lumbar spine. For this prop option, you can loop the strap around the ankles to deter the feet from rolling out to the sides. You can also loop a strap around the thighs for more support.

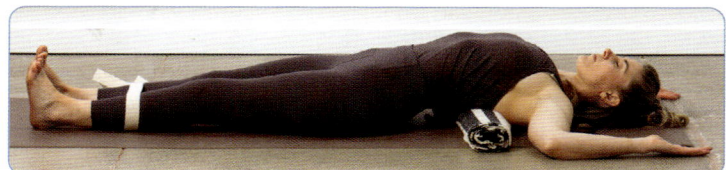

Use a strap to open and engage through your chest.

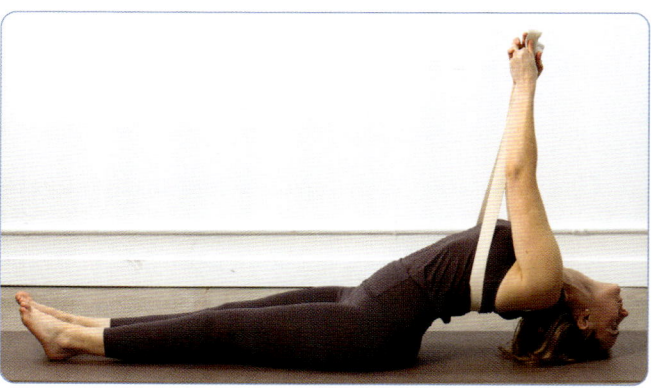

This variation requires more muscle action and will offer a feel-good self-assist! Before entering the full version of the posture, lay a strap under your shoulder blades. Release your head back to the mat, grasp the strap in both hands, and position it just behind the bottom of your shoulder blades. Gently pull the strap up toward the sky, reaching through both arms. This will help you to open your chest and shoulders. Press your sitting bones and thighs firmly into the floor and engage through your core muscles to shift weight-bearing away from the crown of the head.

Sit on a chair.

This is a great option if getting up from and down to the floor is difficult or weight-bearing on the head and neck is not accessible. It also is a nice way to execute fish pose on the go or while sitting at your desk. Scoot your hips to the edge of your chair and place your hands at the back of the seat. Plant your feet firmly into the floor or have them on blocks if you need to bring the floor to you. Press through your hands and ascend through your chest as if an imaginary string were attached to your sternum and lifting it toward the sky. If it does not cause strain, gently lift your chin and your gaze, extending the stretch into your cervical spine.

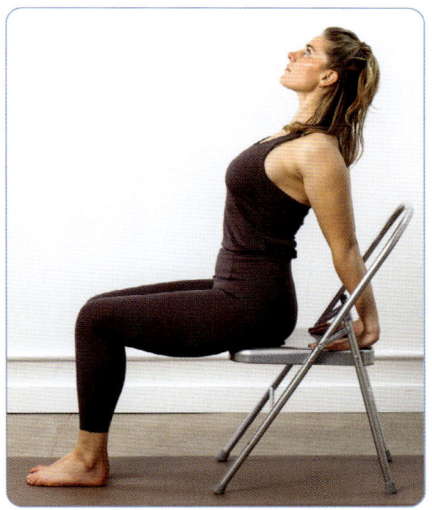

Camel Pose

Ushtrasana

उष्ट्रासन

Camel pose is a dynamic and invigorating posture that involves a deep backbend. This pose actively strengthens the muscles of the back while providing a profound stretch to the throat, chest, abdomen, and psoas. Camel pose stimulates the adrenal glands, contributing to an energizing effect. Here are some prop-supported variations to enhance your practice and fully experience the strengthening and revitalizing benefits of camel pose.

Place blocks under your hands to raise the height of the floor.

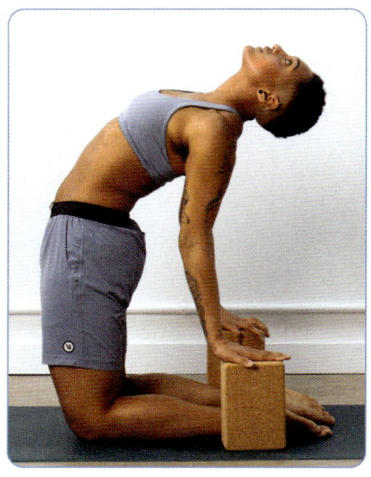

Using blocks in camel pose is a great middle ground if you are not quite ready to reach for your heels but want to deepen further into the pose. Blocks reduce the distance between your hands and the floor and offer the support to walk your hands back while still finding thoracic spine extension. Kneel with the knees hip-width apart, the shins parallel to one another, and the thighs perpendicular to the mat. Place blocks on their tallest height outside your ankles. Rest your palms, facing up or down, on the back of the pelvis where the buttocks and low back meet. Use your hands to lengthen your tailbone toward the backs of the knees as you lift your heart and sternum up toward the sky. Trace your gaze back and wrap your shoulder blades around the back of your ribs. Walk one hand at a time onto the blocks while keeping your thighs perpendicular to the mat. Some gluteal engagement is good, but if your buttocks are hardening into the low back, try to soften a little by rolling the inner thighs up and in. Soften through the muscles of the throat. You can drop your head back fully, but if it becomes difficult to breathe or you feel dizzy or have any cervical spine injuries, keep the back of your neck elongated and your gaze toward the tip of your nose.

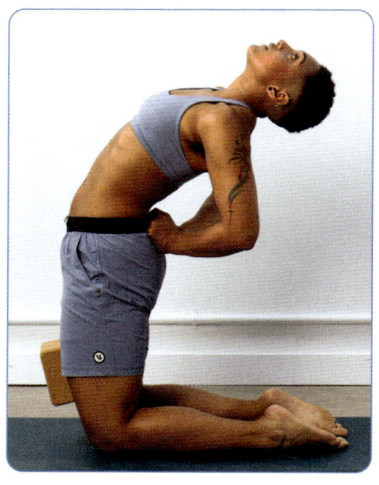

Squeeze a block between your inner thighs to support the lower back.

Using a block helps you to soften through the gluteal muscles and find more space in the low back and engage through your inner thighs and hamstrings. The block also helps direct the positioning of the pelvis. Kneel with the knees hip-width apart, the shins parallel to one another, and the thighs perpendicular to the mat. Place a block between your upper thighs, as close to the pubis as is comfortable. Squeeze the block inward slightly and toward the pubis, encouraging a neutral pelvis and creating space in the low back. Rest your hands, with palms facing up or down, on the back of the pelvis where the buttocks and low back meet. Use your hands to lengthen your tailbone toward the backs of the knees as you lift your heart and sternum up toward the sky.

Trace your gaze back and wrap your shoulder blades around the back of your ribs. If you feel open enough through the front line of the body, reach for the heels; your fingers will point toward the toes. You can tuck your toes so that your heels are a little higher off the mat. If your buttocks are hardening into the low back, try to soften them a little by rolling the block in and up.

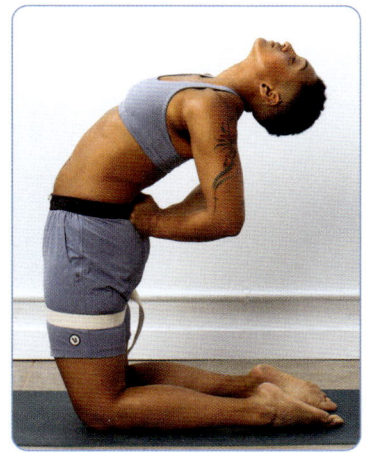

Loop a strap around your thighs to support the lower back and pelvis.

Using a strap around your thighs will help you to firm through your legs and hips, stabilize your pelvis, and keep your legs parallel to one another. Measure the loop of your strap so that it is taut when your legs are about hip-width apart. As you enter the posture, imagine splitting the mat in half with your shins, pressing your outer thighs into the strap. As you do so, simultaneously think about lengthening your tailbone toward the back of your knees and lifting your pubic bone toward your navel.

Press your hips against a wall to open into the chest and support alignment.

A wall is a point of contact to refine hip-over-knee alignment (keeping in mind that this is a common alignment cue, but may not apply to all bodies) and keeps the low back free of unnecessary strain or stress. It also lends feedback to support thoracic spine extension. Using the wall also keeps you honest! If you are feeling a little too eager to reach back for your heels, the separation between your hips and the wall will indicate that you may be doing so at the compromise of this alignment. Facing a wall, kneel with your knees hip-width apart and your shins parallel to one another. Bring your thighs to touch the wall so they are perpendicular to the mat. Bring your hands to your lower back as if to put your hands into your pockets. Slowly lift your chest away from the wall and lift your gaze. Draw your shoulder blades around the back of your ribs. Lift your ribs up and out from your pelvis as you are bending backward, keeping the bend mainly in your middle and upper back and. Stay here and press your hips into the wall. Then, you can walk your hands back, one at a time, toward your heels. Maintain contact between your legs and the wall, pressing your thighs and hips toward the wall.

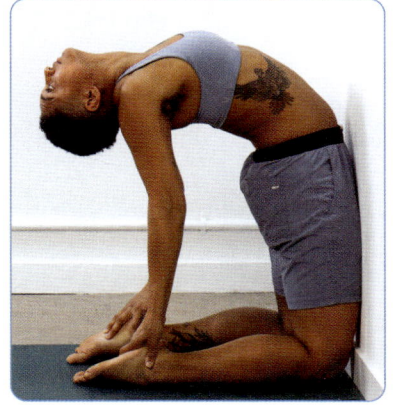

Fold a blanket under your knees for added comfort.

Using a folded blanket takes some of the pressure off the knees and adds extra comfort. If you have tight ankles and extension is challenging, you can also try rolling the end of the blanket under the ankles to fill in the space between your ankle and the floor.

Camel Pose *(continued)*

Use a chair to raise the height of the floor.

You can use the seat of a chair or the legs of a chair to reduce the distance between you and the floor. Slide your shins under the chair with your back facing the seat of the chair. You may even find added support by bringing the front edge of the seat of the chair all the way to your thighs or seat depending on your height. Begin to come into your camel pose. When you reach back for your ankles, extend your arms toward the back of the seat or legs of the chair. Gently press into the chair to guide the chest higher.

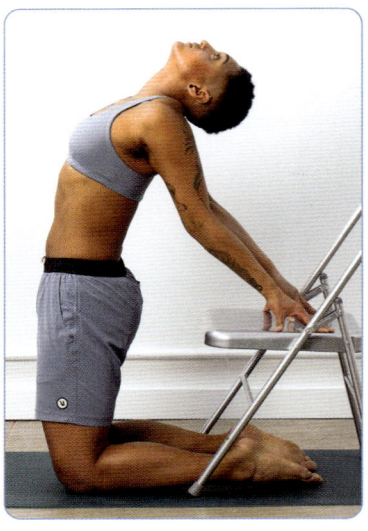

Use a chair to release through the head, neck, and jaw.

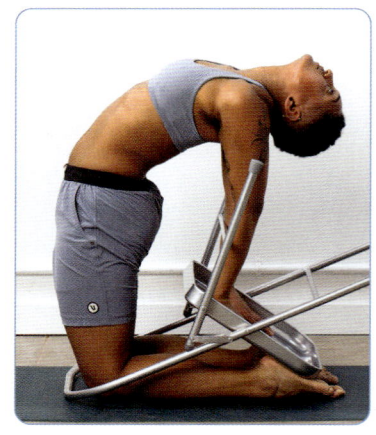

You can use a chair in this pose to support your head, neck, and jaw. For this variation, kneel back-to-back with the chair and bring your ankles just inside the legs of the chair as shown in the photo. As you enter the backbend, rest your neck on the top of the back of the chair; this will allow you to release fully through the head, neck, and jaw. If you need more height, or for added comfort, roll blankets over the top railing of the chair.

Invert a chair for alignment support.

In this variation, invert a chair with the top of the back rail of the chair on the floor closest to you. With your back to the chair, walk your legs inside the top railing, so that the seat of the chair is resting either behind the toes or on the feet and heels. Align your knees with the outer railings of the chair and have your shins directly behind them. As you enter the pose, hold the legs of the chair directly behind you or walk your hands onto the bottom side of the seat of the chair behind you.

Invert a chair and add a bolster to support the head and neck.

For this variation, invert a chair so that the seat and back rail of the chair is touching the floor. The back rail is facing away from you. With your back to the chair, tuck your toes under your heels inside the seat of the chair as shown in the photo. Place a bolster (or two) vertically between your ankles so that it is propped up against the chair railing behind you. Hold the legs of the chair and bend back. Once your head contacts the bolster, release through the muscles of your neck and jaw. Continue to reach your hips forward to stack over your knees.

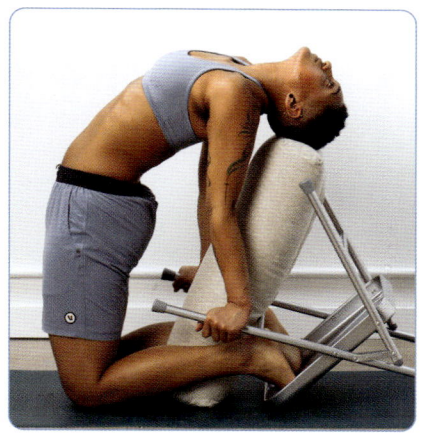

Use a chair to find extension through your spine.

For this variation, fold the chair so that it rests flat. Wedge the legs of the chair in the crease where a wall meets the floor and then distance yourself enough from the wall so that you can place the back railing of the chair at the bottom of your shoulder blades. Hold the sides of the chair as you enter camel pose. The chair should assist you in finding extension through your spine.

Sit on a chair.

This variation is best for those who have trouble getting on the floor. Have your sitting bones near the edge of the chair seat and reach for the railings behind you. Puff up through your chest and extend fully through your arms if possible.

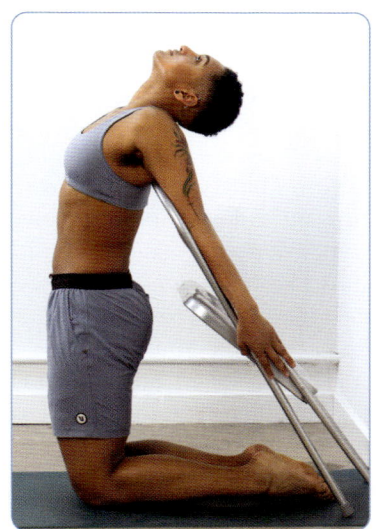

Pigeon Pose

Kapotasana

कपोतासन

Pigeon pose is a deep, backbending posture that engages the back muscles, providing strength and support. This pose also delivers a deep stretch to the throat, chest, backs of arms, abdomen, and psoas. Additionally, pigeon pose stimulates the adrenal glands, promoting an energizing effect. To enhance your practice, explore some prop-supported variations that amplify the strengthening and revitalizing benefits of pigeon pose.

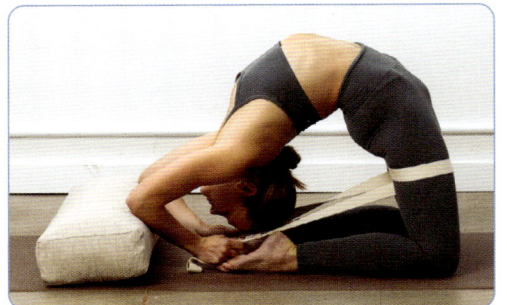

Loop a strap around your thighs and a bolster under your elbows.

In this variation, the bolster will play the role of bringing the floor toward your elbows, and the strap will assist you in walking your hands closer to your feet. The strap will also help to align the pelvis by gently pulling the inner thighs back as you press your hips forward. Place a bolster behind your feet with a little room between the prop and your feet as shown in the photo (you may have to adjust this later). In your kneeling position, slide a strap directly behind your knees and loop the ends around the front of your thighs. The straps should loop all the way around and thread back through between your thighs so that the ends are pointing back toward the bolster. Sit back for a moment and extend the ends of the straps all the way to the bolster so you can reach them later. Kneel on your shins and bring your hands into prayer at heart center. Reach your arms overhead, wrapping your shoulder blades around and firming into the back of the ribs. Press the tops of your shins into the mat and lengthen your tailbone toward the back of the knees. Lead with the sternum up as your reach your hands toward the bolster. Once you have reached it, grab the ends of the straps and walk your hands down the straps closer toward your feet if possible. Gently pull on the straps to draw your elbows down to the bolster. If the elbows still do not reach, you may need to stack a folded blanket or two on top of the bolster. As you pull on the strap, feel your inner thighs gently drawing back to narrow through your hip points and create more room in the lumbar spine.

Place blocks under your hands.

Using blocks raises the height of the floor. If you can *almost* reach your feet, you can position the blocks farther behind your feet to allow for more room in the spine as you enter the backhanding extension. Kneel like you are setting up for camel pose and place two blocks behind the feet. The higher the height of the blocks, the farther back from your feet you should place them. Place the blocks against a wall so that they do not slip or slide

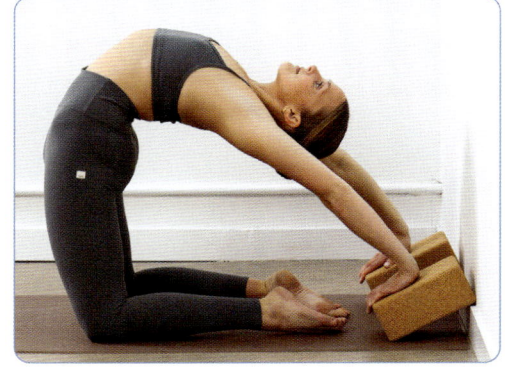

when you press your hands into them. You can also angle the blocks against the wall to support your wrists, as shown in the photo. Bring your hands into prayer at heart center, and reach your arms overhead, wrapping your shoulder blades around and firming into the back of the ribs. Press the tops of your shins into the mat and lengthen your tailbone toward the back of the knees. Lead with the sternum up as you reach your hands toward the tops of the blocks. Once you have contacted them, gently press into them to create more space in the chest.

Use a wall to find support.

A wall is a great way to find support as you build up to coming into the full posture. Kneel with your back to the wall. Start with about a forearm's length between your feet and the wall and adjust the distance as needed. As you enter the posture, your hands will first reach back for the wall. Once they contact it, press into your hands or fingertips to open the space across your chest and shift your hips farther forward (see photo *a*). You can try walking your forearms down the wall directly under your elbows and press into the wall with your forearms to create space again (see photo *b*). Note that if you are walking forearms down the wall, you will need to adjust your distance from the wall accordingly. Over time, your elbows may move lower on the wall and the hands can inch forward on the floor toward your feet.

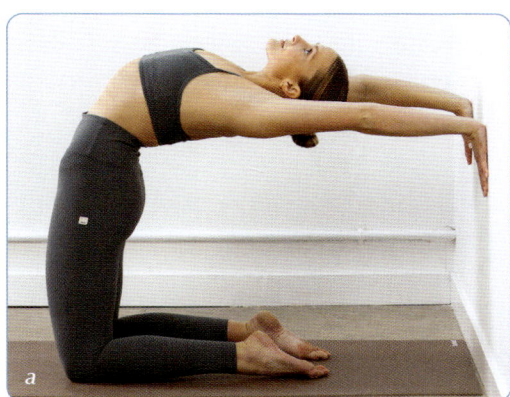 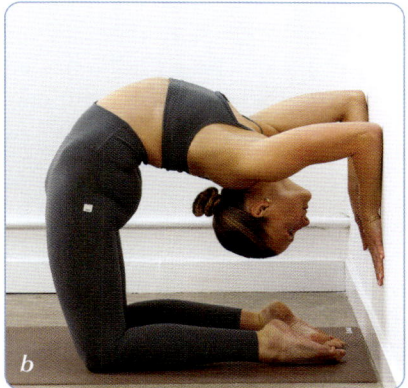

Practice little thunderbolt pose with a block under your head.

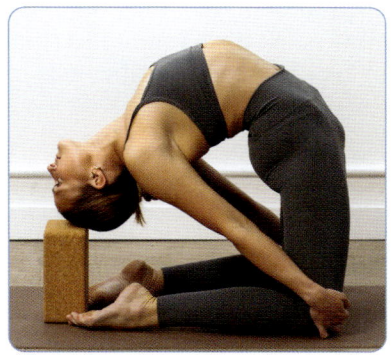

Little thunderbolt pose, supported with a block, is a helpful pose for working toward pigeon pose (kapotasana), which brings your forearms to the mat and your hands to your feet. Using a block brings the height of the floor to your head, lessens the intensity of the backbend, and provides more support for your head and neck. Kneel as you would for camel pose (ushtrasana). Place a block on its tallest orientation between your big toes. Bring your hands to the front of your hips to begin. Draw your shoulders down, lift your sternum, and keep your hips pressing forward as you bend back. Release the crown of your head onto the top of the block. Extend your tailbone toward the back of your knees and press your shins firmly into the mat. Work your hands down the fronts of your thighs to create expansion across your chest and over time work them further down toward the knees (as shown in the photo). Soften the muscles of the throat.

Place a block under your head and arms overhead for a chest expansion.

In addition to raising the height of the floor, blocks also allow support for the head and neck while exploring different arm variations that prepare us for hands on the mat or grabbing the heels with forearms on the mat. Kneel like you are setting up for camel pose. Place a block on its highest height between the big toes. Bring your hands into prayer at heart center, and reach your arms overhead, following them with your gaze. Wrap your shoulder blades around and firm them into the

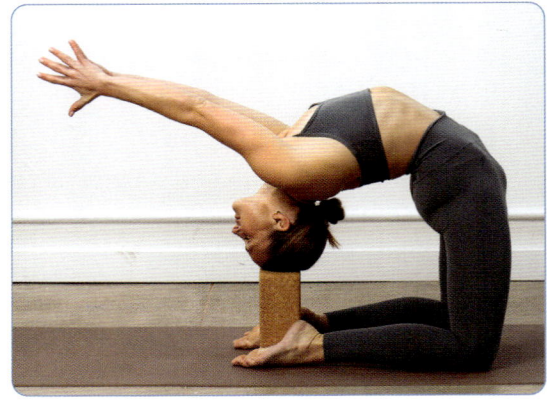

back of the ribs. Keep your hips over the knees as much as possible. Press the tops of your shins into the mat and lengthen your tailbone toward the backs of the knees. Lead with the sternum up as you descend the crown of your head onto the top of the block. Reach your arms straight back, finding a deep stretch along the sides of your body, and breathe into the ribs. Try reaching for the backs of the heels. If you attempt this, keep your elbows drawn in so that your forearms are parallel.

Use a chair for support.

Use a chair for additional support as you build muscle memory getting into this pose! Here are two great ways to get started. In the first variation, kneel with your back to the seat of a chair. Walk your shins back so that your legs are under the chair and your hips are close to the edge of the chair. Before you enter the backbend, place a bolster or rolled blanket or on the seat of the chair for extra comfort and to support a deeper bend in the upper back. Keep your hands in prayer at heart center until your back is all the way on the chair. If needed, add an additional blanket or bolster. Once grounded, extend your arms through the hole in the back of the chair and reach back. You can try to bend your elbows overhead and reach for the legs of the chair or even loop a strap around the legs of the chair and hold the ends in both hands to gently pull yourself farther into the stretch. Relax through your head and neck (see photo a).

In the second variation, sit with your legs through the back of the chair with the soles of your feet on the floor. Hold the back of the chair to lean back while shifting your hips forward. You will eventually reach the point where you are lying all the way back with your shoulder blades just off the seat's edge. You can slide a bolster or rolled blanket under your spine for support. Lengthen your tailbone forward to create more space in your lower back and allow your head and chest to release open. Reach your arms overhead toward the floor. Your hands may contact the floor, or you can bend your elbows and reach for the legs of the chair and grab hold. Once you have a secure grip, you can fire up through your posterior chain, engaging your hamstrings to tuck your feet under the chair, toenail side down, so your shins are diagonal to the floor (see photo b). Try pressing the tops of your feet into the floor to traction the spine (create space in) or try lifting your heels toward the seat of the chair for a fiery hamstring challenge.

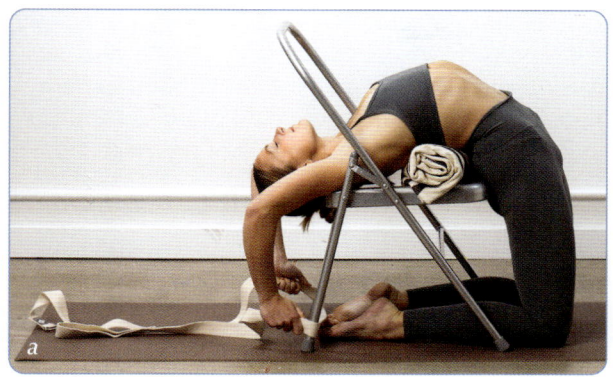 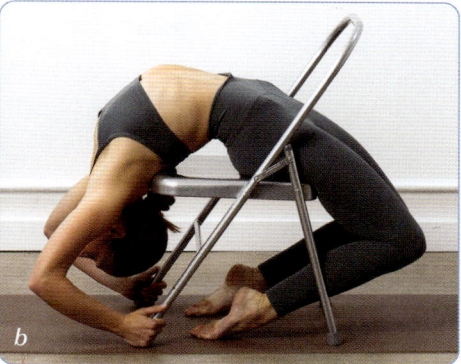

Place a strap around your arms for a chest expansion.

Looping a strap around your upper arms in this pose can facilitate expansion through your chest without allowing the elbows to splay. Loop the strap around the upper arms, just above the elbows so that the strap does not get in the way of your head and neck. As you enter kapotasana, press your outer arms into the edges of the strap to inform the opening across the chest and shoulders without risking internal rotation or compression in the rotator cuff.

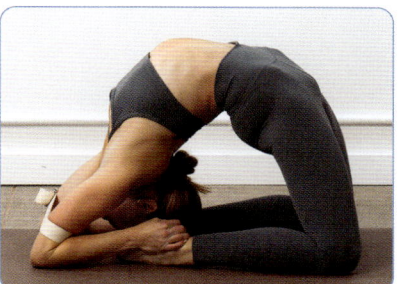

King Pigeon Pose

Eka Pada Rajakapotasana   एक पाद राजकपोतासन

King pigeon pose is a majestic yoga posture that gracefully opens the hips and chest, providing a deep and expansive stretch. It targets the psoas, piriformis, gluteal muscles, hamstrings, and groin, fostering flexibility and release. This pose not only boosts energy, but it may also offer relief from sciatic pain. To enrich your practice, explore some prop-supported variations that enhance the opening and stretching benefits of the pose.

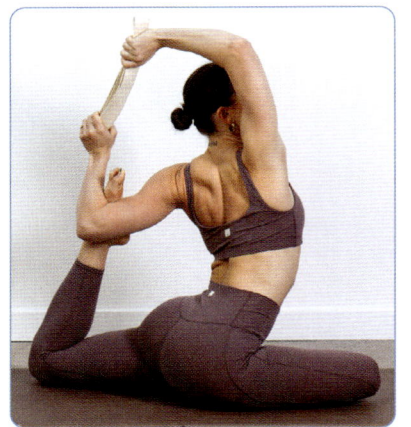

Practice the mermaid variation with the help of a strap.

Using a strap can bridge the gap between your hands! Begin in one-legged pigeon pose, then bend your back knee drawing your heel in toward your gluteal muscles. Grab your back foot with the corresponding hand. Slide your back foot into your elbow crease, bending at your elbow to hold your foot in place. Reach your other arm overhead, holding a strap. Grab the strap with your back hand and kick into your back foot to create space across your chest.

Use a strap to reach your foot overhead.

Just as in the mermaid grip variation, a strap can help you bridge the space between your hands and your back foot in king pigeon pose. It also eliminates the need to reach back and flip your grip (which can irritate the shoulder). Begin in one-legged pigeon pose, with a strap behind your back ankle. Hold the ends of your strap in both hands by your sides. Ensure your hips are level and stable before lifting your hands off the floor. You can draw your front heel closer toward your hips to ease leveling the hips, or you can slide a prop under your sitting bone on the side you tend to roll toward. Bend your back knee, drawing your heel toward your gluteal muscles. Simultaneously lift your arms overhead, bringing the straps together and walking them down the strap enough to maintain tension in the strap (see photo a). Hug your elbows toward each other to offer more space in your shoulders. Continue to walk your hands down the strap over time, making it all the way to your feet. Alternatively, you can loop

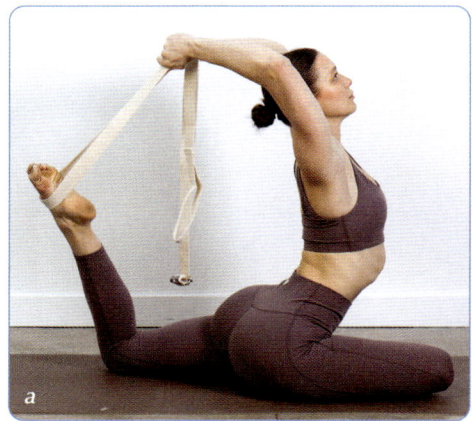
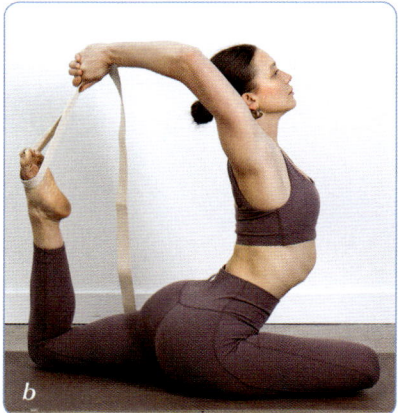

the strap all the way around the back foot or ankle so just one long end of slack remains. As you reach overhead, the strap will be in one hand, then the other hand will join the strap overhead (see photo *b*).

Place your shin in the corner where two walls meet.

In king pigeon pose, when the hips sway off kilter, the back leg will follow. Have you ever reached directly back for your foot, only to discover that it has gone off course? The corner where two walls meet will help guide your back shin toward center and therefore correct the placement of your hips. In this variation, set up as usual but with your back facing the corner of the walls. When you bend your back knee, lifting your shin off the floor, scoot your hips back until you nestle your shin in the corner. The shin should align with the edges of the wall, perpendicular to the floor.

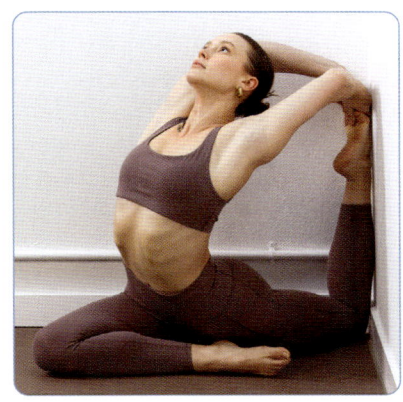

This also shows where you like to shift your weight in your hips as well as what muscles need to lengthen or contract to get you to this same position away from the wall. If it feels accessible, you can reach overhead for your back foot.

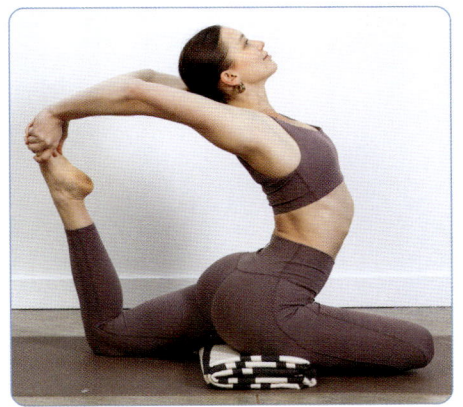

Place a block, blanket, or bolster under your hips.

Using the prop of your choice will help to level your hips and reduce pressure on the front knee if grounding the hips is not otherwise accessible. As you enter one-legged king pigeon pose, slide a block, folded blanket, or bolster under the buttocks of your front-facing leg. This will help prevent rolling off to one side and allow you to relax through the upper body because you have a surface to settle into.

Practice with your back thigh on the seat of a chair.

This variation, while still quite challenging, will support and stabilize the front knee by taking pressure off the joint and removing the external rotation needed in traditional king pigeon pose. It is not quite pigeon pose but rather pigeon *adjacent*. Stand with your back facing the seat of a chair. Bend your back knee, drawing your heel toward your gluteal muscles. Place the knee on the chair seat and slide it back until your back shin is propped up against the back of the chair. You can support the back knee by placing a folded mat or blanket on the chair seat. Hold the chair seat and inch your front foot forward until

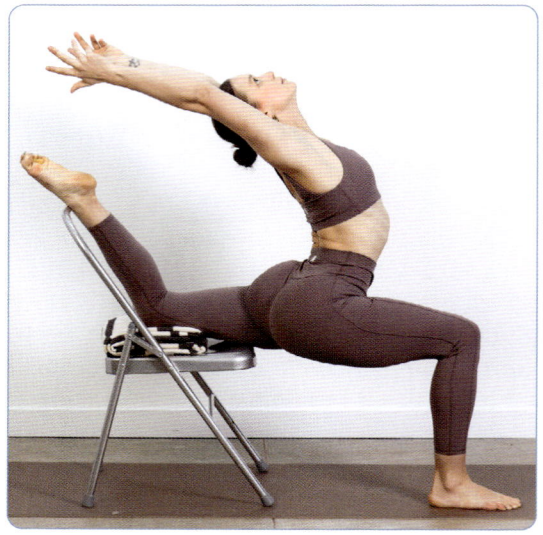

your knee is directly above your ankle. Aim to descend your thigh all the way to the seat of the chair, but if this is challenging, you can slide a bolster to the top of the seat, adding cushion and elevation to the top of your back thigh. Hold the chair as you ascend through your chest and extend through your spine. If you feel comfortable balancing without the support of your grip, try reaching overhead for your back foot.

Fallen Star Pose

Patita Tarasana

पतति तारासन

Fallen star pose, commonly referred to as fallen triangle pose, is a dynamic yoga posture with multifaceted benefits. This pose actively strengthens the arms, shoulders, and the back of the body, providing comprehensive toning. Additionally, fallen star pose opens the chest and shoulders, enhancing flexibility, while engaging core muscles for stability. Explore some prop-supported variations to enrich your experience and fully embrace the strengthening and revitalizing benefits of fallen star pose.

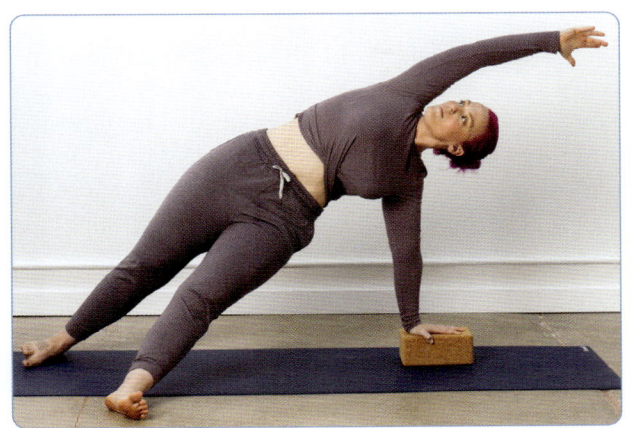

Place a block under your hand to make this posture more accessible.

Placing a block under your hand will take some of the weight from your arm and wrist, shifting weight back toward the lower half of your body. Begin in downward-facing dog, with your hands on blocks. On an inhale, lift one leg up and back into three-legged dog. On your exhale, bring your knee across your body toward the opposite elbow. Now extend your leg out to the side, planting the outer edge of your foot on the floor. Roll to the inner edge of your back foot and imagine reaching the sole of the foot down toward the mat. If you extended your left leg, on an inhale extend your right arm up toward the sky. Press the floor away, through the block, with your left hand, and draw your shoulder blade around the back of the ribs. Lift your hips toward the sky, and open across your chest. Repeat on the other side.

Use a chair to reduce weight on your arms and wrists.

Placing a block under your hand will take some of the weight from your arm and wrist, but if that is not enough, a chair is your next best option! Lunge with your shin against the front edge of a chair seat. Place the chair on a yoga mat or against a wall to ensure that it does not slide when you put weight on it. Place your hands firmly on the seat of the chair and start to wiggle your front foot across the body and continue to the other side. Roll to the inner edge of your back foot and imagine reaching the sole of the foot down. Once the front leg is fully extended, lift your opposite arm. Press into the chair with

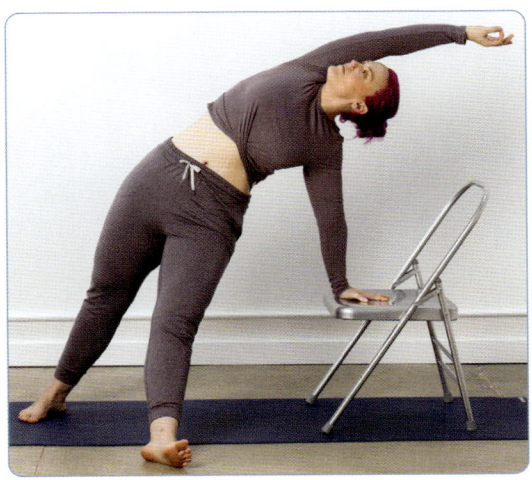

your other hand, drawing your shoulder blades around the back of the ribs. Lift your hips and open across your chest. If you notice your grounded hand shoulder rolling inward, imagine turning a lightbulb with your grounded hand on the chair to guide the shoulder back and away from the direction of your ear facing the floor.

Tiger Pose

Vyaghrasana

व्याघ्रासन

Tiger pose is a dynamic yoga posture that engages multiple muscle groups, offering a range of benefits. This pose actively involves the back and hamstring muscles, providing comprehensive toning. It strengthens core stabilizing muscles, shoulders, arms, and wrists, contributing to overall body strength. Tiger pose also offers a deep stretch to the hips, psoas, shins, and quadriceps. Additionally, this pose stimulates the nervous, lymphatic, and reproductive systems. Let's explore some common prop-supported variations.

Use a strap to reach your back foot.

A strap will bridge the gap between your back foot and your hand. To best utilize a strap, loop the strap around your back foot or ankle so it won't slide when you lift your back leg. Begin in a table top position and have the excess strap over the opposite shoulder. Lift your right leg and left arm simultaneously into balancing table pose (as discussed in chapter 3). Bend your back knee and reach back for the strap with your left hand as close to the foot as you can. Turn your left hand facing out, thumb side up, to facilitate opening across your chest. Once you have a firm grip on the strap, kick into it with your back foot. Resist the kicking motion with your arm and the expansion across your chest and shoulders. Try to square your shoulders forward and keep your weight shifted forward so that your shoulder is stacked over your grounded wrist. If you have wrist pain or injury, having the weight shifted slightly back toward your hips is OK. Stay in this position (see photo a) or eventually try to flip your grip, entering king tiger pose. To do this, draw your elbow to point forward and the palm of your hand that is reaching back to face inward, thumb pointing down. You may need to slide your hand farther down the strap to make room for the switch (see photo b). Repeat on the other side.

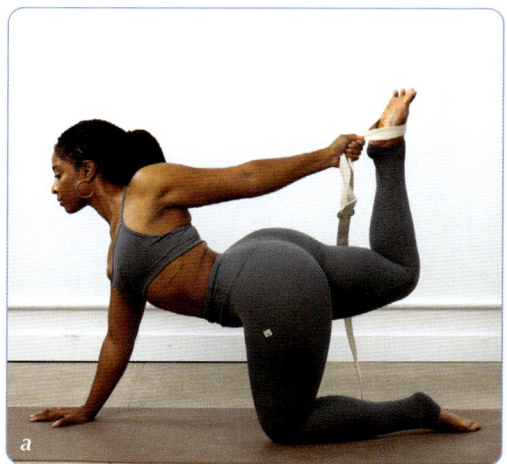 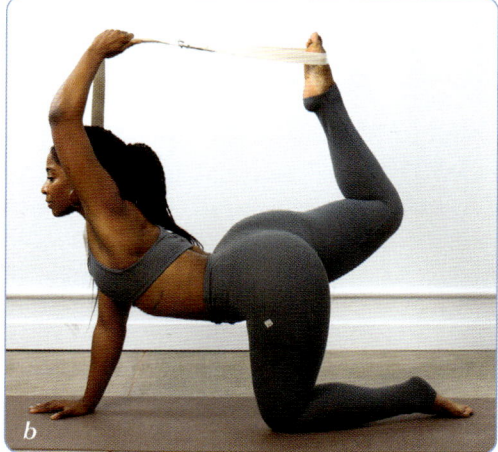

Support your knee with a blanket.

A great way to modify this posture is by kneeling on a blanket. To cushion and protect the knee, place a folded blanket under it. If you do not have a blanket, try folding your mat in half under your knee to double down on support.

The Complete Guide to Yoga Props

Stabilize your hips with a wall.

A wall is a great tool for keeping the hips level. Practice this variation by stabilizing the outer hip of the leg that is lifting against a wall. This way, the wall can also help inform the direction of the back shin, from your knee to your ankle. You will notice if your hip rotates externally as a form of compensation for reaching the back leg higher. You will notice because the shin will try to move away from the wall. As you kick the back leg up, continue to press the outer shin and thigh into the wall. You will feel muscles you never even knew you had to engage!

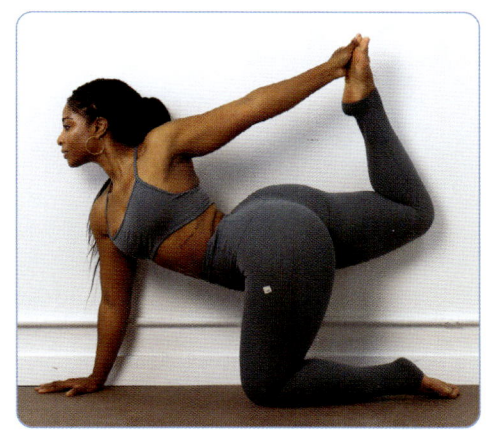

Support your back leg with a chair.

This variation offers a great deal of support and allows you to relax the back leg a little, but you must first be able to lift the back knee to the seat of a chair. If you can support this action, once the back knee or thigh makes it to the chair, you can focus on activating through your chest and shoulders. Practice with a wall in front of you and your back leg supported on the chair. To enhance chest opening, place your hand opposite the leg resting on the chair against the wall and press gently. Alternatively, bring the hand on the same side as the lifted leg to the wall and reach back with the other hand towards your foot (refer to photo a). The wall's support elevates the chest and facilitates reaching towards the foot. Eventually use the chair to stabilize your back leg as you aim to reach your foot without the wall's aid (refer to photo b).

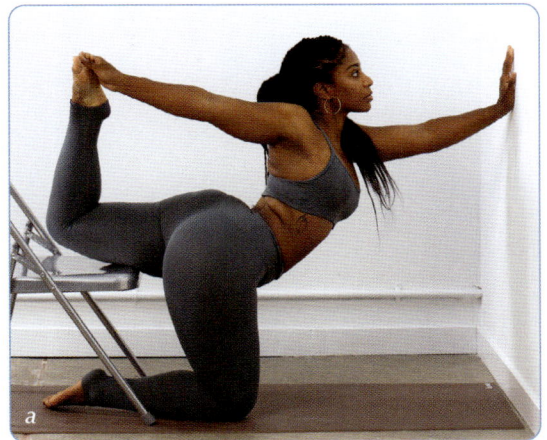
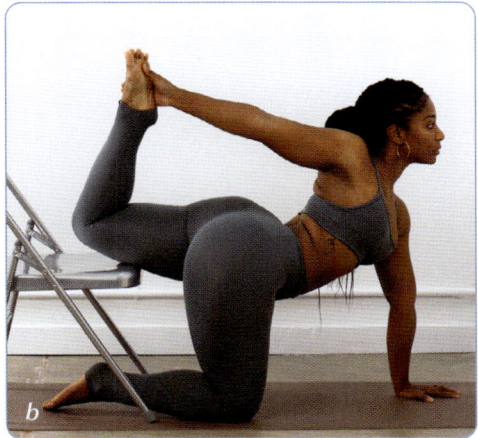

Place your back shin in a corner where two walls meet.

There is a chance you will not be able to get your shin flush against the wall in this variation, which is OK! Be sure to wedge the foot, toenail-side facing the wall, into the corner where the two walls meet. The corner will help guide your back shin toward the center and therefore level your hips. While the full shin does not need to contact the wall, it should align with the edges of the wall, perpendicular to the floor. In this photo, both hands are grounded, but you can also play with reaching your arm, opposite the lifted leg, back toward the foot. Since the foot is pressing into the wall, the reach will be energetic, as if you were going to grab the back foot but without actually grabbing it. This version of tiger pose requires more active mobility

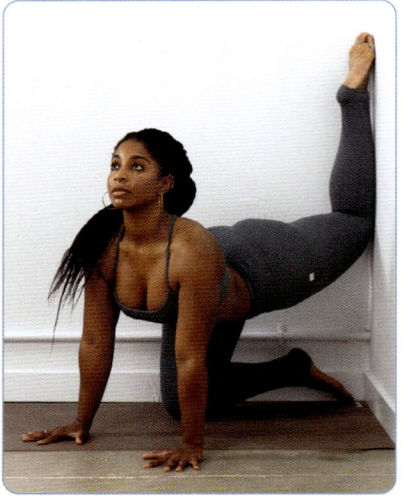

and strength, because you do not leverage the hold on the back foot to stretch deeper. If you desire more space across the back of your body, gently kick into the wall behind you to engage through the muscles along the front of your body.

Partridge Pose

Kapinjalasana

कपञ्जिलासन

Partridge pose is a dynamic yoga posture that actively stretches the abdominal muscles, hip flexors, and thighs, fostering flexibility and release. This enriching pose also strengthens the wrists, arms, shoulders, hamstrings, and core stabilizing muscles, contributing to overall body strength. Beyond the physical benefits, partridge pose engages the mind, creating a meditative aspect to the practice. Furthermore, this pose brings an energizing effect, adding vitality to your routine. Let's explore some common prop-supported variations.

Place the edge of your foot against a wall.

Using a wall can inform activation through the leg muscles and help to prevent collapsing in on your inner ankles in the posture. As you enter the posture, have your grounded foot against a wall and pressing into the wall to engage through the leg and core muscles. You may begin with your foot flush against the wall, but as you build strength and ankle mobility, work the inner edge of your foot closer to the wall and the sole of your foot closer to the floor.

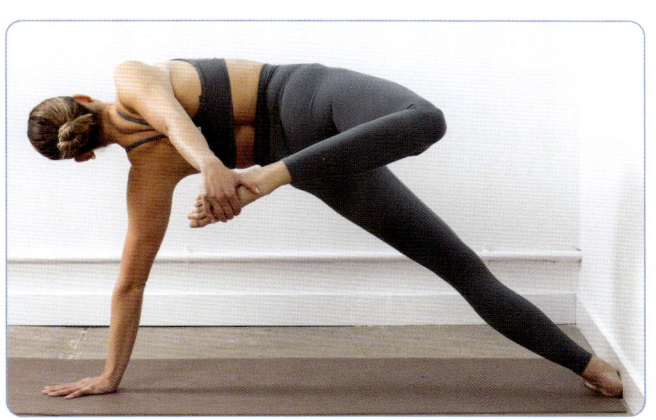

Stand with your hand against a wall.

The wall is great if you have trouble getting up from and down to the floor or need to limit weight-bearing on your wrists! Use two walls if you have room and want additional reference to your hip and shoulder alignment as well. Stand with your side facing a wall and extend the arm closest to the wall placing your hand on the wall at shoulder level. Step your feet away from the wall, creating a line with your body angled toward the wall. If you are using two walls, have your hips and shoulders up against the wall in front of you (if this makes you claustrophobic, then stepping away from the wall in front of you is OK). Squeeze the heel of the foot farthest away from the wall your hand is on toward your gluteal muscles, firing up through your hamstring. If you would like to go further, reach back for your foot with your hand farthest from the wall and kick back into the hand. If you are using the second wall, try to keep your hips and chest grounded to the wall.

Use a strap to bridge your foot and your hand.

A strap will bridge the gap between your back foot and your hand. To best use a strap, loop the strap around your back foot or ankle to ensure it won't slide when you bend your top leg. Begin in a side plank position and have the excess strap over your top shoulder, supported by the neck. Bend the knee of your top leg and reach back for the strap with your top hand, as close to the foot as you can. Ensure your hand is facing out, thumb side up to facilitate more opening across your chest. Once you have a firm grip on the strap, kick into the strap with your back foot. Resist the kicking motion with your arm to expand across your chest and shoulders (see photo *a*). Try to square your hips and shoulders, keeping them stacked on top of each other—especially if that top hip likes to fall back! You can

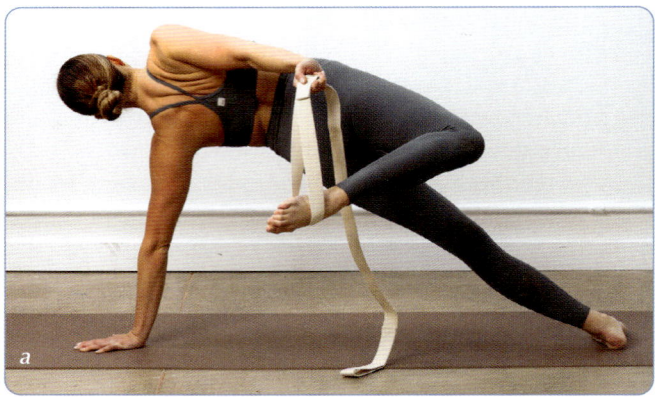

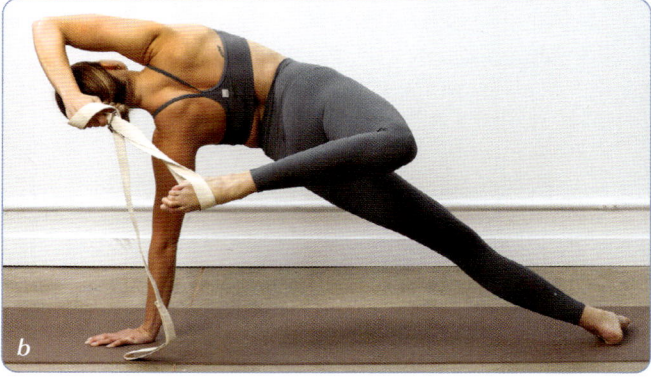

eventually flip your grip, coming into an overhead position. To do this, draw your elbow toward your top hip then up overhead, so your biceps muscle comes toward your top ear (see photo *b*). You may need to slide your hand farther down the strap to make room for the switch.

Place your hand on a block or the seat of a chair.

Placing a block or chair under your hand will take some of the weight from your arm and wrist and shift it toward the lower half of your body (see photo *a* for an example with the hand on a block and photo *b* for an example with the hand on the chair seat). This is great if you are still working up the strength for lateral weight-bearing or if you have wrist pain or injury.

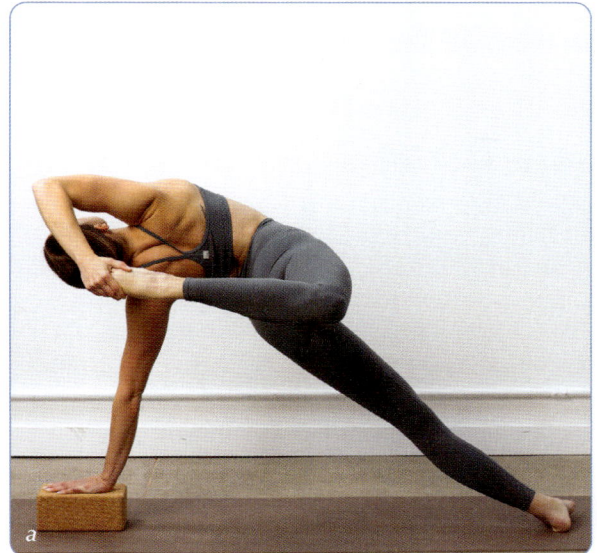

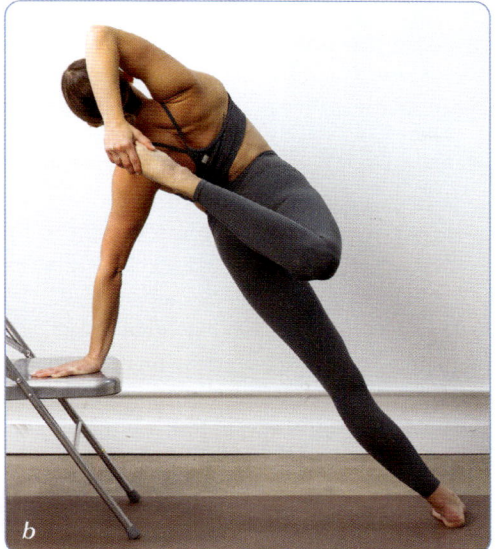

Use blocks to support your hips in a forearm variation.

This option is good if you want more stability through your hips as you enter the backbend. It is also a great modification if you are still building up the strength to support the foundational posture for this pose—side plank. How many blocks you use will depend on your height, and you can even play with slanting a block. You can also add height and comfort by folding a blanket over the top of the blocks. For this variation, practice either a modified version with your knees grounded (see photo *a*) or with the knees lifted in supported forearm side plank (see photo *b*).

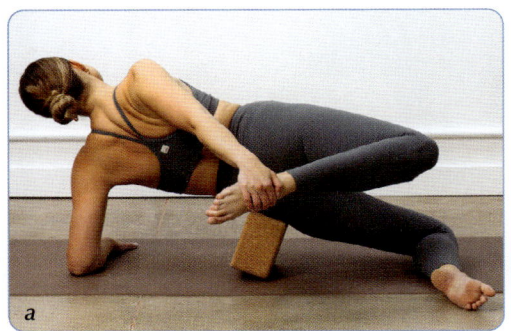

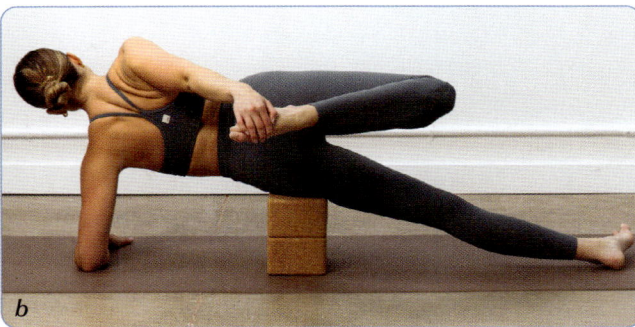

Wild Thing Pose

Chamatkarasana

चमत्कारासन

Wild thing pose is a dynamic yoga posture that opens the chest and lungs, stretches the front of the body and hips, and strengthens shoulders and back muscles. This energizing pose brings a vibrant boost to your practice. Explore prop-supported variations to enhance your experience and fully embrace the expansive benefits of wild thing pose.

Use a block or chair to take weight out of your wrists.

Placing a block or chair under your hand will take some of the weight from your arm and wrist, shifting weight toward the lower half of your body. This is great if you are still working up the strength for lateral weight-bearing or if you have wrist pain. Begin in a chair or block-supported side plank, then step your top foot back. Roll the barrel of your ribs and your hips up toward the sky. Reach your top arm overhead and switch your gaze toward that hand. Press into your bottom hand to create more space across your chest (see photo *a* for an example with the hand on blocks and photo *b* for an example with the hand on the chair seat). This variation can also be used in flip-dog, a slightly deeper version of wild thing, where you begin in a block- or chair-supported three-legged dog, rather than plank, bend the top knee, and step the foot behind you, rolling your chest up.

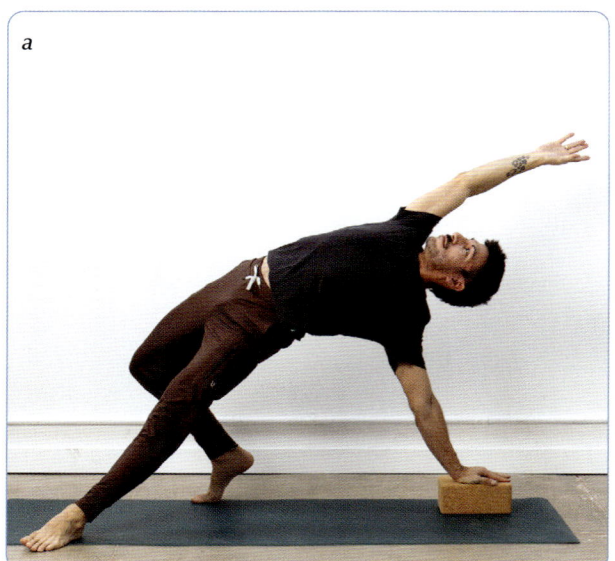

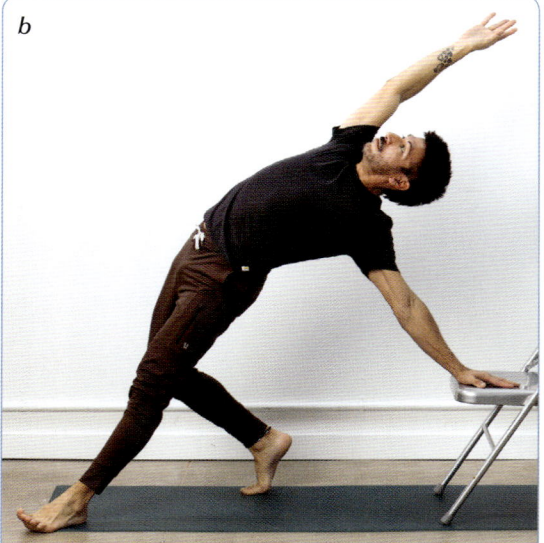

Place a block under the foot to raise the height of the floor.

Placing a block under your foot reduces the distance to the floor, which allows a gentler backbend. For this variation, try finding where your foot will land. A teacher can help place the block under your foot as you step back. This variation can also be used in flip-dog, where you begin in a block- or chair-supported three-legged dog, rather than a plank, bend the top knee and step the foot behind you, rolling your chest up.

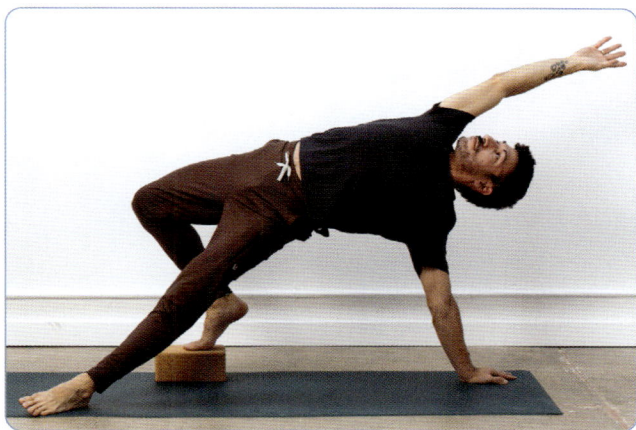

Sit on a chair for more stability.

This is a nice alternative for those who have difficulty getting up from and down to the floor and want more stability in the posture. Sit on the edge of a chair. Ensure the chair is on a grippy surface or against a wall so it does not slide. Bring your right hand behind you on the seat, with your fingertips pointing toward the back of the chair. Extend your right leg in front of you and bring your left heel to the leg of the chair, as shown in the photo. Press through your hand and your heel to lift your hips off the seat. Reach your left arm overhead and try to switch your gaze toward your hand if it does not strain your neck. When you are ready to come out of the posture, gently lower your hips to the seat and repeat on the other side.

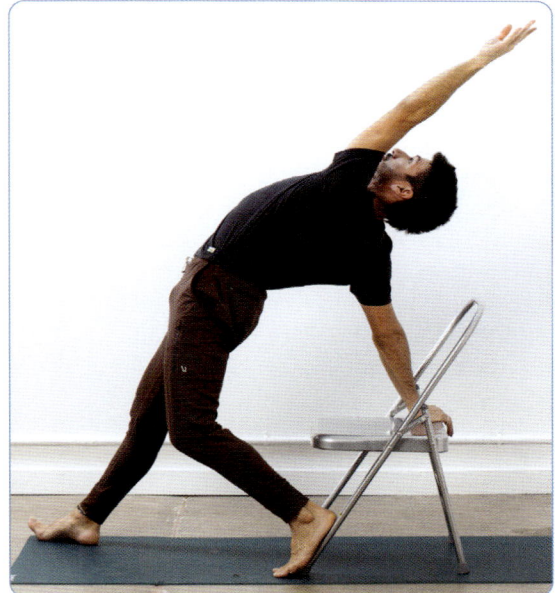

Upward Plank Pose

Purvottanasana

पूर्वोत्तानासन

Upward plank pose is a transformative yoga posture that tones the abdomen, chest, and back while strengthening the triceps, wrists, back, and legs. If you are still working toward upward-facing plank, consider trying these variations in reverse tabletop to build strength and mobility leading up to this posture. This pose also provides a deep stretch to the toes, ankles, and wrists. Explore prop-supported variations to enhance your experience and fully embrace the toning and stretching benefits.

Place blocks or a chair under your hands.

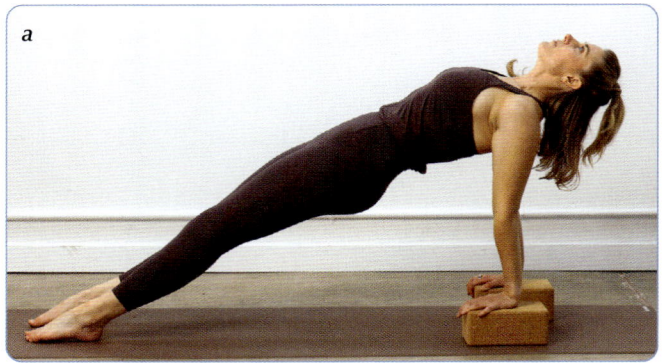

a

Raising the height of the ground will make it less difficult to lift through your hips because you have more space in your shoulders and chest and less gravity to counter because you are at a higher angle from the floor. This means the legs won't have to work as hard! It also makes for a less intense stretch through the ankles and shins. Finally, it will take some of the weight from your wrists, alleviating strain associated with wrist pain. In the first variation, sit with your legs extended in front of you. Place your hands on blocks behind you, shoulder-distance apart, pointing your fingertips toward your backside. Press into the block to lift through your hips. Feel the stretch across the front of your body (see photo a). For even more support and height, especially if you have difficulty getting up from and down to the floor, try a chair instead. Sit on the edge of a chair with your hands

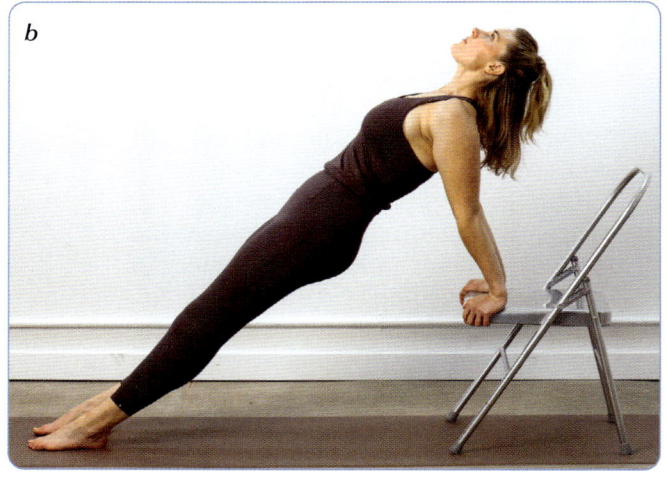

b

behind you on the seat, fingers pointing toward the back of your hips. If this flexion still causes wrist pain, hold the sides of the chair seat instead. Plant your feet in front of you, then extend your legs so that your heels are down and your toes are pointing straight up. On an inhale, press into the chair to lift your hips. Reach the soles of your feet down toward the floor (see photo b). If you want to take weight off your wrists completely, you can also practice standing with your hands face-down on the back of a chair behind you. Walk your feet away from the chair and puff up through your chest.

Place a block between your thighs.

Squeezing the block between your legs engages your thighs and relaxes the gluteal muscles to release tension in your lower back. Sit with your legs extended in front of you. Place a block, on its narrowest orientation, pointing up, between your thighs. Place your hands behind you, shoulder-width apart, fingers pointing toward your hips. Press your hands into the mat and straighten your arms as you squeeze the block. Lift your hips while squeezing the block and broaden through your chest. Press your feet to the mat. Turn your thighs in slightly,

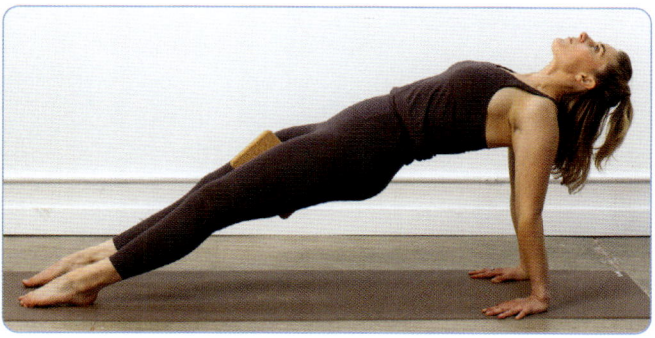

narrowing through your hip points. In reverse plank, it may be tempting to externally rotate your thighs, pushing the block up, which can strain your lower back. Instead, roll your inner thighs down just enough so the block remains in a neutral position between your thighs.

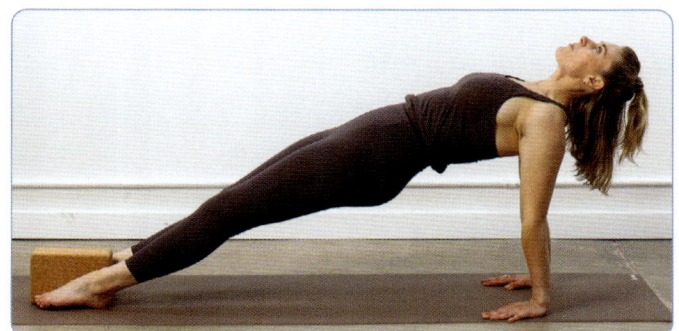

Place a block between your feet to align.

Just as with utilizing a block between your thighs, placing one between your feet can be a helpful tool to engage through your legs and find healthy leg and pelvic alignment. Place the block on its most narrow width, lengthwise between your heels. As you enter the posture, try to ground the inner edge of the big toes into the mat while squeezing the block. The challenge is not rolling to the outer edge of the feet, away from the block in the center.

Place a strap around your thighs to align.

Just as with utilizing a block between your thighs, looping a strap around your thighs will help enforce parallel leg alignment so you can redirect your focus to your breathing and opening through the chest. Having the legs tied together supports healthy leg and hip alignment by preventing external rotation of the thighs, which will also ease tension in the lumbar spine.

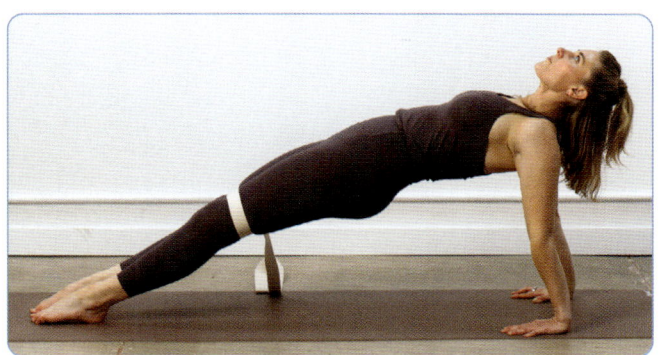

Upward Plank Pose (continued)

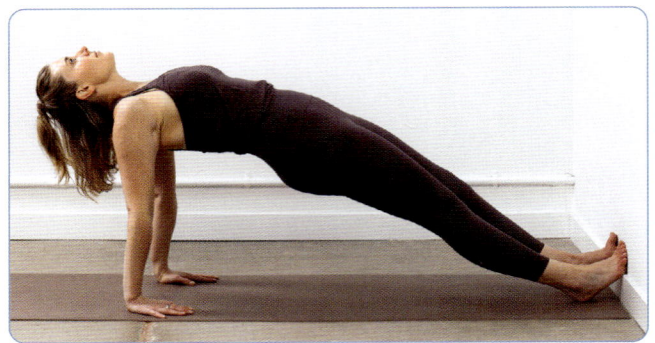

Place your feet against a wall to fire up your muscles and maintain alignment.

For this version, set up the same as in prior variations but bring your feet up against a wall in front of you. For your first attempt, bring the feet flat against the wall. When you lift into the posture, drive your heels straight down to engage through your posterior chain. Then adjust the starting position of your heels—starting back an inch or two (2.5-5 cm) and coming into the posture again. This time extend through your ankles and press into the wall with the balls of your feet. This will engage the muscles of the legs and build muscle memory, and it will also provide something for your feet to bear down on if they cannot reach the floor.

Practice a reverse elbow plank standing against a wall.

This variation is great for those who are still building strength and body intelligence as it relates to one's own body. This variation also diminishes the need to bear weight on the wrists or get up from and down on the floor. Stand with you back against a wall, aligning your head over your shoulders and hips. Walk your feet forward about six inches (15 cm) to a foot (30 cm) away from the wall, keeping the pelvis grounded. Bend at your elbows, creating a 90-degree angle, keeping the backs of the arms pressing into the wall and your palms facing one another. Drive the backs of the arms into the wall to peel the hips and ribs away from the wall. Keep the back of the head and neck grounded, lengthening through the neck. Engage through the muscles of the posterior chain, down the back of the body.

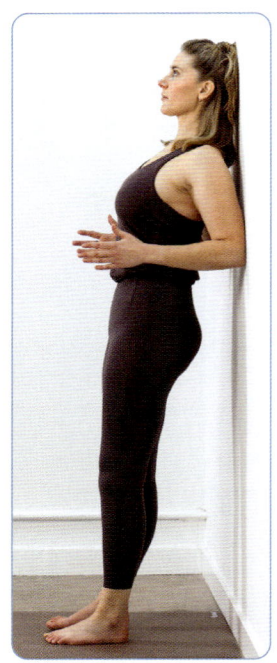

Chapter 6

Arm Balances

It always seems impossible until it's done.

Nelson Mandela

In this chapter, we explore various arm balance yoga postures, providing adaptable variations using props. There's a common saying about "standing on your own two feet," which implies self-sufficiency. But what happens when both feet are out of the equation? Embracing assistance from props isn't a sign of weakness; rather, it allows us to surpass previous limitations. Props sometimes introduce unexpected challenges into our practice. Within yoga, props serve a multifaceted role, enriching poses by enhancing challenge, relaxation, inclusivity, or deviation from traditional alignment. The key is to approach challenges with curiosity and from various angles. To establish a solid foundation for balance, we must dismantle mental and physical barriers through shifts in perspective and attitude. A pose isn't diminished by the use of props; rather, it flourishes in its various expressions. As you delve into this chapter, keep an open mind. Arm balances cultivate strength and determination while requiring focused, compassionate attention infused with a playful spirit. They challenge us to trust ourselves and confront fears methodically, rather than recklessly. With challenging arm balance postures, breath is a very useful tool—a guide for finding the balance between effort and ease. When the breath wanes, it is time to lessen the difficulty and consider experimenting with new props. When breath flows effortlessly and the mind remains calm, take your next step—whether on or off the ground. In addition to the arm balances found in this chapter, certain arm balances can be found in chapter 7, Inversions, due to the head being positioned lower than the heart.

Mantra: I embrace gratitude for the strength I possess and the hidden reservoirs of strength yet to be discovered.

Crow and Crane Pose

Kakasana and Bakasana   काकासन and बकासन

Crow pose and crane pose (the straight arm variation of this arm balance) are empowering yoga postures that actively strengthens the arms, wrists, and abdominals while providing a deep stretch to the upper back. These poses also contribute to toning the chest. Explore prop-supported variations to enhance your experience and fully embrace the strengthening and stretching benefits of crow and crane pose.

Place blocks under your feet to practice shifting your weight forward in crow pose.

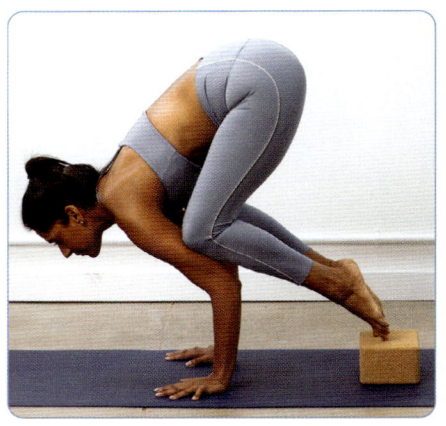

Using a block will help you be more comfortable shifting your weight forward. With the added height, you can enter crow pose without lifting your feet off the floor. Start in a forward fold with your hands on the mat, shoulder-width apart, and your feet on a block on its lowest height and your big toes touching. Bend your knees enough to get your hands firmly planted on the mat in front of you and bring the knees as high up on the back of the arms as possible, toward your armpits. Bend your elbows straight back toward your shins and shift your weight forward, keeping the gaze ahead in the direction you are shifting. Shift your elbows to stack directly over the wrists, coming onto the balls of your feet. Press your hands firmly into the mat, protracting through your shoulders. If you feel up to it, you can eventually try lifting one or both feet from the block. If both feet are lifted, fire up through the backs of the thighs (hamstrings) to try to get the heels as close to the buttocks as possible.

Place a block in front of you to direct your gaze in either crow or crane pose.

I think one of the most challenging things to remember in this pose is to keep the gaze in front of you. As in driving a car, keep your gaze on the horizon in the direction you are heading. (If you were to gaze at your feet or behind you while driving, you wouldn't be very successful!) Your weight will shift where your gaze goes, so place an object such as a block slightly in front of you to remember where to look while shifting forward into the

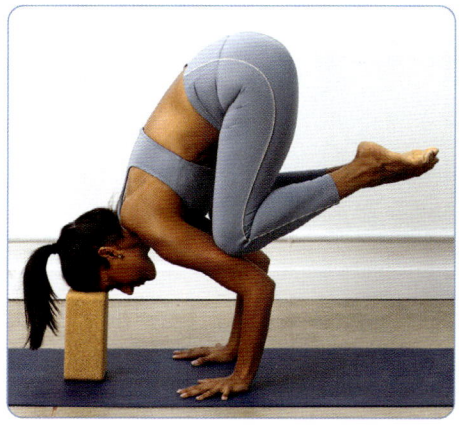

arm balance. If you gaze down or back at your feet, you likely will have trouble shifting forward enough to stack your elbows over your wrists.

Place a block under your forehead for stability and to conquer fear in crow pose.

Using a block will help you to get more comfortable with shifting your weight forward, eliminating the fear of falling forward onto your face; you can have the block against a wall as well, for reassurance. Set up for crow pose with your feet parallel on the mat. Place a block on its tallest height about one foot (0.3 m) in front of the hands (a good measure is the distance from your head to your elbows in chaturanga). Enter crow pose, shifting your weight forward, keeping your gaze on the block. Keep shifting forward until your forehead meets the block. Your elbows should be directly above the wrists and your forearms perpendicular to the mat. Start with your knees close to your elbows to counterbalance your weight for this variation, because the shoulders will need to shift farther forward, like the arms do in chaturanga. This way, the weight is more evenly distributed into the wrists rather than loading into the shoulders and upper arms.

Place blocks under your shoulders for stability in crow pose.

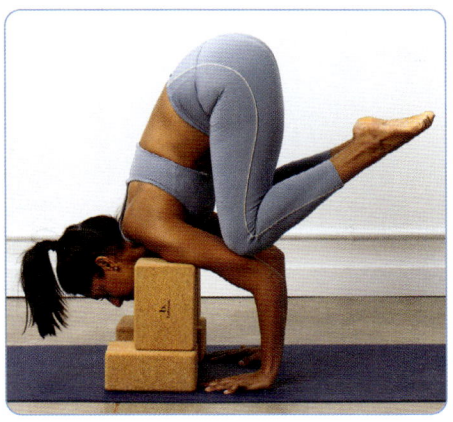

Using blocks helps you to get more comfortable with shifting weight forward, eliminating the fear of falling forward onto your face. This version allows the shoulders to be slightly higher than the elbows—more than in the version with the block under your forehead. Set up for crow pose but with two blocks on the lowest height in front of the hands and two more blocks stacked on top of them, as shown in the photo. Enter the arm balance, shifting your weight forward and keeping your gaze forward and down. Keep shifting forward until your shoulders come to rest on top of the blocks, adjusting the height of the blocks if needed. Your elbows should be directly above the wrists so that forearms are perpendicular to the mat. Keep firmly pressing through the hands as if you were going to lift the shoulders off the blocks to hover.

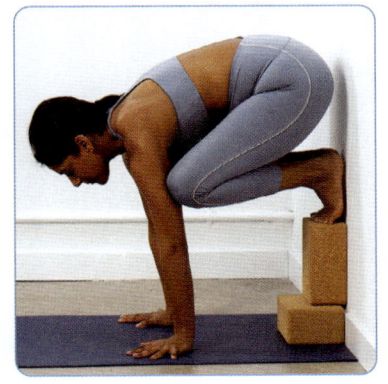

Practice using a wall and blocks to shift into crane pose.

This prop-supported take on crane pose creates the feeling of crane with support. It aids in taking strain out of the wrists when moving from bent to straight elbows by starting with straight elbows. It also increases wrist strength and mobility needed for crane without the help of the blocks and wall. Start by placing two blocks against a wall, the bottom being on the lowest height and the top turned to the tallest height. You can also stack three blocks on the lowest height if you have them. Face away from the wall and place your hands, shoulder-width apart, on the floor in front of you (about a foot [0.3 m] in front of the blocks but adjust as needed) and walk the toes up onto the top block. Walk the hands back until the knees contact the backs of the upper arms. Try to press the tops of your thighs up into the torso and protract through the shoulders, rounding the upper back up. Press into the tiptoes, shifting the weight forward just enough to feel the shoulders pass the wrists. Try lifting one or both feet toward the buttocks.

Place a bolster in front of you for a softer fall.

It is good to practice falling out of poses, just as it is good to practice coming in and out of them. The more control over the situation you have, the more confidence you will have. Practice falling by bringing your knees out to the sides and your shins on the mat. Sometimes it doesn't go as planned, though, and the cushioned surface of a bolster in front of your face can add comfort to unexpected dismounts!

Place a strap around your arms to strengthen alignment in crow and crane pose.

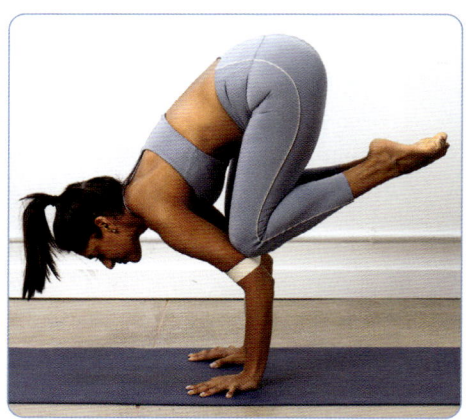

Using a strap in either arm balance pose is helpful for guiding the positioning of your elbows and shoulders. The strap will help you to avoid splaying your elbows and losing stability, and it will help prevent unnecessary strain on the rotator cuff. To avoid pinching your skin with the strap, position the strap away from your knees. Just above the elbows works well, because the knees will be higher up on the arms. Adjust according to your own needs, though! As you enter your arm balance, press the arms out into the strap. If you measured correctly, the strap will not allow the elbows to splay. When you press into the strap, it reinforces actions in other parts of the body, such as the force of your hands into the floor and protraction of the shoulders, gliding your scapula around your ribs. Alternatively, if you want to strengthen the feeling of hugging your elbows in and keeping the arms parallel to one another, use the strap as a guide rather than something to press into. Try to keep the strap free of tension, like you are pulling away from the strap rather than leaning into it.

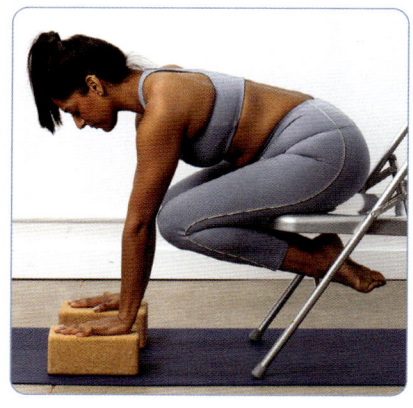

Practice seated on a chair, with your hands on blocks in front of you to prep for either arm balance.

Try taking flight on a chair! A chair is a great tool for those who require more stability and grounding as well as those who need to limit weight-bearing on the wrists. Sit on the front edge of a chair and place two blocks about a foot (0.3 m) in front of you on the lowest height needed. Lean forward, place your hands on the blocks, and press your arms in front of or just inside your knees. Lift your feet and move them back underneath the chair, squeezing your hamstrings. Point through your feet and try to bring the big toes to touch. Gently hug through your inner thighs and puff up through your upper back. Over time, try rocking your weight forward, pressing down through your hands, and lifting your seat to hover over the chair.

Practice with your shins on a chair for support to prep for these arm balances.

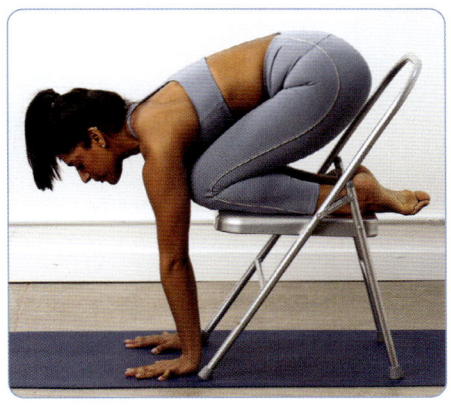

The chair offers support in several ways, such as supporting those who want to work on the muscle actions of the posture without too much weight on the wrists, and those who want to lessen the body weight-bearing on the backs of their triceps. Kneel on a chair, facing away from the back of the chair. Your chair should preferably be backless or have a hole in the back for your feet to slide through. You may need a folded blanket or mat under the shins for cushioning. Imagine you were in child's pose, bringing your big toes to touch and folding over your thighs, with your knees slightly forward off the chair seat. Hold the sides or legs of the chair for support as you enter this pose. Place your hands, one at a time, shoulder-width apart, on the floor or on blocks in front of you. Press your hands into the floor or blocks and hug your knees toward the back of your arms—it is OK if they do not contact the arms. You may eventually try alternating lifting the shins off the chair, at first one at a time and eventually both shins!

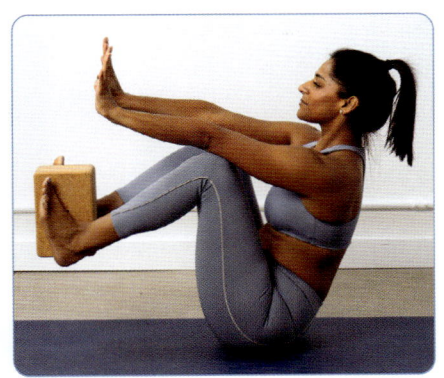

Practice hugging a block between your feet while seated to prep for these arm balances.

This is a great core challenge and a wonderful alternative if weight-bearing on your wrists is not an option. It is also a great way to build strength until you feel confident to take flight! Sit on your mat with your feet planted on the floor in front of you, knees pointing up toward the sky. Place a block on its narrowest width between your feet and hug the block, engaging through your adductors. Start with a foam block if the cork block is too heavy. Reach your arms out in front of you, shoulder-width apart, and flex through your hands. Imagine you are pushing into an invisible wall in front of you. As you push, draw your navel into your spine and gently protract through your shoulders (think about cat pose in your upper back). Continue to squeeze the block between your feet and try to lift your knees toward your upper arms or armpits! Bend your knees and attempt to hug the block in.

Baby Crow Pose

Bala Kakasana

बाला काकासन

Baby crow pose is a challenging pose, despite the cute name. In this pose, you actively strengthen the arms, wrists, and abdominal muscles while experiencing a deep stretch in the upper back. This pose also contributes to toning the chest. Explore prop-supported variations to enhance your practice.

Practice with blocks under your forearms to bring your head farther away from the floor.

Baby crow pose is deceptively harder than crow pose because your center of gravity is so close to the floor. Using blocks can help move you a little bit farther away from the floor as you are learning, giving your head and neck more room if necessary. The front edges of the blocks also give you something to grip. This helps you to ground through your forearms, palms, and fingertips. Begin in garland pose with blocks lengthwise and shoulder-width apart in front of you, on the lowest height. Bring your forearms down to

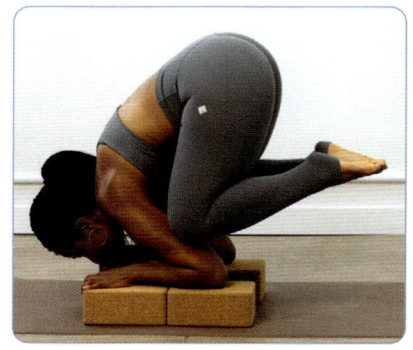

the blocks by shifting your body weight forward and lifting your heels off the mat. Place another set of blocks behind your elbows if this is uncomfortable. Bring your knees into your upper arms as close to your armpits as you can. Shift your weight forward, gazing toward your fingertips. Lift one foot at a time off the mat, squeezing your heels in toward your buttocks. Expand across your upper back and press down through your forearms. Hug your elbows in, resisting splaying them. Draw your abdominal wall in and up to help support the weight of the body in the arm balance.

Practice with blocks or a bolster under your chest to support chest elevation.

It is not hard to feel the weight of gravity pulling on you in this arm balance, so until you work up the strength to resist it, use props for support! If you are using blocks, place them side by side on the medium height and place your forearms alongside them. As you enter the posture, allow your chest to rest on the blocks, preventing collapse toward your hands. There should be enough room for your head and neck in front of the blocks. Hug your forearms into the blocks to counteract elbows splaying. Once in position, press down into the outer edge of your elbows and inner edges of your wrists and try to hover with your chest off the blocks (see photo a). You can also practice with a bolster, which offers more cushion and gives your feet something to step onto. In this variation, ensure there is still room for your

head and neck in front of the bolster. Begin in garland pose, with your feet framing the bolster, then bring your forearms down to frame it in front of you. Bring your knees high up

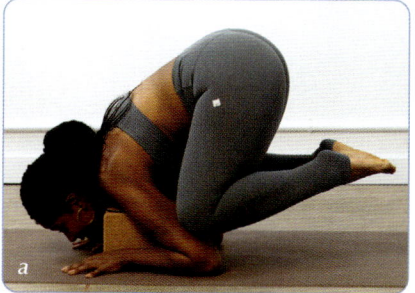

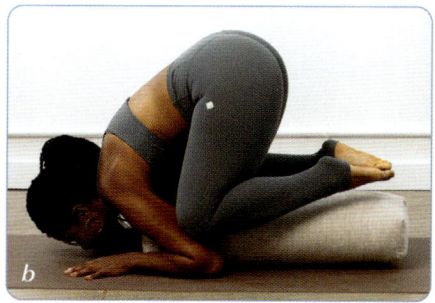

into the back of your armpits. Shift your weight forward, resting your chest on the bolster, then step your feet onto the bolster behind you, big toes touching. Try to lift your feet, chest, or both off the bolster (see photo *b*).

Practice with a block under your feet to build muscle memory of lifting the feet.

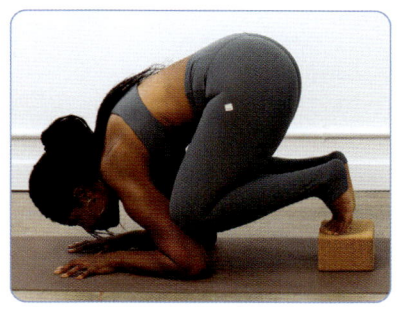

This works like the example with the bolster but without the support of a prop underneath your chest. This means more weight-bearing in the upper body, so be ready to fire up through your arms, shoulders, chest, and deep core muscles! Enter the posture as usual but leave a block on the lowest height between your feet as you shift your weight forward. When you are ready to lift your feet, bring them together at the top of the block. To increase the challenge, turn the block to medium height (or stack two blocks for added height with more stability). This will bring your heels closer to your buttocks, making the hamstrings contract a little more! Try lifting your feet off the blocks altogether—first alternating, then work your way up to lifting both heels toward your gluteal muscles to hover.

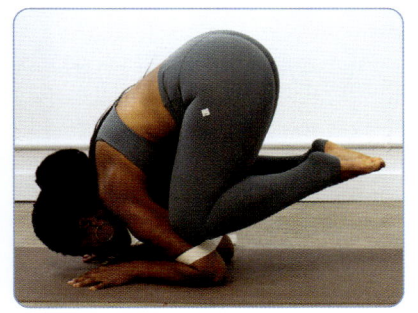

Practice with a strap to strengthen alignment.

Using a strap in crow pose helps in guiding the positioning of the elbows and shoulders. It has the same effect as in your baby crow pose. Sometimes the elbows will want to splay, which can make finding your balance more challenging and bring you closer to the floor, which may already be uncomfortably close. For detailed strap instructions, refer to crow pose in this chapter.

Flying Pigeon Pose

Eka Pada Galavasana   एकपाद गलवासन

Flying pigeon pose is an advanced yoga posture that brings a combination of stretching and strengthening benefits. This pose actively stretches the hips and legs while simultaneously strengthening the shoulders, wrists, arms, core, and chest. Explore prop-supported variations to enhance your experience and fully embrace the expansive benefits of flying pigeon pose.

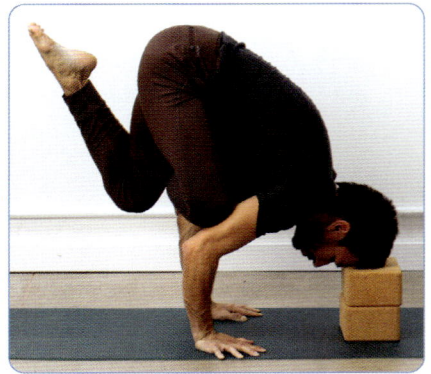

Practice with blocks under your head for balance and support.

Being supported by blocks helps minimize the fear of falling as you become more comfortable with shifting your weight forward. You can place the blocks against a wall if needed. Stand a block placed a foot or two (0.3-0.6 m) in front of you, in its tallest position or stacked on a second block. Transfer your weight to your left foot and lift your right knee toward your chest, bringing your right foot to your left thigh in the shape of a figure four. Move your hips down and back as if you were sitting on a chair. Bring your palms together at your chest, lean forward, and place your hands on the mat, shoulder-width apart. Adjust the block's position if necessary. Bend your elbows and shift your weight forward onto your hands, creating a platform for your right shin with your upper arms. Flex your right foot and wrap your toes around your left arm, placing right knee as high as possible on your right arm. As you lean forward, position your forehead on the block, lifting your back toes off the mat and drawing your left heel toward your buttocks. Try to distribute your weight evenly between your hands, avoiding placing too much pressure on the block. Try pushing into your hands to lift your forehead off the block, hover, and then lower yourself. Also try extending your left leg straight behind you, reaching from the crown of your head through the ball of your left foot. Repeat on the other side.

Place blocks under your hands to bring the floor closer to you.

Getting your hands flat on the floor in flying pigeon pose can be challenging, especially if you have tight hips and hamstrings. Using blocks under your hands is a helpful variation that can assist in achieving the pose. As you bend forward to place your hands down, the blocks will reduce the distance between you and the floor.

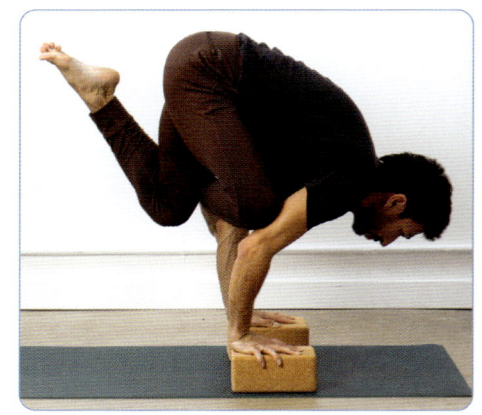

Place your back foot or shin down on a block to prepare for flight.

These are two great options if you are struggling to take flight, or if you want a stepping stone to help build up to extending your back leg. The first variation gives the back foot a little height, helping you to shift your weight forward and stack your elbows over your wrists. The tricky part is deciding which way you want to get into this. You could either start by standing on the block, requiring more balance and flexibility to start, or by hopping your back foot onto the block once your hands have contacted the floor. In this second variation, place a block on its tallest height just in front of your standing leg toes (a cork block is sturdier in nature). As you shift your weight forward into your hands, shift your standing leg shin onto the block and lift your back foot off the mat. Try hovering the leg over the block by pressing down with your hands and hugging your knee to your chest, engaging the psoas (hip flexor). Simultaneously try to squeeze your back heel toward your buttock to fire up your hamstrings (see photo *a* for an example with the back foot on a block and photo *b* for an example of the back shin on a block). Eventually, as hovering becomes more accessible, try extending the back leg fully.

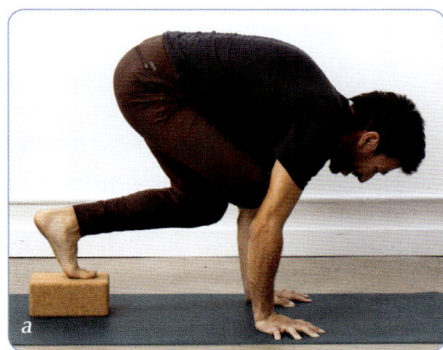 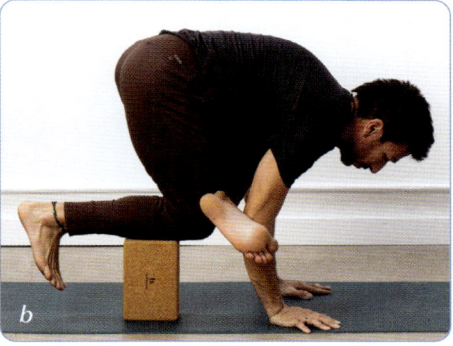

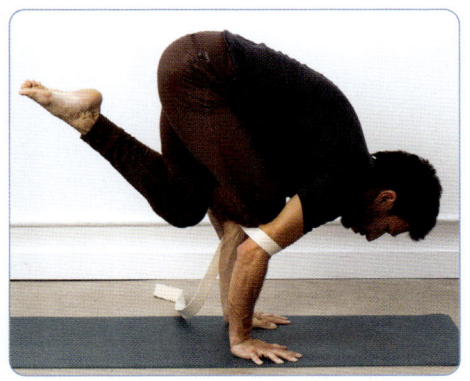

Loop a strap around your arms to align and engage.

Looping a strap around your arms can be a useful technique for improving arm balances such as this, because it helps to engage and stabilize the muscles in the upper body. By drawing the arms toward each other using the strap, you create a strong foundation and a sense of connection between the arms, shoulders, and core. This stability allows you to better control your balance and weight distribution, making it easier to hold challenging arm balances. The strap also provides a physical cue that helps to properly align the arms, preventing them from splaying or collapsing inward. This alignment is crucial for maintaining proper form and preventing injury. Additionally, using a strap in arm balances can provide extra support and confidence for those who may be hesitant or fearful of falling. Because the strap provides more stability, you can feel more secure and confident in your practice, allowing you to explore and deepen into the posture with greater ease and comfort.

Flying Pigeon Pose *(continued)*

Use a wall to support the transition of lifting your back foot off the floor.

If you're having trouble lifting your bottom foot off the floor in flying pigeon pose, using a wall can be a helpful variation. Set up the pose as usual but with your back to the wall. Sit back in chair pose, ensuring that your butt is close enough to the wall to almost touch it. You may need to adjust your distance from the wall depending on your weight distribution. Begin to transition into the pose and when it comes time to lift your back foot, place the ball of your foot on the wall at hip height. You can keep your foot

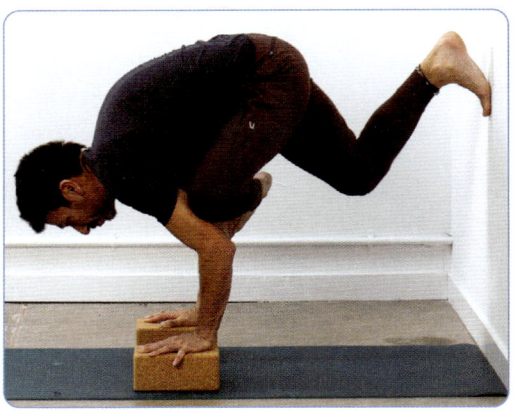

on the wall or try shifting your weight forward to lift your toes away from the wall. Once you feel comfortable, try practicing farther away from the wall and extend your leg behind you, placing your foot on the wall. This variation is particularly useful if you struggle to hold the pose with your leg extended, even if you can lift your bottom foot off the floor.

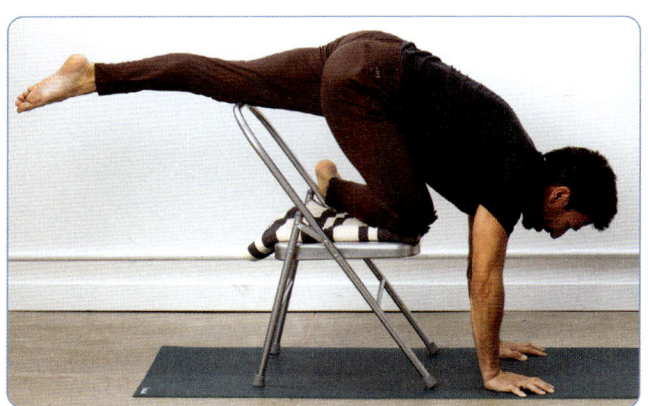

Use a chair to minimize weight-bearing on your wrists and to build muscle memory.

To decrease the weight-bearing load on your wrists and build muscle memory, you can practice flying pigeon pose on a chair. Place a folded mat or blanket on the seat of the chair to cushion your shin. Stand to the side of the chair with your back facing the back of the chair, then lift the leg closest to the chair as if you were going into tree pose. Slide your shin on the chair as shown in the photo, then fold forward and walk your hands in front of the chair. If needed, you can use blocks under your hands to bring the floor closer to you. Once your hands and shin are firmly grounded, lift your back leg behind you over the top of the chair. You can choose to rest your back leg on the chair or lift it to hover. Focus on stacking your shoulders over your wrists and pressing down through the shin of your bent leg to take weight from your arms and wrists. This variation allows you to modify the pose while still building strength and muscle memory.

Shoulder-Pressing Pose

Bhujapidasana

भुजपीडासन

Shoulder-pressing pose is a dynamic yoga posture that actively strengthens the shoulders, arms, and wrists while toning the abdomen. This pose also engages and strengthens the adductor muscles of the inner thighs. Explore prop-supported variations to enhance your practice.

Practice with blocks under your hands to bring the floor closer to you.

By placing blocks beneath your hands, you reduce the distance between you and the floor and make it easier to lift your thighs higher on your arms. This can be a challenging pose, particularly if your hamstrings are tight. Using blocks can also assist you in lifting your feet off

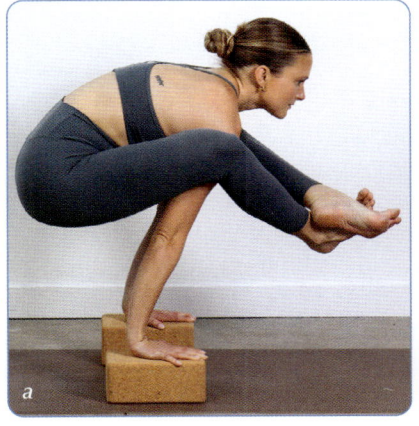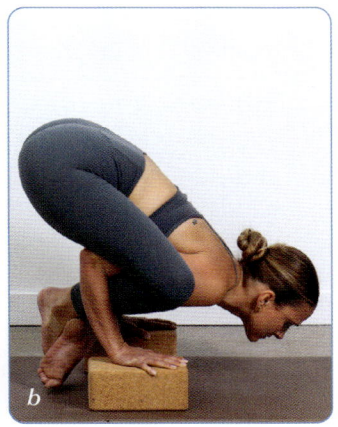

the floor and shifting weight back into your hands. Assume a wide-legged squat stance and position two blocks behind your heels. Lift your hips while keeping your knees bent and bring your chest toward your thighs. With your right hand, grasp the back of your right ankle and move your right shoulder as close to the back of your right knee as you can. Repeat on the opposite side. Bring your feet closer together so that your inner thighs are snug against your sides. Place your hands on the blocks with your fingers pointing forward and bend your elbows. Press your hips against your upper arms and hug your inner thighs toward your body. Move your feet closer until they lift off the floor and hook one ankle over the other. Straighten your elbows by pushing your hands into the blocks (see photo a). Look ahead. Try bending your elbows and squeezing your heels toward your seat while bringing your chin toward the mat (see photo b). Have a bolster or folded blankets nearby for added comfort and peace of mind.

Use blocks to raise the height of the floor in elephant trunk variation.

Elephant trunk pose (eka hasta bhujasana) is similar to shoulder-pressing pose but involves extending one leg in front, making finding your center of gravity and lifting off the floor more challenging. Using blocks to increase the distance of the hips from the floor makes it easier to lift the extended leg, reducing the effort required for air time compared to being closer to the floor, which engages various muscle groups such as hip flexors, abdominal muscles, quadriceps, and shoulder protractors more intensely. To begin, assume a wide-legged squat stance and position two blocks behind you, one behind your right heel and the other behind and between your feet. Fold forward,

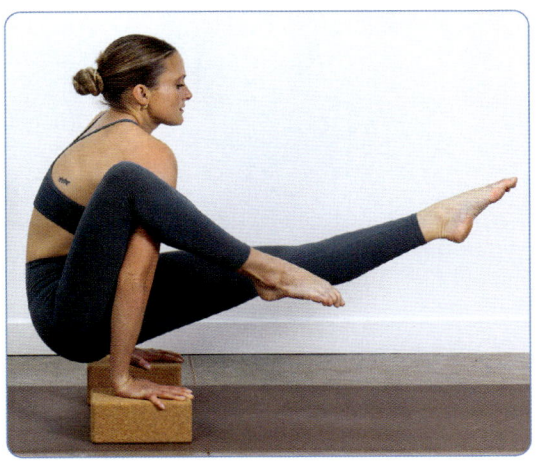

hinging at your hips, and bring your hands to frame your right foot. With your right hand, grab your right ankle and shift your right shoulder only behind the right knee, replacing the right hand outside the foot. Move your feet a little closer together by toe-heeling and place your hands on the blocks behind you. Sit back on your right arm, hugging your right thigh into the upper arm. Extend your left leg between your hands. Aim to lift your left heel off the floor. Repeat these steps on the other side.

Support your hips using a chair and blocks.

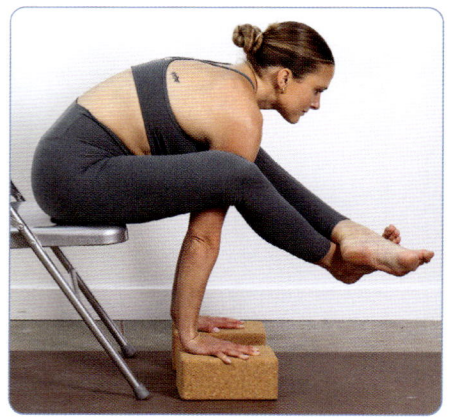

By using a chair for support, you can focus on engaging your legs without worrying about balancing on your hands or placing too much weight on your shoulders and wrists. To practice shoulder-pressing pose using a chair, sit on a chair with your feet flat on the floor and your feet outside of two blocks placed horizontally in front of the chair legs. Lean forward and place your hands, fingertips pointing forward, on the blocks (or the floor if you can reach). Next, slide your arms under your thighs so that your inner knees come high up on your upper arms. You can help with this action by grabbing the backs of your ankles and shimmying your arms under before placing your hands back on the blocks. Then, bend your elbows and squeeze your legs into your arms and your arms into your legs. Move your feet closer together. Push into your blocks or the floor, straighten your arms, and widen your upper back (shoulder protraction). Slide your hips back in the chair and cross your ankles.

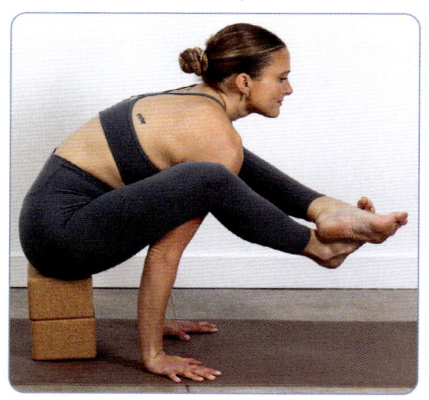

Support your hips on blocks.

This is another great variation to reduce weight-bearing on your wrists or for building the strength to shift your weight into your hands. It also provides peace of mind if you are worried about falling back on your bum! To begin, assume a wide-legged squat stance and position two or three blocks behind you, stacked on their lowest height. To have a better understanding of where the blocks should be positioned, sit back as if you were going into garland pose. The blocks should intersect your sitting bones on your way down. Enter the pose, similar to what was described in the blocks under hands variation (the first variation of shoulder-pressing pose), noting that as you place your hands on the floor behind you, it is OK if your full hand is not on the floor—once you sit back, your weight will shift back into your hands simultaneously. Note that once your hands are placed, bring your feet closer together so that your inner thighs are snug against your sides. Sit your hips back toward the blocks and hug your thighs toward your body. Once the sitting bones are grounded on the blocks, move your feet closer until they lift off the floor and hook one ankle over the other. Try bending your elbows and shifting your weight forward, as if your arms were mimicking shifting into chaturanga and perhaps raising the hips off the blocks. The blocks will be there for you when you need to lower.

Firefly Pose

Tittibhasana   टिट्टिभासन

Firefly pose is a dynamic yoga posture that brings a unique combination of stretching and strengthening benefits. This pose actively stretches the inner groin, back of the torso, and hamstrings while toning the abdomen, wrists, and arms. Firefly pose also engages and strengthens the adductor muscles of the inner thighs. Let's explore prop-supported variations to diversify your practice.

Practice with blocks under your hands.

Blocks can be helpful for those working on their arm balances because they can bring the floor closer to the hands which helps alleviate pressure on the wrists. Blocks are useful for those with tight hamstrings because they assist in getting the inner thighs higher up on the arms. Blocks can also make it easier to lift the feet off the mat, which can be beneficial for those who are not quite ready to straighten their arms. Overall, incorporating blocks into your firefly pose practice can aid in building strength and confidence. To begin, assume the shoulder-pressing pose with your hands on blocks, described earlier. Extend your elbows and tense your chest muscles to create more space between your shoulder blades. Strive to lift your inner thighs onto the backs of your arms as far as possible. As you straighten your legs, maintain pressure on your inner thighs toward your body. When your arms are straight, try to lower your hips, elevate your heart, and look ahead (see photo a). You can also try moving your legs parallel to the mat (see photo b) or bending your elbows, working on your bent-arm strength (see photo c).

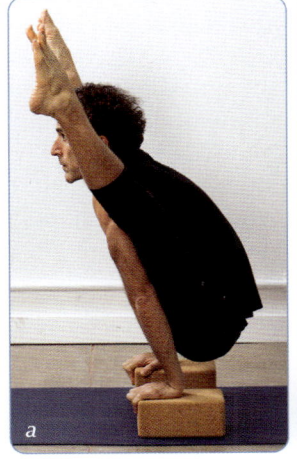
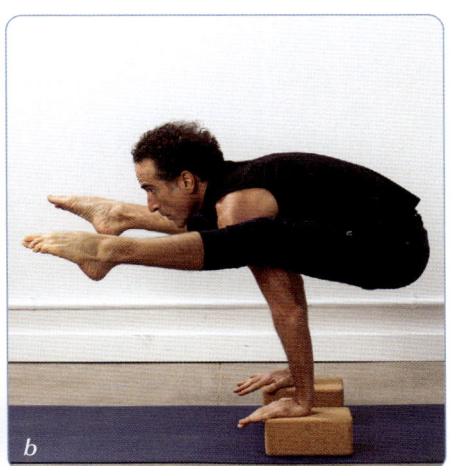
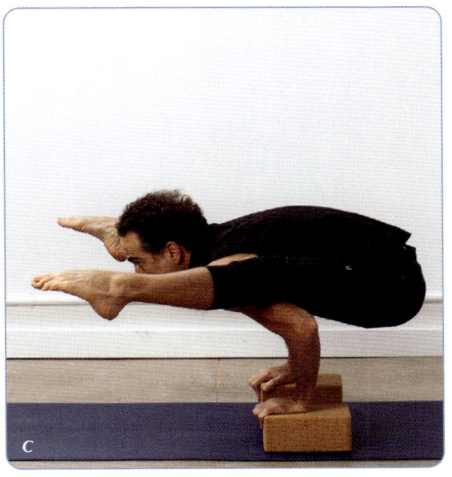

Support your hips using a chair or by stacking blocks.

Using a chair or blocks to support your yoga practice is an excellent way to modify poses, especially for beginners or those needing extra support. This approach is beneficial for building strength and flexibility while fostering confidence in challenging poses like firefly pose. By incorporating a chair, you can focus on engaging your legs without balancing on your hands or placing excessive weight on your shoulders and wrists. To practice firefly pose with a chair, sit on it with feet outside two horizontally placed blocks placed in front of the chair legs. Lean forward, placing your hands on the blocks or floor, and walk your feet in front of the blocks to slide your arms under your thighs. Try to get your knees high up onto your upper arms. Straighten your arms, engage the core, and lift your feet off the floor, extending through your legs. As you do, squeeze your inner thighs into your upper arms (see photo a). Keep your gaze forward. You can also use blocks to support your hips during this pose. To do this, assume a wide-legged squat stance and position two or three blocks behind you, stacked on their lowest height. Lift your hips while keeping your knees bent and bring your chest toward your thighs. Grab behind your ankles to shimmy your arms and shoulders as close to the back of your knees as you can. Place your hands on the floor behind your ankles with your fingers pointing forward and bend your elbows. Bring your feet closer together so that your inner thighs are snug against your sides. Sit your hips back toward the blocks, shifting more weight into your hands, and hug your inner thighs toward your body. Once the sitting bones are grounded, move your feet closer until they lift off the floor and extend through your legs, lengthening your hamstrings (see photo b). Try shifting your weight forward to raise the hips off the block. The blocks will be there for you when you need to lower.

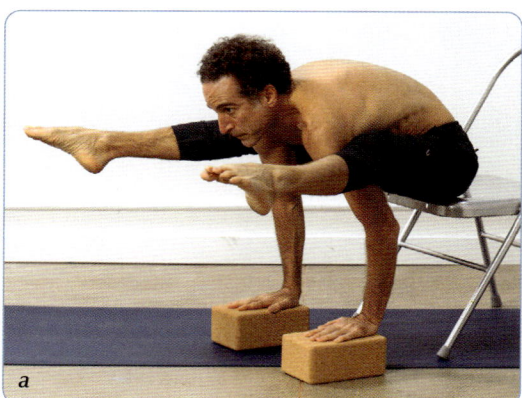
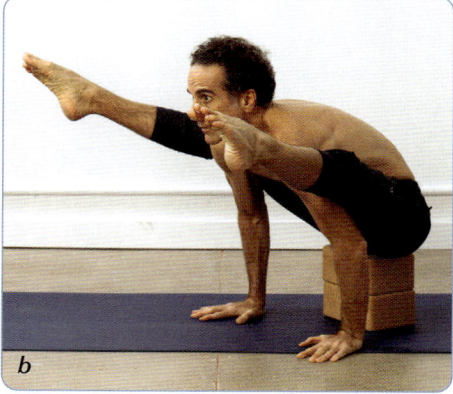

Practice with your hands on blocks, a bolster behind the lower back against a wall, and your feet on two chairs.

To set up, you will need a mat against a wall, with a bolster standing tall on it against the wall. You will also need two blocks, about shoulder-width apart in front of the bolster. Place two chairs in front of you angled slightly beyond your shoulders. Practice on a hard surface so that the chairs can slide as you shift into the pose and put towels under the chair legs if needed for sliding. Enter a squat, placing your hands behind your feet on the blocks and wiggling your shoulders as far under your knees as you can manage comfortably. Sit your hips back until your sitting bones contact the bolster. Walk your

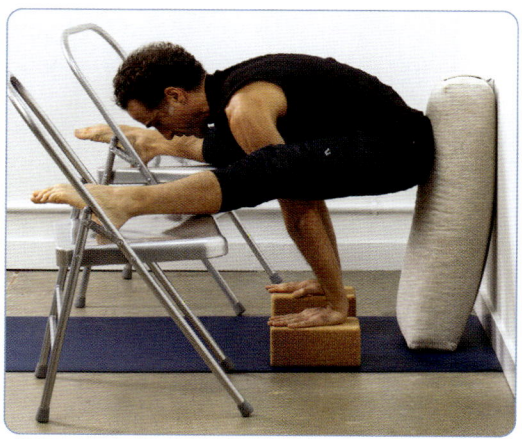

feet onto the chairs. If your chair has a back bar between the legs of the chair, step onto that first, then bring your heels to the top of the seat, one at a time. Now it's action time! Slowly straighten your arms, pressing your hands into the blocks and lifting through your hips, sliding them up the bolster. As you do this, straighten through your legs, pressing the chairs forward.

Practice with a strap around your feet.

A strap is a great tool for engaging both the inner and outer thighs in this pose! It also helps to prevent your legs from sliding farther down your arms. Stand at the top of your mat with your feet mat-distance apart. Place a yoga strap around your ankles and make sure it's a little wider than the distance between your feet. Bend your knees and squat, bringing your palms to the floor behind your feet. Keep your feet firmly planted. Lift your hips and shimmy your shoulders further behind your legs, then squat again. Press your outer ankles into the strap to extend through the legs and lift the feet off the floor. As you continue this motion, straighten through your arms, lowering your hips closer toward your wrists. With the strap around your ankles, press your ankles into the strap and draw your thighs toward

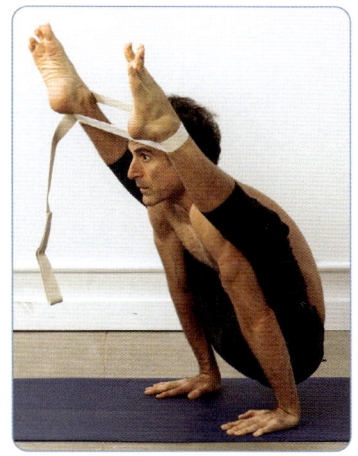

each other. This will help you engage your inner thighs and create stability in the pose. Lift through your chest, finding length in your spine. Keep your gaze forward and avoid rounding your shoulders.

Practice with a strap around your full body.

This is a great aid for learning to lower your hips toward the back of your wrists and for learning to press up into a handstand eventually! To begin, measure the loop of your strap to be the length from about your ankle to your hip point. Not every body is the same, so adjust the loop if necessary once you come into the pose. Loop the strap around your thighs just above your knees, then grab hold of both sides of the loop with your hands and pull them forward so that you have to walk your feet closer together to squatting distance. Sit back and pull the straps over your head. One strap side should go over the shoulders and the other should slide down

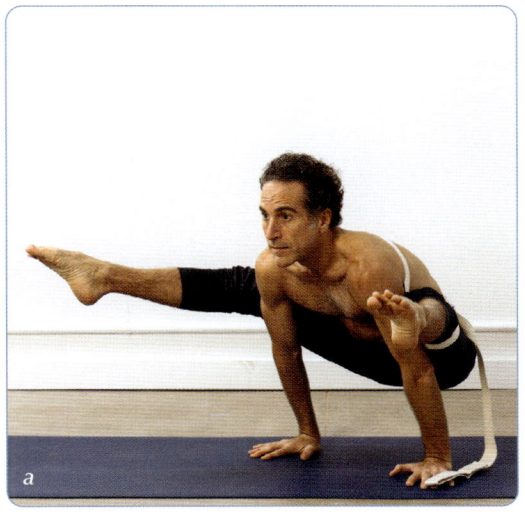

behind the lower back, just above the hips. Walk your hands behind your feet and enter the pose. The strap will hold the legs up as you lift your feet off the floor. Practice lowering the hips; the strap will help to pull the legs back and keep them from sliding (see photo a). If you are working toward lifting your hips into the handstand, try pressing your thighs

Firefly Pose *(continued)*

into the strap while simultaneously pushing your hamstrings down into the strap (see photos *b* and *c*). This will cause your hips to lift, and the strap support across your back will help reinforce lengthening through your spine. Press down into the floor with all your arm and shoulder strength!

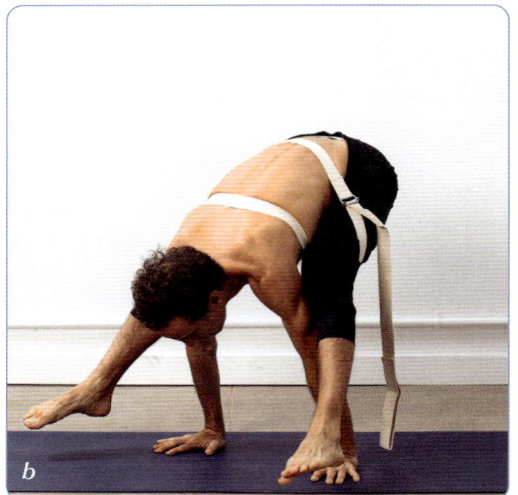

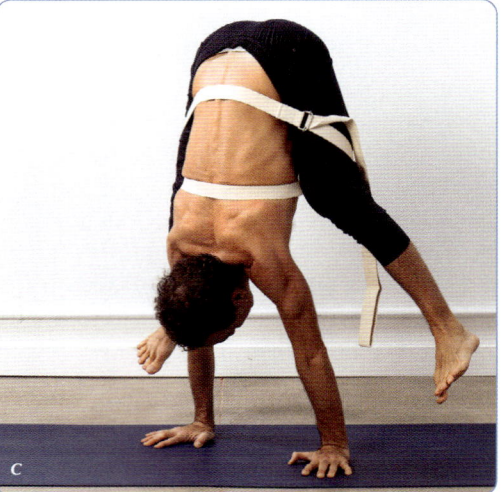

The Complete Guide to Yoga Props

Pendant Pose

Lolasana   लोलासन

Pendant pose is a dynamic yoga posture that actively strengthens the wrists and arms while toning the psoas and abdomen. This pose also provides a deep stretch to the upper back. Explore prop-supported variations to enhance your experience and fully embrace the strengthening and stretching benefits of pendant pose.

Practice with blocks under your hands to support elevation.

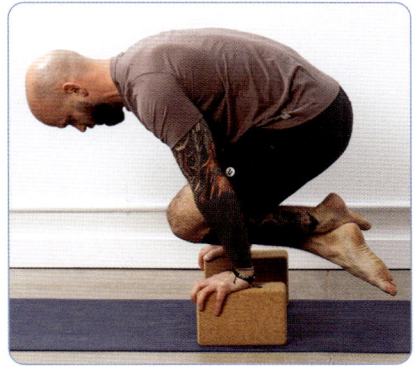

This posture involves the use of blocks to create more space between the torso and the floor, which, in turn, makes it easier to lift the feet off the floor. Start in a forward fold with your hands on blocks placed shoulder-distance apart and just in front of the feet. Bring your feet together to touch and find a toe squat, bending your knees into the chest and sitting on the heels. Allow the upper back to round over the thighs. Shift your weight forward into the hands and press into the blocks while straightening the arms. Hollow through the chest and protract (round) through the shoulders. Keeping the thighs and knees together, bring the left heel toward the right sitting bone and then lift the right heel toward the left sitting bone, crossing the ankles and shins. Once the feet are lifted off the mat, try to draw the tops of the thighs closer to the torso by engaging the psoas. Contract through the backs of the thighs and calf, working the heels closer to the sitting bones. Repeat by crossing the ankles the opposite way.

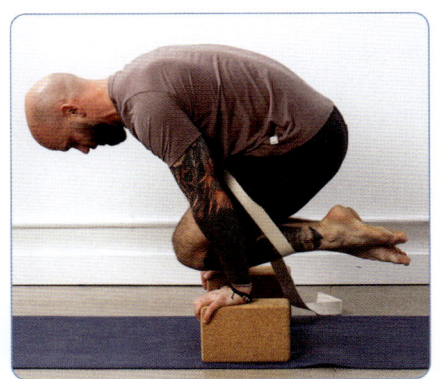

Feel lighter with the help of a strap.

You can use a strap to bind the upper and lower legs together to create a unit that allows you to lift yourself into pendant pose with greater ease and a stronger connection to the core. Sit on your heels in thunderbolt pose (vajrasana) with your knees together. Add a blanket if you need extra cushioning under your knees. Loop a strap around the tops of your thighs, close to the hip creases, and around the tops of your ankles. Make sure that the strap is snug but not too tight. Place your hands on the floor beside your hips with your fingers pointing forward. Round forward and press the floor, protracting through your shoulders. Hug your knees into your chest, keeping your heels close to your seat. The strap will help in bringing your heels closer to your seat, reinforcing the action of the hamstrings and easing their workload. The strap will also help to create more distance between your legs and the floor. Engage your core and lift your feet off the floor, bringing your shins parallel to the floor.

Pendant Pose (continued)

Practice seated on a chair.

This variation is great if getting up from and down onto the floor is challenging. It also modifies the posture to be more accessible if you are still working up the strength for the traditional version. Sit on a chair with your hands holding the sides of the chair seat. Round your chest forward, and press down to lift the hips up. If you are feeling confident here, try lifting your feet off the floor as well and hugging your knees to your chest.

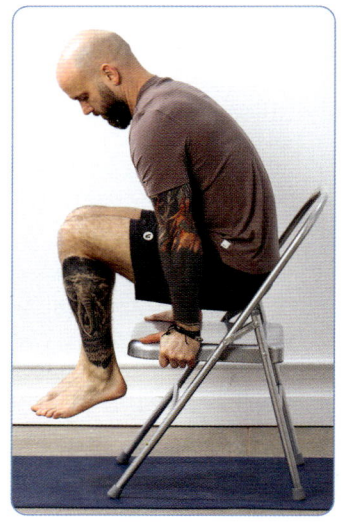

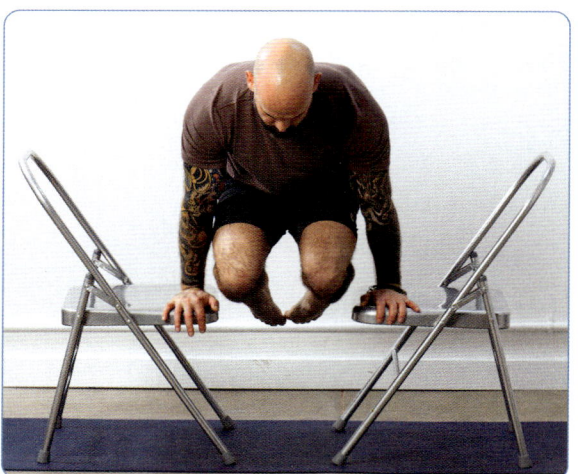

Practice between two chairs.

This variation is great if getting up from and down onto from the floor is challenging. It also modifies the posture in a way that makes it more accessible if you are still working up the strength for the non-prop supported posture. The chairs serve in a similar way to the variation with blocks under your hands, providing more space between you and the floor. If you are working on hamstring and psoas strength, this added space will also make lifting the feet off the floor easier to do. Kneel between two chairs that are facing one another. Add a blanket if you need extra cushioning under your knees. Place your hands on the seat of the chairs and forcefully press into them. As you press, draw your knees toward your chest and your heels toward your seat.

Celibate's Pose

Brahmacharyasana
ब्रह्मचर्यासन

Celibate's pose, also known as floating stick or an L-sit, is a dynamic yoga posture that actively strengthens the wrists and arms while toning the psoas and abdomen. This pose also offers a deep stretch to the upper back and contributes to the strength of the legs. Explore prop-supported variations to enhance your experience.

Practice with a block under your heels to help lift off the floor.

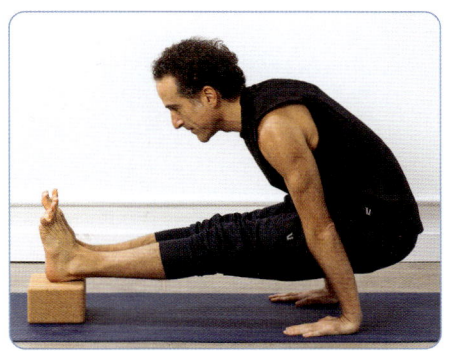

Celibate's pose is a challenging yoga pose that requires strength, flexibility, and balance. By adding a block, the benefits can be enhanced and the pose can be more accessible to those of varying levels of experience and flexibility. Start this variation in staff pose (dandasana), sitting with your legs extended in front of you. Place a block on its lowest height underneath the feet. Walk your hands forward on the mat to the outsides of the thighs, rounding through the torso so that your chest is hovering over the thighs. As you press the hands into the mat, you will feel the hips lift off the floor. This is where the block comes in. By using the block, you can support the lift of the hips without sacrificing alignment in the pose. As you continue to round through the upper back and hollow out through the belly and chest, you will create a deeper stretch in the hamstrings while also engaging the core muscles. Firming through the thighs and squeezing the inner thighs toward each other can also provide additional stability and support. If you are feeling strong in the prop-supported posture, you can try to lift the heels from the block so that they are parallel with the hips. This further challenges you and helps to create muscle memory when both hips and feet are lifted. By practicing the pose with a block, you can gradually increase flexibility and strength, making the pose more accessible over time.

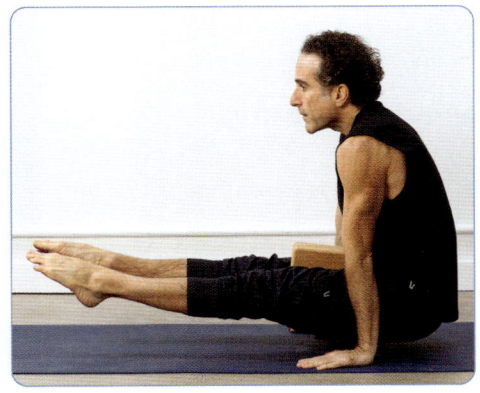

Practice with a block between your thighs to align and engage.

Squeezing a block between your thighs can help when practicing celibate's pose. Doing so can help to engage the inner thigh muscles, providing added support and stability in the pose. Squeezing the block helps create a muscular connection between the inner thighs, which helps to activate the adductor muscles. Engaging the adductors helps to draw the thighs toward the midline of the body, providing a firm foundation for the pose. This can help to prevent the legs from splaying, which can cause the hips to drop. Squeezing the block can also help to activate the core muscles, creating a deeper engagement of the entire body. As you squeeze the block between your thighs, imagine hugging your sitting bones toward one another and engaging root or pelvic lock (mula bandha).

Celibate's Pose (continued)

Practice seated on a chair.

This variation is great if getting up from and onto the floor is challenging. It also modifies the posture in a way that makes it more accessible if you are still working up the strength for the traditional version. Sit on a chair with your hands holding the sides of the chair seat. Extend your legs out long in front of you, with the toes pointing toward the sky. If you need extra height, place blocks under your heels. Round your chest forward and press down to lift the hips up. If you are feeling confident, try lifting your feet off the floor and hugging the sitting bones toward one another, engaging your deep core muscles.

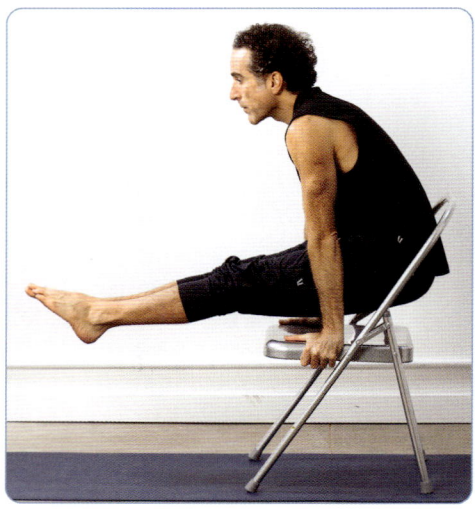

Loop a strap around your thighs.

Looping a strap around your thighs can be a helpful modification for celibate's pose, particularly for those who may have limited strength in the legs or those who want to refine parallel leg alignment. This technique can help to activate the outer thigh muscles, providing additional support and stability in the pose. To use a strap in this pose, sit with your legs out long in front of you and place a strap around the middle of your thighs. Adjust the strap so that it is snug but not too tight. As you lift the hips off the floor and round through the torso, press outward into the strap with your thighs. By pressing out into the strap, you activate the muscles of the

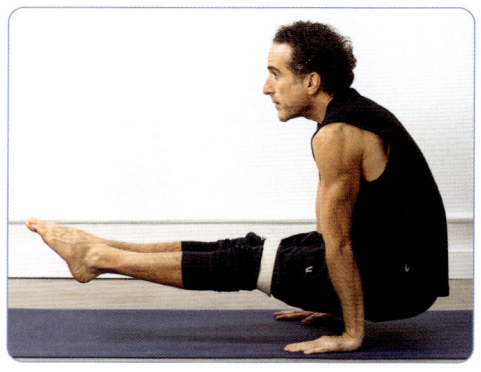

outer thighs, particularly the tensor fasciae latae. These muscles play an important role in stabilizing the pelvis and thigh bones, helping to maintain stability in the pose.

Loop a strap around your shoulders and feet or behind the thighs.

Try these strap variations for an extra boost when trying to lift your legs off the floor. In the first variation, the strap will act as a lift for your legs as you press your upper back into the other side of the loop. To set up, sit on your mat with your feet planted firmly on the floor in front of you, as if you were setting up for boat pose. Loop the strap around your shoulder blades and under your thighs, just above the knee. Make sure the loop is snug and secure so that when you straighten your legs in front of you, your torso will be pulled forward to hover over the thighs. Place your hands on the mat outside your thighs, closer to your knees than your hips, then press down forcefully into the floor, lifting your hips. Expand your upper back into the strap to add tension to the loop, pulling the legs off the floor. Squeeze your inner thighs together and breathe (see photo a). The second variation functions similarly, but with slightly less support. Rather than the strap pulling the legs up from underneath, place the loop around the balls of the feet. As you come into the posture, press your feet into the strap. The opposing force to your shoulder protraction should help to lift the legs and encourage lengthening in the hamstrings (see photo b).

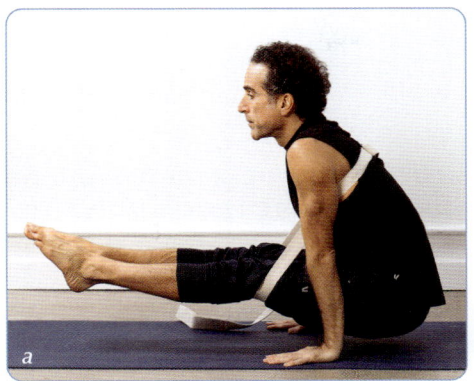

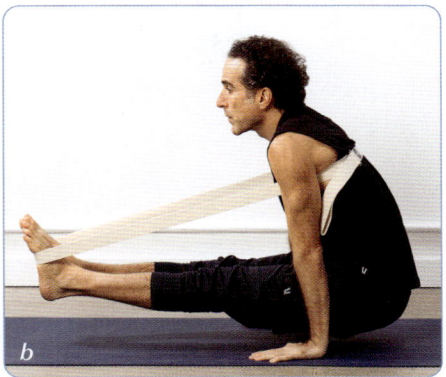

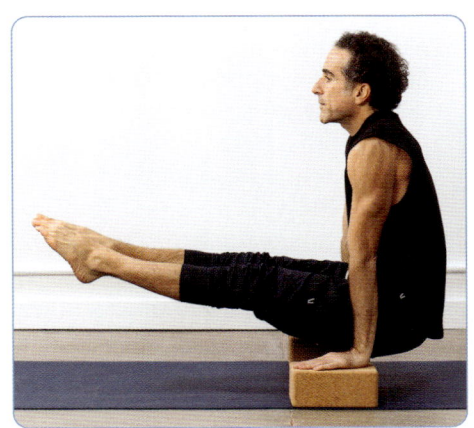

Practice pressing your feet into a wall.

To practice celibate's pose with your feet against a wall, find a clear wall space to enter staff pose (dandasana) with your feet against the wall and your hands framing the outer thighs. The wall will help you reinforce the pose by providing muscular feedback and aid in leg alignment by keeping the toes and knees pointing up and the legs parallel. The first step to practice celibate's pose with your feet against the wall is to start with your heels grounded, your feet flexed against the wall, and your hips lifted. As you exhale, press your feet into the wall and engage your core muscles to lift your hips. Focus on pressing into the hands as you expand through the upper back, protracting the shoulders. The second option is to start with your feet a few inches up the wall and lifting your hips from there. This variation is a bit more challenging and requires more core strength. Keep your legs straight and strong as you hold this position.

Practice with blocks under your hands to raise the height of the ground.

Blocks under your hands provide a few benefits to the L-sit pose. First, they help to elevate your hands, making it easier to engage your shoulder muscles and lift your body off the floor. This is especially helpful if you have a long torso and short arms! Second, placing blocks under your hands during this pose could help alleviate discomfort or tightness in your wrists, because it can reduce the pressure on them and make the pose more accessible. Sit with your legs straight out in front of you and with your hands on blocks framing the thighs. Press down into the blocks and lift your hips off the floor, straightening your arms and legs. Keep your core engaged and your shoulders down and away from your ears. First try lifting your hips, and over time, lift both legs fully off the floor.

Eight-Angle Pose

Ashtavakrasana अष्टावक्रासन

Eight-angle pose is a challenging and engaging yoga posture that actively strengthens the wrists, upper arms, core, and inner thighs. This pose also requires spinal rotation, adding to the dynamic elements taking place. Let's explore some common variations with the help of props.

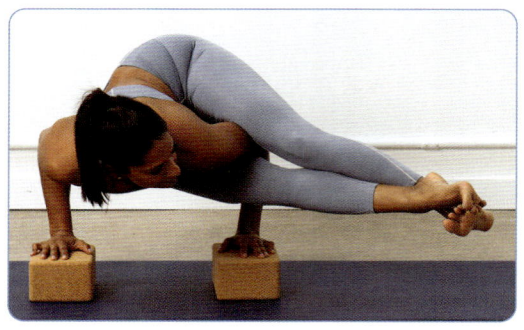

Practice with blocks under your hands to support lifting your hips off the floor.

To get into eight-angle pose with blocks under your hands, start by sitting cross-legged with blocks at their lowest height on the outer edges of your hips. The blocks will provide enough space for you to lift your hips off the mat and work your chest forward. Cradle your left shin in your arms, bringing your left knee inside the left elbow crease and the sole of your left foot in the right elbow. Transfer the sole of your left foot into your right hand, reaching under for the left ankle with your left hand. Guide the left knee behind your torso and nudge your left shoulder under the left knee, treating your left leg like a backpack strap hooked over your shoulder. Aim to get the leg as high up your left arm as possible if it doesn't make it over your shoulder. Release your left hand from the ankle, placing it on the left block. Squeeze your left knee toward your upper body, engaging the inner thigh's adductor muscles. Put your right hand on the right block. Hook your right ankle over the left, keeping your feet flexed. Move the blocks toward your outer hips, then slightly forward. Round your torso forward, facing the mat. When you can't shift forward farther, press your hands into the blocks to lift your hips. Think about entering a chaturanga arm shape and extend your legs out to the left, hugging the inner thighs toward one another around the upper left arm. Repeat on the right side.

Practice with three blocks stacked under one shoulder to help lift the hips.

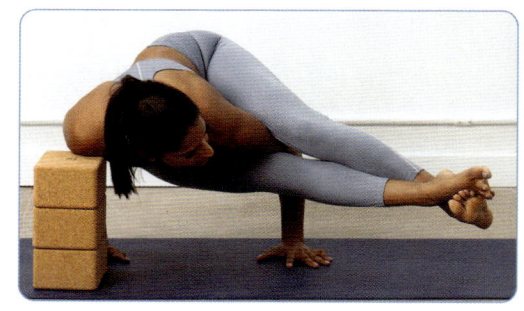

This variation of the pose involves using three blocks to support your shoulder opposite the arm that is supporting your legs. The blocks help you achieve the right angle needed for the pose, similar to your arm position in chaturanga. However, you may find that using two blocks works better for you. Start in the same way as described in the previous variation, but this time place the three blocks in front of your hand (opposite the hand attached to the arm supporting the legs), making sure the stack is stable and secure. Next, shift your weight forward, bringing your shoulder on top of the stacked blocks. Engage your inner thighs, straightening your hooked legs. As you lift your hips off the floor, focus on pressing your shoulder into the blocks to create an opposing force, helping you to lift into the pose.

Practice with blocks under your hips for added support.

The blocks will give your hips the height they need without compromising support. Start by positioning two blocks on their lowest height, side by side with the short edges of the blocks touching on the floor or mat. Sit on one block so that the other block is to the right of you and cross your legs. Enter the pose as described in 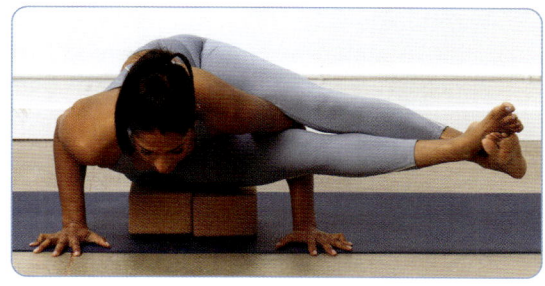 more detail in the previous version with the left leg hooking over the left arm, then the right ankle hooking over the left, then place your hands down in front of your blocks. Shift your weight forward into your hands and bend through your elbows. As you do, roll your right hip onto the second block to your right. Straighten your legs and squeeze your inner thighs. As you get more comfortable shifting your weight into your hands, practice lifting your hips to hover over the block, then lowering. Repeat on the other side.

Formidable Face Pose

Ganda Bherundasana

गण्डभेरुण्डासन

Formidable face pose, commonly known as chin stand, is an arm balance that requires a lot of spinal mobility and strength! It also requires some amount of caution when approaching this pose. This pose actively expands the chest, tones the upper arms and back, and stretches the abdomen. Explore prop-supported variations for a well-rounded experience.

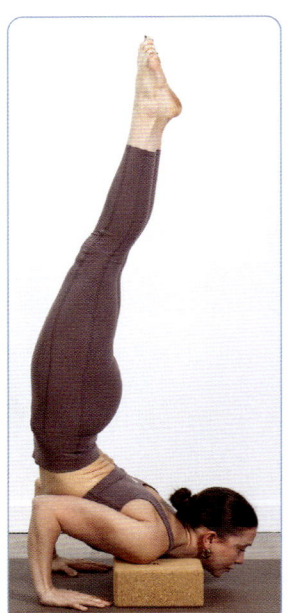

Practice with blocks under your chest and shoulders to protect your neck.

The use of blocks in this posture creates space between the chin and mat, protecting your neck. Start in a block-supported chaturanga with two blocks on medium height under your shoulders (as you progress with this pose, you might want to have the blocks on the lowest height). Walk your feet toward your hands, piking the hips, like the shape of downward dog. Lift your chin, extend the front of your neck, and keep your gaze slightly forward. The blocks elevate your shoulders, reducing strain on the rotator cuffs for those building strength. When your feet reach as close as they can to your hands, hug your elbows to your sides. Lift one leg toward the sky, aiming for the highest possible foot position. To raise the second leg, come to the tiptoes of the foot on the mat. If lifting both legs is challenging, start by alternating legs. Stacking your bones to make your legs perpendicular to the mat reduces muscle effort against gravity, making it easier to maintain the posture. When your legs are overhead, squeeze the inner thighs. Press your hands into the mat to lift your torso weight off the arms, ensuring your torso and belly don't sink below the elbows. Over time, as your back and arms strengthen, you'll rely less on the blocks, making the posture more accessible without them. Without the blocks, engage the muscles similarly to avoid putting downward pressure on the chin and neck.

Practice by walking your feet up a wall.

A wall can help you achieve one of the hardest steps in chin stand—lifting your legs overhead. It helps by giving your feet a walking path to the destination so that it doesn't feel like such a big step from grounded to lifted. Start with a wall behind you. Place the blocks on the medium or lowest height. Instead of starting in chaturanga, begin in table top pose and lower your chest and shoulders onto the blocks. This position allows you to get closer to the wall, so there is room to bend your knees as you walk your feet up the wall without feeling like your feet are going to slip off the wall. Once you're in position, walk your feet up the wall behind you, piking your hips up. Step one foot back onto the wall, then the other, and

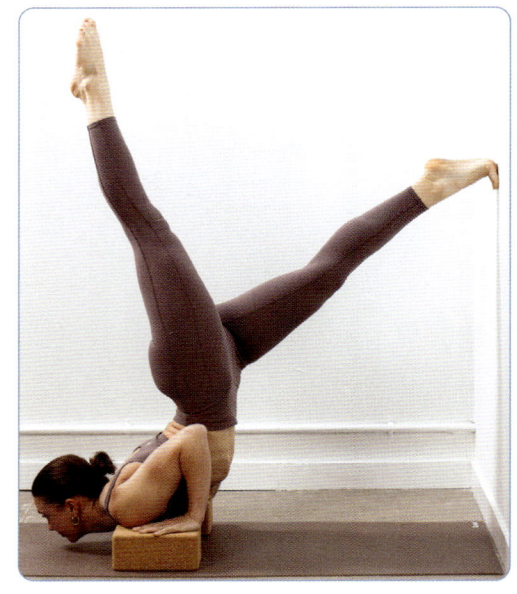

press your feet into the wall to lift your hips higher over your shoulders. Be careful not to strain your back more than necessary. Try alternating lifting the legs overhead until you are ready to try lifting them both. When you lift both legs, squeeze the inner thighs down through your hands, and try not to let your torso and belly sink below the elbows.

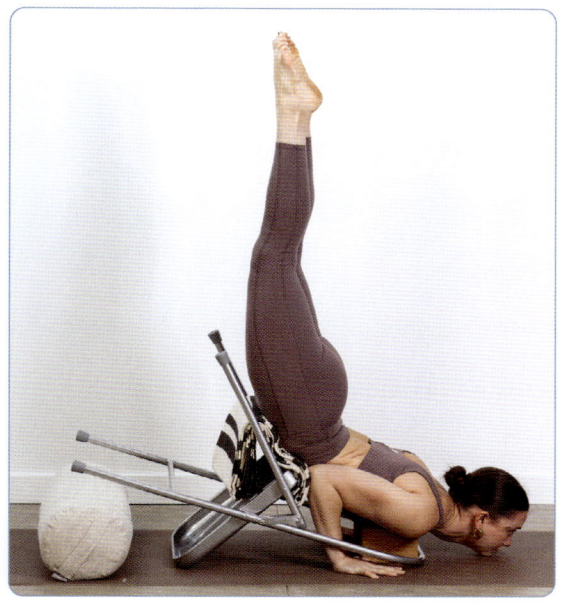

Practice using an inverted chair, blocks, a blanket, and a bolster.

This variation offers the ultimate support for you as you journey into learning the mechanics of this pose! Start by turning a chair upside down so that the back support railing and front edge of the seat are down on the mat. Place your blocks inside the railing because that is where your chest and shoulders will be. If this does not fit your proportions, you can move the blocks in front of the railing or use a firm bolster on top of the railing. Fold a blanket over the railing that connects the back legs of the chair; this is where your hips will fold over. You can use additional blankets if needed. Place the bolster behind the front edge of the chair seat and kneel on it. Place your hands on the mat behind the blocks and lower your hip creases onto the blanket. Bring your chest onto the blocks and straighten your legs. The railing your hips are on should help to support you in lifting the legs as the hips are grounded in the elevated position. You can keep them grounded on the chair or over time lift your hips away from the chair and shift more weight into your chest and arms.

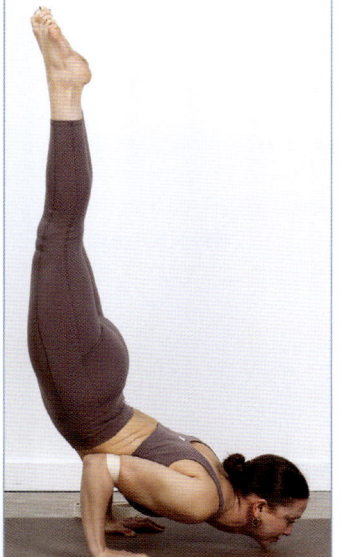

Practice with a strap around your upper arms to support alignment.

Using a strap around your arms just above the elbows can help support hugging the elbows toward the ribs and prevent the belly from collapsing between the arms. Loop the strap around your arms shoulder-width apart. Then, enter a table top position with your hands and knees on the floor. Shift your weight forward to lower your chin to the mat, pressing firmly into the strap with your arms. Tuck the back toes under to lift the knees and hips, walking your toes toward your hands. As you lift your legs to enter the posture, let your torso rest against the strap, causing the elbows to be pinned into your sides. Engage your core muscles to prevent your belly from collapsing. Work gradually to reduce the bodyweight resting on the strap over time.

Side Crow Pose

Parshva Kakasana   पार्श्व काकासन

Side crow pose is a dynamic yoga posture that effectively strengthens the arms, shoulders, and wrists while toning the abdominal muscles. This pose also provides a beneficial stretch to the hips and contributes to improved spinal rotation. Other physical benefits include enhanced digestion, balance, and coordination. Explore prop-supported variations for a well-rounded experience.

Practice with a block under your feet to get your legs higher up on your arms.

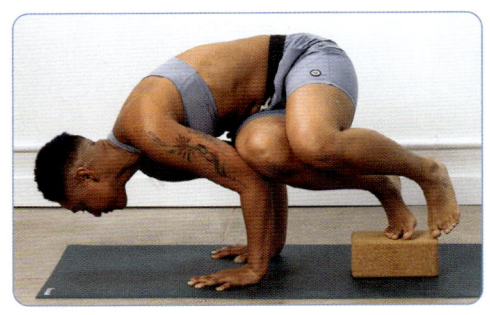

Using blocks to support your practice can make getting into side crow pose more accessible. By placing your feet on the blocks, you can easily lift your legs onto your arms without the need for a full liftoff. To get started, step onto a block turned on its lowest height with both feet. Next, bring your feet and knees together in a squatting position and your hands in prayer at heart center. Twist to the right until the imaginary line between your shoulders is perpendicular to the imaginary line between your hips. Place your hands on the mat, shoulder-width apart. Bend your elbows to create a shelf for your right thigh with your upper arms. Shift your weight forward into your hands and lean until your right thigh rests on the back of your upper arms. Finally, start lifting your feet while actively squeezing your thighs. Repeat on the other side.

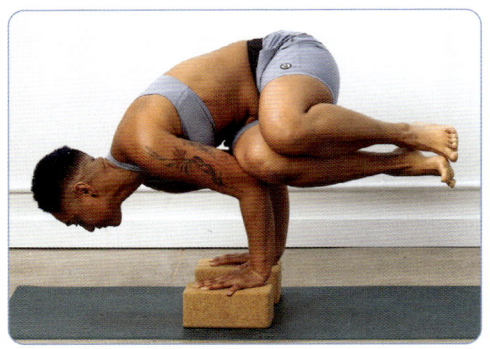

Practice with blocks under your hands to bring the floor closer to you.

When you place blocks under your hands, the blocks bring the floor closer to you, which can be particularly helpful if you have limited mobility in your hips or ankles, which hinders squatting low. A higher starting point lets you work on building strength and flexibility in your upper body and worry less about your lower body mobility. By adding height with the blocks, you can also reduce the amount of twisting required in the pose. This can be beneficial for those who have limited range of motion in their spine or for those who are still working on building the strength and flexibility required to twist deeply.

Practice with blocks under your shoulders for stability.

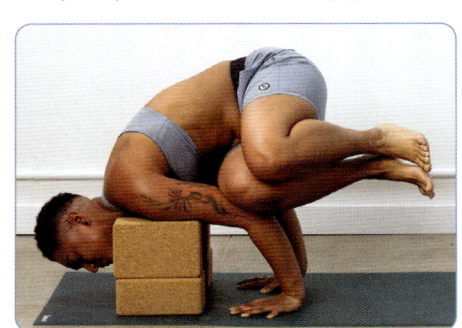

Using blocks helps you to get more comfortable with shifting weight forward, eliminating the fear of falling onto your face. This version also allows the shoulders more stability as you take flight! Depending on your body proportions, you might require three blocks under each shoulder, but start with stacking two. As you enter the arm balance, keep shifting your weight until your shoulders come to rest on top of the blocks. Your elbows should be directly above your wrists so that your forearms are perpendicular to the mat. Keep firmly pressing your hands as if you were going to lift the shoulders off the blocks to hover.

Practice using a wall to capture the feeling of flying.

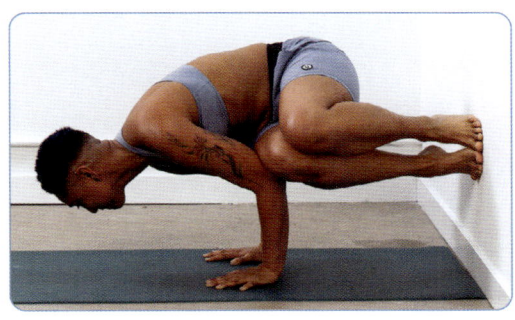

This wall-supported side crow variation gives you the sensation of flying while offering support from the wall. It can help you understand how to use your legs for liftoff eventually. Face the wall in a squatting position with your feet together and your left shoulder about two to three inches (5-7.6 cm) away from the wall. Twist your torso to the right and place your hands on the floor, shoulder-width apart. Lift your hips a little to get your thigh higher onto your arms and shift your weight into your hands, creating chaturanga arms. When you feel the weight in your arms, raise your left foot and press the ball of your foot onto the wall. Move closer to or farther from the wall if needed. Once you feel comfortable, lift your right foot. Keep your legs active and your shoulders steady by pushing your hands into the floor. Hold the pose with your feet on the wall and gradually lean forward until only the big toes rest on the wall. If you feel steady, try floating the remaining toes off the wall. Repeat on the other side.

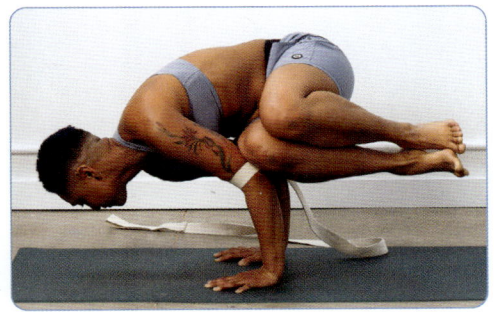

Place a strap around your arms to strengthen alignment.

Using a strap in side crow pose is helpful for positioning the elbows and shoulders. To avoid pinching your skin with the strap, be sure to have the strap looped around the upper arms in a place the thigh will not be resting. Try just above the elbows, because the thigh will ideally be higher up on the arms. Adjust according to your own needs though! Sometimes the elbows will want to splay, which can make finding your balance more challenging and puts unnecessary strain on the rotator cuff. Rather than thinking about hugging the elbows in, you will counterintuitively press the arms out into the strap. If you measured correctly, the strap will not allow the elbows to splay. When you press into the strap, it eventually stops you from pressing out any more. That energetic force will instead travel into other parts of your body, reinforcing the actions such as the downward pressing force of your hands into the floor and the protraction of your shoulders, gliding your scapula around your ribs. To strengthen the feeling of hugging your elbows in and keeping the arms parallel to one another, use the strap as a guide rather than something to press into. Try to keep the strap free of tension, like you are pulling away from the strap rather than leaning into it.

Side Crow Pose *(continued)*

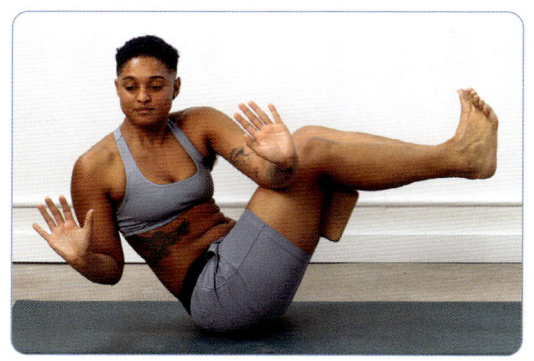

Practice hugging a block between your thighs while seated.

This is a great core challenge and a wonderful alternative if weight-bearing on your wrists is not an option. It is also a great way to build strength until you feel confident to take flight! Sit with your feet planted on the floor in front of you, knees pointing up toward the sky. Place a block on its narrowest width between your thighs and hug the block, engaging your adductors. Reach your left arm up, lengthening through your spine, then twist to the right, hooking your elbow outside the right thigh. Lift your right hand off the mat and hug your elbow into the side of your ribs. Flex through both hands and mimic chaturanga arms. Imagine you are pushing into an invisible wall in front of you. As you push, draw your navel into your spine and gently protract through your shoulders. Try not to round too much though because the thoracic spine needs extension to facilitate the twisting motion. Continue to squeeze the block between your thighs, engaging your pelvic floor, and try to lift your feet off the floor! Repeat on the other side.

Practice with a looped strap for flight support.

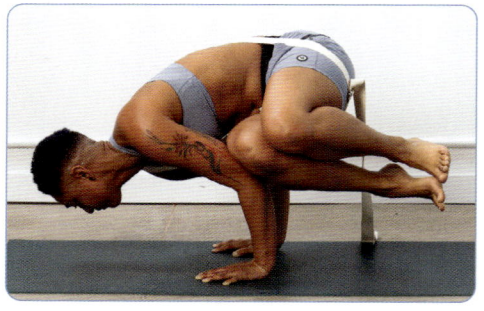

For added support and to deepen your twist, practice side crow with a looped strap. The strap will help you feel the necessary twist as you move into the pose. The more you twist, the greater the resistance from the strap, which ultimately makes side crow more accessible. This version also provides support as your lower body lifts. Grab a large, looped strap and step your left foot into it, pulling it up to your left thigh from a standing position. Squat and loop the strap over your right shoulder and tighten it to draw your left thigh close to your torso. Find a balance between the strap being too tight (preventing easy twisting) and too loose (which is ineffective). Twist to your right and set up your side crow arms, leaning into your hands. Begin by trying to lift the left leg with the encouragement of the secured strap helping to lift the thigh. Then play with lifting your right leg up to meet your left. Hold the pose, maintaining steadiness in your shoulders, pressing your hands down firmly, and hugging your elbows in toward each other. Repeat on the other side.

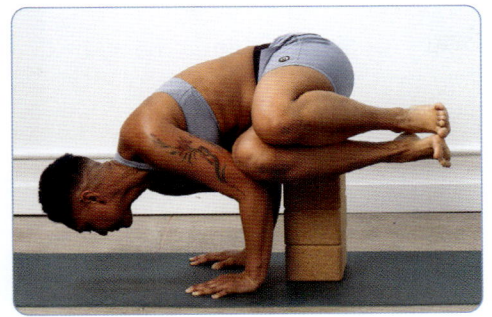

Practice with blocks supporting the weight of your hips.

This technique offers additional support to the hips, allowing for an easier connection between the arms and legs. Stack two or three blocks on their lowest height. Sit on the blocks with your right sitting bone on top, keeping your knees bent and your feet on the floor. Bring your legs together tightly. Rotate your torso to the right and hook your left elbow on the outside of your right thigh, creating a firm connection between your arm and leg. Lean to the right, making sure that your left sitting bone is not on the block and that you are stable on the outer right hip. Place both hands on the floor, about shoulder-width apart, and shift your weight forward into your hands. As you lean forward onto your hands, bend both elbows and lift your feet off the floor to enter side crow pose. Continue to roll the barrel of your ribs so that the chest is working to face down toward the floor. Repeat on the other side.

Practice seated on a chair, with your hands on blocks to remove weight-bearing from the wrists and shoulders.

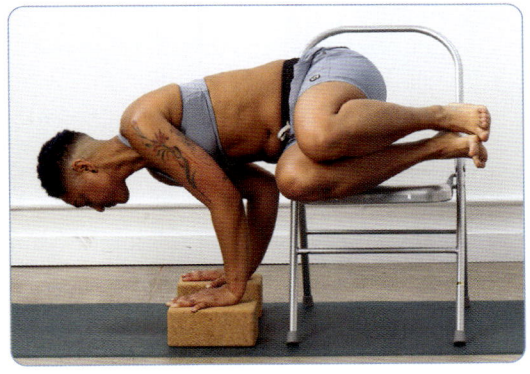

Take flight on a chair! This is a great option for those who need more stability or want to limit wrist weight-bearing. Sit on the chair and firmly plant both feet on the floor. Place two to four blocks on the right side of the chair, about shoulder-width apart and on the lowest height for added stability. You can stack more blocks for a gentler twist and to raise the height of the floor. Start by twisting your torso to the right and reaching your hands toward the blocks. Once your hands contact them, roll onto your outer right hip and thigh, lifting your feet off the floor and to the left. Place a folded blanket on the chair seat for more cushioning. Most of your weight will be on the chair, so your wrists won't bear much weight. Still, actively press into the blocks and work to level your left ribs with your right. Squeeze your thighs together. Repeat on the other side.

Peacock Pose

Mayurasana   मयूरासन

Peacock pose is a powerful yoga posture that actively strengthens and stretches the wrists, while also building strength in the arms, shoulders, and muscles supporting the spine. Toning the abdominals, peacock pose contributes to improved digestion and circulation. Explore prop-supported variations to enhance your experience.

Practice with a block under your hands to feel a different grip in the fingers for control.

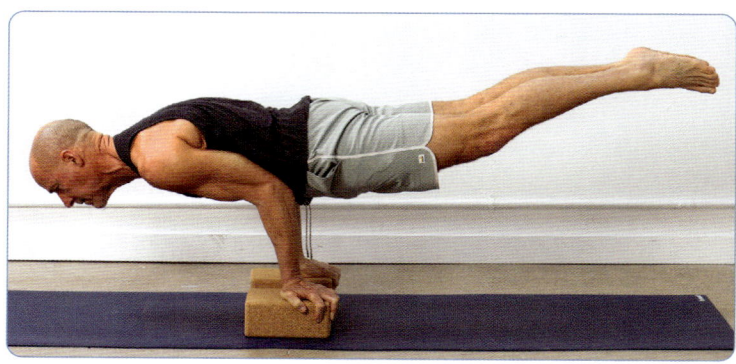

Utilizing a block under your hands enables you to explore improved grip and control in this pose. Kneel with your knees hip-width apart and your toes pointing back. Place a block horizontally on the mat in front of you on the lowest height. You can also use two blocks, lengthwise (as shown in the photo), for more space between the wrists. Experiment with the block's placement; position it between your knees and move it forward or backward as needed. Position your hands on the block with your fingers pointing back toward your body, ensuring a wide spread and a firm grip around the back edge of the block. Bend your elbows and place them just below your front ribs. Walk your feet back until your legs are straight and your hips are lifted. Keep your elbows bent and your belly resting on the backs of your upper arms. Shift your weight forward to lift your feet off the floor, keeping your gaze forward and engaging your core to elevate your hips. As your legs ascend, squeeze your thighs together, reach through the legs, and maintain parallel alignment for better balance. For an alternative grip, consider holding the outside edges of the block with your fingers pointing to the sides, offering reduced wrist flexion and potential comfort.

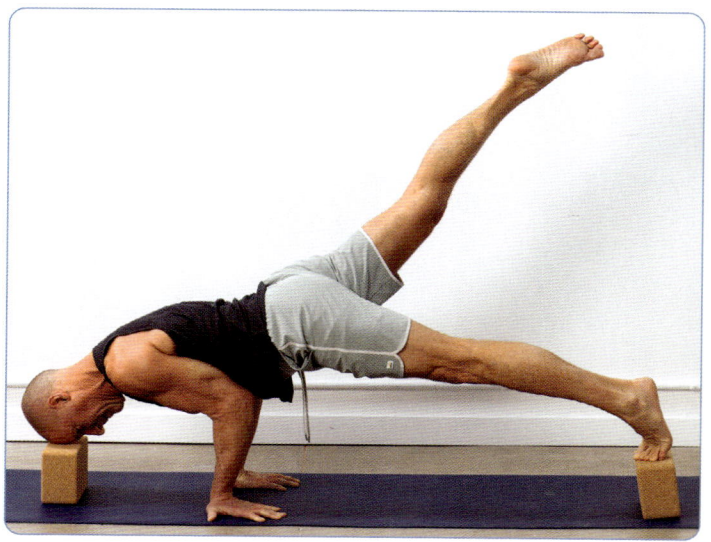

Practice with blocks under your feet or head to take flight without leaving the floor.

To find balance and stability in this pose, using blocks under your head, feet, or both can provide structural support. This can help build muscle memory and strength without leaving the ground, giving you the feeling of taking flight. To use this variation, measure the distance between the blocks to ensure one block is under your head and the other under your feet. If using both blocks, step back onto the block behind you, then lean forward to rest either your chin or your forehead on the second block in front of you. Resting the chin teaches you to gaze slightly forward, but it may feel safer on the neck to first learn by resting the weight on the forehead and keeping the back of the neck elongated. Press into your hands, engage your posterior chain muscles, and practice lifting off the blocks. Start with both blocks on the lowest height and experiment with what works for you. Try removing one of the blocks and supporting either the upper or lower half of the body on your own. This can be a bit of a teeter-totter game but can help identify which muscles need strengthening. If you want to break it down even further, try lifting one leg at a time as shown in the photo.

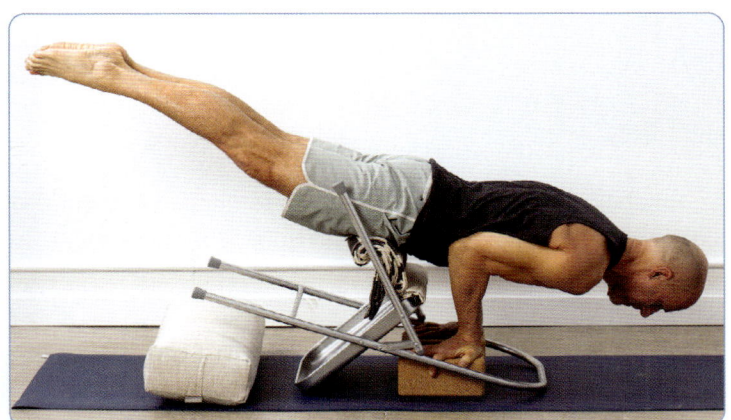

Practice using an inverted chair, blocks, a blanket, and a bolster.

This chair-supported variation of peacock pose offers pelvic support, aiding in lifting the legs for those still developing strength and stability for the traditional version. It also provides increased stability, making it more accessible to try different leg positions during the pose. The pelvic support also allows for refining actions such as bringing the elbows closer together and core engagement. Open your yoga chair and flip it upside down on your mat so that its legs are up. Place a folded blanket or two on the crossbar between the back chair legs, then place a bolster up against the edge of the seat so you have something to kneel on as you enter and exit the pose. Place the blocks close together on the floor, inside or on top of the railing of the back of the chair in front of you. To enter the pose, kneel on the bolster, then bring your hip creases to fold over the blanket on the crossbar. You might need to grab the legs of the chair and lift your knees off the bolster to do so. Turn your fingers to point back toward you and bring your hands onto the blocks. Bend your elbows toward your abdomen, hugging them closely together, while tucking your toes under and pressing through the balls of your feet to lift your knees and extend your legs. Shift your weight forward until the backs of your arms are nestled under your ribs and abdomen. With chair support, lift your legs away from the floor as if entering locust pose. Hug your inner thighs together and lift through your chest.

Peacock Pose (continued)

Practice with a strap around your arms to stabilize your arms and hug your elbows closer together.

Fastening a strap around your arms in peacock pose can be beneficial in several ways. First, it can help to improve your alignment and stability in the pose. It requires a lot of strength and balance in your arms, core, and upper body. By using a strap to secure your

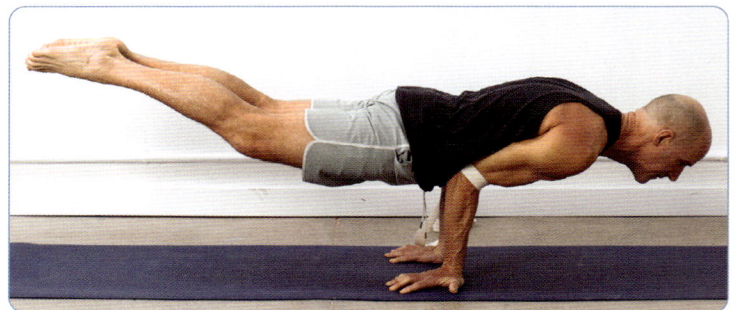

arms together, you can create a more stable foundation for the pose and ensure that your elbows are directly over your wrists, helping to distribute the weight evenly and prevent strain on your joints. Second, the strap can help to deepen the stretch in your wrists and shoulders. Peacock pose requires a lot of flexibility and mobility in these areas, which can be challenging. By using the strap to gently pull your arms toward each other, you can create a gentle stretch in your wrists and shoulders, which can help to improve your range of motion. Finally, using a strap in peacock pose can also help to build strength in your arms and upper body. By pressing your arms into the strap and engaging your core and upper body muscles, you can create a powerful isometric contraction that can help to build endurance and strength.

Practice with your feet against a wall.

A wall is a free and easy prop to create a stable foundation for this pose! Pressing your feet into a wall is beneficial in more ways than one! First, it can help to create a stable foundation for the pose. Peacock pose requires a lot of strength and balance in

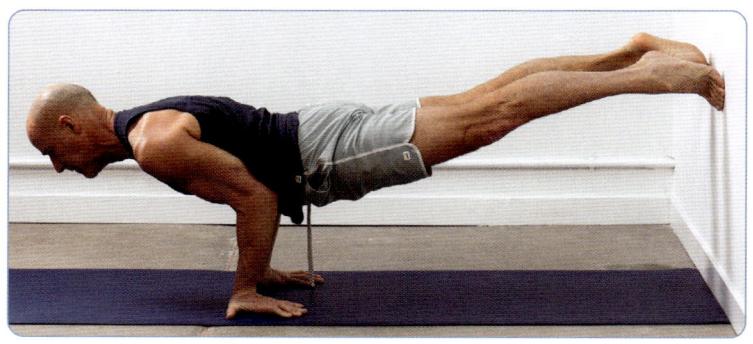

your upper body, but it's important not to neglect your lower body. By pressing your feet into a wall behind you, you can create a stable foundation that helps you balance and distribute your weight evenly. Second, pressing your feet into a wall can help to engage your leg muscles, including your quadriceps, hamstrings, and calves. These muscles support your lower body and can also help you to maintain a supportive alignment in the pose. For added height, step your feet onto blocks placed against the wall. This can help to elevate your hips and create a more vertical line with your torso, for ease in balancing. It can also help to deepen the stretch in your wrists and shoulders by creating more space between your hands and feet. Finally, having your feet, toes pointing down, pressing into the wall aids in informing leg alignment. With your legs parallel, you will resist the urge to externally rotate in the hip sockets, which can free up some space in the lower back.

Place a bolster between your elbows and belly to add comfort and stability.

Peacock pose can be challenging due to the amount of direct pressure it places on your abdomen and elbows. However, a bolster variation can add comfort and stability to the pose. To practice the bolster variation, place a bolster between your elbows and your belly. This will help to distribute the weight more evenly and create a more stable foundation for the pose. While you may not feel the same intensity of direct elbow pressure into your belly, you will still gain all the benefits of stimulating blood circulation in your abdomen. Over time,

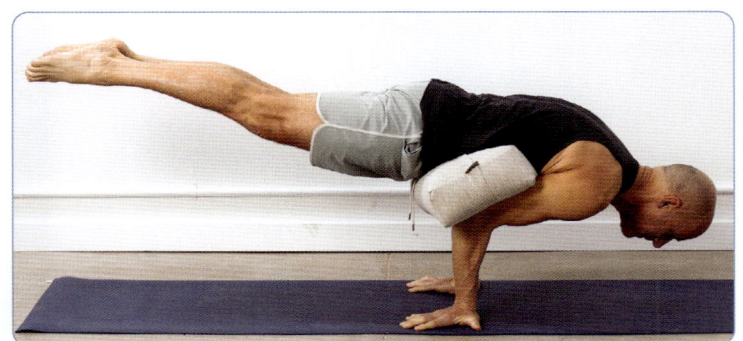

as your core strengthens, the discomfort should decrease. The bolster also provides added comfort and support so you can hold the pose for longer periods. If you prefer even more grip and stability, you can swap the bolster for a folded sticky mat. The added traction and support can help you to maintain alignment and balance in the pose.

Scorpion Pose

Vrishchikasana   वृश्चिकासन

Scorpion pose, also known as scorpion forearm stand, is an invigorating yoga posture that actively strengthens the arms, shoulders, core, and posterior chain muscles. This pose not only improves spinal flexibility but also brings a revitalizing boost of energy. Explore prop-supported variations to enhance your experience and fully embrace the strengthening and energizing benefits of scorpion pose.

Use a chair to support your feet.

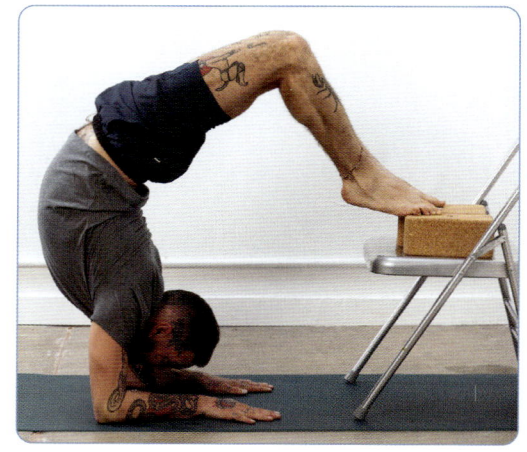

Utilizing a chair for a scorpion forearm stand offers multiple benefits. It helps build core and leg strength—crucial for balance—by bringing your toes overhead to the chair seat. The chair serves as a reference point, aiding alignment and form development—particularly helpful for those new to the pose. Practicing with a chair also fosters confidence, provides stability, eases anxiety associated with inverting the body, and helps build flexibility. Position a chair with a sturdy back against a wall, facing away from the wall, with the seat facing you. Enter the forearm stand by placing your forearms on the floor, either with your hands gripping the chair legs or with your forearms framed by the legs of the chair, pressing outward. You may want to start further back from the legs of the chair though (as shown in the photo), and work your way closer over time. In all cases, ensure your elbows are straight back from the wrists. Walk your feet toward your elbows, coming into dolphin pose. Press down firmly through your forearms to resist sinking into your shoulders. Work your way into forearm stand pose, gradually bending your knees toward the chair seat. Extend your head and chest forward, shifting your gaze in front to counteract the actions of the legs in the backbend. To add an extra challenge, bring your toes toward the front edge of the chair seat and hover them off the seat, holding

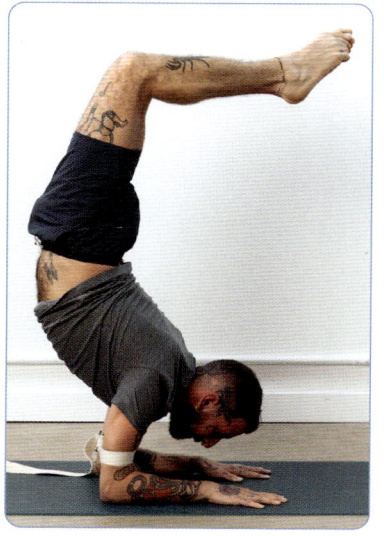

for a few seconds before lowering them. If the chair seat feels too low, try adding blocks to raise the height of the chair (as shown in the photo).

Practice with a strap around your biceps to stabilize and engage.

Practicing scorpion forearm stand with a strap around your biceps can be beneficial for two reasons. One reason is that it can help to improve your alignment and form in the pose. When you bring your legs overhead in a scorpion forearm stand, the elbows tend to splay, which can cause the shoulders to collapse inward and compromise the stability of the pose. Using a strap around your biceps creates resistance that helps to keep your elbows hugged toward your body, promoting a healthier alignment and form in the pose. Another reason is using a strap can help to engage the muscles of the upper body. As you press down with your forearms and engage your core, the strap can provide a challenge that helps to build strength and stability in the upper body.

Practice with a block or two between your hands.

Practicing with blocks between your hands provides a reference point and support for your body, helping you to keep shoulder alignment and form as you move into the pose. It can also help to prevent the elbows from sliding apart, which can cause instability and compromise the integrity of the pose. To do this variation, place one block between your hands on the lowest height, turned to the widest orientation. If this is too narrow, try using two blocks on their lowest height, side by side and lengthwise. You can frame the blocks with your thumb and index fingers creating two L shapes around the edges of the blocks. Using two blocks instead of just one gives you more room for the chest to pull forward than a regular forearm stand would. As you find your way into scorpion, engage the upper body muscles. Work to build strength and stability in the shoulders, arms, and chest as you press down and hug into the blocks.

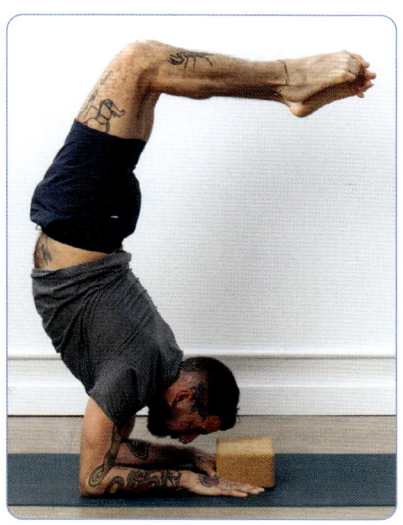

Practice bringing your feet to a wall and walking your toes toward your head.

Descending into scorpion forearm stand by walking your feet down the wall is a rewarding challenge, elevating your practice with a blend of focus, determination, and resilience. This variation not only cultivates strength and stability in your upper body—activating shoulders, arms, and chest muscles—but it also promotes enhanced flexibility and mobility in a more accessible and controlled manner as you progress. As you progress further into the pose, you stretch and lengthen the front of your body while engaging the posterior chain. This contributes to overall flexibility and range of motion, and the support of the wall allows for controlled movement, reducing the risk of injury. Another advantage of walking your feet down the wall in scorpion is the improvement of balance and proprioception. Shifting your weight and adjusting your body position challenges your body to maintain balance and stability in a changing environment. As you work toward moving your feet away from the wall toward your head, try alternating bringing one foot in at a time to build hamstring strength and focus!

Scorpion Pose *(continued)*

Practice with your belly against a wall for structural support.

This wall variation intensifies the challenge in your scorpion forearm practice but comes with the benefits of enhancing alignment, form, and providing essential support for the belly to prevent strain on the lower back. Your belly serves as a reference point, promoting a healthier alignment and minimizing injury risks. The wall also contributes to stability, ensuring a more controlled and supported progression in the pose. For this variation, the trickiest part is getting into it. Possibly the easiest—but still not easy—way to get set up is by walking your feet up the wall behind you with your belly facing the wall. Once you have made your way to a forearm stand, walk your elbows back enough to put your belly on the wall. The distance between your elbows and the wall is different for every body. It will even change as your relationship to the posture changes over time regarding

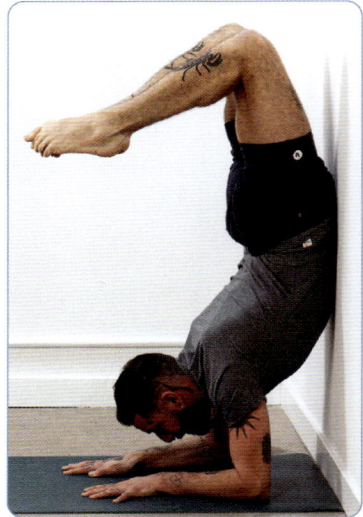

mobility. The second tricky part is exiting the pose, so you may want a teacher present to assist you out if you get stuck. You will want to save enough energy to reverse your steps and work your way back out, so be mindful of that.

Pose Dedicated to the Sage Koundinya I

Eka Pada Kaundinyasana I   एक पाद कौण्डिन्यासन I

Pose dedicated to the sage Koundinya I is a dynamic yoga posture that actively strengthens the wrists, arms, shoulders, chest, and core muscles. Simultaneously, it provides a deep stretch to the muscles of the legs and hips, enhancing flexibility. Additionally, this pose improves spinal rotation! Let's explore some ways you can support this arm balance with props.

Practice with a block or two under your feet to get your leg higher up on your arms.

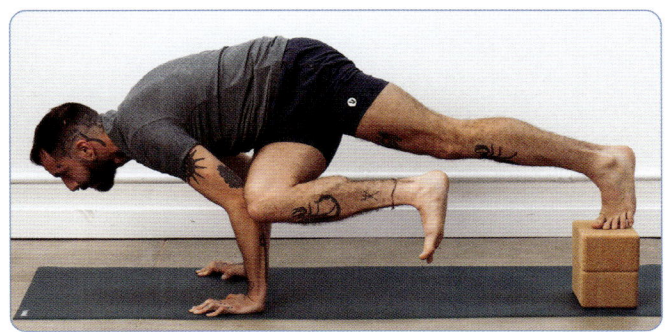

Using blocks to support your practice can make getting into sage I pose more accessible. With your feet on the blocks, you can more easily lift your leg onto your arms without a full liftoff. One way of coming into this posture is by stepping onto a block, or two stacked blocks, on their lowest height with both feet. Bring your feet and knees together in a squatting position and join your hands together at your chest. Twist to the right until your shoulder line is perpendicular to your hip line. Place your hands on the mat, shoulder-width apart. Bend your elbows to create a shelf for your right thigh with your upper arms. Shift your weight into your hands and lean until your right thigh rests on the back of your upper arms. Start lifting your feet while actively squeezing your thighs. Finally, extend your legs, scissoring the left leg back. In an alternate variation, as shown in the photo, you can place the back foot onto a block or a stack of blocks while bringing the opposite knee across the body. This elevation provides additional support and allows you to shift your weight forward into the pose. Consequently, you can raise the back leg without the need to lift it off the ground, mimicking the posture's traditional execution but with added stability. Repeat on the other side.

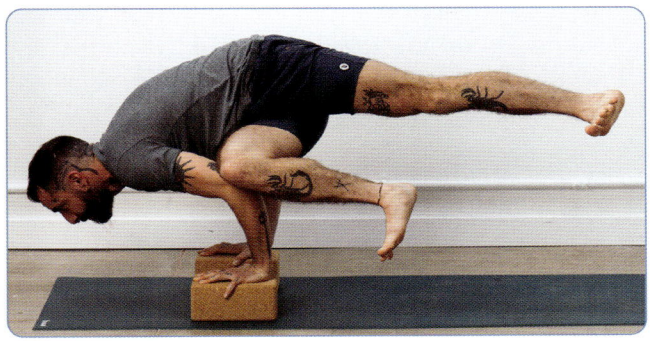

Practice with blocks under your hands to bring the floor closer to you.

When you place blocks under your hands, the blocks bring the floor closer to you, which can be particularly helpful if you have limited mobility in your hips or ankles, which hinders squatting low. A higher starting point lets you work on building strength and flexibility in your upper body and worry less about your lower body mobility. By adding height with the blocks, you can also reduce the amount of twisting required in the pose. This can be beneficial for those who have limited range of motion in their spine or for those who are still working on building the strength and flexibility required to twist deeply.

Practice with blocks under your shoulders for stability.

Using blocks helps you to get more comfortable with shifting weight forward, eliminating the fear of falling onto your face. This version also allows the shoulders more stability as you take flight! Depending on your body proportions, you might require three blocks under each shoulder, but start with stacking two. As you enter the arm balance, keep shifting your weight until

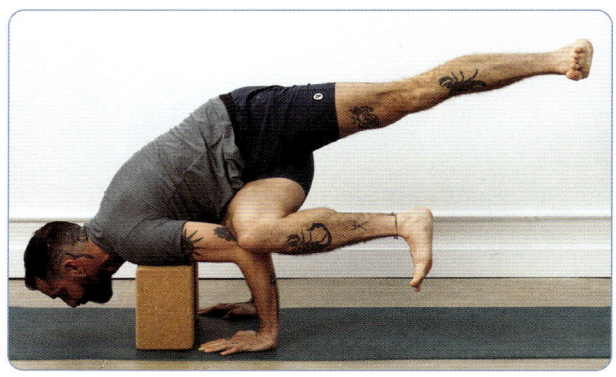

your shoulders come to rest on top of the blocks. Your elbows should be directly above your wrists so that your forearms are perpendicular to the mat. Keep firmly pressing your hands as if you were going to lift the shoulders off the blocks to hover.

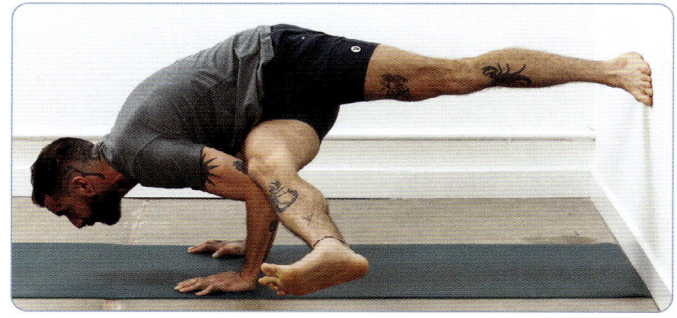

Practice using a wall to capture the feeling of flying.

This wall-supported sage I variation gives you the sensation of flying while getting support from the wall. Squat with your left side to a wall with your feet together and your left shoulder about a leg's length away from the wall. Twist your torso to the right and place your hands on the floor, shoulder-width apart. Lift your hips a little to get your thigh higher onto your arms and shift your weight into your hands, creating chaturanga arms. When you feel the weight in your arms, raise your left foot, extend the leg back, and press the ball of your foot on the wall. Move closer to or farther from the wall if needed. Once you feel comfortable, lift your right foot as well, extending the leg parallel to the wall so the legs are in a scissors shape. Keep your legs active and your shoulders steady by pushing your hands into the floor. Press into the wall with the back foot to engage the muscles of the back leg and be more stable in this arm balance. Hold the pose with your foot on the wall and gradually lean forward until only the big toe rests on the wall. If you feel steady, flex your big toe off the wall. Repeat on the other side.

Place a strap around your arms to strengthen alignment.

Using a strap in sage I pose is helpful for guiding the positioning of the elbows and shoulders. To avoid pinching your skin with the strap, be sure to have the strap looped around the upper arms in a place the thigh will not be resting. Try just above the elbows, because the thigh will ideally be higher up on the arms. Adjust according to your own needs though! Sometimes the elbows will want to splay, which can make finding your balance more challenging and put unnecessary strain on the rotator cuff. Rather than thinking about hugging the elbows in, you will counterintuitively press the arms into the strap. If you measured correctly, the strap will not allow the elbows to splay. When you press into the strap, it eventually stops you from pressing out any more. That

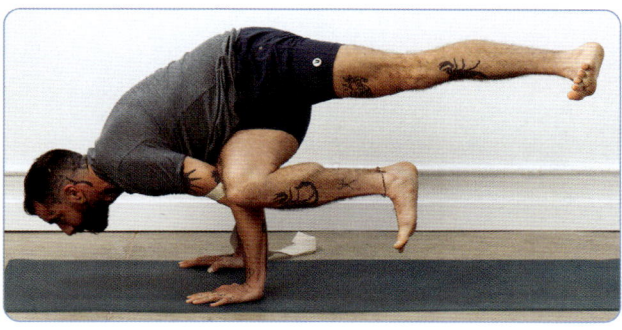

energetic force will instead travel into other parts of your body, reinforcing the actions such as the downward pressing force of your hands into the floor and the protraction of your shoulders, gliding your scapula around your ribs. To strengthen the feeling of hugging your elbows in and keeping the arms parallel to one another, use the strap as a guide rather than something to press into. Try to keep the strap free of tension, like you are pulling away from the strap rather than leaning into it.

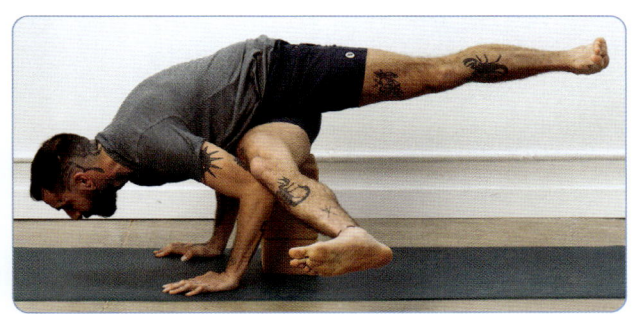

Practice with blocks supporting the weight of your hips.

This technique offers additional support to the hips, allowing for an easier connection between the arms and legs. Stack two or three blocks on their lowest height. Sit on the blocks with your right sitting bone on top, keeping your knees bent and your feet on the floor. Bring your legs together tightly.

Rotate your torso to the right and hook your left elbow on the outside of your right thigh, creating a firm connection between your arm and leg. Lean to the right, making sure that your left sitting bone is not on the block and that you are stable on the outer right hip. Place both hands on the floor, about shoulder-width apart, and shift your weight forward into your hands. As you lean forward onto your hands, bend both elbows and lift your feet off the floor to enter side crow pose. Continue to roll the barrel of your ribs so that the chest is working to face down toward the floor. Extend your legs, scissoring the left leg behind you and reaching the crown of your head forward in the opposite direction. Repeat on the other side.

Practice seated on a chair, with your hands on blocks to remove weight-bearing from the wrists and shoulders.

Take flight on a chair! This is a great option for those who need more stability or want to limit wrist weight-bearing. Sit on the chair and firmly plant both feet on the floor. Place two to four blocks on the right side of the chair, about shoulder-width apart and on the lowest height for added stability. You can stack more blocks for a gentler twist and to raise the height of the floor. Start by twisting your torso to the right and reaching your hands toward the blocks. Once your hands contact them, roll onto your outer right hip and thigh, lifting your feet off the floor and to the left. Place a folded blanket on the chair seat for more cushioning. Once you have lifted your feet off the floor, scissor the legs open, with your right leg extending past the front of

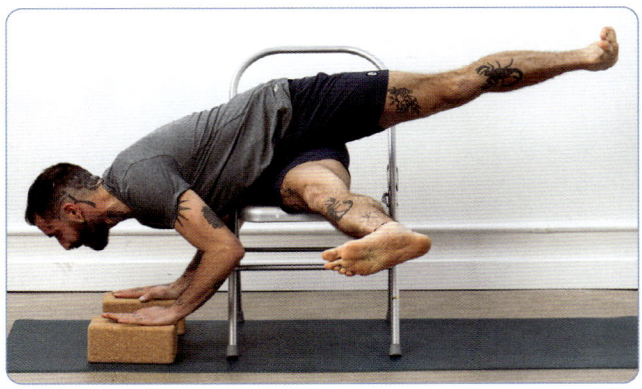

the chair seat and your left leg extending back over the side of the chair seat. Continue to activate the inner thighs as you do so. Most of your weight will be on the chair, so your wrists won't bear much weight. Still, actively press down into the blocks and work to level your left ribs with your right. Repeat on the other side.

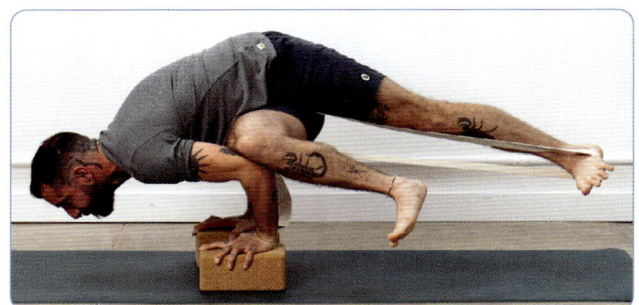

Loop a strap around your back foot, front leg, and hip to engage and align.

Using a looped strap in this pose will reinforce the actions of the legs. This action engages the muscles of the back leg by pressing the foot into the strap, which will offer more lengthening through the side of your body. As you press into the strap with your back foot, the front of the loop will gently draw your bottom hip back, rooting the femur bone into your hip socket. Resisting the pull of the strap on the bottom leg will also help to inform the muscle actions needed in that leg. You may need to experiment and adjust the size of the loop depending on the length of your legs and distance between your feet. Start in a high or low lunge with the strap around the front of your front leg hip and the ball of the back foot. Have your back toes tucked under to keep the strap secure on the foot. If you are beginning from a low lunge, there will be some slack in the loop, but this will tighten up as soon as you extend through the legs. Come into your twist, placing your hand on the mat or blocks with your fingertips perpendicular to the body. Shift your weight onto your arms and extend through your legs. Your back leg will need to shift so that it is perpendicular to the right. Actively kick into the strap with the back foot and notice your legs starting to feel lighter!

Pose Dedicated to the Sage Koundinya II

Eka Pada Kaundinyasana II   एक पाद कौण्डिन्यासन II

The pose dedicated to the sage Koundinya II is a confidence-boosting yoga posture that actively strengthens the wrists, arms, shoulders, chest, and core muscles. Simultaneously, it provides a deep stretch to the muscles of the legs and hips, enhancing flexibility. Explore prop-supported variations to enhance your practice.

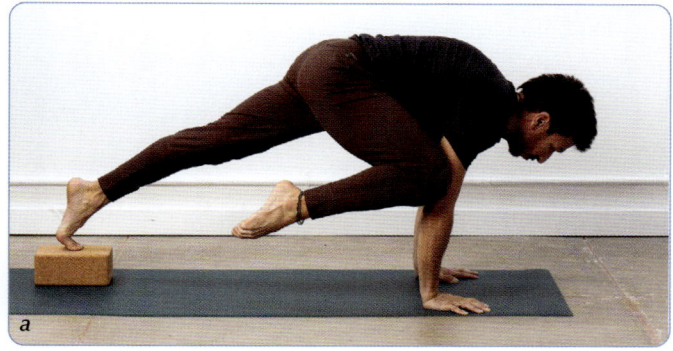

a

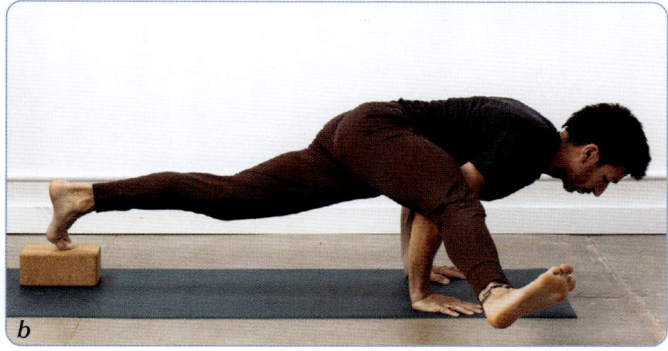

b

Practice with your back foot on a block.

This is a challenging yoga pose that requires strength, flexibility, and balance. Elevating the back foot on a block during practice offers several benefits, including increased hip flexibility, improved core strength, and better balance. Placing the foot on a block forces engagement of the back leg and core muscles, resulting in overall stability and strength in the pose. The lifted leg also benefits from the challenge, with improved strength and tone in the quadriceps, hamstrings, and gluteal muscles. Elevating the back foot can also reduce strain on the lower back and hips that accompany trying to lift the back leg with sheer strength, making the pose safer and more accessible. You may want to start with a little bend in the back knee or with the knee fully grounded and the toes tucked on a block behind you, so that when you shift your weight forward into chaturanga arms and straighten the back leg, the foot will remain on the block (see photos a and b). Finally, if you want to try lifting the back foot off the block, you may find that it is an easier takeoff position!

Practice with blocks under your shoulders and your back foot aligned with a wall for stability.

This sage II variation gives you the sensation of flying while offering support from a wall. As discussed with similar variations in other poses, using blocks helps you eliminate the fear of falling on your face and provides more shoulder stability as you take flight! You may require three blocks under each shoulder, but to start, try stacking two as shown in the photo. You may want to start with a little bend in the back knee or with the knee fully grounded and the back foot flexed against a wall (you have the option here to place it on a block for more support). This is so that when you shift your weight forward into chaturanga arms and straighten the back leg, the foot will remain on the wall. As you enter the arm balance, keep shifting your weight until your shoulders come to rest on the blocks. Your elbows should be directly above the wrists, not behind them, so that your forearms are perpendicular to the mat. Keep firmly pressing through the hands as if you were going to lift the shoulders off the blocks to hover.

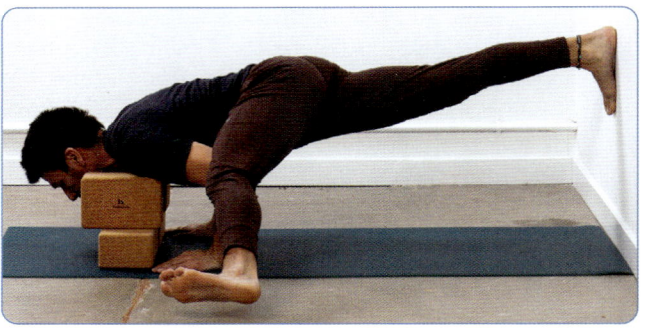

Press into the wall with the back foot to engage the muscles of the back leg and be more stable in this arm balance. Hold the pose with your foot on the wall and gradually lean forward until only the big toe rests on the wall. If you feel steady, flex your big toe off the wall. Repeat on the other side.

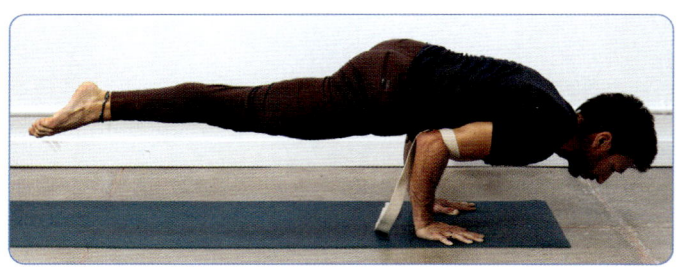

Place a strap around your arms to strengthen alignment.

Using a strap in sage II pose is helpful for positioning of the elbows and shoulders. To avoid pinching your skin with the strap, be sure to have the strap looped around the upper arms in a place the thigh will not be resting. Try just above the elbows, because the thigh will ideally be higher up on the arms. Adjust according to your own needs though! Sometimes the elbows will want to splay, which can make finding your balance more challenging and put unnecessary strain on the rotator cuff. Rather than thinking about hugging the elbows in, you will counterintuitively press the arms into the strap. If you measured correctly, the strap will not allow the elbows to splay. When you press into the strap, it eventually stops you from pressing out any more. That energetic force will instead travel into other parts of your body, reinforcing the actions such as the downward pressing force of your hands into the floor and the protraction of your shoulders, gliding your scapula around your ribs. To strengthen the feeling of hugging your elbows in and keeping the arms parallel to one another, use the strap as a guide rather than something to press into. Try to keep the strap free of tension, like you are pulling away from the strap rather than leaning into it.

Practice on a chair with your hands on blocks to reduce weight-bearing on the wrists and shoulders.

Take flight on a chair! This is a great option for those who need more stability or want to limit wrist weight-bearing. Step your back leg through the back of a chair so that you can get your hips onto the chair or a rolled blanket (for added comfort). Walk your front foot just outside of the front leg of the chair (use a block under the foot if needed). Fold forward, bringing your arms and chest over the front edge of the seat of the chair and place your hands down on the mat or blocks. Draw your front knee in toward your shoulder and lift the front foot off the floor. Continue to shift your weight forward until the belly is on the seat of the chair and the back leg is lifted and extended behind you. You can invite a slight bend in the elbows, mimicking the actions of the arms in the classical arm balance. Because most of your weight will be on the chair, your wrists won't bear much weight, giving you more freedom to focus on the actions of the legs and posterior chain, finding spinal extension, and activating through the inner thighs. Repeat on the other side.

Invert a chair for hip and wrist support.

This chair-supported variation of sage II provides the pelvic support necessary to lift the legs from the floor for those still building up the strength and stability to do the traditional version. It also offers less weight-bearing on the wrists.

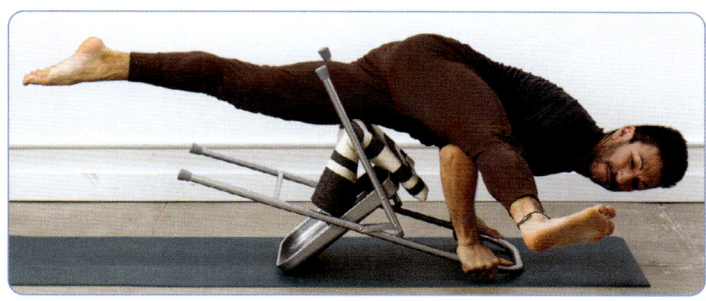

Pelvic support helps so you can switch your focus to refining the actions of the arms by hugging the elbows toward the ribs and engaging the core. Flip your chair upside down so that its legs are up. Place a folded blanket or two on the crossbar between the back chair legs, then step over the crossbar and come into a wide pyramid pose with your front foot outside the back of the chair railing. Place your hands on the railing in front of you and bend your front knee until your hips rest comfortably on the crossbar and blankets. Gently bend at your elbows and hug your front knee into the front shoulder, adducting the inner thigh. Shift your weight forward to lift the back leg off the floor. As you come into this pose, consider starting the practice with your front foot grounded or extended to adjust the challenge. Repeat on the other side.

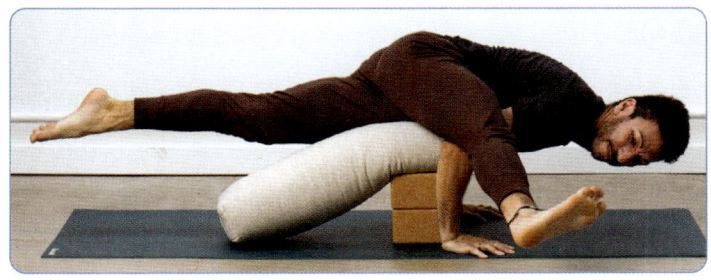

Prop yourself up with a bolster and two blocks.

This option is another great tool for providing pelvic support while taking flight. Stack two blocks on the lowest height horizontally on top of one another. Then place the bolster on top of the blocks, creating a ramp with the bolster. Enter lizard pose with your pelvis grounded on the bolster where it rests on the blocks. Your hands will be on the mat, just inside your front leg. Walk your hands back toward the blocks, bending the elbows so that the hand closest to your front leg is just behind the front foot. Work your front knee high up onto your front shoulder and squeeze the knee into your shoulder to lift the front foot. Squeeze your front foot toward your buttocks, bending at the knee. Continue to shift your weight forward, finding chaturanga arms, and float your back leg off the mat. Your hips should be resting on the blocks and shoulders. Try not to let your head and neck collapse while gazing forward. To continue expanding the actions of your legs, try extending your front leg. Repeat on the other side.

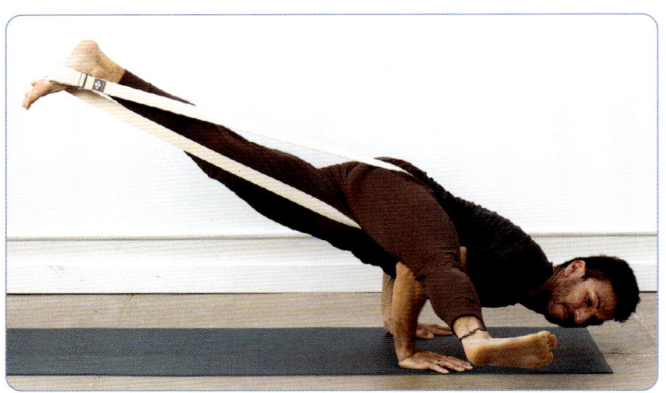

Use a strap to engage and align.

Using a looped strap here will reinforce the actions of the legs. This action engages the muscles of the back leg by pressing the foot into the strap, which will provide more lengthening through the side of your body. As you press into the strap with your back foot, the front of the loop will gently draw your front hip back, rooting the femur bone into your hip socket and stabilizing the sacroiliac joint. Resisting the pull of the strap on the front leg will also help inform the muscle actions needed in that leg. Experiment with the size of the loop and adjust as needed. Enter this pose by starting in a runner's lunge with the strap around the front of your front leg hip and the ball of the back foot. Tuck your back toes under to keep the strap secure on the foot. From here, toe-heel your front foot to the outside of your hand, coming into lizard pose. Hug your front knee into your shoulder, adducting through the inner thigh, and lift your front foot off the mat. Shift your weight forward, coming into chaturanga arms, then press into the strap with your back foot to lift the back leg. Kick into the strap with the back foot and notice your legs starting to feel lighter. This kicking action will also help to bring the feeling of locust pose into the lower half of your body, necessary to lifting the back leg. To expand from here, try extending the front leg.

Parshva Bhuja Dandasana पार्श्वभुजदण्डासन

Side arm staff pose, commonly referred to as grasshopper pose, can be a challenging yet rewarding yoga posture that strengthens the wrists, arms, shoulders, chest, and core muscles. This dynamic pose also increases flexibility in the hips and hamstrings while enhancing overall balance, coordination, and range of motion in the spine. In addition to the variations discussed in the following pages, place a bolster in front of you to practice falling. Let's explore some of the ways you can prop up this pose and support your determination!

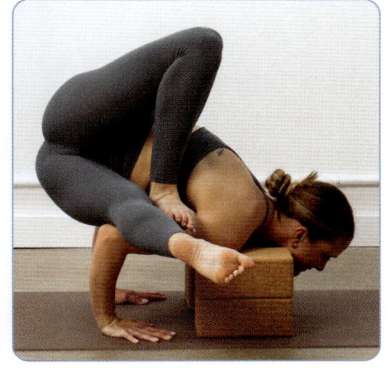

Practice with blocks under your shoulders for stability.

Using blocks helps you to get more comfortable with shifting weight forward, eliminating the fear of falling on your face. This version also gives the shoulders more stability as you take flight! Other benefits include deepening the stretch in your chest and shoulders, improving your posture, reducing tension, and reducing strain on the neck and upper back, making the pose more comfortable overall. You may require three blocks under each shoulder, but to start, try stacking two as shown in the photo. As you enter the arm balance, keep shifting your weight until your shoulders rest on top of the blocks. Your elbows should be directly above the wrists, not behind them, so that your forearms are perpendicular to the mat. Keep firmly pressing your hands as if you were going to lift the shoulders off the blocks to hover.

Practice with blocks under your hands to bring the floor closer to you.

When you place blocks under your hands, it can be easier to reach the floor, which can be particularly helpful if you have limited mobility in your hips, ankles, or hamstrings, which hinders squatting low. A higher starting point lets you work on building strength and flexibility in your upper body and worry less about your lower body mobility. By adding height with the blocks, you can also reduce the amount of twisting required in the pose. This can be beneficial for

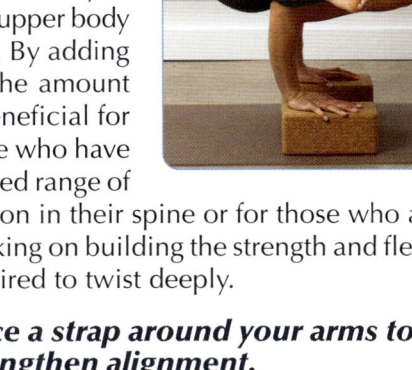

those who have limited range of motion in their spine or for those who are still working on building the strength and flexibility required to twist deeply.

Place a strap around your arms to strengthen alignment.

Using a strap in grasshopper pose is a helpful tool in guiding the positioning of the elbows and shoulders. To avoid pinching your skin with the strap, ensure the strap is looped above the elbows, ideally placing it just above the elbows.

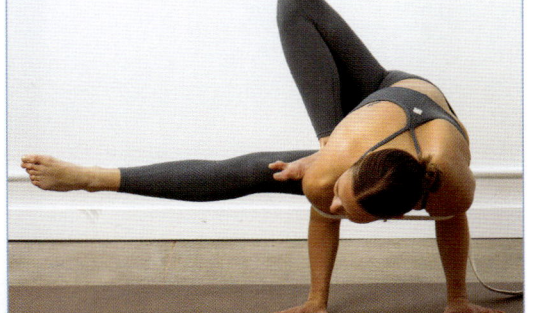

The strap will keep your elbows from splaying as well as provide a force to press into, promoting better balance and avoiding unnecessary strain on the rotator cuff. Engaging with the strap in this way reinforces other essential movements, such as the force of your hands into the floor and the protraction of the shoulders, guiding your scapula around your ribs. Alternatively, if you want to strengthen the feeling of hugging your elbows in and keeping the arms parallel to one another, use the strap as a guide rather than something to press into. Try to keep the strap free of tension, like you are pulling away from the strap rather than leaning into it.

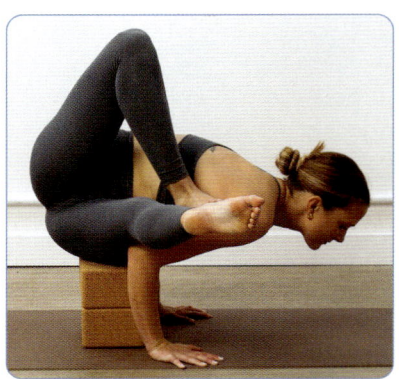

Practice with two blocks supporting the weight of your hips.

This technique offers additional support to the hips, allowing for an easier connection between the arms and legs. Stack two blocks on their lowest height. Sit on the blocks with your left sitting bone on top, keeping your knees bent and your feet on the floor. Cross your right ankle over your left knee, bringing your legs into a figure four position. Rotate your torso to the left and hook your right foot inside your right armpit (or as close as you can manage), creating a firm connection. Lean to the left, making sure that your right sitting bone is not on the block and that you are stable on the outer left hip. Place both hands on the floor about shoulder-width apart and shift your weight forward into your hands. As you lean forward onto your hands, bend both elbows and lift your other foot off the floor to enter grasshopper pose. Continue to roll the barrel of your ribs so that the chest is working to face down toward the floor. Extend through your bottom leg, activating your thigh. Repeat on the other side.

Practice seated on a chair with your hands on blocks to remove weight-bearing from the wrists and shoulders.

Take flight on a chair! This is a great option for those who need more stability or want to limit wrist weight-bearing. Sit on the chair and firmly plant both feet on the floor. Place two to four blocks on the left side of the chair, about shoulder-width apart and on the lowest height for added stability. Stack more blocks for a gentler twist and to raise the height of the floor. Cross your right ankle over your left knee, bringing your legs into a figure four position. Rotate your torso to the left and hook your right foot inside your right armpit (or as close as you can manage), creating a

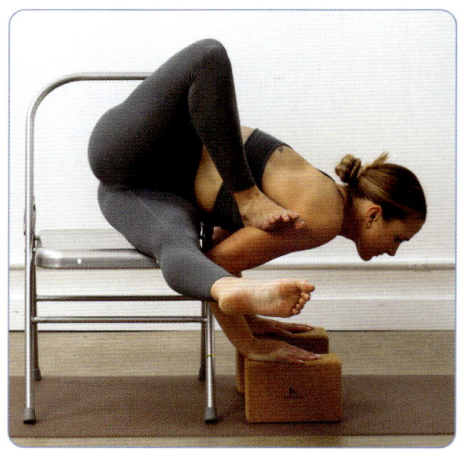

firm connection. Reach for the blocks with your hands, then roll onto your outer left hip and thigh, lifting your bottom foot off the floor and extending that leg. Most of your weight will be on the chair, so your wrists won't bear much weight, and you can focus on the subtle actions of the legs and the spine. Still, actively press into the blocks and work to level your right ribs with your left. Repeat on the other side.

Place your foot on a block to reduce the weight on your arm.

This is a wonderful option for those with limited hip mobility or those who are working up to the demands of having the full weight of their foot on the back of their arms. Stand with one, two, or three stacked blocks to the right of you (two shown in the photo). Come into a figure four position and twist to the right. Rather than hooking your foot onto the back of your arm, bring the back of your right thigh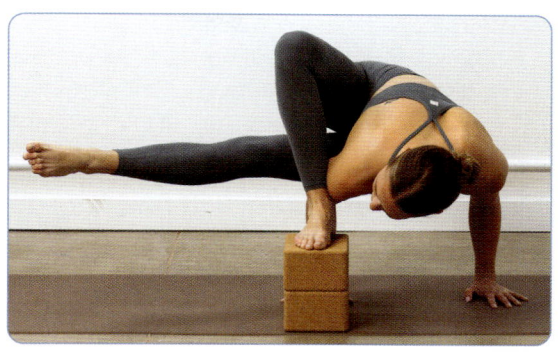

(just inside the foot) high up onto your left triceps. Place your hands on the mat and position them so the right hand is just inside and slightly behind the blocks. Shift your weight forward into your hands and lean until your right thigh rests on the back of your upper arms, coming into chaturanga arms. Place your right foot on top of the blocks and firmly press down to take some of the hips' weight off the arm. Extend fully through your right leg and breathe. Notice that if you add more blocks, the need for hip mobility increases, and therefore so does the challenge. Conversely, if you would like to make the pose more accessible, start with just one block. This helps you to build up mobility and eventually have your foot shoulder high without compromising alignment or chest and shoulder integrity. Repeat on the other side.

Sit with your hands pressing into a wall.

This is a great option for those who want to minimize weight-bearing on their wrists and focus on increasing the mobility needed to execute this posture. Sit with your left hip about a foot (0.3 m) away from the wall. Cross your right ankle over your left knee, creating a figure four. Reach your right arm across your left thigh, trying to get your foot onto the back of your arm, near your armpit. Grasp your left shin or ankle with your hand and place your left hand on the floor behind you to deepen into the twist. Take a few breaths. When you

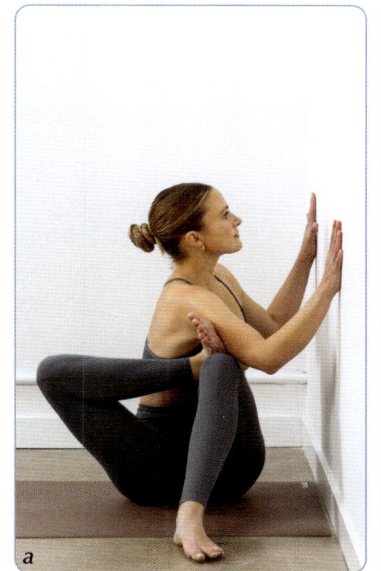
a

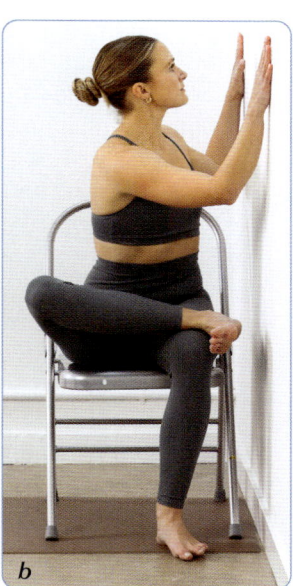
b

are ready, place your left hand on the wall, then the right hand, shoulder-distance apart, like chaturanga arms with a slight bend in the elbows. Press your left hand into the wall to open the left side of the chest, bringing it level with the right. Continue to lengthen through your spinal column as you anchor your sitting bones into the mat (see photo a). Repeat on the other side. To modify this pose even more, come into a figure four position seated on a chair and work on thoracic rotation without hooking the foot (see photo b).

One-Legged Crow Pose

Eka Pada Kakasana   एक पाद काकासन

One-legged crow pose can initially seem challenging, especially compared to crow pose, but with the support of props, it becomes achievable! This yoga posture builds balance and coordination while actively strengthening the arms, wrists, back, and abdominal muscles. Additionally, it opens and stretches the groin and upper back. Try prop variations for a balanced and strengthened one-legged crow pose experience.

Practice with a block in front of you to direct your gaze.

As with the crow and crane pose, it is important in this pose to remember to keep the gaze in front of you. Your weight will shift where your gaze goes, so place an object such as a block slightly in front of you to remember where to look while shifting forward into the arm balance. If you gaze down or back at your feet, you likely will have trouble shifting forward enough to stack your elbows over your wrists.

Practice with a block under your forehead for stability and to conquer fear.

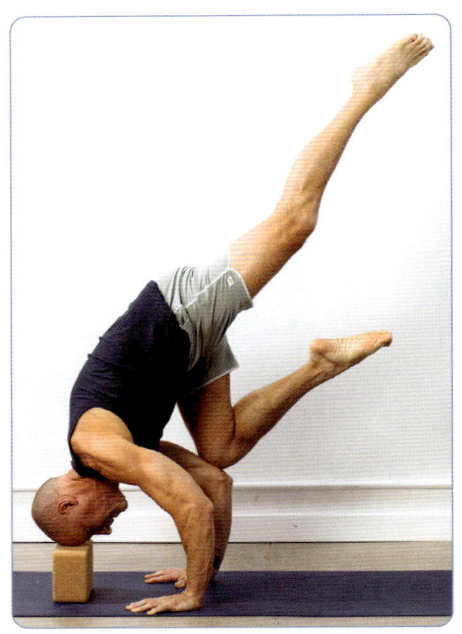

Using a block will help you to get more comfortable with shifting your weight forward, eliminating the fear of falling on your face; you can have the block against a wall as well if you need the reassurance. Start with your feet parallel on the mat. Place a block on its tallest height about one foot (0.3 m) in front of the hands (or the distance from your head to your elbows in chaturanga). Enter crow pose by shifting your weight forward, gazing toward the block. Feel your toes lifting off the mat, bring the big toes to touch, and raise the heels toward the buttocks. Continue shifting forward until your forehead meets the top of the block, ensuring your elbows are directly above your wrists for perpendicular forearms. To distribute your weight evenly into the wrists and avoid strain on the shoulders and upper arms, start with your knees closer to your elbows, gradually working them higher over time due to the deeper bend in your elbows. Once you feel stable, draw one knee off the back of your arm to hover between your elbows. If you feel comfortable, try extending your leg.

Practice with blocks under your shoulders for stability.

Using blocks helps you to get more comfortable with shifting weight forward, eliminating the fear of falling on your face. This version allows the shoulders to be slightly higher than the elbows—more than in the version with the block under your forehead. Set up for the pose, but place two blocks on the lowest height in front of the hands and an additional two blocks stacked tall on top of them as shown in the photo. Enter the arm balance, shifting your weight forward and keeping your gaze forward and down. Keep shifting forward until your shoulders come to rest on the blocks, adjusting the height of the blocks if needed. Your elbows should be directly above the wrists, not behind them, so that your forearms are

The Complete Guide to Yoga Props

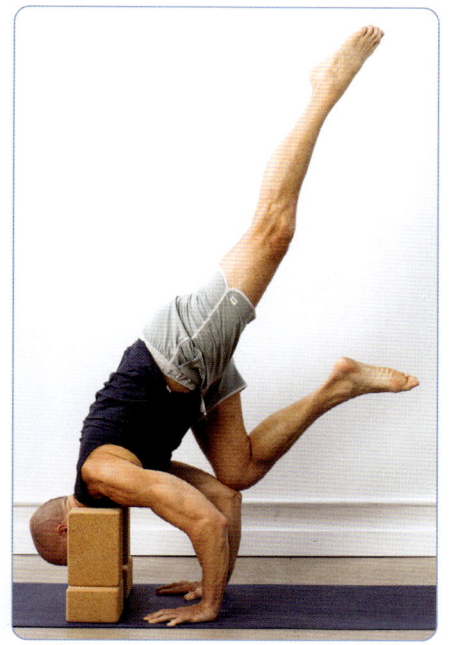

perpendicular to the mat. Once you feel stable, draw one knee off the back of your arm to hover between the elbows. If you feel comfortable, extend your leg. Keep firmly pressing the hands as if you were going to lift the shoulders off the blocks to hover. Repeat on the other side.

Place a bolster in front of you for a softer fall.

As mentioned earlier in this chapter, it is good to practice falling out of poses. The more control over the situation you have, the more confidence you will have. Practice falling by bringing your knees out to the sides and your shins on the mat. If the dismount doesn't go as planned, the cushioned surface of a bolster will make for a more comfortable landing.

Place a strap around your arms to strengthen alignment.

To enhance stability in one-legged crow pose, use a strap looped around your arms for crucial support during the transition. Keeping your arms close with the strap allows you to concentrate on core activation, balance, and strength. Stand at the front of your mat with feet hip-width apart, looping the strap around your upper arms, just above the elbows. Transition into a squat, placing your hands on the mat, and bring your knees onto the backs of your upper arms. Initially, stacking your knees on your elbows provides stability, aligning the downward force of your femur bones directly over the forearms. This alignment distributes weight evenly, easing the battle with gravity. Over time, work the knees higher up the arms,

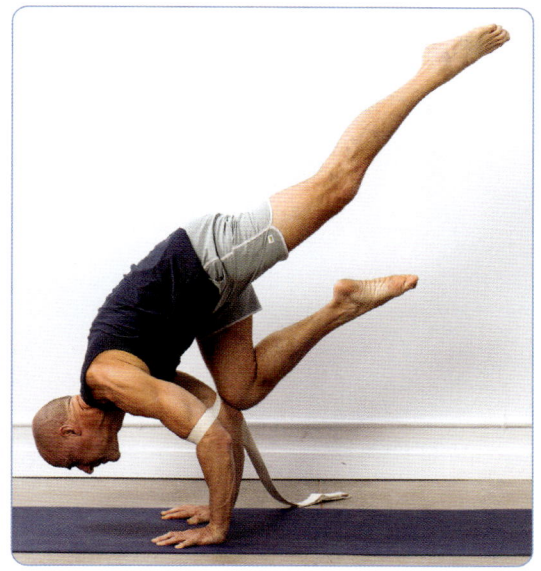

shifting your weight forward to lift your feet off the floor and balance on your hands. Once you feel stable, draw one knee off the back of your arm to hover between the elbows. If you feel comfortable, extend your leg. Press your outer arms into the strap to reinforce shoulder protraction and core engagement. Keep your gaze slightly forward as you hold the pose for a few breaths. Repeat on the other side.

Practice standing to take weight-bearing from your shoulders and focus on the actions of the hips.

This is a great option for those who cannot bring weight into the wrists due to pain or injury. It will also help to strengthen and lengthen the psoas—necessary muscle actions to accomplish this pose. Measure your standing distance by stretching your arms out in front of you and placing your hands on the wall as if you were in plank pose. Release your hands from the wall and grab your prop of choice—a block, a folded blanket, or maybe even a towel for a lighter challenge. Lift your right knee into your chest, coming into one-legged mountain pose, and place your prop into your hip crease. Hug the thigh into the chest to stabilize the prop and engage your deep pelvic and abdominal muscles. Place your hands back on the wall to inform postural alignment and aid in stability. Repeat on the other side.

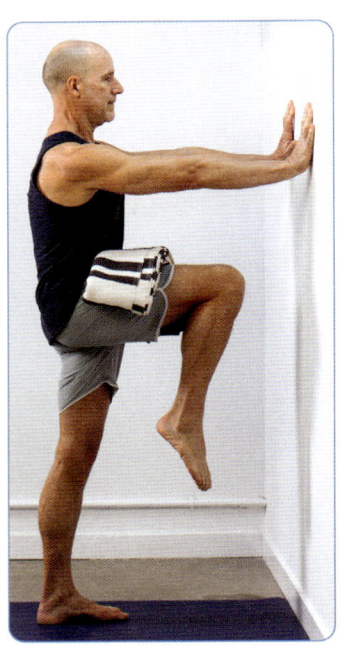

Practice knee lifts from a block.

This variation can be thought of as a drill that will help you build the strength needed to effortlessly perform the one-legged crow pose in the future. To start, place a block on its tallest height and medium width in front of your toes and behind your hands as you set up for crow pose. Lift your hips and bring your knees toward your triceps, keeping one knee on the upper arm while sliding the other off so that the shin of that leg rests on the block between and slightly behind your hands. As you shift your weight into your hands, lift your toes off the floor sense the posture with structural support. To challenge yourself further, lift your shin to hover over the block for a few seconds before lowering it. Eventually, you might gain the strength and confidence to extend your leg all the way back, balancing your opposite knee on just one arm.

Place a foot on a block to practice shifting your weight forward.

You would approach this similarly to the way you would enter a crow pose with your feet on a block. Using a block will help you to feel comfortable with shifting your weight forward. With the help of a block, you can come into one-legged crow pose without having to lift your foot off the floor. Enter crow pose with your feet on a block, then practice sliding one knee off your upper arm and bringing it to hover below your chest. Try hugging the top of that thigh toward your chest and engaging your hamstrings to squeeze your heel toward your buttock. If you are feeling strong and stable here, you can eventually attempt to lift the toes of the grounded leg from the block. Another option

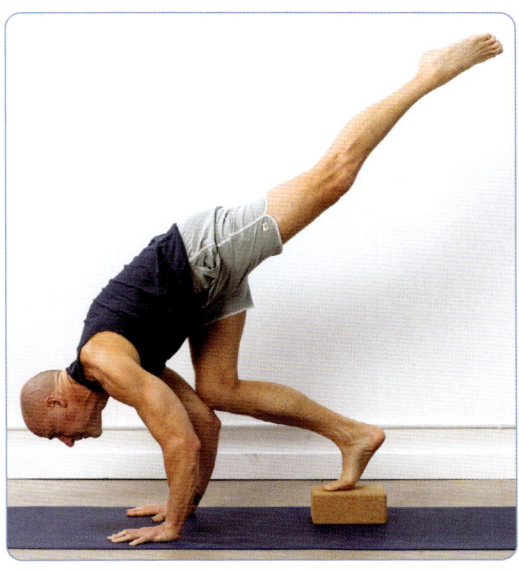

is keeping the toes grounded on the block and focusing on extending the hovering leg back. Over time, you can put these variations together to build your one-legged crow pose.

Practice with a wall to build confidence and strength.

Mastering one-legged crow pose demands strength and balance, achievable through a wall-supported approach. This variation fosters confidence and strength by providing stability. The wall helps ensure a solid foundation for the extended leg, while enhancing muscle engagement. The practice also enhances core strength and overall body awareness, fostering concentration and mental focus. Set up for crow pose with your back facing a wall. Bring your knees toward your triceps, keeping your elbows bent and your palms firmly pressed into the floor. Once you feel stable, extend one leg back behind you toward a wall, eventually pressing the ball of your extended foot into the wall. As you press the

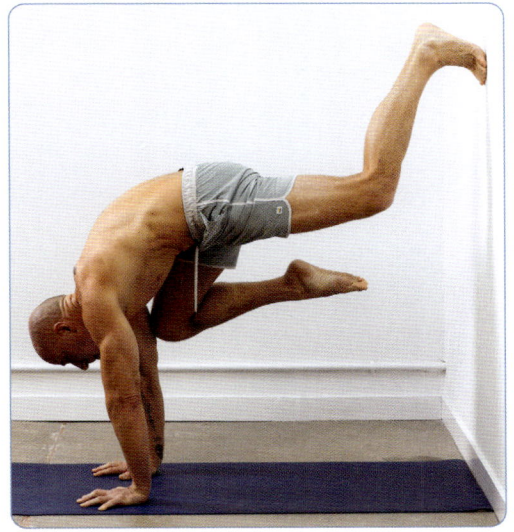

foot into the wall, you should feel a sense of grounding and stability. With the leg firmly anchored to the wall, try lifting your other foot off the ground, shifting your weight forward into your hands. As you engage your core and arm muscles, you have the option to try and straighten your arms into crane pose and lift your hips higher, as shown in the photo. Hold the pose for a few breaths, then release and repeat on the other side.

One-Legged Crow Pose *(continued)*

Practice with blocks or a chair under your back foot to support the feeling of flying.

This variation with blocks or a chair can help you get the feeling of flying into one-legged crow pose while providing support and stability. It can also help you build strength and balance in your core and leg muscles, as well as enhance overall body awareness. Place a block or chair behind you. Measure the distance between your hands and feet so that when you step onto your props, you can find chaturanga-like arms without your feet sliding off the props. To do this, enter a plank position and step your feet onto the seat of the chair or your blocks. Measure the distance between your back feet and your hands in plank pose, then walk your hands back about a foot (0.3 m), piking your hips slightly. This is about the distance needed to shift forward into chaturanga arms. Draw your right knee toward your triceps and shift your weight forward onto your bent arms. Press your knee into your triceps and squeeze your heel toward your buttock, engaging your core and leg muscles. Keep your shoulders protracted and your back leg firm (see photo *a* for an example with blocks and photo *b* for an example with a chair). When you feel stable, try hovering your foot off the prop. Repeat on the other side.

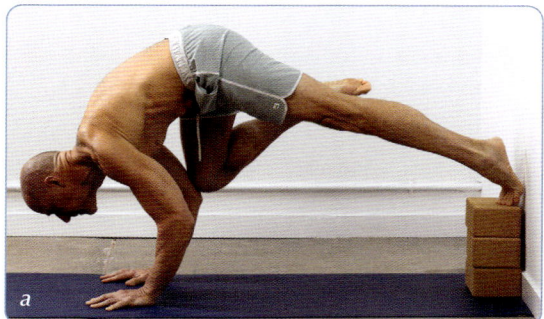 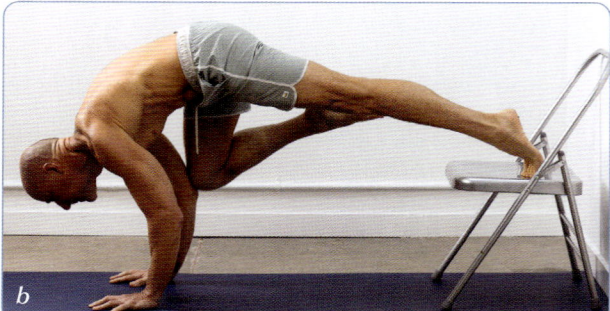

Flying Lizard Pose

Udayana Utthan Prishthasana   उदयन उत्थान पृष्ठासन

Flying lizard pose is a dynamic yoga posture that effectively strengthens and tones the arms, legs, and core, while simultaneously improving flexibility in the legs, hips, and groin. Let's explore some ways you can support this arm balance with props.

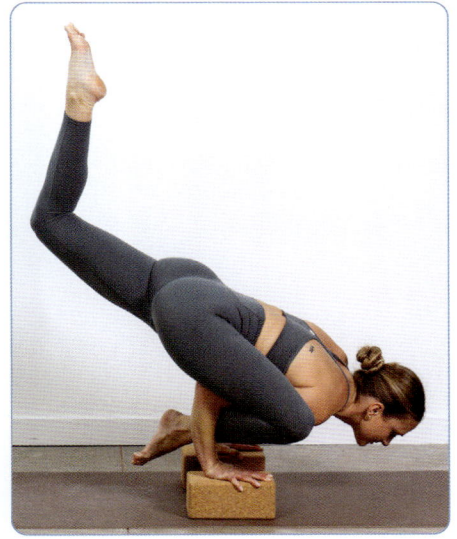

Practice with blocks under your hands to raise the height of the floor.

Flying lizard pose, a challenging arm balance necessitating strength and flexibility, benefits from block support. The elevation achieved with a block is helpful for those who are uncomfortable with their face so close to the floor and the elevation creates more space to wrap the front leg around the forearm. Begin in lizard pose, then shimmy your right shoulder under your right knee, reaching your right arm under the leg and placing your hand down just outside the foot. Place two blocks on their lowest or medium height under the hands, keeping your fingers spread wide and your palms firmly pressed down. Rock your weight forward, as if you were approaching chaturanga, simultaneously lifting your right toes off the mat. Focus on hugging your right inner thigh into your arm while wrapping and hugging your right outer shin into the arm at the same time. As you continue to shift forward, your back foot will naturally lift off the mat. Engage through the posterior chain muscles to lift the leg higher. Remember to breathe deeply and hold for a few breaths before repeating on the other side.

Practice with your back thigh on a chair or stacked blocks to reduce weight on the wrists and take flight in a supported way.

This variation is an effective way to establish muscle memory with added structural support. With the back leg supported, accessibility increases, allowing you to focus on the actions of the front leg and upper body. It significantly reduces weight-bearing on the wrists, making it

ideal for those with wrist pain or injury. Place your back knee on a chair, sliding it back until the thigh is fully on the chair. The back shin can go through the chair's backrest opening or rest on the back rail. Alternatively, you can use stacked blocks for height and support instead of a chair. Move your hips forward until you can firmly plant your front foot on the floor, then fold forward and place your hands inside the front foot to enter lizard pose. Wiggle your shoulder under your knee, reaching your arm beneath the leg, and place your hand just outside the foot. Shift your weight forward while simultaneously lifting your right toes

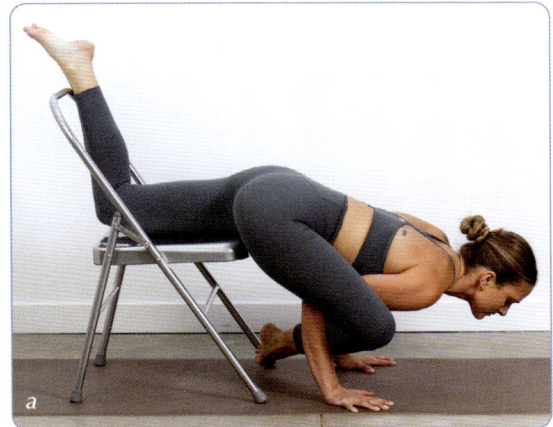

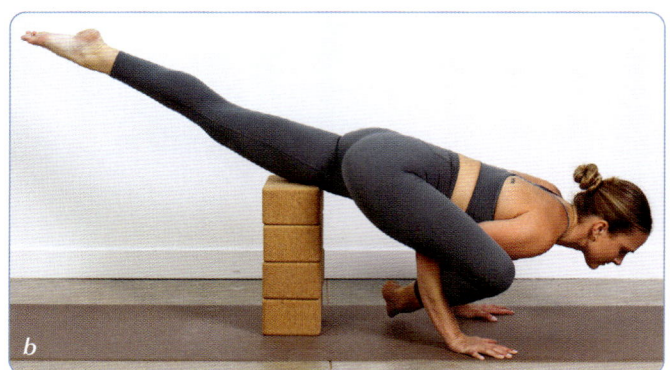

off the mat. Be cautious if you have a wrist injury while experimenting with rocking your weight forward. Concentrate on hugging your right inner thigh into your arm and wrapping your right outer shin into the arm simultaneously. Contract the thigh muscles of your back leg (see photo *a* for an example with a chair and photo *b* for an example with blocks). Repeat on the other side.

Chapter 7

Inversions

When I initially ventured into yoga, I mistakenly lumped arm balances and inversions into the same category. However, inversions don't always necessitate defying gravity. In their essence, inversions are postures that position the heart and hips above the head, effectively inverting one's typical upright stance. By embracing an orientation that is unnatural, we can use these upside-down positions to rebalance both body and mind by shifting into a new perspective, both literally and metaphorically. The act of courageously going upside down can also serve as a significant confidence booster. Furthermore, inversions are known for their potential benefits in aiding circulation and venous return, directing deoxygenated blood back to the heart and oxygen-rich blood to the brain. Additionally, by stimulating lymph movement, certain inversions may alleviate pain or swelling in elevated areas. While increased blood flow to the heart can be invigorating, some inversions are believed to have a calming effect on the nervous system. With the support of props, we can safely explore these postures, whether our aim is intensifying, easing, or adapting the traditional pose. In addition to the inversion poses in this chapter, you'll discover other inversions featured in other chapters, strategically placed where they align more seamlessly with the overall flow.

Mantra: On certain days, my heart guides me, rising above the chatter of the mind.

Downward-Facing Dog Pose

Adho Mukha Shvanasana अधोम्‌खश्वानासन

Downward-facing dog pose is a foundational yoga posture that offers a myriad of benefits. This pose actively lengthens hamstrings and calves, elongates the spine, improves circulation, and strengthens the upper body. To enhance your practice, let's explore a few prop-supported variations.

Place blocks under your hands to reduce pressure on the wrists.

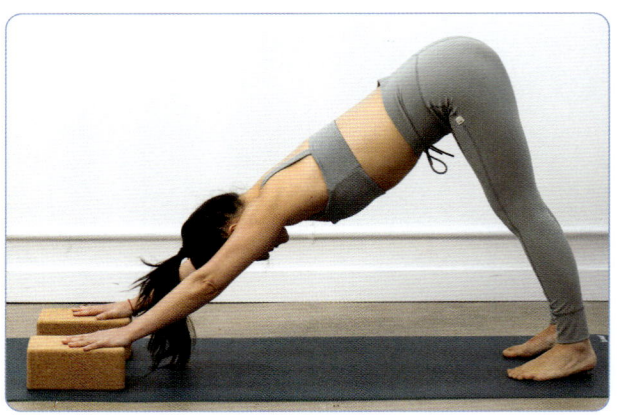

Utilizing blocks beneath your hands in downward-facing dog offers numerous advantages, such as redistributing weight toward the lower body and alleviating pressure on the wrists. This is particularly beneficial for individuals experiencing wrist pain. Start in a plank position with your hands on the blocks at their lowest height. This will help you measure the appropriate distance between your hands and feet for downward dog. On an exhale, lift your hips up and back into downward dog, bending the knees as necessary to lengthen through your spine. Ground through your knuckles on the blocks and wrap your upper, outer arm bones toward the mat. Firm through your thighs, lifting your femur bones into the hip sockets as you lengthen your heels toward the mat. To get the feeling of flexing through the fronts of your legs, try flexing your toes up while keeping the rest of your foot rooted firmly on the mat. Contracting through the fronts of your thighs aids in lengthening the hamstrings and alleviates additional pressure from the upper body.

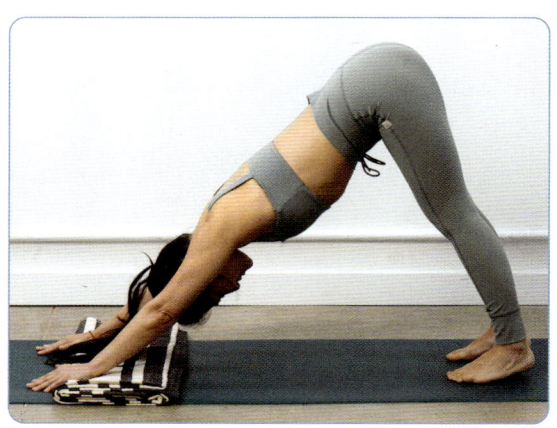

Fold a blanket or mat under the heels of your hands to decrease wrist flexion.

A great way to support your wrists during yoga practice is by folding a blanket or mat under the heels of your hands. This modification can be particularly helpful for those who have discomfort in their wrists during weight-bearing postures such as downward-facing dog. By elevating the heels of your hands, you can decrease the amount of wrist flexion required in these poses, which can reduce the strain on your wrists and make the postures more accessible. Additionally, this modification can help to distribute your weight more evenly through your hands and arms, which can help to prevent strain and injury. To practice this modification, simply fold a blanket or mat into a small, even rectangle and place it under the heels of your hands when entering weight-bearing poses such as this. Make sure to adjust the height of the blanket or mat to a level that feels comfortable and supportive for your wrists.

Place a block or bolster under your forehead to extend and release through the neck.

Placing a block or bolster under your forehead in downward-facing dog is a great way to extend and release tension in the cervical spine (neck). This modification provides a reference point for where to rest your head, allowing for greater extension through the spine. Starting in a plank position, measure the appropriate distance between your hands and feet for downward dog. On an exhale, lift your hips up and

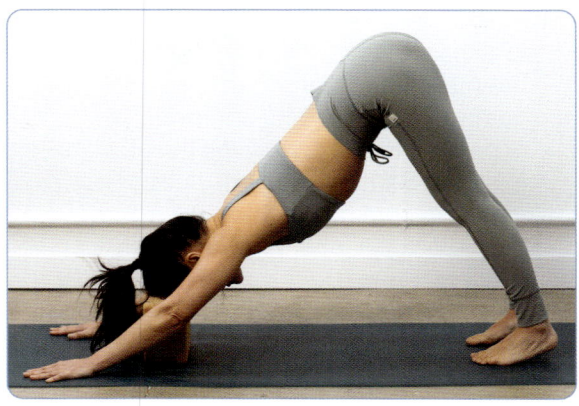

back into downward dog. Slide a block on medium height under your forehead to relax through your head and neck. The height of the block or bolster will vary based on your height, so you may need to adjust the level, stack two, or use a thick bolster. Make sure to place the prop so that when you rest your forehead, your ears are in line with your biceps. This modification allows for the facial and neck muscles to release any strain or tension, creating a more comfortable and enjoyable downward-facing dog pose.

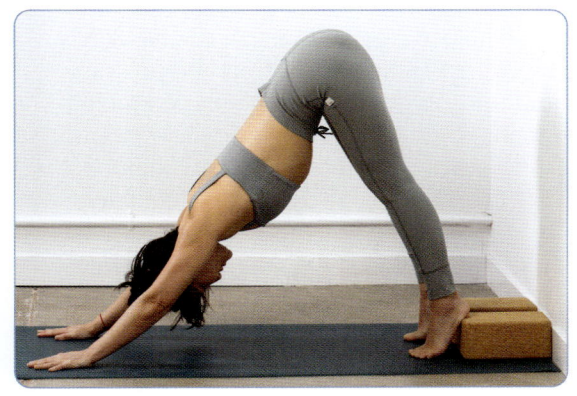

Place blocks under your heels to bring the floor to you and to engage your leg muscles.

Using blocks in downward-facing dog is an excellent variation for those who cannot reach their heels to the mat. The blocks stabilize the feet and legs, keeping the heels from turning in or out and helping to keep the legs parallel. For added stability, you can place the blocks against a wall. Begin by placing the blocks on their lowest height, hip-width apart and against a wall. Enter your downward dog, resting the heels of your feet on top of the blocks and the balls of your feet on the mat. Direct your heels straight back and press them into the blocks. This helps to activate the muscles on the front of your body. Use the feedback from the blocks to firm your thighs and engage your quadriceps (fronts of thighs). If you prefer not to use blocks, you can bring your heels directly to the wall. By engaging your legs and lifting your quadriceps, you can take some weight off your hands, making the pose more comfortable and accessible.

Place a block between your thighs to stabilize your core and pelvic muscles.

Using a block between your thighs in downward-facing dog can be a great way to stabilize your core and pelvic muscles while also engaging and lifting your groin and thighs. Place a block on its narrowest width between your thighs, high up near the pubis, and then enter downward dog. Once in the pose, hug the block up and in toward the pubis, engaging your inner thighs. For those with tight hip flexors and hamstrings, the feeling of a slight internal rotation of the thighs can help to combat pelvic tucking and bring you back to neutral. Imagine pressing the block back in space slightly. This will help to narrow the frontal hip points and widen across the lower back, lengthening the hamstrings and deepening the psoas stretch. Remember to keep your toes and knees pointing forward.

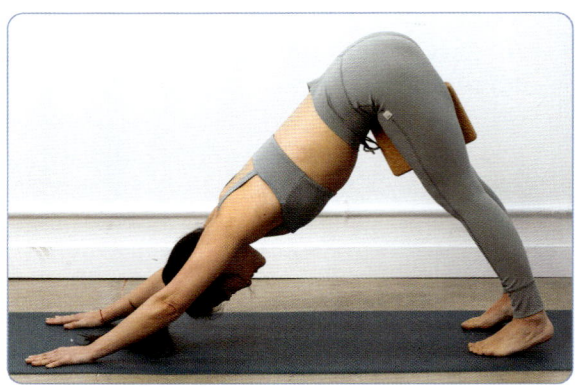

Align and engage by looping a strap around your thighs.

Practicing downward-facing dog with a strap looped around the thighs has many benefits. By engaging the abductor muscles of the legs, you encourage a widening between the sitting bones and a lifting action through the inner legs from the arches of the feet to the pubic bone. This can help to create more space in the pelvis and low back, relieving tension and pressure. In addition, engaging through the abductors can help to bring greater stability and support to the hips, which can be particularly helpful for those with hip pain or instability. This can also improve overall balance and alignment in the pose, helping to ensure that both sides of the body are equally engaged and active.

Align and engage by looping a strap around your arms.

Looping a strap around the arms, shoulder-width apart, can provide several benefits during the downward-facing dog pose. It helps to inform weight distribution in the upper body, from hands to shoulders. By engaging the muscles around the upper arms, it encourages a balanced weight distribution, taking pressure off the wrists and reducing the risk of injury. In addition, looping a strap around the upper arms or forearms can encourage a broadening

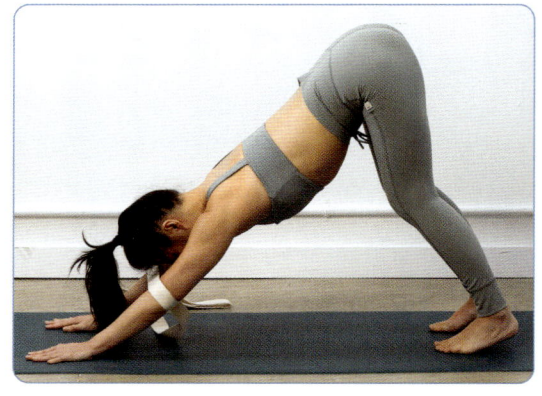

action in the upper back. As you glide the scapula around the sides of the ribs, it helps to open the chest and shoulders, reducing tension and stiffness in the neck and shoulders. This can be particularly beneficial for those with tightness or limited mobility in the upper body, because it provides support to help maintain proper form. It also helps to bring awareness to any imbalances or asymmetries in the body, allowing for greater balance and alignment during the pose.

Create a do-it-yourself rope wall to support you and apply traction to the spine.

This variation does involve a slightly unconventional prop—a door with handles! Once hooked up to the door, a strap in your hip creases will lift and support, taking most of the weight from your upper body. The strap will also help to traction (create space in) the spine and lengthen the hamstrings. Create a large loop with your strap, then

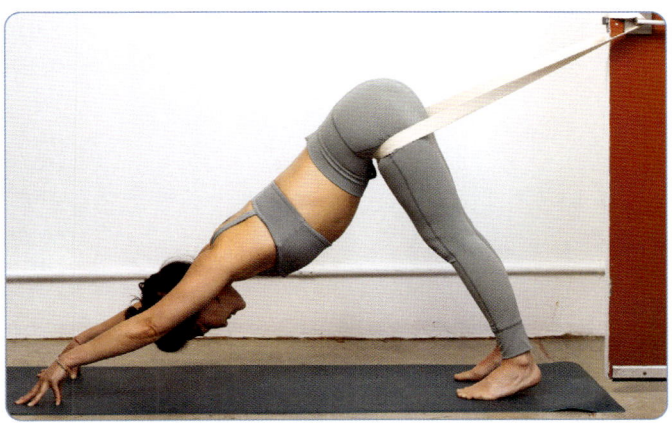

open the door and loop one end of the strap around the handles on both sides. Take the other half of the loop over your body with your back facing the door. Put the strap over your thighs, just below the hip creases. Fold forward, over the strap, then walk your hands forward into downward dog. If your hands do not reach the floor, you can use blocks under them. Feel the gentle pull of the femur bones into the backs of the hip sockets as the spine lengthens.

Place your hands on a wall or chair to reduce weight on the upper body.

Practicing downward-facing dog with your hands on a wall or chair is a great way to increase accessibility for those with limited mobility or injuries. This variation reduces the amount of weight-bearing on the hands and wrists, making the pose more approachable. Using the wall removes weight-bearing from the upper body almost entirely while still asking you to engage the muscles supporting extension of your spine (see photo a). To gradually increase weight-bearing, you can prop the back of the chair against a wall, bring your hands to the seat of the chair, and walk your feet back slightly behind the hips (see photo b). If your hands start to slide, you can grab onto the sides of the seat or the sides of the back railing.

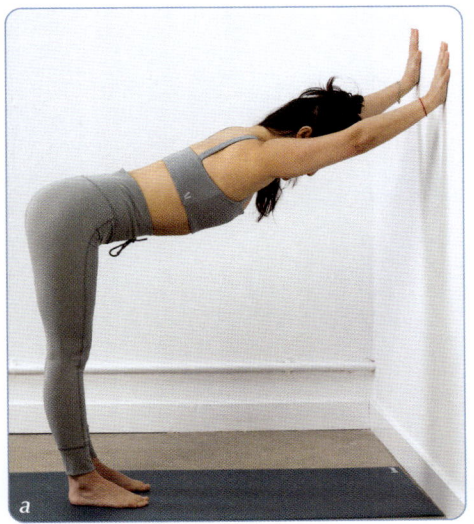

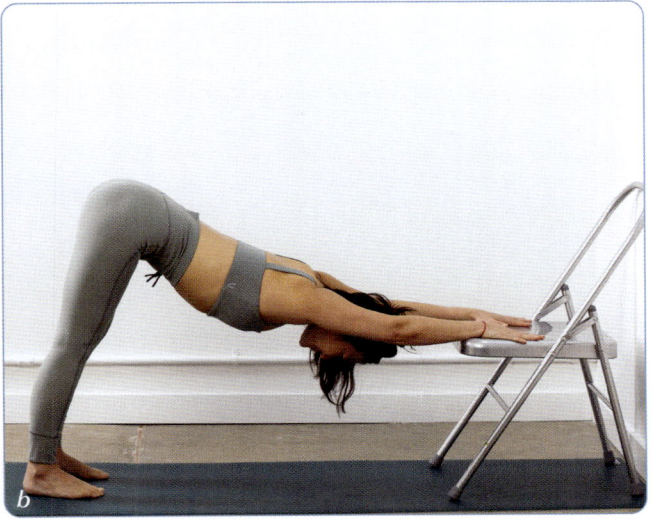

Downward-Facing Dog Pose (continued)

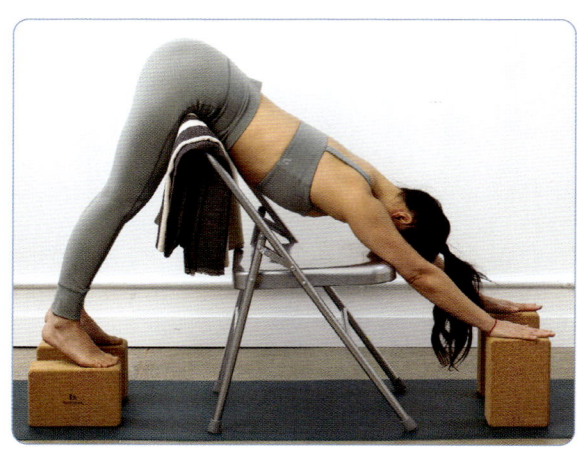

Support your hips on a chair to apply traction to the spine.

For those looking to minimize weight-bearing on their wrists while still enjoying the benefits of downward-facing dog, practicing with a chair can be an excellent option. By resting your groin on the chair's rail, you can focus on elongating and stretching your spine. For more comfort, place a folded blanket over the back rail. Position the chair on a sticky mat to prevent it from sliding. Stand behind the chair and fold your body over it, placing your hands on the seat. Gradually walk your feet backward until your hip creases rest against the chair's back rail. Allow your torso to release forward and bring your hands toward the floor in front of the seat of the chair. Depending on the size of your torso, the chair seat may rest behind your arms or armpits. If your limbs aren't long enough to reach the floor, use blocks under your hands and feet as needed.

Use a strap to engage and align in three-legged dog.

This variation takes a little bit of strap measuring, but it is so worth it! The strap encourages leveling the hips, anchoring the front thigh back, and engaging the leg muscles and core stabilizing muscles. By pressing the back foot into the strap, you also reinforce a lengthening action in the spine, creating space from your tailbone to the crown of your head.

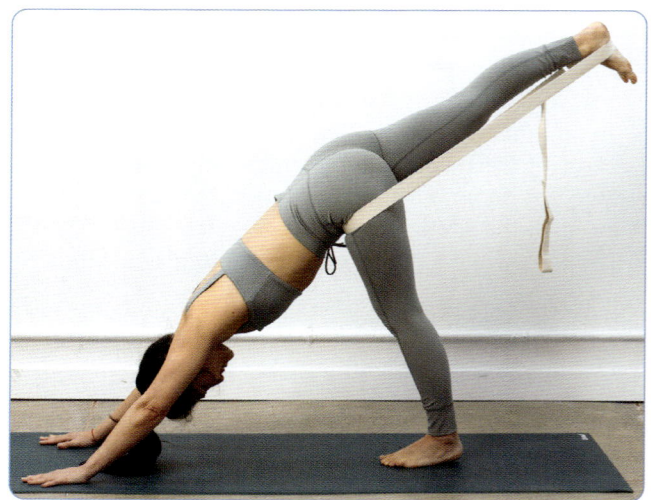

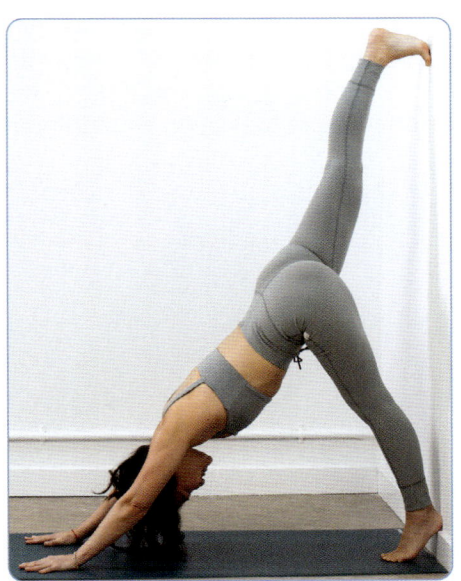

Use a wall to engage and align in three-legged dog.

This wall variation is great for maintaining balance while working on alignment, leveling the hips, and integrating muscle memory for taking the posture off the wall. Place the ball of your extended leg's foot on the wall, at your preferred height (adjust your distance from the wall as needed). Gaze back to ensure all your toes are pointing toward the floor. Press your foot into the wall to contract the quadriceps muscle of that leg to lengthen the hamstrings.

Dolphin Pose

Ardha Pincha Mayurasana   अर्ध पञ्चि मयूरासन

Dolphin pose is a challenging yoga posture that simultaneously strengthens and stretches the shoulder girdle, arms, upper back, and legs. Offering benefits such as improved overhead mobility, thoracic extension, and flexibility in the hamstrings and calves, this pose also enhances circulation. Explore prop-supported variations to deepen your dolphin pose experience and embrace its holistic benefits.

Place a block between your hands to activate muscle engagement and inform posture.

When practicing this pose, squeezing a block between your hands helps to enhance external rotation of the shoulders, which fosters a healthy shoulder alignment by preventing the elbows from splaying and the shoulders from collapsing inward. Squeezing the block also provides more stability, allowing for a better extension of the 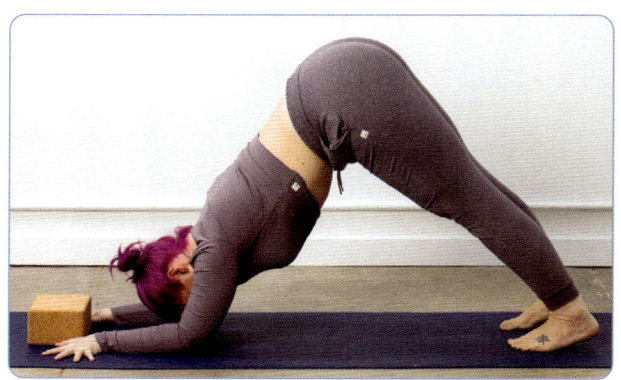 thoracic spine. To enter dolphin pose, begin in a table top position with the block turned to its widest orientation between your hands. Create an L shape with your thumbs and index fingers, framing the bottom corners of the block. For some wrists, it may feel better to have the block between the thumbs with the wrists slightly turned out (as shown in the photo). Play around and see what feels better for you! Walk your elbows in until they are shoulder-width apart. Tuck your toes and lift your hips up and back, moving into dolphin pose. Ground down through the outsides of both elbows and the insides of both wrists while maintaining your gaze on the block. Tiptoe forward to deepen the hamstring stretch. Press your forearms into the mat to create space between the tops of your shoulders and ears. Focus on gliding the shoulder blades away from the spine to add space in the upper back.

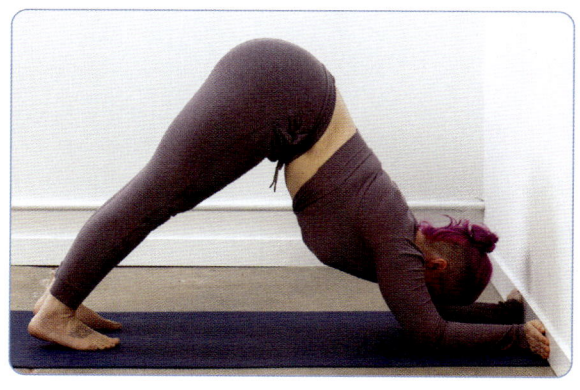

Practice with your hands against a wall to encourage external rotation of the shoulders.

To encourage external rotation of the shoulders, try a variation of dolphin pose where your forearms are grounded but your hands are against a wall with your fingers turned out. As you turn your fingers outward, this reinforces the rotation of your shoulder blades, creating space in the upper back. This also aids in hugging your elbows inward to align them behind your wrists. This variation also helps to engage your upper body muscles—particularly the serratus anterior—and create length in your spine through the pressing action of the hands into the wall.

Loop a strap around your arms to inform and align.

Using a strap around your arms in dolphin pose can help you to engage and strengthen your upper body muscles, particularly the shoulders and triceps. Additionally, the strap can help you to maintain a healthy alignment in your shoulders and spine, which can reduce the risk of injury or your elbows splaying open to the sides. To enter dolphin pose with a strap, get onto your hands and knees. Then, place your forearms

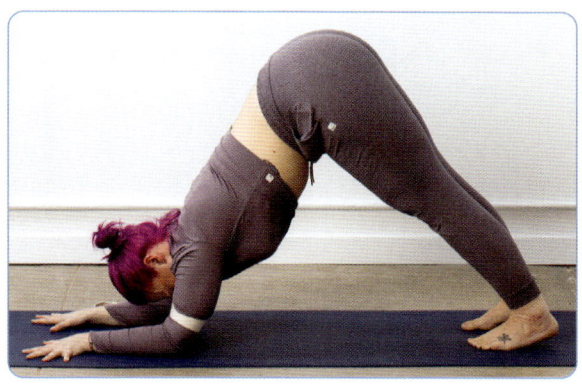

on the floor, making sure that your elbows are directly under your shoulders. Wrap a strap around your arms, just below or above your elbows—whichever is most effective for you. Ensure the loop of the strap is snug but not too tight. Tuck your toes under and lift your hips up and back, straightening the legs as much as you can without compromising length in the spine. As you hold the pose, focus on pressing your forearms and hands into the floor, engaging your upper body muscles.

A fun exercise you can add here is practicing transitioning between dolphin pose and downward-facing dog. As you transition between the two, the strap will inform the muscle actions of the shoulder girdle and keep the elbows from going rogue on you. This exercise also helps to strengthen muscle memory connecting the similar actions needed to perform both asanas.

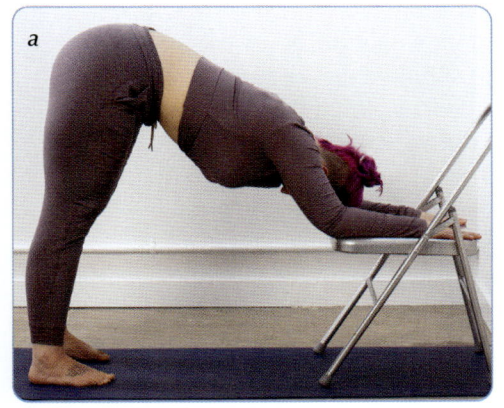

Use a chair or wall to transfer weight from your upper body.

These variations are great if getting up from and down on the floor are challenging. It also modifies the posture in a way that makes it more accessible if you are still building up the strength for dolphin pose. The first two variations involve the use of a chair. Have the chair on a sticky mat or the back of the chair up against a wall to ensure it does not slide as you enter the posture. In the first variation, you will modify the pose by bringing your forearms down onto the seat of the chair, just as you would the floor (see photo *a*). This version also requires less flexibility in the hamstrings. In the second variation, place a blanket on the seat of the chair to cushion your elbows. You can also loop a strap around the upper arms just above the elbows so that they don't slide out. Lift your forearms to grab the top rail of the back of the chair (see photo *b*). If it is out of reach, stack more blankets to elevate your elbows higher. In both variations, you can gradually increase weight-bearing and axial extension of the spine by walking your feet away from the chair. The third variation is similar but uses a wall. Bring your forearms shoulder-width apart on a wall in front of you. Align your

Dolphin Pose *(continued)*

wrists over your elbows and walk your feet back, working toward a flat back and a long spine. Press down through the outer edges of your elbows and inner edges of your wrists simultaneously and soften your shoulders away from the ears (see photo *c*).

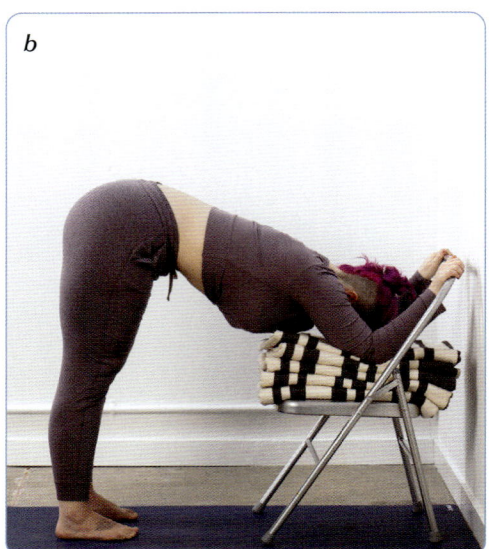

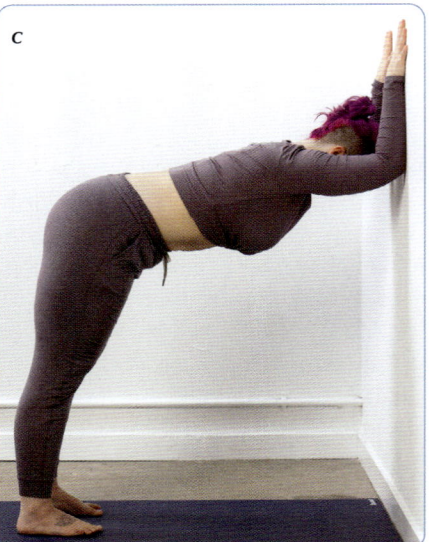

Practice with your heels against a wall or pressed into a rolled-up blanket to bring the floor to you.

These options are great for those who cannot reach their heels to the mat. Without compromising traction and extension in your spine, you can still reap the benefits of pressing your heels into a surface. Both options help to stabilize the feet and legs, keeping the heels from turning in or out, and they help to keep the legs parallel. Enter dolphin pose, resting the heels of your feet on top of the rolled blanket or against a wall and the balls of your feet on the mat. Direct your heels straight back and press them into the blanket or wall. This helps to activate the muscles on the front of your body. Use the feedback from the surface to firm your thighs and engage your quadriceps. By engaging your legs and lifting your quadriceps, you can take some weight off of your upper body, making the pose more comfortable and accessible (see photo *a* for an example with a blanket and photo *b* for an example with a wall).

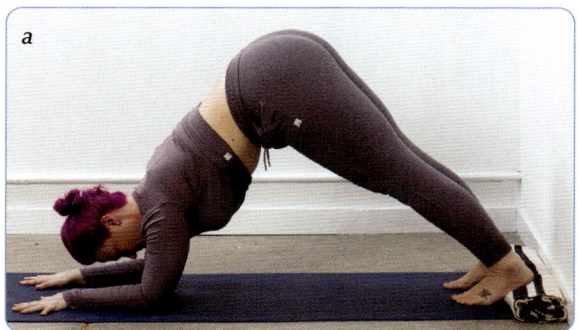

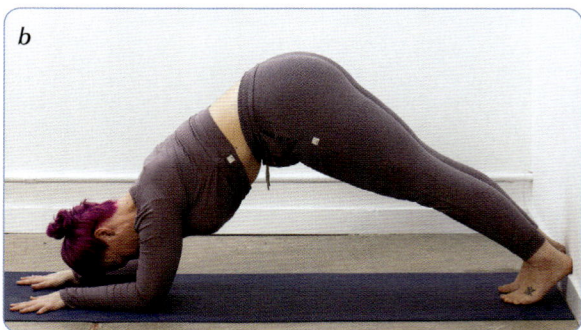

Standing Forward Bend Pose

Uttanasana

उत्तानासन

Standing forward bend pose is a revitalizing yoga posture that actively stretches the calves, hamstrings, and hips. This pose goes beyond flexibility, releasing tension in the low back, spine, and neck. Additionally, it contributes to the strengthening of thighs and knees. Elevate your practice by exploring prop-supported variations for an enriched standing forward bend experience.

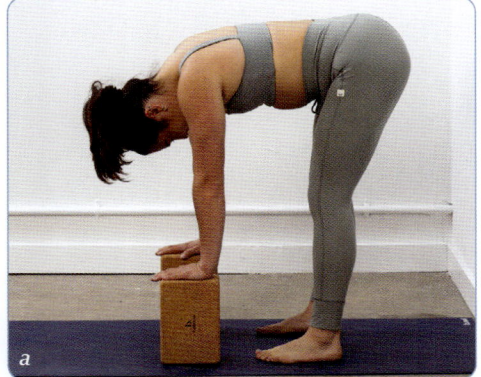

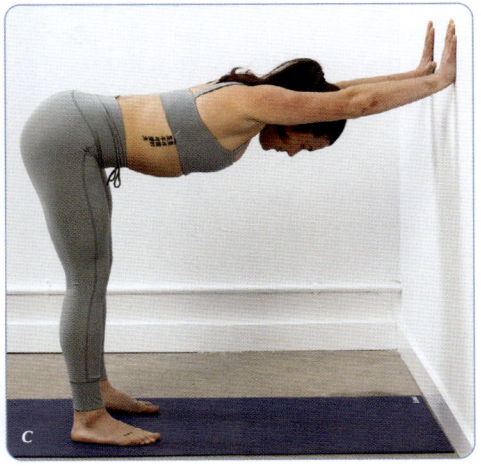

Place blocks or a chair under your hands or use a wall to bring the floor to you.

Using blocks in a standing forward fold variation can offer several benefits. By bridging the gap between you and the mat, you can access better balance and release tension in your upper body. Placing your hands on the blocks also helps to distribute weight more evenly through your feet. This relieves pressure on your knees and hips while creating a safer stretch through the backs of your legs. For this variation, start in mountain pose with your feet hip-width apart and hinge forward at the hips, rather than the waist. If this is difficult to do, try bending your knees. Place your hands on the blocks at a comfortable height and soften your belly, head, and neck. Draw the tops of your shoulders away from your ears to lengthen through your neck while firming your shins and thighs. Imagine your brain resting heavy in your skull. Breathe deeply into your lower back to deepen the stretch (see photo a). Stack blocks or use the seat of a chair if you need more height (see photo b). For the least intense fold, practice with your hands extended out on a wall in front of you (see photo c).

Place blocks under your feet to deepen the stretch.

Using block in a standing forward fold can provide a more challenging stretch that targets the hamstrings and helps to open and lengthen the back on a deeper level. This is because standing on blocks makes the mat harder to reach with the hands, requiring more hamstring flexibility. To practice this variation, start in

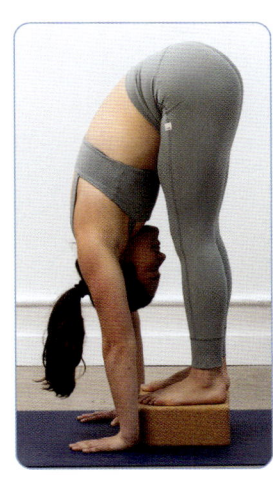

mountain pose with your feet on a block. If you need a wider stance, use two blocks at their lowest height. Hinge forward at the hips and fold over your thighs, bending your knees enough to place your hands on the mat in front of the blocks. Straighten your legs again while keeping your weight even in your feet and hands and lifting through the arches of your feet. Focus on lengthening through your low back and reaching your heart toward your shins. You can also try to round through your upper back and lift your heels to simulate the feeling of pressing into a handstand. Breathe deeply into your lower back to deepen the stretch.

Practice with a strap to gently lengthen the spine.

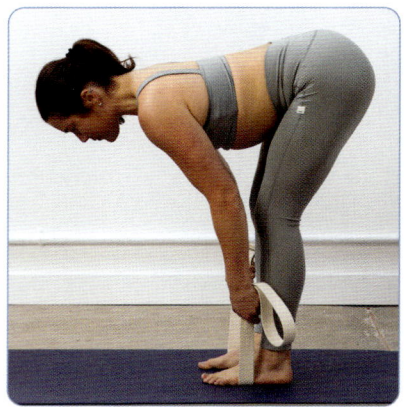

Using a strap can help to deepen your forward fold in standing forward bend pose by aiding in lengthening the spine. Begin by standing in mountain pose with your feet hip-width apart. Place the strap around the balls of your feet and hold one end of the strap in each hand. On an exhale, hinge forward at the hips and fold over your thighs, keeping your knees slightly bent if necessary. Gently pull on the strap to lengthen your spine and draw your chest toward your thighs. If you feel comfortable, you can try straightening your legs while maintaining a long spine. Breathe deeply and hold the pose for several breaths, allowing your upper body to release further with each exhale. To release the pose, gently release the tension on the strap and slowly roll up to standing.

Practice seated in a chair.

These variations of the pose can be beneficial for those with limited mobility or trouble balancing. Practicing while seated can help to stretch the entire back, from the neck and shoulders down to the hamstrings and calves. It can also help to calm the mind and relieve stress. Practicing in a chair can also help to improve posture and spinal alignment, because it encourages lengthening through the spine and opening through the chest. These variations of the pose are accessible for a wide range of individuals. In the first variation, begin sitting tall at the edge of the seat of the chair with your feet planted firmly on the floor or blocks and enter your fold (see photo *a*). In the second variation, deepen the stretch by extending your legs and placing your feet against a wall. You may need to measure this distance beforehand to get your feet all the way to the wall. You can also place blocks under your heels if your legs do not comfortably reach the floor or if you are ready to deepen the stretch. Having contact with the wall informs the direction of the legs, pointing your knees and toes straight up. As you fold forward, you can hold the seat of the chair for support or walk your hands down your thighs or to blocks framing your thighs (see photo *b*). The third variation is like the first variation but with an added prop and benefit! Roll a blanket to your desired firmness and thickness and place it in your lap at your hip crease. This will encourage lengthening the waist up and over the blanket, finding extension away from the hips before you round through the spine (see photo *c*). It also gently stimulates the digestive system. In the fourth variation, you can also practice a standing rolled-blanket variation as you build balance and mobility (see photo *d*).

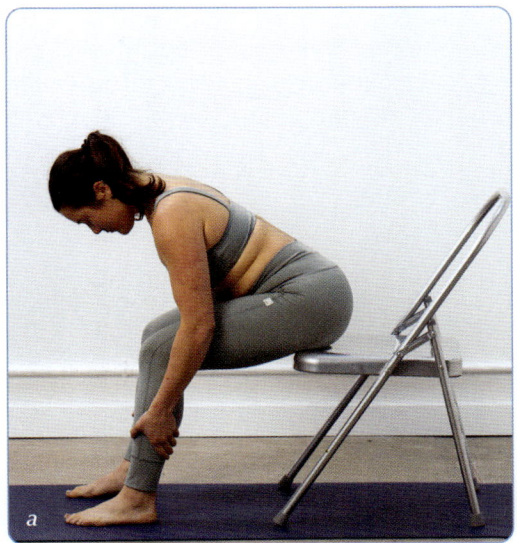

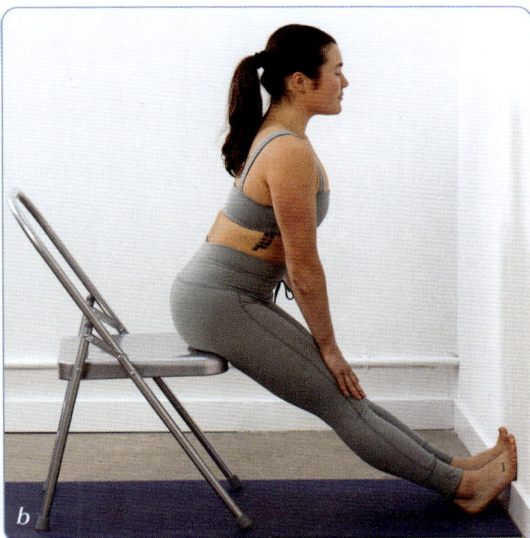

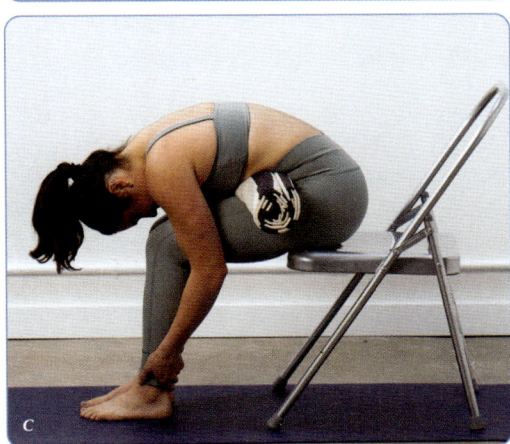

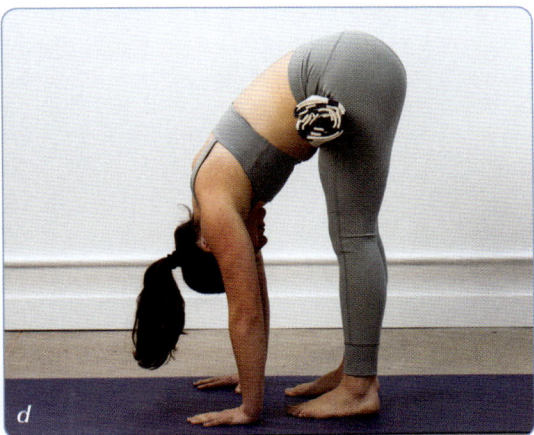

Practice with a strap around your shins to encourage lifting through your inner ankles.

In this variation of standing forward bend pose, using a strap around your shins can help you to engage your inner ankles and lift through the arches of your feet. By focusing on lifting through the inner ankles and engaging the inner thighs, you can create greater stability and balance. This variation can be particularly helpful if you tend to pronate or experience knock-knees. This variation can also be beneficial for individuals who have discomfort or tightness in the hips, inner thighs, or lower back. To perform this variation, start by standing comfortably with your feet hip-width apart and loop a strap around your shins. Adjust the tension of the

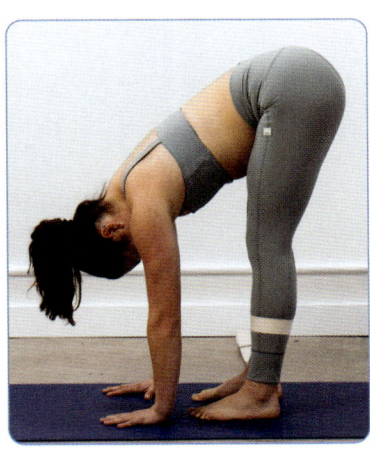

strap so that you feel a gentle pull toward the midline of your body. As you fold forward, press your outer legs into the strap, engaging the muscles of the outer hips and thighs. Imagine the feeling of trying to split your mat in two with your feet. To further deepen the stretch, focus on lifting through the arches of your feet and grounding down through the big toe mounds.

Practice with your butt against a wall to ground and challenge you.

By grounding your hips against the wall, you can create a more stable foundation. The first variation is especially beneficial for those who are transitioning from practicing the pose in a chair. To perform this variation, stand with your back facing the wall with your feet hip-width apart or touching. Lean your sitting

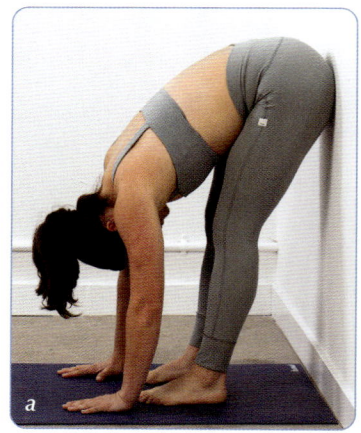 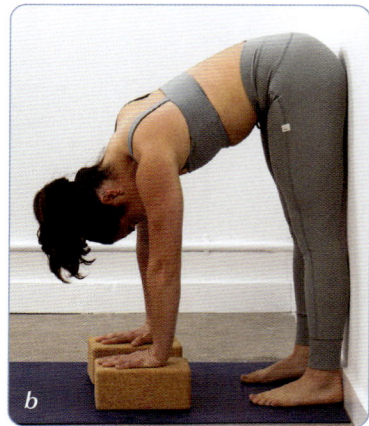

bones into the wall, with a gentle bend in your knees. Position your feet about a foot (0.3 m) away from the wall and fold forward (see photo *a*). Over time, work your feet closer to the wall to deepen the stretch. For a more challenging variation, bring your heels all the way to the wall. This is ideal for individuals who tend to shift their weight toward their heels during forward folds, which can cause pain often referred to as yoga butt or, in medical terms, proximal hamstring tendinopathy, which is an irritation or inflammation of the hamstring tendons at their attachment site on the sitting bones. In this variation, you'll need to engage your thighs to resist gravity and maintain balance as you fold forward. Place your hands on a chair or blocks and press the back of your legs into the wall (see

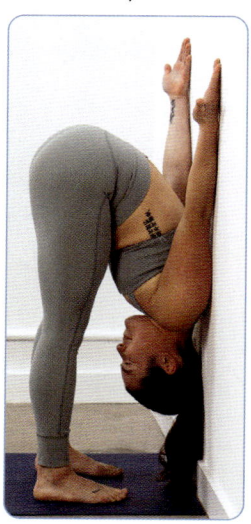

photo *b*). Over time, you can progress to bringing your hands to the floor. Overall, both variations of standing forward bend pose can help improve flexibility in the hamstrings, calves, and hips while also promoting proper alignment and posture.

Practice with your back against a wall to support your upper body.

This variation of standing forward bend pose involves using the wall as a prop to promote greater opening and release in the lower back. This variation can be particularly beneficial for individuals who spend a lot of time sitting or have a sedentary lifestyle, and those who have tightness or discomfort in the lower back. By leaning forward and pressing your shoulder blades against the wall, you can deepen the stretch and create a stable base. To perform this variation, face the wall and lean forward, pressing your shoulder blades against the wall, and lift through your sitting bones. Lower your arms toward the floor, bending your knees if necessary to support your hamstrings and spine. Alternatively, you can reach your arms overhead (as shown in the photo) to gently open through the chest. Use the support of the wall to release into the stretch, feeling a gentle opening and lengthening in your lower back, which can alleviate pressure and tension, promoting greater comfort and ease of movement.

Practice folding over a chair to release the upper body.

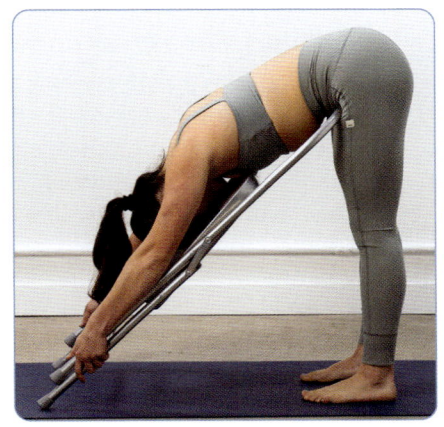

This variation of standing forward bend pose involves a folded chair to help enhance the stretch and relaxation of the hips and groin. It is an adaptable pose that can be modified to the height and mobility of individual practitioners. By adjusting the angle of the chair or standing on blocks, you can customize the pose to align with the height of your hip creases. To perform this variation, position the back of the chair against your groin and hinge forward at the hips, draping your torso over the chair. Allow your body to fully relax into the support of the chair. Feel free to grasp the legs of the chair for added stability. This pose promotes deep stretching in the hips and groin, which can be especially beneficial for people who spend a lot of time sitting or have tightness in this area. It can also help improve posture and relieve tension in the back and neck.

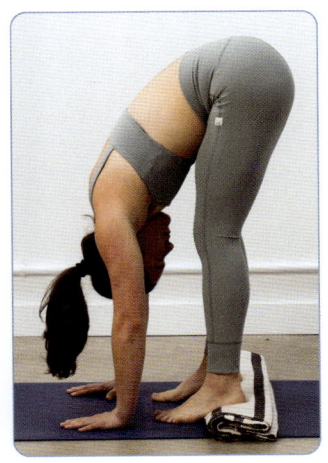

Practice with your heels on a folded blanket to lessen the intensity in your hamstrings and calves.

This variation of standing forward bend pose involves using a folded blanket to support the heels and reduce the intensity of the stretch in the hamstrings and calves. This can be particularly helpful if you have tightness or discomfort in these areas or if you are looking for a gentler way to ease into the pose. The blanket also helps to prevent shifting your weight back into the heels. Fold a blanket and place it on the floor, then stand with your heels on the blanket. This heel elevation will create a gentler angle for the stretch. As you fold forward, focus on maintaining a soft bend in the knees to further lessen the intensity in the hamstrings and calves. You can also use props to support your hands if you can't reach the floor comfortably.

Standing Half Forward Bend Pose

Ardha Uttanasana

अर्ध उत्तानासन

Standing half forward bend pose is a staple for your sun salutations that effectively stretches the hamstrings, calves, and both the front and back torso. Simultaneously, it strengthens the muscles of the back and spine. Elevate your practice by exploring prop-supported variations to enhance the stretching and strengthening benefits of standing half forward bend pose.

Place blocks or a chair under your hands or use a wall to bring the floor to you.

Using blocks in a halfway lift can offer several benefits. By bridging the gap between you and the mat, you can access better balance as you extend through your spine. Placing your hands on your prop of choice also helps to distribute weight more evenly through your feet. This relieves pressure on your knees and hips while creating a safer stretch through the backs of your legs. For this variation, start in mountain pose with your feet hip-width apart and hinge forward at the hips, rather than the waist. Place your hands on blocks at a comfortable height and lift your torso away from your thighs. Draw the crown of your head away from your tailbone and engage through the posterior chain muscles along the spine. Slightly tuck your chin to lengthen through the back of your neck (see photo a). Stack blocks or use the seat of a chair if you need more height (see photo b). For more spinal extension, practice with your hands extended out on a wall in front of you (see photo c).

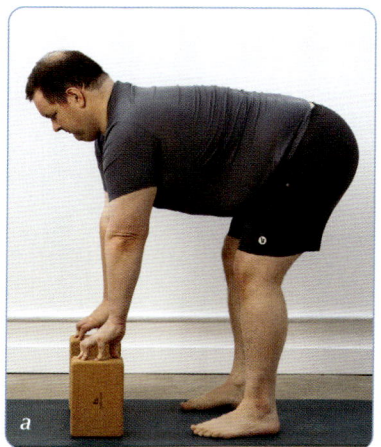
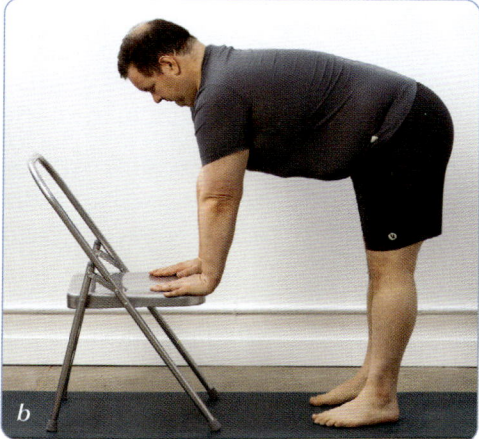

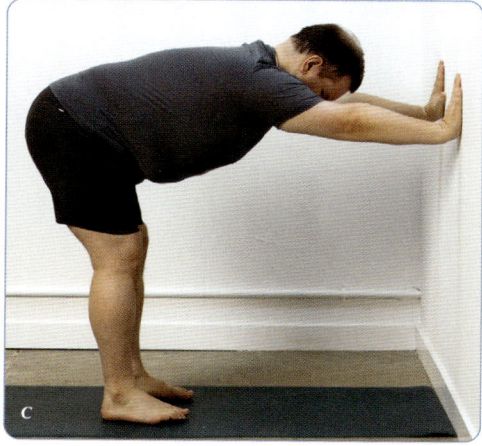

The Complete Guide to Yoga Props

Use a strap to gently lengthen the spine.

Using a strap can be a helpful way to deepen engagement of your posterior chain muscles as you enter your halfway lift. Begin by standing in mountain pose with your feet hip-width apart. Place the strap around the balls of your feet and hold one end of the strap in each hand. On an exhale, hinge forward at the hips and fold over your thighs, keeping your knees slightly bent if necessary. Gently pull on the strap, bending the elbows, using it to lengthen your spine and draw your chest toward your thighs. On an inhale, lift your chest up and away from the thighs, straightening the arms. Use the gentle resistance from the strap to engage the back of the body.

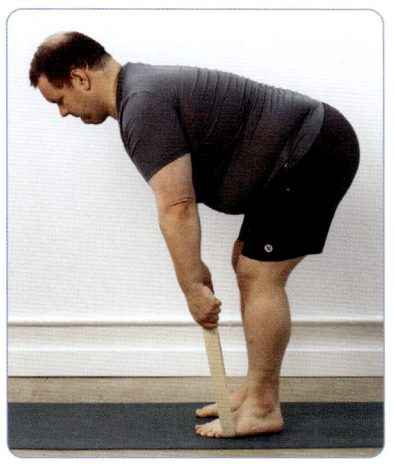

Place a block between your thighs to stabilize your core and pelvic muscles.

Using a block between your thighs in this pose can be a great way to stabilize your core and pelvic muscles while also engaging and lifting your groin and thighs. Place a block on its narrowest width between your thighs, high up near the pubis, and then enter a forward fold. On an inhale, lift your chest away from your thighs and elongate through your spine. Once in the pose, hug the block up and in toward the pubis, engaging your inner thighs. For those with tight hip flexors and hamstrings, the feeling of a slight internal rotation of the thighs can help to combat pelvic tucking and bring you back to neutral. Imagine pressing the block back in space slightly. This will help to narrow the frontal hip points and widen across the lower back, lengthening the hamstrings and deepening the psoas stretch. Remember to keep your toes and knees pointing forward.

Practice grounding your hips in a chair or against a wall.

Whether you have limited mobility or difficulty balancing, or if you simply find it hard to get up from and down on the floor, these variations of standing half forward bend pose can be helpful. Plus, they're accessible for a wide range of individuals. For those who prefer practicing in a chair, the first variation can help improve posture and spinal alignment by encouraging lengthening through the spine and opening through the chest. Sit tall on the chair with your feet firmly planted on the floor or on blocks. Place your hands on your thighs near your knees, and as you exhale, fold your torso toward your thighs by bending your elbows. On an inhale, press your hands down and slightly forward to lengthen your spine and broaden your chest (see photo a). To create a more stable foundation for the pose, try grounding your hips against the wall. This variation is especially beneficial for those transitioning from practicing in a chair. Since your hips will be elevated higher than your knees in this version, start practicing with the torso at an angle that requires more core engagement to halfway lift. To perform this variation, stand with your back to the wall with your feet hip-width apart or touching and lean your sitting bones into the wall. Position your feet about a foot or two (0.3-0.6 m) away from the wall, and with bent knees, fold forward. On an inhale, press your hands into the tops of your thighs to lift and lengthen your spine (see photo *b*). Feel the connection of your sitting bones with the wall and press into that connection to encourage more traction in the spine.

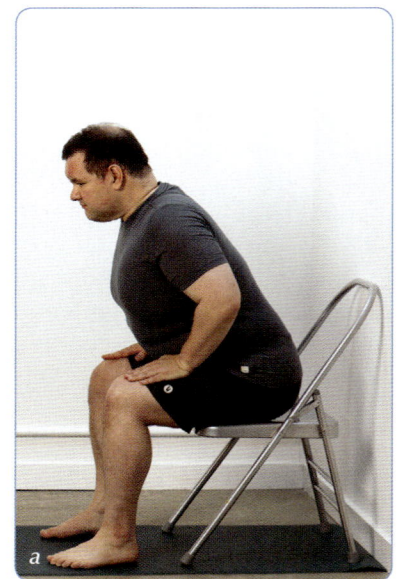
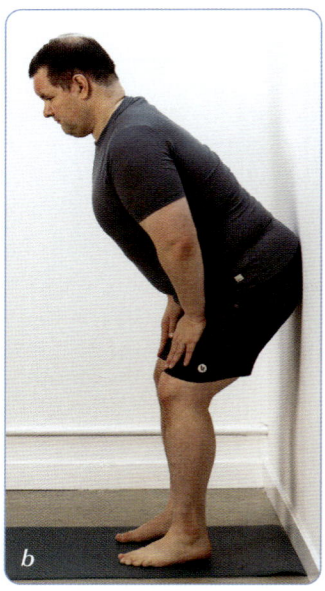

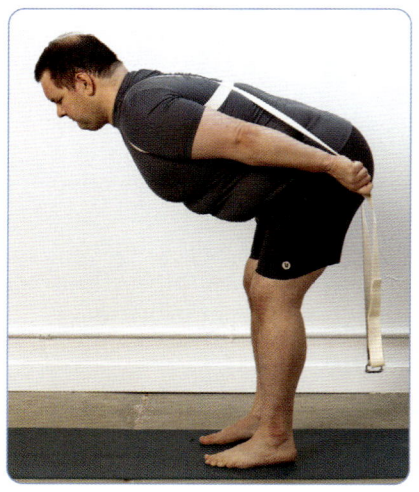

Improve postural alignment with the help of a strap.

This posture trick is something you can use to train your body into healthier postural patterns by anchoring your shoulders back and down and to open across your chest. Thread a strap around your back at your shoulder blades and wrap them under your armpits. Then loop the ends of the strap over your shoulders to drape down behind you again. Cross the two ends of the strap over your upper back, creating the letter X. Hold the ends of the straps in your hands and enter your halfway lift. Extend your arms straight back and slightly out as shown in the photo. Have the strap tight enough that you feel your shoulder blades being drawn down and back, resisting any postural urge to slump or hunch!

Wide-Legged Forward Bend Pose

Prasarita Padottanasana   प्रसारति पादोत्तानासन

Wide-legged forward bend pose is a standing yoga posture that actively stretches the calves, hamstrings, and hips. Other than flexibility, it releases tension in the low back, spine, and neck. This pose also contributes to firming the thighs and knees. Elevate your practice by exploring prop-supported variations to enhance the stretching and strengthening benefits of this pose.

Place blocks or a chair under your hands or use a wall to bring the floor to you.

Using a chair, blocks, or a wall in wide-legged forward bend pose can offer several benefits. Using props raises the height of the floor to meet your hands, which means that balance is more accessible, and the upper body can release more deeply. Practicing these supported variations also allows you to shift weight from the heels and more evenly into the feet while reducing the fear of falling, taking the pressure out of the knee and hip joints, and creating a safer stretch through the backs of the legs. Stand in a wide-legged stance with feet three to four feet (0.9-1.2 m) apart, ensuring that they are parallel or slightly pigeon-toed but not turned out. Fold forward, hinging at your hips, and place your hands on the seat of a chair (see photo a), perhaps even resting your head on the chair seat. Alternatively, you can place your hands on blocks at your preferred height if the chair is too high. For a less-intense fold, practice with your hands extended on a wall in front of you (see photo b). Soften the belly and relax the head and neck, releasing the crown of your head toward the floor. Firm the front of the shins and thighs to open the muscles down the backs of the legs. This muscular contraction will also help prevent you from feeling like you are going to fall—especially if you are working toward hands-free variations. Draw the inner thighs toward the pubis as you simultaneously press down through the outer edges of the feet.

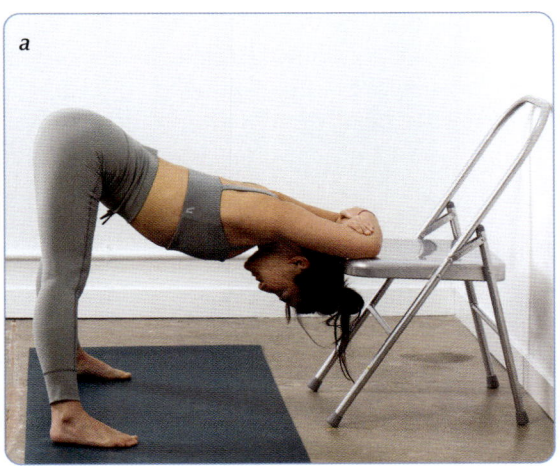
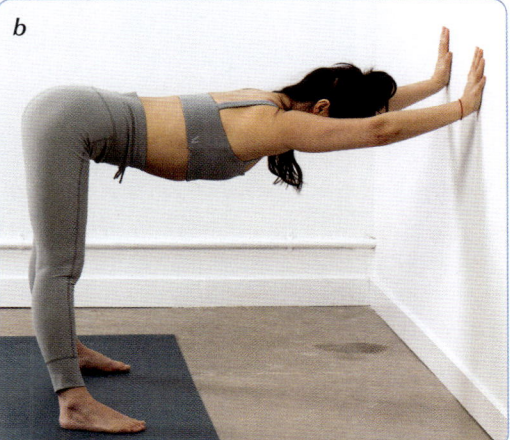

Place blocks under your feet to deepen the stretch.

Using blocks in wide-legged forward bend pose can offer unique benefits. Standing on blocks makes the mat harder to reach with the hands, making the stretch more challenging and requiring more hamstring flexibility. This also helps to open and lengthen through the back on a deeper level. To practice this variation, start in a wide-legged forward fold with your feet directly in front of the blocks on the lowest height. Walk your hands back so that you can step onto the blocks, one at a time. Keep your weight evenly distributed through your feet and bring your hands to the mat, either in front of you or to the sides. Remember to breathe deeply into the lower back to open deeper through the hips, and if you are gazing toward the mat, try shifting the gaze back between the thighs, so that the crown of the head releases toward the mat.

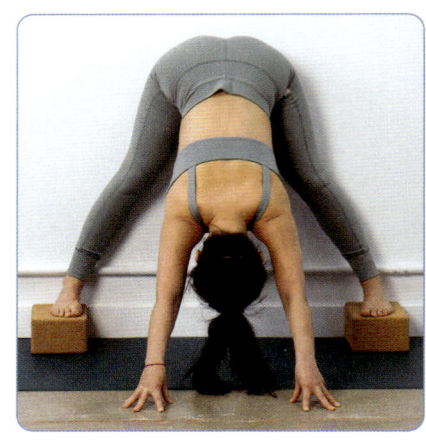

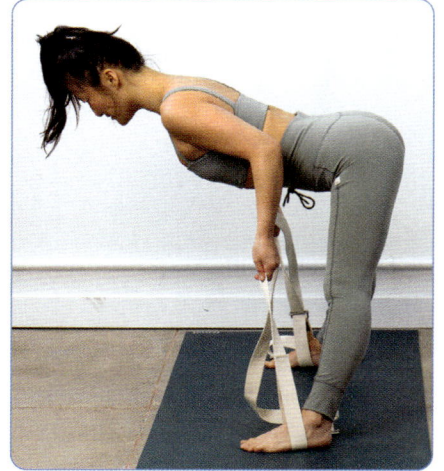

Practice with straps around your feet and in your hands to gently lengthen the spine.

Using straps can be a helpful way to deepen your forward fold and open through your lower back! Loop a strap around each foot and hold the ends of each strap in the corresponding hand. On an exhale, hinge forward at the hips and fold over your thighs, keeping your knees slightly bent if necessary. Gently pull on the strap, using it to lengthen your spine and draw your chest toward the space between your thighs. If you feel comfortable, experiment with straightening your legs while maintaining a long spine. Breathe deeply and hold the pose for several breaths, allowing your upper body to release further with each exhale. To release the pose, gently release the tension on the strap and slowly roll up to standing.

Sit on a chair to stabilize the pelvis.

If you have difficulty getting up from and down on the floor, balancing, or are looking for a gentler stretch, try wide-legged forward bend pose in a chair. The chair offers a platform to stabilize the pelvis, freeing up more of your attention to focus on postural alignment and the actions of the legs. While seated, step your feet out to the sides, opening through your hips and inner thighs. You may use sheer muscle strength to do so or use your hands to guide each leg, one at a time. If your chair feels too wide to comfortably bring the legs out to the side, try sitting on the corner of the seat instead of facing forward. Sitting on the corner also gives more room to eventually extend the legs. Enter your fold, placing

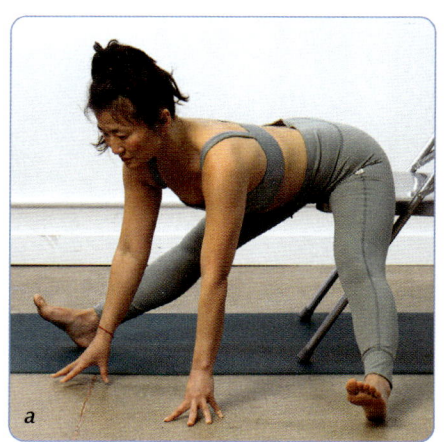

a

your hands on the mat (see photo *a*). If you can't reach the floor, you can use blocks (see photo *b*). For a deeper stretch, reach for the back legs of the chair and release through the crown of your head (see photo *c*).

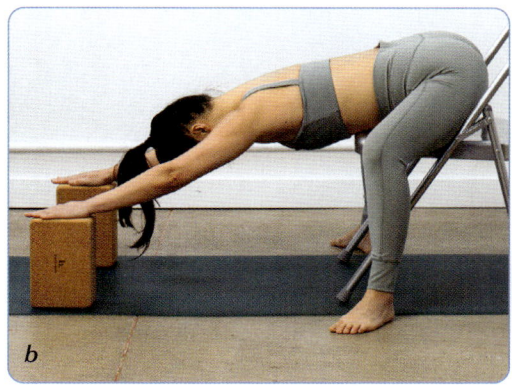

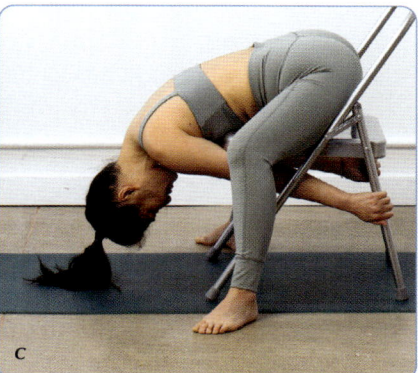

Practice with a strap around your feet to encourage lifting through your inner ankles.

In this variation, using a strap around your feet can help you to engage your inner ankles and lift through the arches of your feet. This variation can be particularly helpful if you tend to pronate or experience knock-knees. By focusing on lifting the inner ankles and engaging the inner thighs, you can create greater stability and balance in the body. To perform this variation, start by measuring the loop of the strap to match the distance between your feet. Slide the feet through both ends of the loop so the strap is flat on the floor and over the tops of the feet. Adjust the tension of the strap so that you feel a gentle resistance as the outer edges of the feet press into the strap. As you come into the fold, press into the strap,

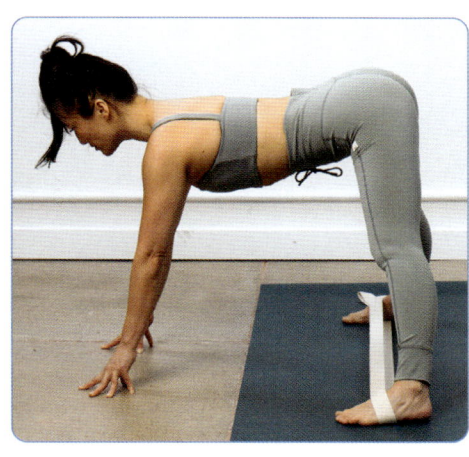

engaging the muscles of the outer hips and thighs. To further deepen the stretch, focus on lifting the inner arches of your feet and grounding down through the big toe mounds.

Practice with your legs against a wall to ground and challenge you.

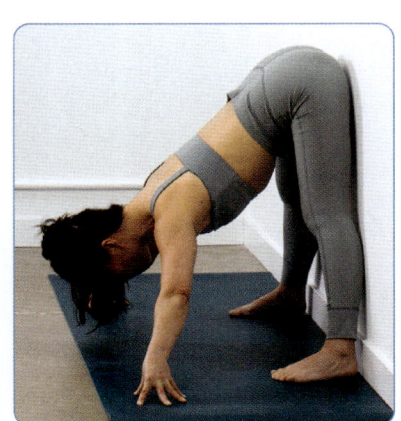

This variation will offer quite the challenge! Contact the wall with your heels and the backs of your thighs. Engage your thighs to resist gravity and maintain balance as you fold forward. This variation is ideal for those who tend to shift their weight toward their heels during forward folds. Place your hands on a chair or blocks and press the backs of your legs into the wall. As you become more comfortable over time, progress to bringing your hands to the floor.

Wide-Legged Forward Bend Pose (continued)

Practice with your back against a wall to support your upper body.

Utilizing the wall as a prop can enhance your stretch and amplify the sensation of release and relaxation. By pressing your shoulder blades against the wall, you create a secure foundation, making this variation especially beneficial for individuals with lower back tightness or discomfort. To perform this variation, face the wall and lean forward, placing your shoulder blades against the wall. As you lower your arms toward the floor, allow the wall's support to help you sink deeper into the stretch, feeling a gentle opening and lengthening in your lower back (see photo a). You can take this stretch even further with a partner-assisted exercise, which should only be attempted with an experienced teacher for safety. Have your partner sit behind you and grasp their hands. The partner will then place their feet at the tops of your hamstrings. As you inhale, elongate your spine and lift your sitting bones. With each exhale, have your partner gently press up with their feet to lengthen your hamstrings while simultaneously pulling your arms down the wall to slide your shoulders even farther down (see photo b). It is crucial to maintain open communication throughout to prevent overstretching or injury.

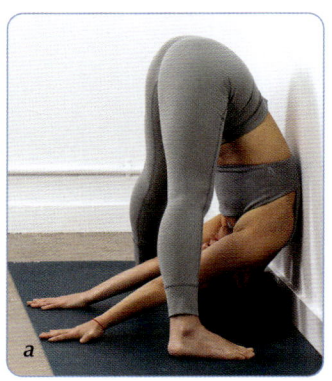
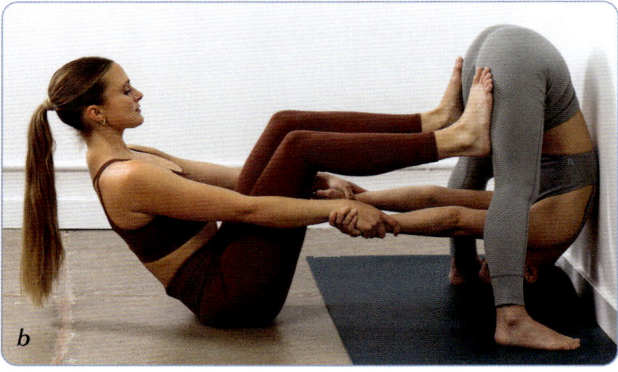

a

b

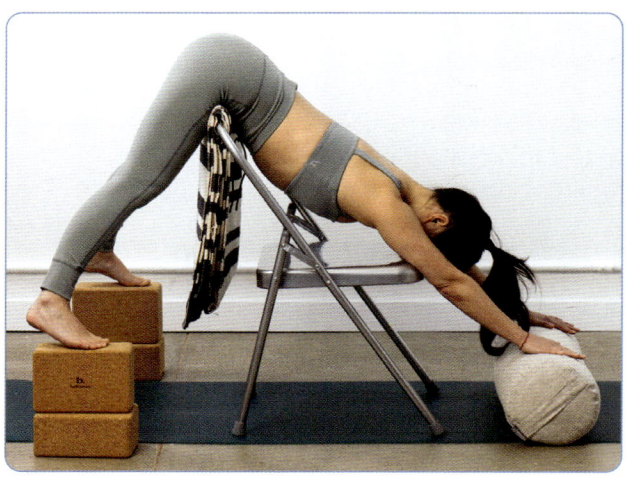

Use a chair, bolster, and blocks to release through the upper body.

Use a chair in this variation of wide-legged forward bend pose to help enhance the stretch and relaxation of the hips and groin. By resting your groin on the chair's rail, you can focus on elongating and stretching your spine. Place a folded blanket over the back rail to make the experience more comfortable and position the chair on a sticky mat to prevent it from sliding. Using blocks under your feet will allow the hips to reach the height of the chair.

Allow your torso to release forward and bring your hands toward the floor. Depending on the length of your torso, you may need to place a bolster in front of the chair to rest the hands. Allow the forehead to rest on the front edge of the chair seat.

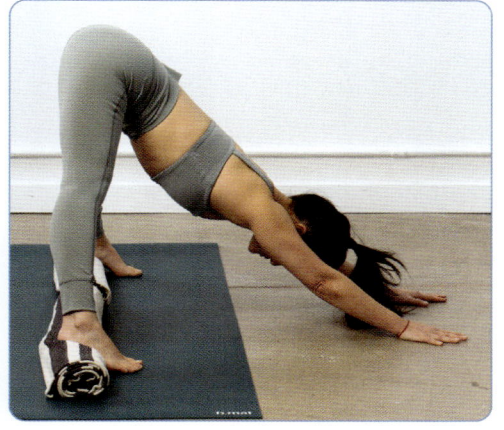

Place your heels on a folded blanket to lessen the intensity in your hamstrings and calves.

Use a folded blanket in this variation of wide-legged forward bend to support the heels and reduce the intensity of the stretch in the hamstrings and calves. This can be particularly helpful if you experience tightness or discomfort in these areas or if you are looking for a gentler way to ease into the pose. This variation also helps to inform not sitting your weight back into the heels. Fold a blanket lengthwise and place it on the floor. Stand with your feet three to four feet (0.9-1.2 m) apart and place your heels on the folded blanket. This will elevate the heels and create a gentler angle for the stretch. As you fold forward, focus on maintaining a soft bend in the knees to further lessen the intensity in the hamstrings and calves. You can also use other props to support your hands if you can't reach the floor comfortably.

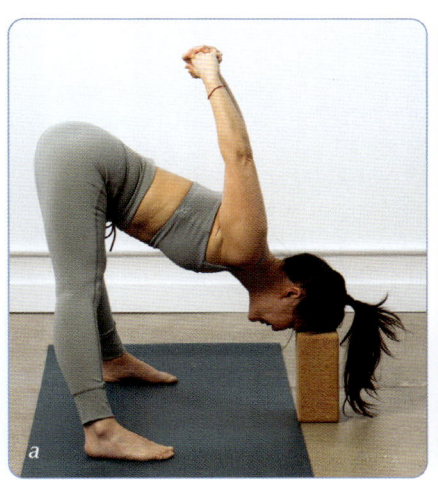
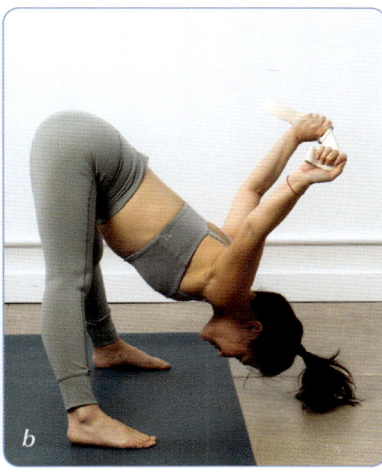

Practice with the help of blocks or a strap.

To practice the challenging variation of wide-legged forward bend pose C, using props like blocks or a strap can be helpful. These props can also assist with some of the limitations that may arise when entering the posture. The first variation involves using a block or stacked blocks under the forehead to shift the weight forward in the feet. This is especially useful for those who tend to overcorrect their balance by sinking weight into their heels. As you reach your arms overhead, it's important to lift through your thighs instead of sinking your weight back. Placing blocks under your forehead helps support your balance and helps develop muscle memory for this alignment (see photo a). The second variation is for those who have limited space in their shoulders. Using a yoga strap can be a great tool for bridging the gap between your hands if needed. It can also alleviate pain or strain from the full clasp. Additionally, the strap can assist in creating enough room in the shoulders to deepen your overhead reach (see photo b).

Tripod Headstand Pose

Mukta Hasta Shirshasana   मुक्तहस्त शीर्षासन

Tripod headstand pose is an empowering yoga posture that offers a multitude of benefits. This pose not only stimulates the pituitary and pineal glands but also actively strengthens the arms, spine, and core. Additionally, it contributes to decreasing fluid buildup in the legs and alleviating symptoms of edema while stimulating the lymphatic system. Let's explore some common ways to prop up this pose!

Place blocks under your shoulders to support your head and neck.

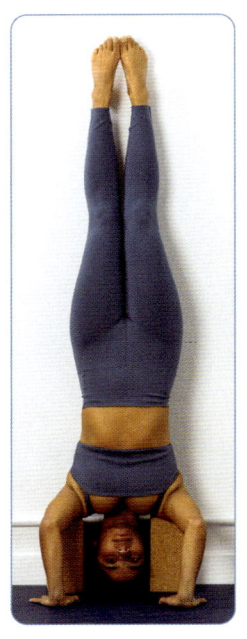

Using blocks while practicing tripod headstand offers numerous benefits, the most important being that they take the weight off the head and neck, unlike traditional headstand pose where weight can be distributed into the forearms to decompress the spine. Tripod headstand, on the other hand, always requires a third of your weight to be in the crown of your head, which may not be beneficial to everyone. To practice tripod headstand with blocks, you will need two to four blocks, depending on whether you want your head to touch the mat. For those with cervical spine issues or pain, use four blocks to find a deep release through the head and neck without weight or strain in those areas. To begin the pose, make a T shape with your blocks against the wall, with the bottom blocks on the lowest height and the top blocks on the tallest height. You can also stack three blocks each if you have six blocks, with the top blocks shoulder-width apart. Start in table top pose with your fingers facing the blocks, lift your hips, and walk your toes in, placing the tops of your shoulders on the blocks. You can place towels on the blocks for extra cushioning. Release the crown of your head toward the mat so that the back of your head is facing the wall. Walk one knee at a time on to the backs of the arms, lifting your feet off the mat and toward the gluteal muscles. Try to lift your knees off the triceps, bringing them in together against the front of the torso and perhaps try lifting your legs overhead. In this tripod headstand variation, ensure your elbows stack over your wrists with your forearms perpendicular to the mat; avoid placing your hands too close or too far from the face, keeping them within your field of vision. As a rule of thumb, channel chaturanga arm measurements with your hands shoulder-width apart and your elbows over your wrists before lifting your torso and legs away from the wall.

Use two chairs against a wall to support your neck.

Headstands can be a great addition to your yoga practice, but they can also put a lot of strain on your neck and head if not done properly. Using chairs and a wall can help take the weight off your neck and allow you to focus on building strength and balance. Set up two chairs on a sticky mat facing each other, with a folded mat on top of each chair for comfort. The chairs should be far enough apart to allow space for your head and shoulders to fit between them, while still providing ample surface area for your shoulders to rest on. Before entering the pose, step onto blocks or kneel on a third chair to bring your feet or knees higher, because the chairs raise the height of the floor significantly. Lower your

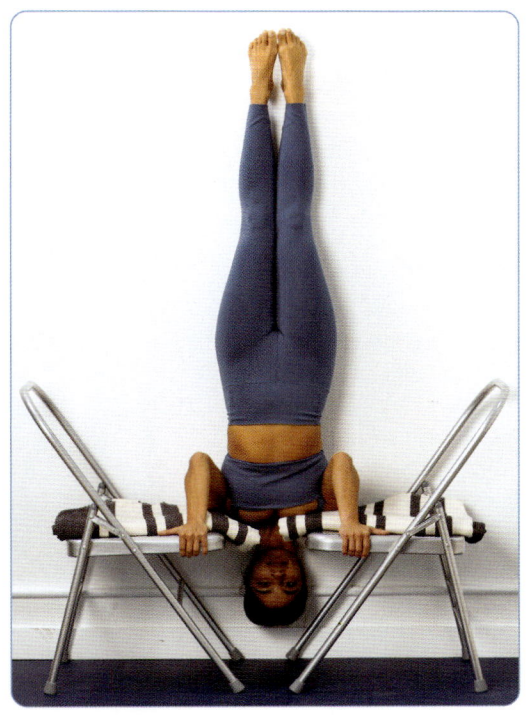

head between the chairs and shift forward until your shoulders touch the wall. The wall serves as a support and prevents you from falling forward. Grab the sides of the chairs' seats with your palms facing you and your elbows straight up. Press into the chairs with your shoulders, lengthening through your spine, and lift your legs.

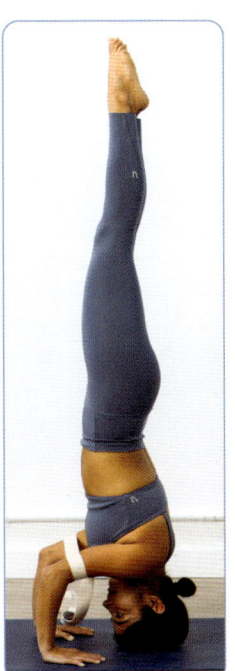

Loop a strap around your arms to stabilize.

This posture requires upper body strength, balance, and focus. One way to acquire more support is by using a yoga strap looped around your arms, just above the elbows. The benefit of using a strap is that it helps to engage and stabilize the shoulders, making the pose more accessible and safer. It also helps to keep the elbows stacked over the wrists, preventing them from splaying. Kneel, then lower the crown of your head to the floor. Walk your hands back away from your gaze until your elbows stack over the wrists, as in chaturanga arms. Using the strap for support, engage your core and press your legs toward the ceiling. Keep your gaze focused between your hands and lift the tops of your shoulders away from your ears by pressing down.

Supported Headstand Pose

Salamba Shirshasana

सालम्ब शीर्षासन

Supported headstand pose (salamba shirshasana) is a transformative yoga posture with a range of benefits. This pose stimulates the pituitary and pineal glands while actively strengthening the arms, spine, and core. It also helps to decrease fluid buildup in the legs and alleviate symptoms of edema, and stimulates the lymphatic system. Moreover, supported headstand pose may offer relief from symptoms of rotator cuff impingement. Elevate your practice by exploring prop-supported variations for a comprehensive experience of these enriching benefits.

Stack blocks against a wall to help stabilize your shoulders and spine.

Using blocks against a wall is a great way to practice headstand poses and stabilize the shoulders and spine. To start, place one block on its tallest height against a wall with the narrowest side facing the wall, then place two blocks on the lowest height on top of that block with the widest side against the wall. Facing the blocks, kneel and place your palms facing each other on the sides of the lowest block. Lift your hips to bring the crown of your head onto the mat with the back of your skull against the block. Tuck your toes and walk your feet as close to your hands as possible, ensuring the back of your head is in full contact with the block and the shoulders and hips are as close to stacking over the head as possible. Drawing one knee into the chest, get the thigh as close to the torso as possible and hug the heel toward your buttocks. Then try to draw the second knee into the chest, lifting both feet off the mat. Work on holding the legs tucked in toward the body without untucking the tailbone and elevating the legs right away. Press the forearms down, lift the shoulders away from the ears, and widen them across the upper back. Once you can comfortably hold the tucked tailbone shape for a few breaths, untuck the tailbone, bringing the tops of the shoulders fully against the top two blocks. Extend the legs overhead, pointing through the toes. Lengthen the tailbone toward the heels and squeeze the inner thighs together. Keep squeezing the block between your hands and pressing the forearms firmly into the mat to lift some weight from the head and neck. Practice exiting the pose with control.

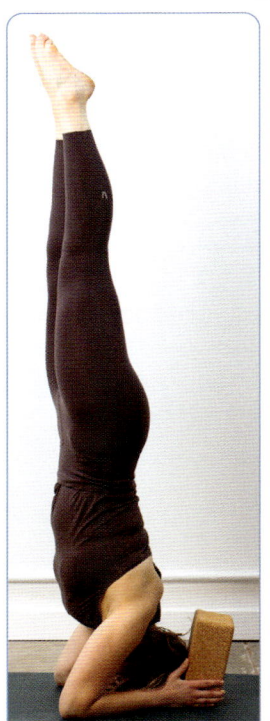

Hold a block behind your head to ground and lengthen.

Holding a block on its tallest setting can benefit you in a few ways! It provides a platform for the back of your skull to align with—as you probably know, finding the crown of your head on the mat can be difficult once you are upside down. Having the back of the head on the block will help provide reference. Also, if you have shorter arms and a longer neck, moving the wrists farther in front of the head can help by bringing your head closer to the upper arms.

Use a blanket to support and lengthen the neck.

When practicing headstand poses in yoga, supporting your head on a folded blanket can provide cushion and support for your head and neck, helping to prevent discomfort or injury. Otherwise, your head and neck would bear the full weight of your body, which can be problematic, especially for beginners. A folded blanket can also help to improve your alignment in the pose. A blanket under your head elevates your head slightly, which can help to lengthen your neck and create more space between your shoulders and ears. This option is good for a student with long arms and a short neck who have the feeling of not being able to lift the shoulders up without also lifting the head off the floor. Folding a blanket just under the head brings the floor to you, so you can refocus on the lifting action of the shoulders.

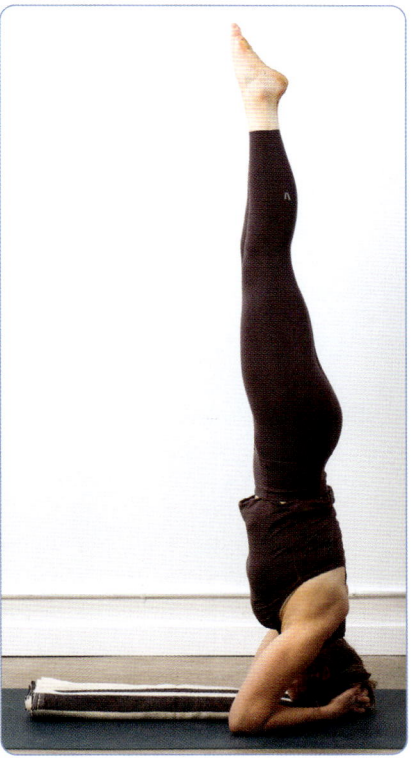

Practice with your back against a chair for support.

By using a chair as a prop for headstand poses, you can build confidence in this inversion and develop the strength and stability needed for a safe and successful practice. The chair helps by stabilizing the shoulders and spine, allowing you to focus on engaging your arms, shoulders, core, and leg muscles. It also eases the fear of falling! Choose a sturdy chair and place it against a wall with the seat facing the wall. Kneel in front of the chair and bring the crown of your head to the floor between the back legs of the chair, setting up as you normally would for headstand pose. Tuck your toes under and walk your feet toward the chair, lifting your hips until they stack over the shoulders. When using a nonfoldable chair with a straight back aligned with the seat's back edge, you can also lean your shoulders against this edge. From here, start raising the legs. Ideally, the sacrum should rest on the back rail of the chair. However, depending on the length of your torso, the back rail may be too high or too low. If needed, you can fold a blanket under your forearms to raise the height of the floor and create a more comfortable position.

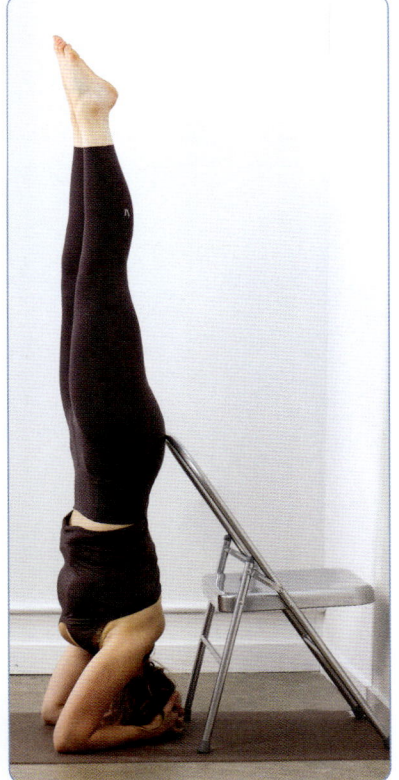

Supported Headstand Pose (continued)

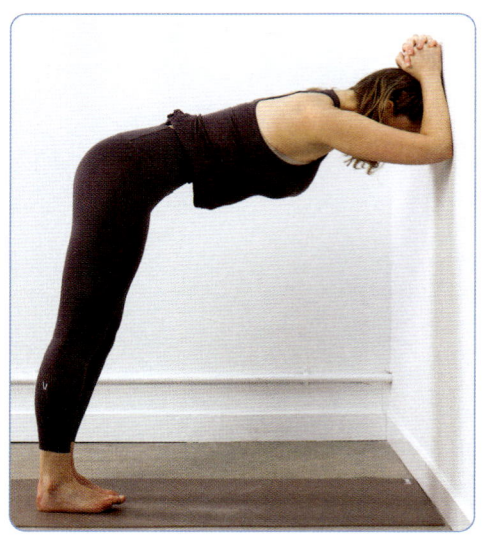

Practice headstand pose at a wall to reduce pain in the shoulders.

Calling all practitioners with rotator cuff injuries and tears! This one's for you. The headstand technique known as triangular forearm support was developed by Loren Fishman, MD, a well-known physician and yoga teacher (and author of the foreword of this book). It is a modified version of the traditional headstand that can be used to treat rotator cuff injuries without surgery. This technique is beneficial because it safely reduces pain of arm abduction and flexion by substituting the action of the subscapularis muscle for the supraspinatus. Those with neck injuries, disc compression, or lack of balance and strength needed for traditional headstand poses can also benefit from this technique by using a wall. Stand with your feet together facing a wall and about a foot or two (0.3-0.6 m) away from the wall. Interlock your fingers and press your palms together, then lean forward to bring your forearms to the wall, with your elbows shoulder-width apart. Then step away from the wall, working your forearms down the wall toward your hips or as close as you can get! Press your forearms into the wall and relax the tops of your shoulders away from your earlobes. Hold the position for about 45 seconds to 2 minutes, then stand up and quickly raise your arms out to the sides, then overhead. Repeat, raising your arms at least twice. Then try raising your arms in front of you and all the way up twice. Fishman's book *Healing Yoga* provides more detailed instructions and guidance on the triangular forearm support technique.

Use a chair to reduce neck compression and build confidence.

This variation allows you more accessibility in headstand pose by placing less weight on your shoulders and neck. Place a sturdy chair against a wall with its back to the wall or on a sticky mat so that it doesn't slide. Kneel on the seat of the chair, facing away from the back of the chair seat, and fold over your thighs, walking your hands to the floor. Slowly lift through your hips to work your forearms down to the floor until you can clasp your hands. If you're trying this for the first time, have a teacher spot you. Place the crown of your head on the floor with your hands clasped behind the skull. Walk your

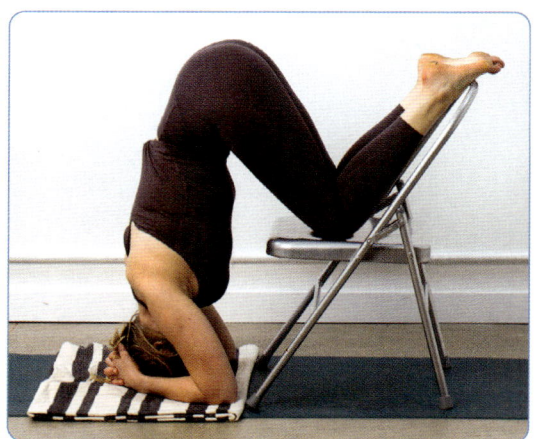

knees back to bring your shins to rest on the back rail of the chair so that your knees are pointing down. If you need extra cushion for your knees, place a blanket on the seat of the chair. With the shins grounded on the back of the chair, walk your knees forward on the seat of the chair, working your hips closer to a vertical stance above the shoulders. By doing this, you can control the amount of weight you place on your shoulders and neck.

The Complete Guide to Yoga Props

Feathered Peacock Pose

Pincha Mayurasana

पञ्चि मयूरासन

Feathered peacock pose, also known as forearm stand, is a dynamic yoga posture that actively strengthens the shoulders, arms, core, and back, offering a comprehensive upper body workout. Simultaneously, it provides a deep stretch to the shoulders, chest, and neck. Feathered peacock pose is also good for testing out your balance upside down! Let's explore some common ways to prop up this pose.

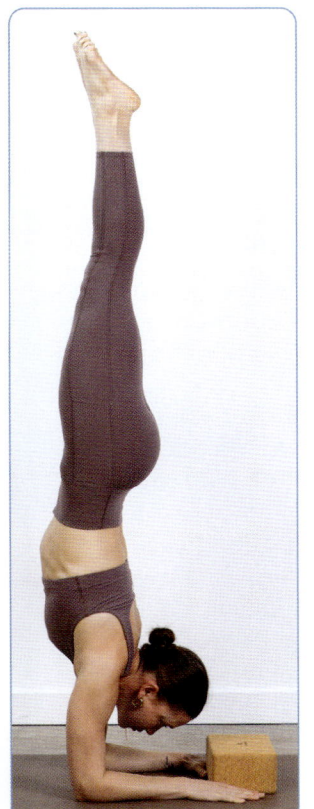

Use a block to inform the shoulders.

Squeezing the block between your hands while in forearm stand pose helps to facilitate external rotation of the shoulders, preventing the shoulders from collapsing toward one another along the upper back. This action also provides more stability, which helps you extend through your thoracic spine and maintain the integrity of the pose. Start in a tabletop position and place a block on its widest orientation between your hands. Create an L shape with your thumb and index finger, framing the bottom corners of the block. Walk your elbows toward each other until they are shoulder-width apart. Tuck your toes and lift your hips up and back, entering dolphin pose. As you hold this pose, focus on grounding down through the outside edges of both elbows and the insides of both wrists. Keep your gaze on the block between your hands and tiptoe your feet forward, working your shoulders over your elbows and your hips over your shoulders. Press your forearms into the mat to lift your shoulders away from your ears. To facilitate external rotation of the shoulders and prevent them from collapsing in, squeeze the block with your hands. This action also helps to provide more stability to achieve thoracic spine extension. Think about rounding through your upper back and contracting through your chest muscles to protract your shoulders. To further strengthen your practice, lift one leg toward the sky and shift your weight forward onto your opposite toes. Practice alternating legs before working toward lifting both legs to meet overhead. Externally wrap through your shoulders, rolling the tops of your upper arms back and hollowing out through your armpits. Squeeze your inner thighs together and lengthen your tailbone toward your heels while drawing your pubic bone in and up toward your navel.

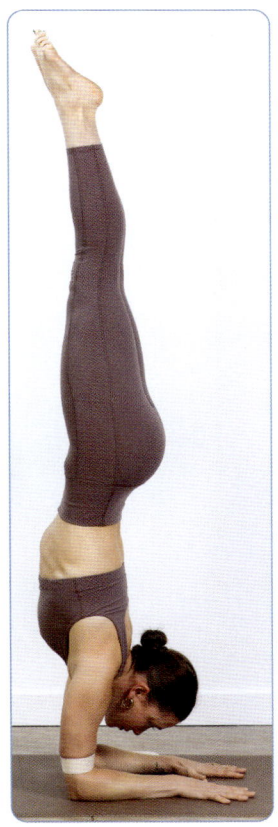

Loop a strap around your arms to inform and align.

Using a strap around your arms in forearm stand can help you to engage and strengthen your upper body muscles, particularly the shoulders and triceps. Additionally, the strap can help you to maintain a healthy alignment in your shoulders and spine, which can reduce the risk of injury or your elbows splaying open to the sides. Start by getting onto your hands and knees. Then, place your forearms on the floor, making sure that your elbows are directly under your shoulders. Wrap a strap around your arms, just below or above your elbows—whichever is most effective for you. Ensure the loop of the strap is snug but not too tight. Tuck your toes under and lift your hips up and back, straightening the legs as much as you can without compromising length in the spine. As

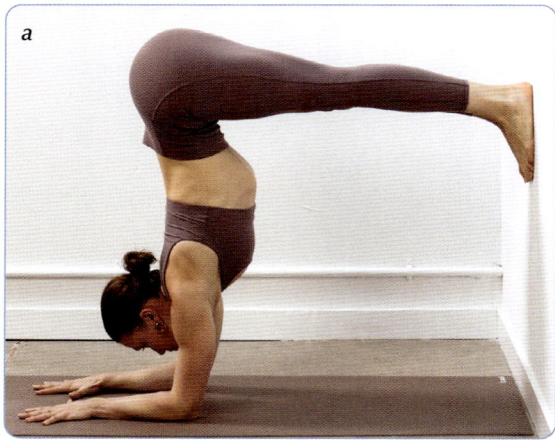

you hold the pose, focus on pressing your forearms and hands into the floor, engaging your upper body muscles. When you are ready, begin to practice alternating lifting the legs before eventually working toward lifting both legs to meet overhead.

Bring your feet to a wall to strengthen your shoulders.

Experience the benefits of a wall-supported forearm stand by strengthening your shoulders and core. This variation is an excellent way to practice the action of shifting your shoulders over your elbows and your hips over your shoulders, while still having more control with your feet on the wall. While it may not be easy, practicing the L shape position against the wall will fire up your core as you work to prevent your feet from sliding down. This is a great core challenge that will help you build the necessary strength and mobility to confidently enter the pose away from the wall. To get started with this variation, first measure your distance from the wall. Begin by sitting in staff pose (dandasana) with your feet flat against the wall and place a placeholder such as a prop where your hips are. Then turn away from the wall and position your elbows where the placeholder is. Enter dolphin pose and step your feet up the wall behind you until they are level with your hips. If you feel like your shoulders are too far forward or too far back, adjust your distance from the wall accordingly. Once you find the sweet spot, hold the L shape position against the wall for 30 seconds or longer to build strength (see photo *a*). Alternatively, you can practice a bending

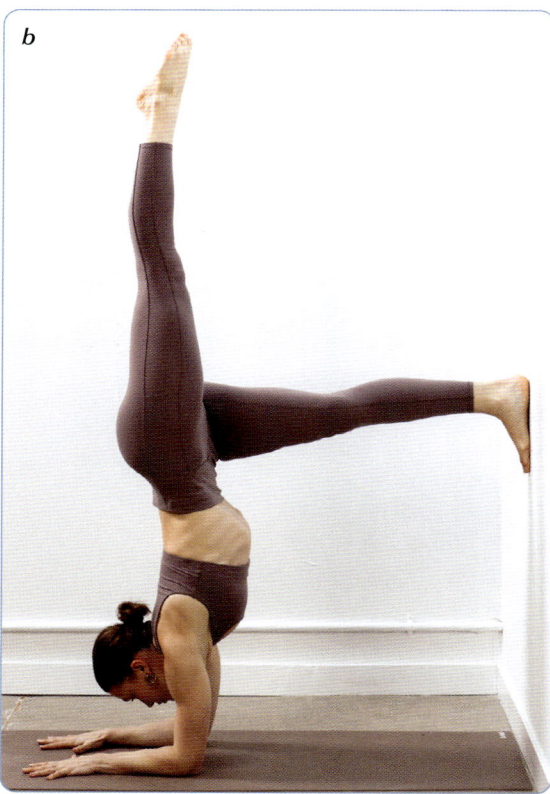

your knees, bringing your hips closer to your heels at the wall, and then straightening your legs several times. As you gain confidence in the hips-over-shoulders position, you can try alternating lifting one leg overhead at a time (see photo *b*). Practicing this variation regularly will not only strengthen your shoulders and core, but it will also help you develop the mobility and confidence to perform the pose away from the wall.

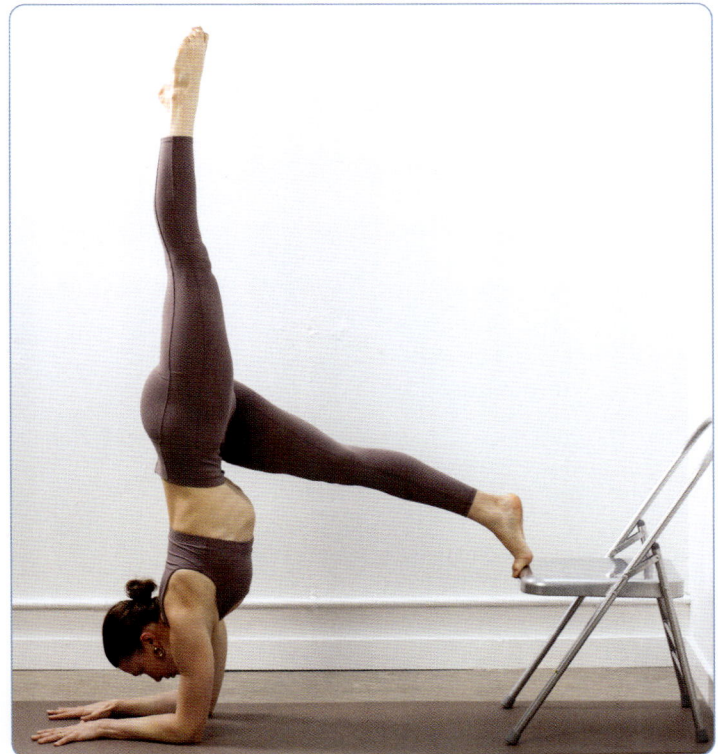

Step on a chair to give your hips a lift.

To practice forearm stand with a chair, place a chair against a wall with the seat facing away from the wall. Make your way into dolphin pose facing away from and in front of the chair. Next, step your feet onto the front edge of the chair seat and press the balls of your feet to shift your hips over your shoulders. Your starting distance from the chair will vary depending on your height and hamstring flexibility. This technique is like using a block in crow pose, where you can experience the pose without lifting your feet off the floor. Stepping onto a chair will encourage your hips to move over your shoulders while providing a stable base to ground into. This variation is particularly useful if you are still working on your balance and strength to lift both feet off the floor. It can also help to build your confidence as you progress. Using a chair also provides more opportunity to focus on building muscle memory. With added support, you can concentrate on the actions of your shoulders, arms, and upper back.

Practice with the backs of your shoulders against the front edge of a chair seat.

Using a chair as a prop during forearm stand can provide a stable base for the shoulders and help to open the chest. Using a chair and a wall during forearm stand can also provide a safer way to practice the pose, especially if you are still developing your strength and balance. Position the chair with its back against a wall to prevent it from sliding. Set up for dolphin pose first, placing your forearms below the seat of the chair, and walk your feet toward the wall until your hips are over your shoulders. Bring the upper back to the front edge of the chair seat, keeping the shoulders in line with the elbows. Having the upper back against the front edge of the chair seat provides a stable surface to push against, which can help to engage the muscles of the upper back and shoulders. This can help to stabilize the shoulders and prevent them from collapsing in, which is a common occurrence when attempting forearm stand without support. From here, try lifting one or both legs.

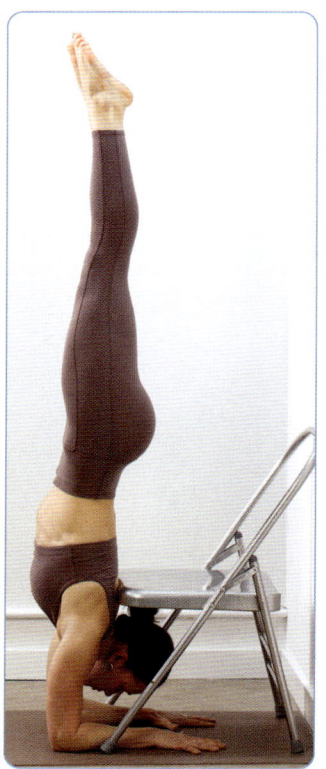

Supported Shoulder Stand Pose

Salamba Sarvangasana   सालम्ब सर्वाङ्गासन

Supported shoulder stand pose is an inversion that requires focus and determination. This pose actively stretches the shoulders and neck while inducing a sense of calm in the nervous system. Additionally, it contributes to reducing fluid retention in the legs and feet, stimulates the thyroid, and diminishes fatigue. Supported shoulder stand pose further enhances digestion. Let's explore this inversion with the help of props.

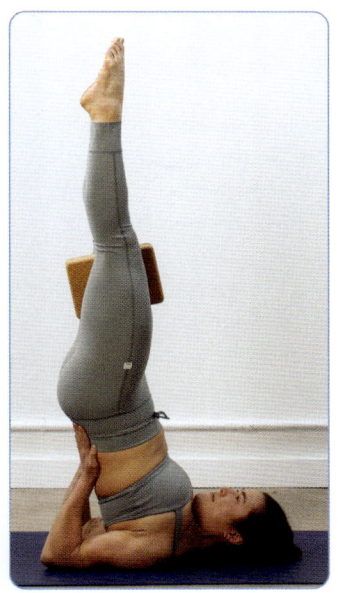

Place a block between your thighs to activate muscle engagement and inform posture.

This block-supported variation increases the engagement of your inner thighs and pelvic floor muscles, which can help to improve stability and balance in the pose while also strengthening these areas of the body. It can also help to keep the legs parallel and hips level. To enter this modified shoulder stand, lie on your back with your knees bent and your feet flat on the floor. Place a block between your thighs at its narrowest width, squeezing it gently to engage your inner thighs. Slowly lift your legs off the floor, bringing your knees toward your chest. Use your hands to support your lower back as you lift your hips off the floor, extending your legs toward the ceiling. Walk your hands down your back, lift your hips, and hug your elbows toward your midline.

Use a chair and bolsters to practice a restorative version.

To perform a gentler variation of the shoulder stand that reduces neck flexion and spinal compression, use a chair and bolsters for extra support. For stability, position the back of the chair against a wall and the legs of the chair on a mat. Place a folded blanket or mat on the chair, followed by a bolster in front of the chair, as well as a second bolster perpendicular to the first one, resting on the back bar of the chair. Straddle the seat on the chair with your chest facing the back of the chair and hold on to the chair back's side rails. Slide the backs of your knees to the top of the back chair rail, framing the bolster on either side. Keep a firm grip on the rail with your hands and slide your hips forward to lower your head, neck, and shoulders. Once you are settled, walk your hands down to the legs of the chair to lower your shoulder blades fully onto

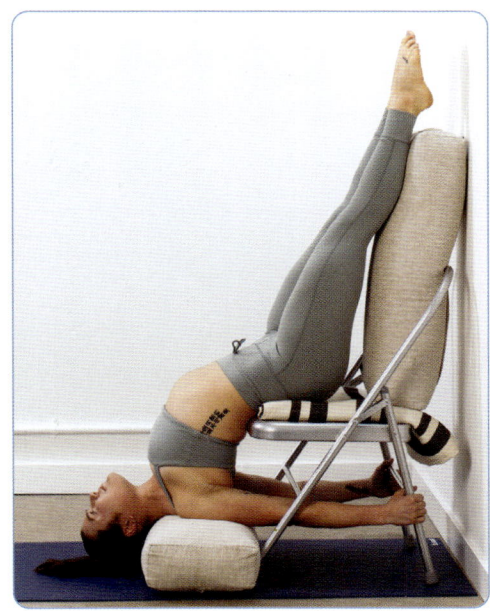

the other bolster and your head toward the floor; this may require adjusting your hips a little. Rest your legs on the bolster on the seat of the chair. Shimmy your shoulders under your chest, sliding your arms through the inside edge of the chair legs, and try to grasp the back legs of the chair to open your chest. Relax your entire body and breathe.

Press your feet into a chair to help lift your hips.

A chair-supported version of the shoulder stand can be a great starting point if you are struggling to build sufficient strength and control to perform the pose. It is also an excellent stepping stone to perform the full pose without support. In this variation, you start by lying down on a mat with your feet on a chair seat and your hands holding the front legs of the chair positioned against a wall on a mat for stability. The chair assists in lifting your body and practicing stability and control. Start by pressing your feet to elevate your hips and chest. As you hold the legs of the chair, wiggle your shoulders further underneath you to open your chest (see photo *a*). To deepen the pose, try coming up onto your tiptoes on the chair. This may create more space in the lower back and allow for a greater range of motion. Breathe deeply and engage your core muscles to maintain balance and control.

To make this chair variation a little more challenging, start with your buttocks on the chair, shoulders on the bolster below the chair, and step your feet onto the top rail of the back of the chair. Have a firm grip on the sides of the chair. Depending on your arm length, your hands may be in different locations; have them high enough up on the side rails as possible so that you can pull down and back to counteract the pressing of the feet into the top of the chair. This variation helps you to work toward getting your hips stacked over the chest (see photo *b*).

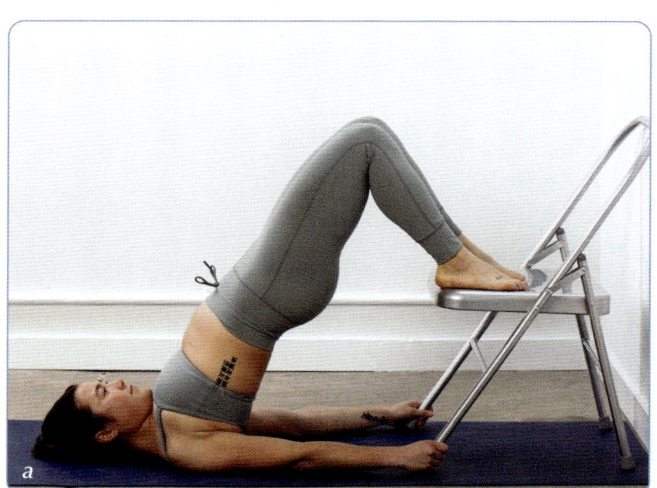
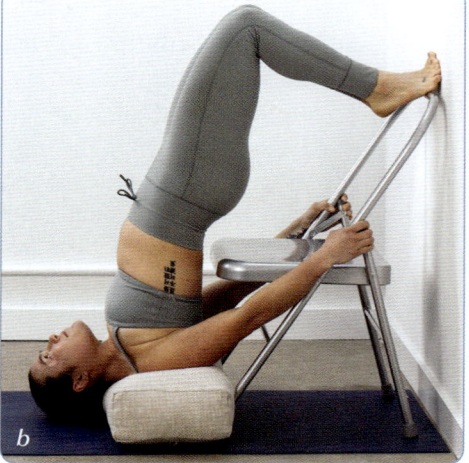

Place folded blankets under your shoulders to decompress the neck and breathe more easily.

By elevating the shoulders, blankets can provide additional cushioning and support, making the pose more comfortable for those with neck or shoulder issues. Blankets can also help create a more aligned posture, reducing the strain on the neck and upper back muscles, and allow for extension in the neck and chest, making breathing easier. Using blankets

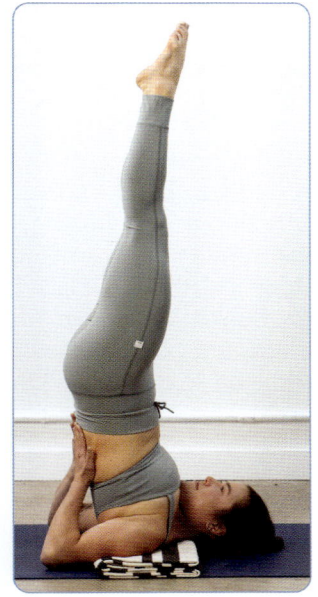

can also create a stable base for the shoulders to rest on, reducing the risk of injury or strain. For beginners or those with limited flexibility, blankets can provide added support and confidence to hold the pose longer and more comfortably. Prior to entering the pose, fold your blanket on the mat to create a few inches of thickness; feel free to add more. Position your shoulder blades on the blankets, resting your head and neck on the mat behind them. While lying on your back, extend both feet up toward the sky and pin your elbows into your sides with your forearms pointing straight up (as if you were holding an imaginary box). Drive your elbows and the backs of your arms into the mat, lifting your hips off the mat, capturing the lower back with your hands for support. Reach and extend through your legs as you press down through the backs of your arms.

Use bolsters to practice a restorative version.

Here are two variations of shoulder stand that can be practiced with bolsters for a restorative experience. The first variation involves opening the neck and shoulders and is ideal for those who want to engage the thyroid glands through throat lock (jalandhara bandha) without having to come into the full posture. To practice this version, lie your spine down on a bolster so that the tops of the shoulders can release off the short edge of the bolster, and the back of your head can rest flat on the floor. This will stretch the back of your neck gently while bringing your chin closer to the top of the sternum (see photo a). The second variation entails stacking one or two bolsters under your sacrum and extending your legs up toward the sky, like the legs up the wall pose (see photo b). This version focuses more on the lower half of the body without requiring you to lift your hips off the mat. Both options help reduce strain in the neck.

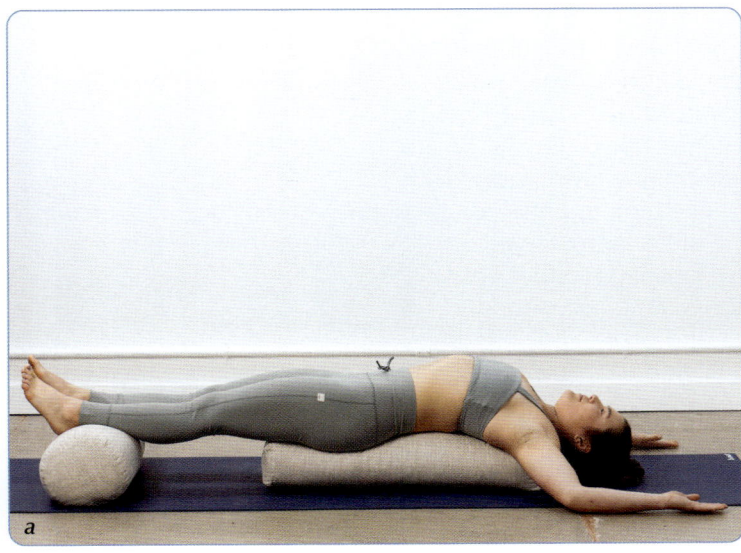

a

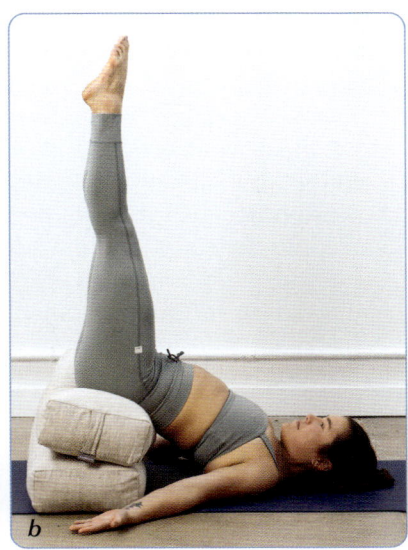

b

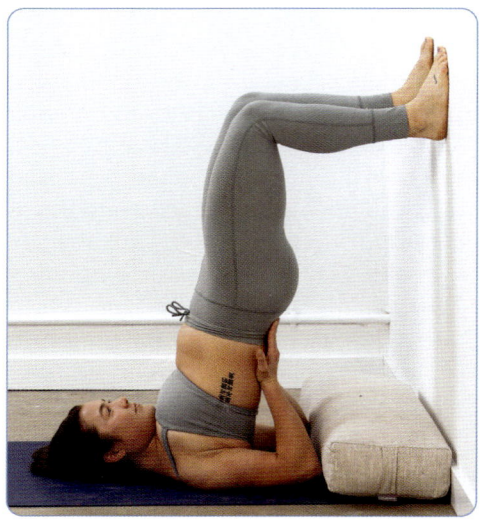

Walk your feet up a wall to gently enter the pose.

You can gently ease your way into the pose by walking your feet up the wall. This variation can be done by starting in the legs-up-the-wall pose with an optional folded blanket under your shoulders and a bolster under your hips. When you are ready, bend your knees and place your feet on the wall, gradually pressing into it to lift your hips off the bolster. For added support, walk your elbows in and place your hands on your lower or middle back. To deepen the stretch and challenge your balance, lift your heels off the wall and press the balls of your feet into it, firming your buttocks toward the pelvis to elongate your spine. For an extra challenge, alternate lifting one leg at a time off the wall.

Loop a strap around the arms.

Using a strap in shoulder stand can offer several benefits to your yoga practice. The strap helps to keep your elbows hugged in toward each other, ensuring that your upper arms and shoulders remain aligned and engaged in the pose. This helps to prevent the shoulders from collapsing and reduces the risk of injury. The strap also allows you to maintain a deeper stretch in your shoulders, upper back, and neck. This can help to relieve tension and tightness in these areas and improve your posture. By hugging your elbows in toward each other, the strap provides increased stability and support to your upper body. This can help you to maintain the pose for longer and with greater ease. For this variation, measure the loop of the strap to be shoulder-width length and place it by your side. Set up for either the chair-supported version or wall-supported version because you will need something to press your feet into for support while adding in the strap. Once the hips are lifted, grab your strap and loop it just above your elbows on your upper arms. Drive your elbows and the backs of your arms into the mat and place your hands

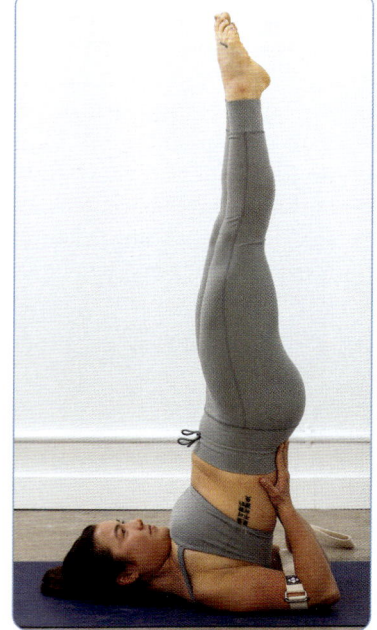

on your lower back for support. With hands in position, try lifting one leg at a time away from the wall or chair. Reach and extend through your legs as you press down through the backs of your arms.

Plow Pose

Halasana

हलासन

Plow pose is a rejuvenating yoga posture known for its fatigue-reducing and thyroid-stimulating benefits. This pose also offers a deep stretch to the shoulders, spine, and hamstrings. Elevate your practice with prop-supported variations for enhanced benefits.

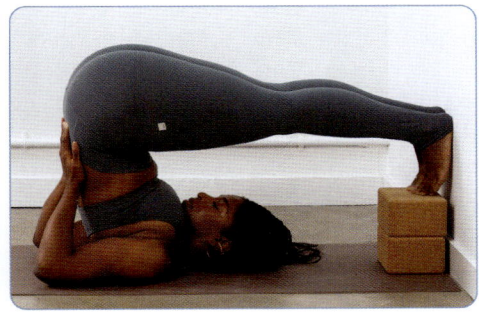

Stack blocks under your feet against a wall to bring the floor closer to you.

Using a block reduces the distance between you and the floor, creating more space for your chest and neck and enhancing stability in the spine. Use two blocks if your feet are hip-width apart or one block if your big toes touch. Place your blocks against the wall and then lie on the mat, away from the wall, aligning your shoulders where your hips would be in staff pose, as if sitting with your feet touching the wall. Measure and mark this spot with a block if needed.

From a supine position, extend both feet upward and pin your elbows into your sides, forearms pointing up (as if holding an imaginary box). Drive your elbows and arms into the mat, lifting your hips into shoulder stand. Gradually bring your elbows closer, slide your shoulder blades beneath the back of the ribs, and hinge at the hips to lower your feet to the wall behind you. Feel free to just use the wall for support, but if you want something to land the balls of your feet on, walk the feet down the wall to the blocks. If the blocks are out of reach, stack more blocks.

Place folded blankets under your shoulders to decompress the neck and breathe more easily.

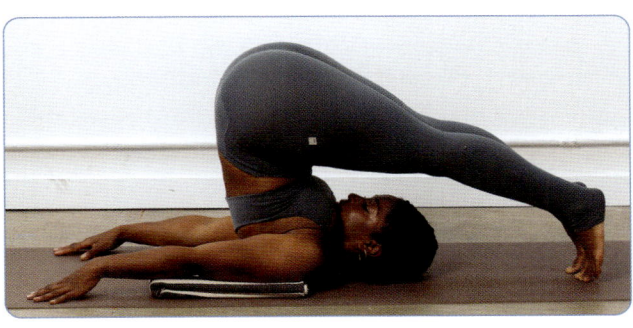

By elevating the shoulders, blankets can provide additional cushioning and support, making the pose more comfortable for those with neck or shoulder issues. Blankets can also help create a more aligned posture, reducing the strain on the neck and upper back muscles, and allow for some extension in the neck and chest, promoting greater ease in breathing. Using blankets can also create a stable base for the shoulders to rest on, reducing the risk of injury or strain. For beginners or those with limited mobility, blankets can provide added support and confidence to hold the pose longer and more comfortably. For this pose, begin in in a blanket-supported shoulder stand described in supported shoulder stand pose, then reach your toes overhead toward the floor.

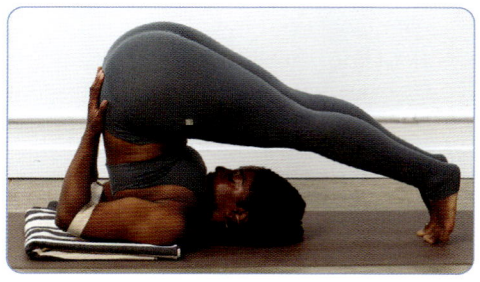

Loop a strap around the arms.

Using a strap in this pose can offer several benefits. The strap helps to keep your elbows hugged in toward each other, ensuring that your upper arms and shoulders remain aligned and engaged in the pose. This helps to prevent the shoulders from collapsing and reduces the risk of injury. The strap also allows you to maintain a deeper stretch in your shoulders, upper back, and neck. This can help to relieve tension and tightness in these areas and improve your posture. By hugging your elbows in toward each other, the strap provides increased stability and support to your upper body. This can help you to maintain the pose for longer and with greater ease. To perform this pose, enter shoulder stand with the strap around your arms, as described for supported shoulder stand pose, then lower your toes overhead toward the floor.

Practice with a chair under your feet or thighs.

These two variations work like bringing your feet to the wall or blocks but provide a higher platform to rest your feet or thighs on. If you are bringing your feet to the chair, set up and practice like the description of the feet walking down the wall option described previously, but this time bringing your feet to the seat of a chair (see photo *a*). If you would like an even more supported option, bring a folded blanket just in front of the front legs of a chair, then lay your shoulders on the blanket, sliding your head under the seat of the chair. Note that the blanket is optional, as you can see in the photo. As you enter the pose, slide your legs through the back of the chair and let the tops of your thighs release fully into the seat of the chair (see photo *b*). This will also allow the hip flexors to release. To help prevent sliding, try placing a sticky mat on the chair.

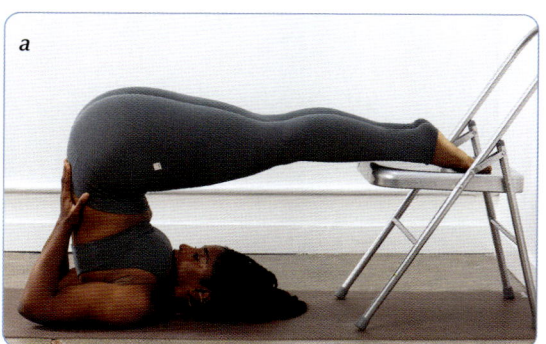

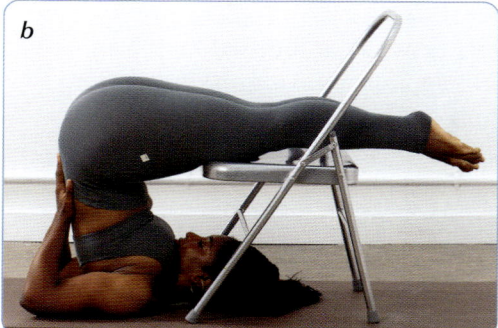

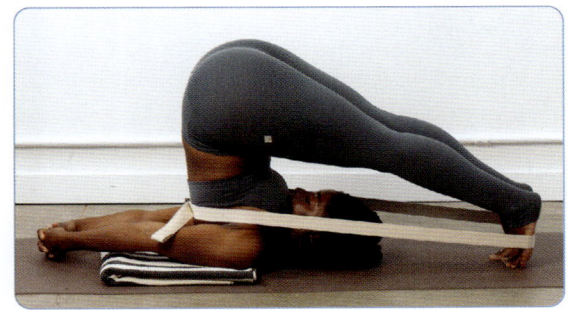

Loop a strap around backs of your shoulders and feet.

You can use a strap to assist in bringing the shoulders forward and creating more space in the front of the torso. Make a loop in the strap that fits comfortably around your shoulder blades and the balls of your feet when lying on your back with your legs extended up. Place the backs of your arms by your sides, with your elbows hugged in, forearms pointing up, and palms facing each other. Drive your elbows into the mat to lift your hips and use your hands to support your low back. Press the balls of your feet into the strap to help pull the backs of your shoulders forward.

Place a bolster under your low back for a more grounded take.

This variation helps reduce neck tension and flexion. It allows for a gentle elevation in the hips and allows you to stretch through the backs of the legs and spine. Begin in a supported bridge pose with your hips on top of a bolster (or two). Lower your legs toward your body, keeping them extended and engaged. Reach for your feet or ankles with your hands or slide a strap over your feet, holding both ends of the strap in your hands to gently draw the legs to you.

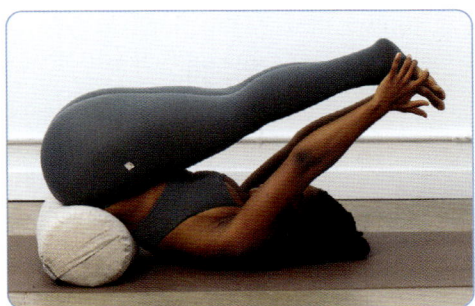

Ear Pressure Pose

Karnapidasana   कर्णपीडासन

Ear pressure pose, a dynamic yoga posture, brings rejuvenation as it actively stretches the spine and posterior chain muscles. With benefits such as improved digestion, a calm mind, increased blood circulation, and boosted energy levels, this pose offers a holistic experience. Explore prop-supported variations for an enhanced practice.

Place blocks under your knees or shins to bring the floor to you.

Using blocks under the knees or shins in ear pressure pose can be beneficial for practitioners who have limited flexibility in the spine, hips, or hamstrings. Placing blocks under the knees or shins reduces the distance between you and the floor which can help to make the pose more accessible. It also helps to release any tension in the hips or hamstrings and allows you to focus on deepening your upper body

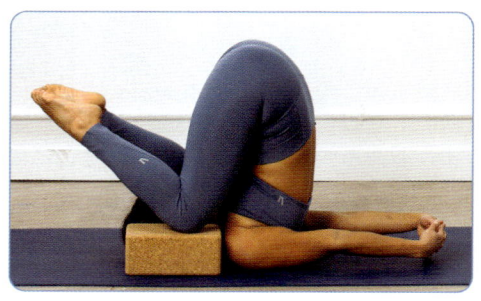

stretch. Placing the blocks beside the ears can also provide additional support and stability. This helps to ensure that you are properly aligned and can maintain the posture without straining your neck or shoulders. From plow pose, lower your knees onto the blocks.

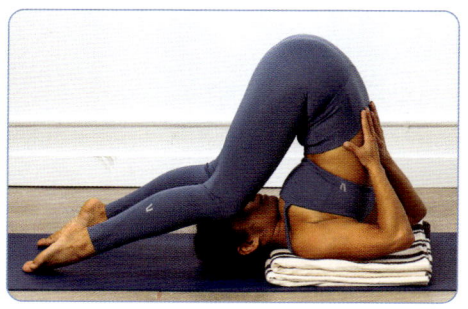

Place a folded blanket under your shoulders to decompress the neck and breathe more easily.

Blankets can elevate the shoulders, provide additional cushioning and support, and make ear pressure pose more comfortable for those with neck or shoulder issues. Blankets can also help create a more aligned posture, reducing the strain on the neck and upper back muscles, and allow for some extension in the neck and chest, promoting greater ease in breathing.

Using blankets can also create a stable base for the shoulders to rest on, reducing the risk of injury or strain. For beginners or those with limited mobility, blankets can provide added support and confidence to hold the pose longer and more comfortably. For this pose, enter a blanket-supported shoulder stand, as described previously for the supported shoulder stand pose. Place folded blankets under your shoulders to decompress the neck and breathe more easily, then lower your knees toward the floor, framing your ears.

Bring your knees or thighs to a chair seat and allow your shins to rest on the back of the chair.

This variation works like bringing your knees or shins to blocks but provides a higher platform to rest your knees on. Bring a folded blanket just in front of the front legs of a chair, then lay your shoulders on the blanket, sliding your head under the seat of the chair. As you enter the pose, release the knees toward the seat of the chair and if you can, slide the tops of your thighs onto the chair to fully release the hips and groin. Allow your shins to relax and rest on the back of the chair. To help prevent sliding, place a sticky mat on top of the chair.

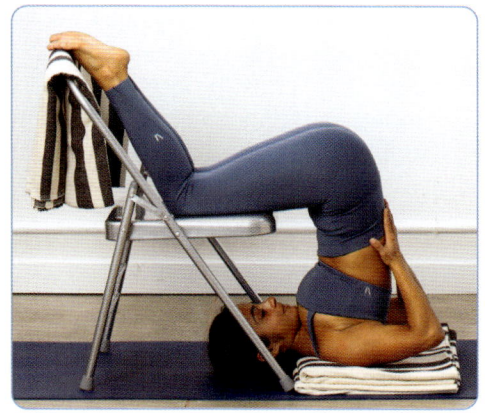

Downward-Facing Tree Pose

Adho Mukha Vrikshasana

अधोम ुखव ृक्षासन

Downward-facing tree pose, or handstand, is a dynamic yoga posture that powerfully strengthens the shoulders, arms, core, and back. With its stretching benefits for the shoulders, chest, and neck, this pose enhances flexibility and relieves tension. It also improves balance, making it an invigorating addition to your practice. Explore prop-supported variations for a more comprehensive and fulfilling experience.

Hug a block between your torso and your thigh to practice confidence and control.

This variation of handstand involves hugging a bent knee into a block to help keep you from arching your back and falling over. It also teaches you how to engage the required muscles in this pose, including the deep core muscles such as the hip flexors. Start in mountain pose, place a block on the left thigh, and bend forward at the hips, securely holding the block between the chest and the leg. Place your hands on the mat, shoulder-width apart, fingers forward. Maintain shoulder alignment over your wrists and gaze between them. Lift your right leg toward the ceiling, squeezing the block into the body with the left thigh. Shift your weight forward and press your hands into the mat to lift into handstand; use small hops if needed. Keep squeezing the block, trying not to drop it, to maintain length in your lower back! Repeat on the other side.

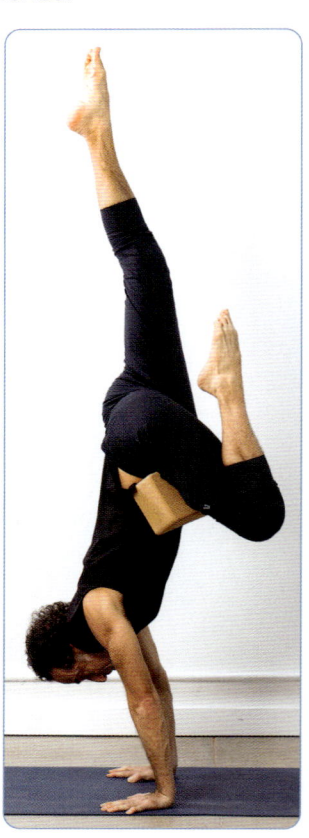

Stand on a block to assist in shifting your weight forward.

Starting a handstand from a standing position on a block helps shift your weight forward and makes stacking your shoulders directly over your wrists easier. It also helps to work the hips over the shoulders, making it easier to enter handstand with minimal momentum, which can be destabilizing. Stand on a sturdy block, then bend forward and place your hands on the floor, shoulder-width apart, directly in front of the block. Bend your knee as much as needed to accommodate tight hamstrings. Lift one leg, entering a standing split, then shift your weight forward into your hands, positioning your shoulders over your wrists. Push with the hands and shoulders to straighten your arms and work your hips as far over your shoulders as you can. Stay here to build strength in the stacked position or try floating your bottom foot off the block coming into an L shape in your handstand. If you feel stable, bring your legs together overhead, focusing on maintaining balance and control.

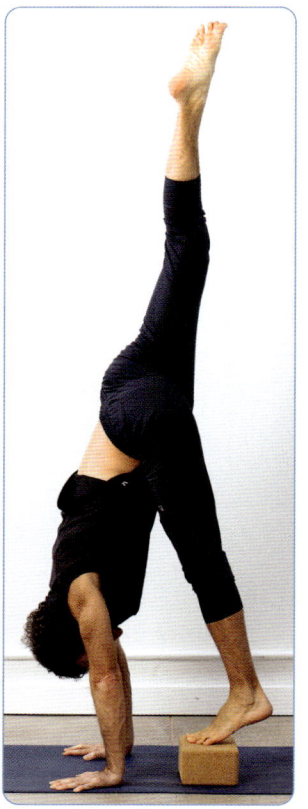

The Complete Guide to Yoga Props

Step your feet onto a chair to stack your hips over your shoulders.

This variation strengthens the posture without lifting your feet off the chair, providing a chance to build muscle memory for future challenges. Place a chair against a wall for added stability, then face away from the chair, fold forward, and position your hands on the floor. Step your feet back onto the chair seat, lift your hips, and extend your legs. Gradually walk your hands toward or away from the chair until your hips are directly above your shoulders and your shoulders are over your wrists. You can work toward handstand by trying one of two exercises. The first is lifting one leg up, directly over your hips (see photo a). If you're feeling confident, press your hands firmly into the floor and lift your toes off the chair seat. Then repeat on the other side. The second variation requires a little more core and hip flexor power. Draw one knee into your chest as close as you can. Then, try to draw the other knee into the chest, crossing your ankles. Rather than untucking your tailbone to stack fully, it will be slightly curved to draw the thighs to the chest (see photo b). This means that you will have to work harder to resist gravity, but if you can hold this, you will feel more stable when it is time to lift the hips directly up over the shoulders. It will also help you develop the muscles that counteract the tendency to fall forward past the hands.

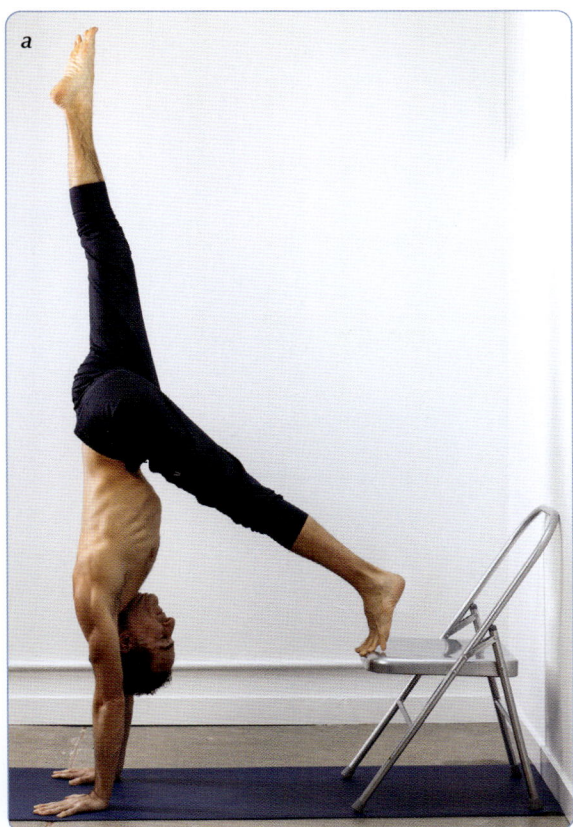
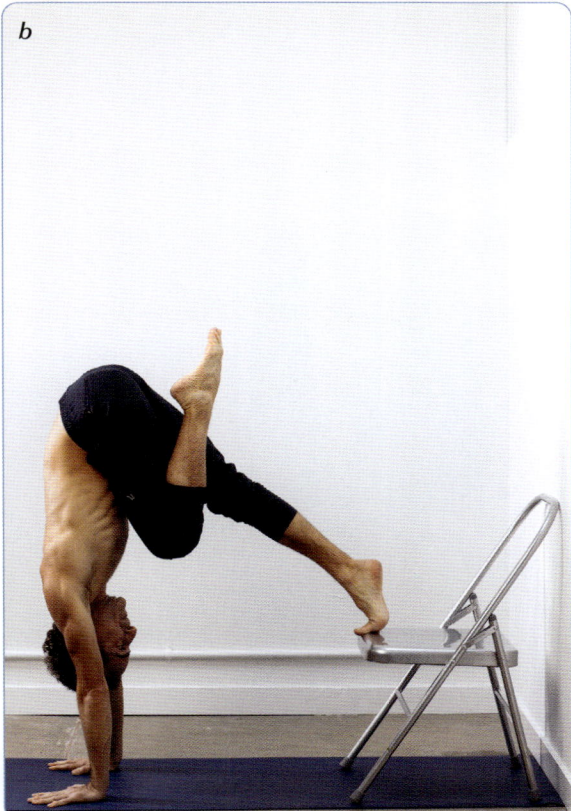

Downward-Facing Tree Pose (continued)

Practice using a wall.

Using a wall to practice handstands can improve posture and alignment and ease the fear of falling. Here are four variations you can try, each with its own advantages and challenges. The first variation is the most common and involves facing away from the wall and practicing handstands with your back against the wall (see photo *a*). This approach provides a safety net and helps build confidence. However, it can also encourage a tendency to kick too hard and rely on the wall for support. To avoid this, start with your hands about a foot away from the wall and focus on not touching the wall with your feet.

The second variation involves facing the wall while on your hands (see photo *b*). Enter a forward fold, then walk your feet up the wall behind you. Walk your hands back to the wall until your legs, hips, and chest are in contact with the wall. Contract your muscles and squeeze your inner thighs together, and, if possible, bring your forehead to the wall. If you can comfortably bring your forehead to the wall, try peeling your hips and legs away from the wall, which requires more shoulder mobility.

The third variation is like the second one, but with your hands a foot or so (0.3-0.6 m) away from the wall. A pair of comfy socks will help protect the tops of your feet from wall burn. Press the tops of your feet into the wall and hollow out through your belly, creating a

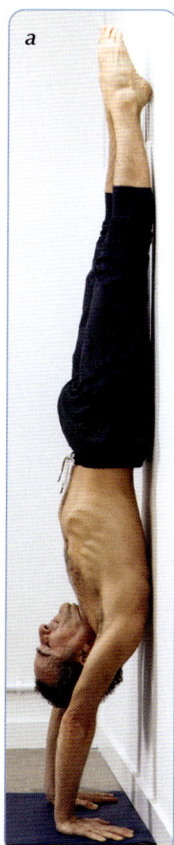
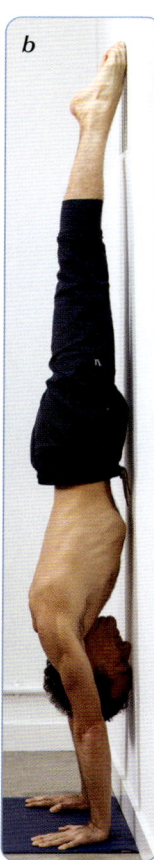
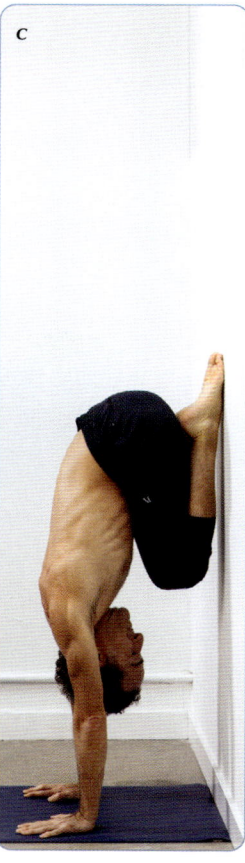
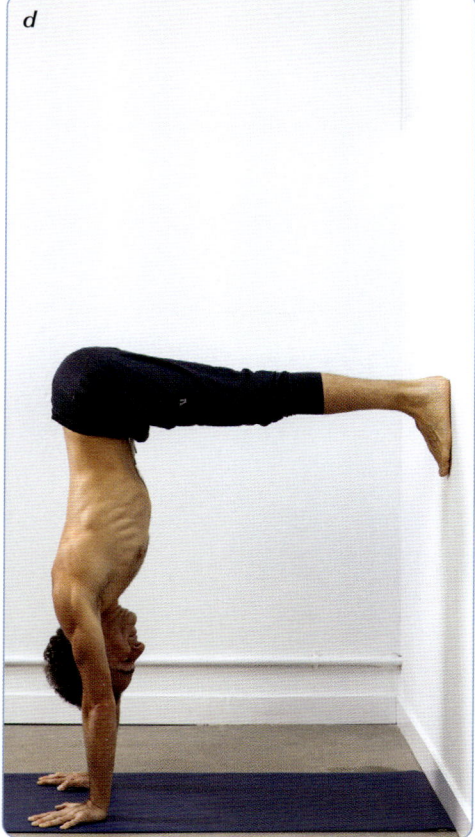

The Complete Guide to Yoga Props

straight line with your body at an angle to the wall. Slide your feet down the wall, drawing your knees into your chest, and then slide them back up to the starting position. Repeat several times; be careful to not collapse your belly and hips toward the wall (see photo c).

The fourth variation involves walking your feet up the wall to create an L shape with your body, like the L-shaped handstand with a chair but with a wall instead of a chair (see photo d). Try to stack your shoulders over your hips and your hips over your shoulders. You can also practice the same drills outlined in the chair example.

Use a strap around your arms to assist in shoulder elevation and protraction.

If you're working toward a press handstand someday, you need strong shoulder muscles for protraction and elevation. A strap can be an effective tool in this process. It prevents the elbows from bending and promotes external rotation of the shoulders. It also helps in the protraction of the upper back by allowing you to forcefully press the floor as the arms fire up, pressing into the strap, which is essential for lifting your feet in the opposite direction. Loop the strap shoulder-width apart around your arms, just above your elbows. Press into the handstand from a tuck, straddle, or L shape. You can also use the strap to press up from crow into the handstand. Have an experienced teacher spot you or use a wall for support to ensure your safety.

Place a folded mat or blanket under your hands to ease wrist tension and flexion.

If you experience wrist tension or have limited wrist flexion, performing handstands can be challenging and uncomfortable. A folded mat or blanket under the heels of your hands is a great modification to alleviate some pressure from your wrists. By elevating your hands, you can maintain a neutral wrist position and distribute your weight more evenly throughout your hands 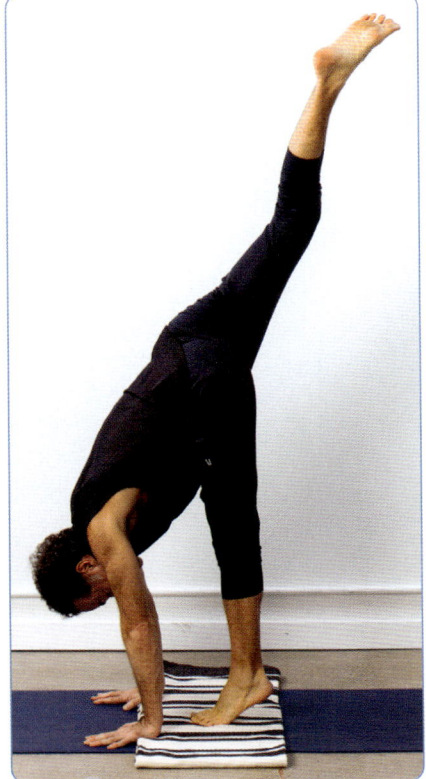 and arms. This position is considered neutral because if your wrists cannot flex back at a 90-degree angle, then the rest of the body most likely will try to compensate in ways that compromise your alignment and stability. This modification can also help you build the necessary strength and stability to progress toward performing handstands without the support of the folded mat or blanket.

Practice tuck handstand by squeezing a block between your thighs.

This variation can help you engage your inner thigh muscles and adductors, which are important stabilizing muscles for maintaining balance in the handstand. This engagement can also help you maintain proper alignment in your legs and prevent them from splaying. The block can provide a tactile cue for keeping your legs together and maintaining a healthy alignment in your hips and pelvis. This can help you improve your form and control in the handstand. The block can also provide an additional challenge to your core and hip flexor muscles, because you'll need to use them to hold the block between your thighs. Begin the tuck handstand with a block between your thighs. Fold forward, placing your hands on the mat, and begin taking small hops with your knees toward your chest while squeezing the block with your thighs for stability (see

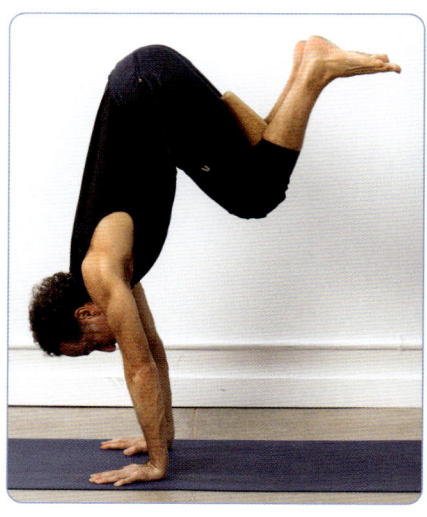

photo for an example mid-hop). Practice controlled descents to refine your technique and build strength.

Practice with your hands on blocks to work on your claw grip.

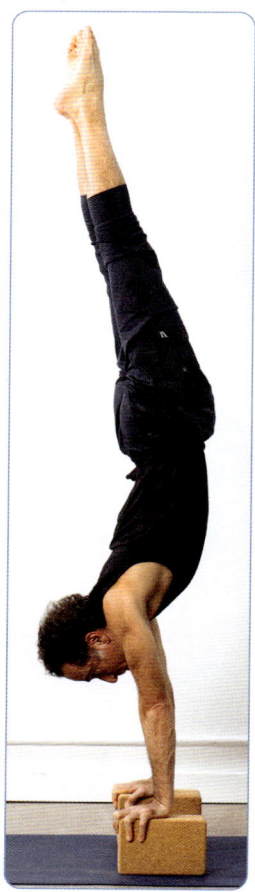

Improve your claw grip by practicing with your hands on blocks. Just as the front part of the feet sometimes work as brakes when we are standing and shift our weight forward, the hands also need a good braking system to maintain balance in the handstand. By gently bending your fingers and pressing the pads of your fingers into the mat, you create a better braking system for when you feel your weight shifting forward and don't want to fall. However, this requires significant finger strength, which you can build by using blocks. You can use small blocks specifically designed to fit in the palm of your hand or simply flip regular blocks to their narrowest width. Cork blocks are recommended for their sturdiness and weight. Use a wall or have a teacher spot you to prevent the blocks from falling over. To find the grip, bring your pointer and middle fingers over the front edge of the blocks and grab the outside edges with your thumbs, ring, and pinky fingers. Your hands will be higher than your feet, so you may need to stand on a block or stack a few blocks to raise the height of the floor under your feet. As you enter handstand, contract all your muscles so that the weight shift happens in the wrists and hands. Focus on pressing on the front knuckles as your weight shifts forward and pressing on the heels of your hands as the weight shifts back.

Use a rolled-up blanket or mat to practice "floating" to handstand.

Achieving a soft and quiet hop to the top of the mat, resembling a float on a cloud, is a playful exercise. To work on floating into handstand without the intimidating leap, use a rolled-up blanket or mat. Instead of attempting a full handstand on the first go, place the prop just in front of your toes in downward dog. Practice hopping over the prop with straight legs by focusing on lifting your hips up and down, not just moving forward and back. Bend your knees on an exhale and straighten them on an inhale to clear the prop. This technique trains your hips to lift higher. This sounds simple, but keeping your legs straight in the air might initially feel unfamiliar. It may take a few attempts not to bend your knees while hopping

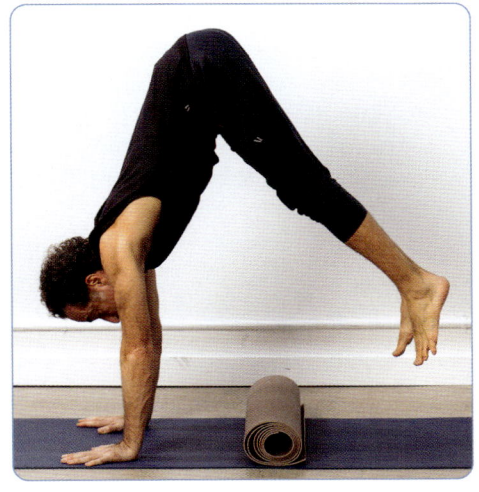

over the rolled prop. Once the brain grasps this action, ensure you bend the knees upon landing to absorb the shock, preventing a straight and locked position. Once you can successfully do this 10 times in a row, move the prop a few inches closer to your hands and continue to practice until it is right in front of your wrists. This way, you incrementally build the strength, flexibility, and confidence needed to float into a handstand. Be patient with yourself and do not rush progress. With consistent practice, you will eventually be ready to float into a handstand from downward dog with ease.

Practice toe taps with blocks or a wall.

Here are five fun ways to practice tapping your toes to your wrists! The first option involves leaning your head or shoulders into a wall. Place your hands about half a foot (15 cm) from the wall, then shift your weight forward to bring the back of your head to the wall. Lean into the wall to bring the backs of the shoulders to the wall and lift your hips. Try to tap both toes to the wrist, hold, then release (see photo *a*). Over time, you will need to rely less on the wall.

The second option will help you to build the flexibility needed to bring your toes to your wrists. Begin in an L-shaped handstand with your feet on the wall. Try alternating one foot down at a time to tap your wrists (see photo *b*). If they cannot reach the wrists just yet, go as far as you can while keeping the hips stacked over the shoulders. In the third option, bring your butt to the wall in a forward fold, then come up on to your tiptoes to elevate your sitting bones higher up the wall. Press your sitting bones back into the wall, flex your feet, and lift your legs away from the wall to tap the backs of your wrists (see photo *c*).

The fourth option involves blocks. Place two blocks to frame your feet in a standing forward fold. Shift your weight forward into your hands and protract through your shoulders. Lift onto your tiptoes as you shift your weight forward, and just when it feels like your body is going to fall forward, try to float your feet up (without hopping) and on to the blocks (see photo *d*). Then practice the same shifting forward exercise to float the feet back between the blocks. The fifth option is great for those with wrist pain as it takes the

Downward-Facing Tree Pose (continued)

weight off your wrists entirely! Lie on your back, place a block between your thighs to squeeze and stabilize the pelvis, and extend your feet toward the sky. Extend your arms overhead, keeping the backs of your hands flat on the ground or flexing your fingers back to point towards the floor if you want to simulate the wrist actions in a handstand. Bring your toes toward your wrists, using your core to lift the hips off the mat (reverse crunch) (see photo e). Repeat several times.

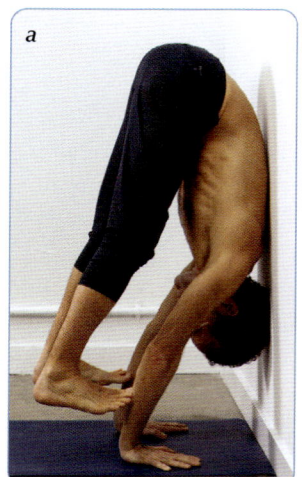

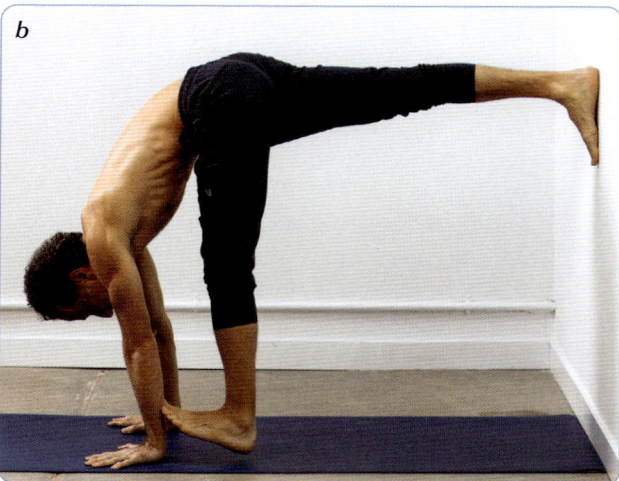

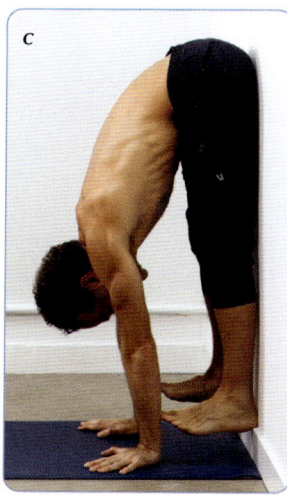

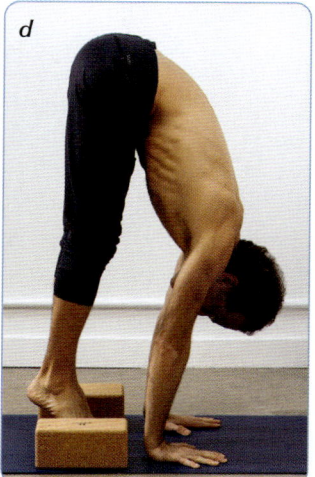

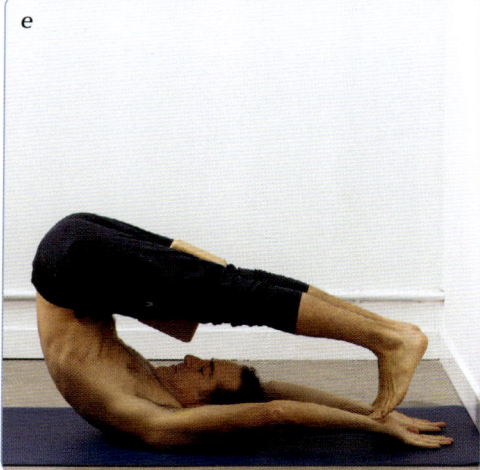

Chapter 8

Prone Poses

Peace is this moment without judgment. That is all. This moment in the Heart-space where everything is welcome.

Dorothy Hunt

In this chapter, we delve into prone postures, exploring flexible adaptations achieved with the assistance of props. While this category of poses is traditionally associated with lying down with the belly resting on the floor, we broaden this definition to encompass poses in which the belly either touches or faces the ground. These postures not only connect us with the foundation beneath us but also serve as a reminder of our roots, allowing us to build with a deeper understanding. Some yoga postures in which the belly connects with or faces the ground can be likened to moments of surrender and grounding. Like a seed nestled in the earth, these poses symbolize a return to the source—a humble acknowledgment of our connection to the earth and its nurturing energy. Just as a seed must surrender to the soil in order to germinate and grow, so too must we surrender to the earth's embrace in these poses, allowing transformation and growth to unfold from within. Prone postures can also draw attention to the belly, digestion, and the flow of energy stemming from and returning to the core. Throughout this section, the versatile use of props enhances the poses, making them more demanding, comfortable, accessible, or creatively expressive. It's important to note that the chapters in part II are organized based on each pose's originally intended form, but in some cases the adaptations alter the orientation of the posture from its initial form. Also, a few ambiguous postures (poses in which the individual is in a sideways orientation) are included here because they flow best with the overall theme of the chapter and because they need a home.

> Mantra: I ground myself, belly down, connecting with the earth's strength and stability.

Child's Pose

Balasana   बालासन

Child's pose is a restorative posture that elicits relaxation and a feeling of calmness. This pose also stretches the low back, hips, thighs, and ankles. It also relaxes and softens muscles along the front of the body. This pose is also known to aid in digestion. Let's look at a few common variations of child's pose using props.

Use a block or folded blanket to support your head and neck.

If your head doesn't comfortably reach the mat in child's pose, consider placing a block or rolled blanket beneath your forehead for additional support and comfort.

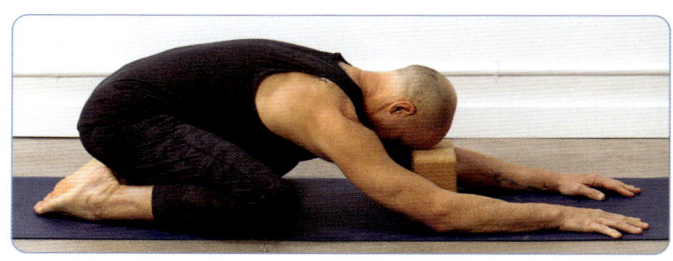

This extra elevation brings the floor closer to you, promoting greater extension in the cervical spine (neck). It also offers a supportive surface for your forehead, helping to release tension in the head and neck as you relax into the pose. Sit on your heels and bring your big toes together so they touch. You can spread your knees wider than your hips for greater thoracic extension and chest expansion or bring them together for more of a release in the back of the body. You can extend your arms in front of you or place them back by your sides. Fill the space between your forehead and the floor by sliding either a block or a rolled blanket underneath. Focus on breathing into the back of your body.

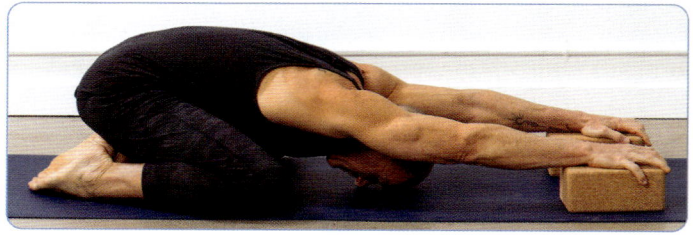

Place your hands on a block for more extension.

By using blocks in this pose, you can create more length in the sides of the body and back, and by descending the head and neck between the arms, you can experience a deeper stretch through the chest. Sit on your heels and bring your big toes together so they touch. Spread your knees wider than your hips and extend your arms in front of you. Place blocks on the lowest height under your palms and ensure that they are shoulder-width apart. Release your head and neck between your arms. If you feel any low back pain, draw your knees closer together, and lengthen your tailbone away from the crown of your head. Taking deep breaths down the back as if you were breathing into the space of the kidneys and adrenal glands can help you to fully relax and deepen the stretch. Lastly, relax your facial muscles and jaw to promote even greater relaxation throughout the entire body.

Place a block or blanket under your head to practice a thread-the-needle variation.

Whether you prefer a table top pose or a child's pose, practicing this technique can be more comfortable if you use a block or folded blanket. The prop provides support for those with stiff neck muscles and shoulders, bridging the gap between the head and the mat so that you can fully relax. Enter a table top position and press down with your left hand

and inhale as you lift your right arm to the sky, opening the chest (see photo *a*). Exhale and thread your right arm under your left arm, bringing your right ear toward the mat. Slide a block or folded blanket under your right ear to bridge the gap between your head and the floor (see photo *b*). You can also walk your left fingertips forward or reach them around for a half bind. Work on keeping your hip points level and equidistant from the mat. Breathe deeply into the space between your shoulder blades, chest, and belly, letting your diaphragm release with every inhale. Remember to relax your head and neck and soften your gaze. Repeat the technique on the other side. You can also do this variation from child's pose by inhaling to lift your gaze forward and coming onto your fingertips (see photo *c*), and then exhaling to thread your arm under (see photo *d*).

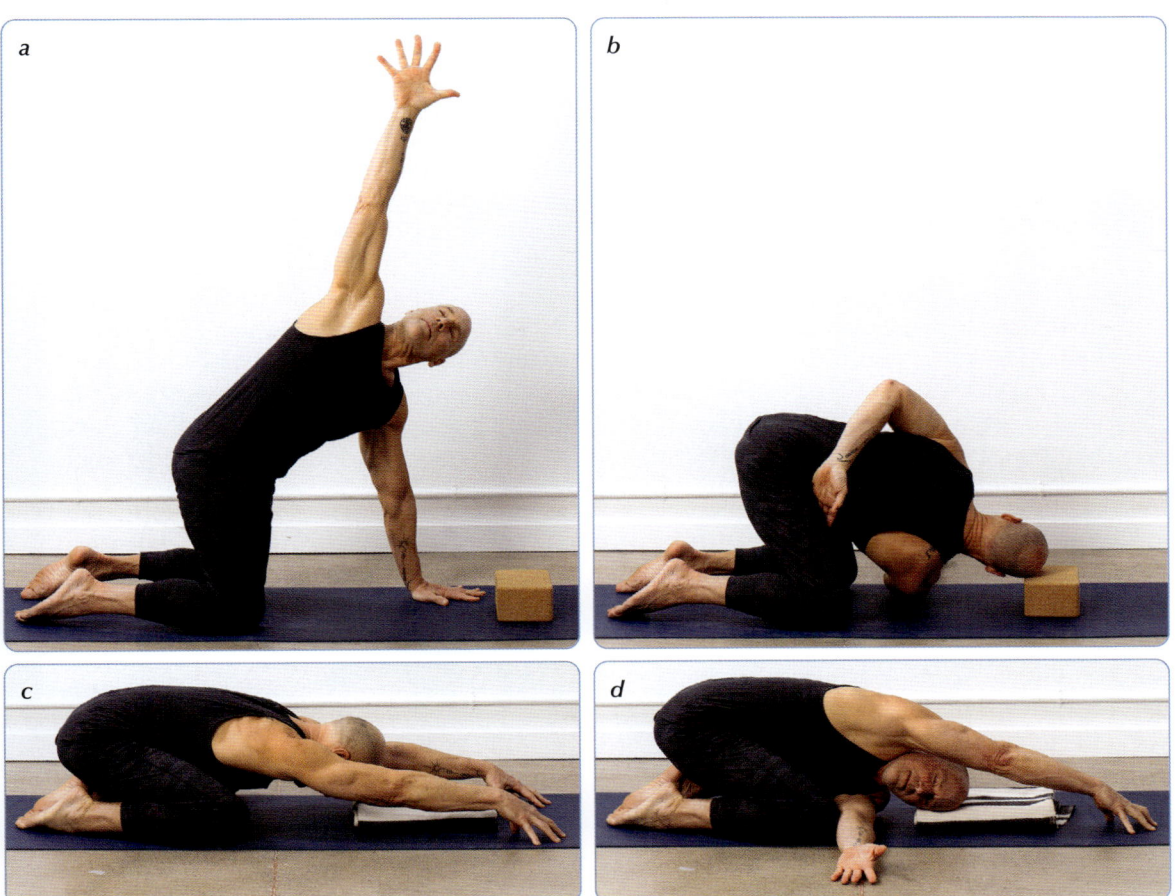

Place blocks under your shoulders to release tension.

Placing blocks under your shoulders in child's pose can help release tension and deepen your breath by allowing your body to fully relax into the pose. Child's pose is a resting pose that can help stretch the hips, thighs, and ankles, while also relieving stress and tension in the back, shoulders, and neck. However, some people find it difficult to fully relax in this pose due to tightness or discomfort in the shoulders. The blocks raise the height of your shoulders, which can help open the chest and shoulders, allowing you to fully relax into the pose. As you release tension in the shoulders and neck, you might also find that you are able to release tension throughout the rest of your body, leading to a more profound sense of relaxation and rejuvenation.

Create a restorative ramp using two bolsters, blocks, and blankets.

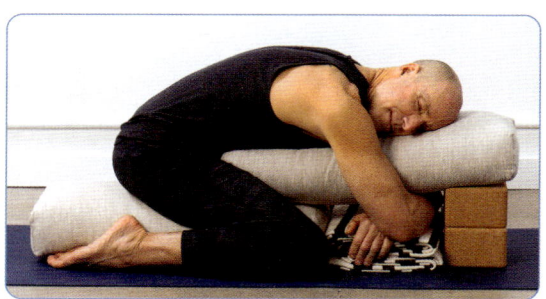

This restorative variation offers cushion and support for longer holds. To set up, place a sturdy bolster in the middle of your mat and stack two blocks about half a foot to a foot (0.2-0.3 m) in front of the bolster. Stack a second bolster on top of the first, supported by the blocks. Fold two to three blankets and place them between the bolster and blocks for arm support. When entering the pose, sit on the bottom bolster and ease your body onto the top bolster, making sure there is no feeling of collapse. Wrap your arms around the bolster and rest them on the folded blankets. Turn your head to one side as it rests on the bolster, fully relax into the pose, and release any tension in your shoulders and upper back. As you settle in, notice any areas of tightness or discomfort and adjust your props as needed. Prioritize your comfort and relaxation during this restorative pose, fully melting into the supporting props and releasing tension. Turn your head to the other side when ready and slowly peel yourself up to sit when complete.

Place a rolled-up blanket under your seat to support your hips and knees.

Child's pose is a calming and restorative pose that can help release tension and reduce stress. However, some people find it difficult to fully relax in this pose due to discomfort or tightness in the hips, knees, or ankles. Rolling a blanket or towel and placing it between your sitting bones and

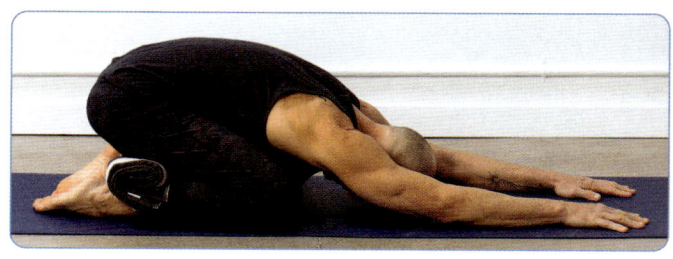

ankles can help create a more comfortable and stable position in the pose. The blanket helps to elevate your hips slightly, providing relief to the lower back and creating more space in the hips. This added space can help to reduce pressure on the knees and ankles, which can be especially beneficial for people with knee or ankle pain. This additional support can allow you to stay in the pose longer, deepening the stretch and promoting relaxation throughout the body. As you breathe deeply and relax into the pose with the support of the blanket, you may find that you experience a deeper sense of physical and mental calm and peacefulness.

Place a rolled-up blanket under your ankles for support.

A rolled blanket placed under your ankles in child's pose can provide many benefits. First and foremost, it can help to relieve any discomfort

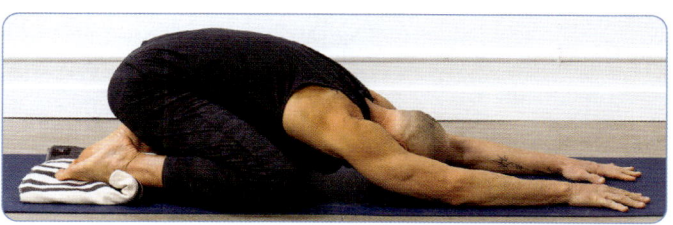

or pain in your ankles by providing extra support and cushioning. This is especially useful for those with sensitive or injured ankles or those with limited ankle mobility (limited plantar flexion—generally referred to as *ankle extension*). By elevating your ankles, it can also help to take some pressure off your knees and hips, making the pose more comfortable overall.

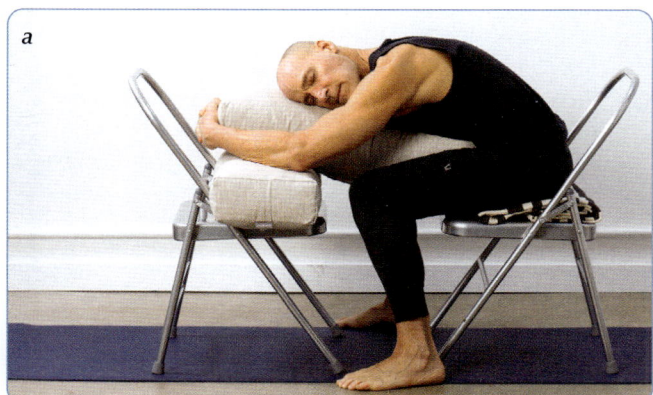

a

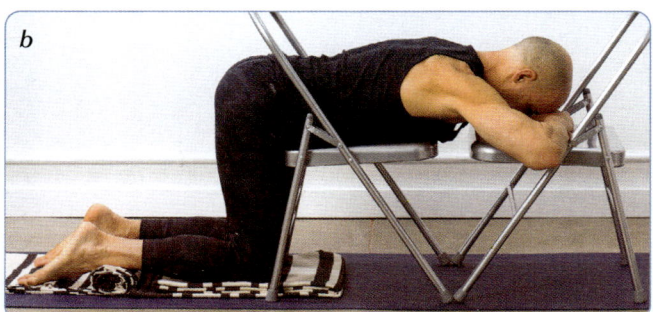

b

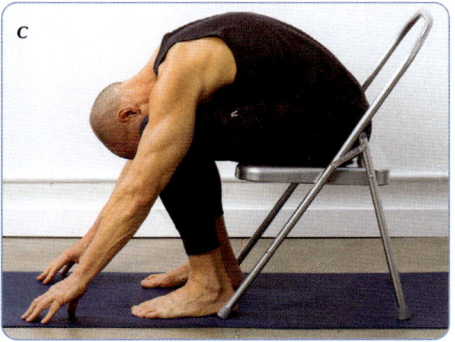

c

Practice with chairs.

One way to practice child's pose with the use of chairs is to sit on one chair with a bolster between the thighs and fold forward while the other chair supports the other end of the bolster (see photo a). You might have to adjust by sitting on a blanket so that your knees are lower than your hips or placing a block under your feet so that you are grounded. You can also prop up the other end of the bolster with blocks, another bolster, or a blanket, to create a ramp. This modified version is a great alternative for those with pain in the knees or ankles.

Another way to practice child's pose with the use of chairs is to kneel on a bolster or a stack of blankets so your hips are level with the height of two chair seats positioned facing each other in front of you. Bring your hips to the edge of the seat and fold forward over the chair. Rest your head and arms on the second chair seat (see photo b). This variation lengthens the entire spinal column.

If getting up from and down on the floor is difficult or if you have knee pain, the final chair-supported variation of child's pose can be an excellent option. Sit on a chair and fold over your thighs, extending your arms toward the floor and relaxing your head and neck (see photo c).

Child's Pose (continued)

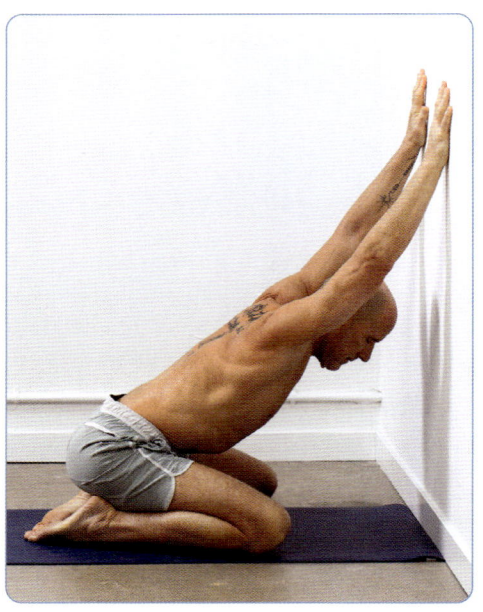

Support the pose with a wall.

By using the wall as a supportive prop, you can deepen the stretch and provide stability to the body, allowing for greater ease and comfort. Practicing this pose regularly can lead to improved flexibility and overall physical and mental well-being. Kneel a little less than arm's-length away from the wall with your knees farther apart than your hips. Rest your hands on the wall so that your biceps are working to frame your ears and allow your chest and shoulders to relax. As you breathe, imagine your whole body melting toward the wall, with only your palms touching it. On each exhalation, soften your neck, shoulders, back, and hips, releasing any tension in your body. You can play with your distance from the wall, having your hands closer to, or further from the floor, to see what feels best in your body.

Practice against a wall by inverting.

This version of child's pose against the wall with a handstand element is an excellent way to challenge yourself and add variety to your yoga practice. Enter a handstand with your belly facing the wall. Draw your knees into your chest, sliding the tops of your feet down the wall until your heels are close to your sitting bones. Your knees can stay together or come a little wider than your torso, mimicking a few variations of child's pose. You may need to adjust the distance between your hands and the wall to find the right amount of space. The wall provides support and stability, allowing you to deepen the stretch and find a comfortable position.

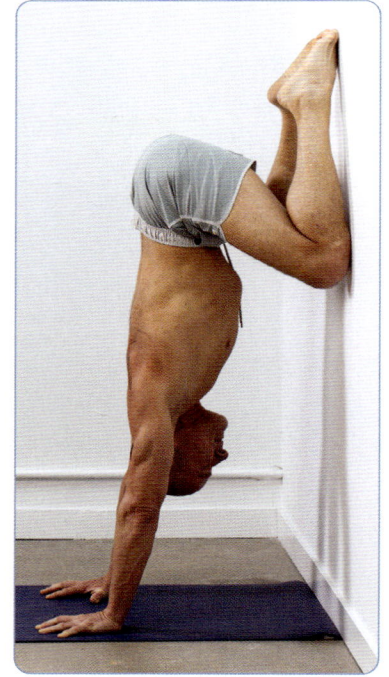

     The Complete Guide to Yoga Props

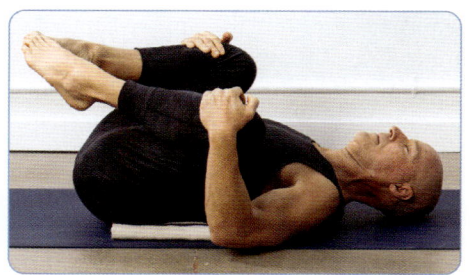

Practice on your back with a blanket under your hips to support your knees.

If you can't bear weight on your knees, there's still an option to practice the mechanics of child's pose. You can lie on your back and draw your knees into your chest or armpits. To increase the rounding sensation through the lower back and spine, roll a blanket under your sacrum to gently elevate your pelvis and stretch the lower back.

This modification allows you to experience the benefits of child's pose without putting any pressure on your knees.

Bind the arms with a strap.

To enhance the stretch in your arms and shoulders, you can find a bind at your low back, traditionally by interlacing your fingers. To create more room in your chest and shoulders, try holding a strap, adjusting the distance between your hands to allow for a range of motion that works for you. Maintain the connection near your hips and reach the hands farther back to move the tops of your shoulders farther away from your ears. Try raising your arms up and overhead. Keep your head and neck relaxed on the mat or props as you do.

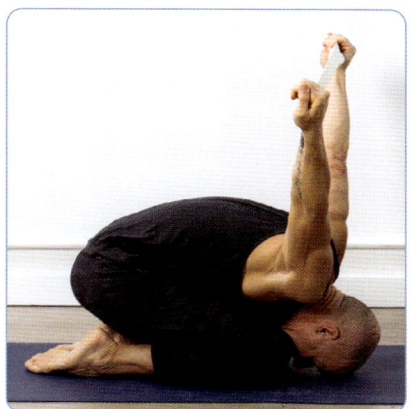

Locust Pose

Shalabhasana   शलभासन

Locust pose is a dynamic yoga posture that targets and strengthens the spine, buttocks, and the muscles along the backside of the body, including the arms and legs. With its stretching benefits for the shoulders, chest, belly, and thighs, this pose also enhances flexibility. Locust pose also stimulates abdominal organs, contributing to a revitalizing practice. Let's look at a few common variations of locust pose using props.

Place blocks under your hands to strengthen your anterior chain.

This variation not only strengthens the anterior chain muscles on the front of the body but also tones the triceps and core muscles. It develops the "hollow-body" muscles necessary for poses like handstand. Lie on your belly and place blocks on any of the three heights, arm's-length distance in front of you. Engage the muscles of the inner thighs, drawing your legs toward one another, and reach your arms forward, placing your palms on the tops of the blocks. Straighten your arms as much as possible. Engage the thighs and begin to press through the hands to lift the head and neck off the mat, followed by the chest. Now for the most challenging part: Engage the backs of the arms to draw your front low ribs off the mat and toward the spine. This core engagement creates more space in the spine and stability around the spinal discs, alleviating potential for injury due to sinking all your weight into the joints. Try the different heights of the blocks for other degrees of challenge.

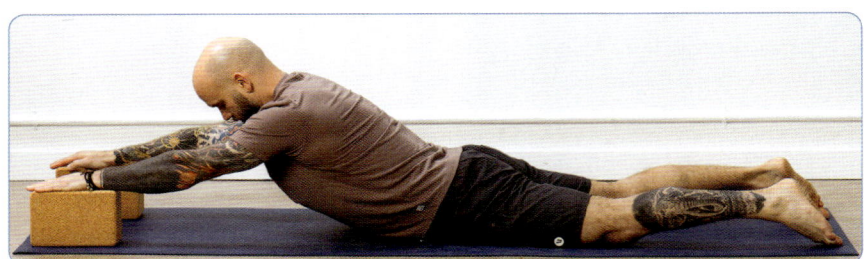

Use a strap to practice bound locust pose.

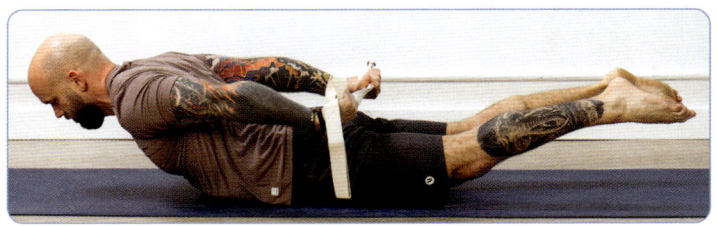

Bound locust pose (baddha shalabhasana) is a great way to enhance your backbend practice and deepen the stretch in your chest and shoulders. Using a strap allows you to bridge the gap between your hands, which can be especially helpful for those with tight shoulders or limited flexibility. Lie on your belly with your arms by your sides and a strap laid out across your lower back. Reach back with your hands for the strap, grabbing hold at a comfortable distance where you can still straighten your arms. Begin to lift your chest and legs off the mat while pressing down with your pubic bone to lengthen the lower back. As you lift, reach your hands away from your buttocks and toward your feet.

Practice shoulder alignment with a strap.

To deepen your locust pose, try using a strap to enhance your chest and shoulder opening. Bring the strap behind your shoulder blades and hold the ends in your hands. Wrap the ends under your armpits and over your shoulders, creating an *X* shape on your back. Once in position, lie on your belly and prepare for locust pose. Make sure the strap is secure around your shoulders. As you move into the posture, gently pull up and back on the strap to lift and broaden your chest, deepening your stretch and strengthening your back muscles. This modification can be especially beneficial for those looking to improve their posture, relieve tension in the upper body, and experience a greater sense of openness and ease in their practice.

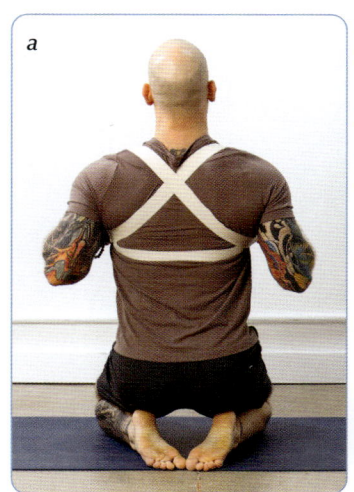
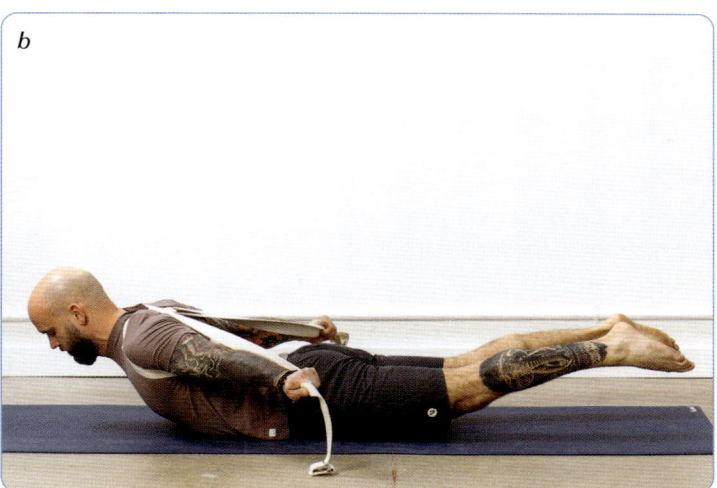

Support your head and arms with blocks and a blanket.

If you're looking for a supported variation of locust pose that will allow you to build muscle memory without straining your body, try using props. Roll a blanket under your forehead for support or fold a blanket over a block on the lowest height and rest your forehead on it. Place blocks by your sides at medium height and extend your hands toward them. Press into the blocks to lift your chest and roll your shoulders down and back. Lengthen your pubic bone toward the mat and extend through your spine, creating space and alignment in your body. Allow your head and neck to fully relax, releasing any tension or tightness in your upper body. With this supportive variation, you can deepen your locust pose practice and experience the benefits of the posture without pushing yourself too hard or compromising your alignment.

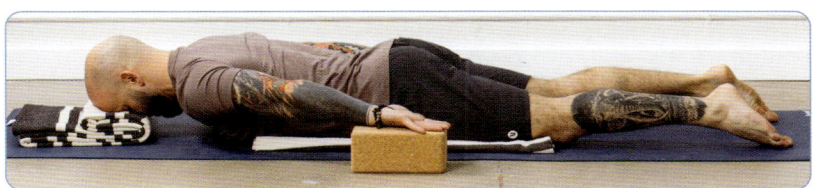

Locust Pose (continued)

Use a blanket and a block or bolster to support your belly.

This variation of locust pose can be helpful for individuals who find it hard to raise their arms off the floor. Lie face-down on a bolster or blocks with a blanket on them, beneath your torso,

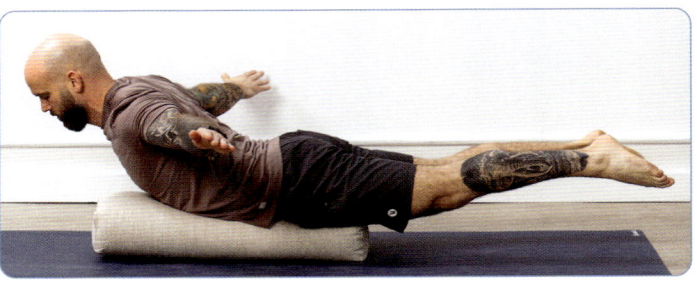

lengthwise. Your head and legs should have room to release toward the floor in front of and behind the props. This added elevation will give room for the arms to move away from the floor. Rest your arms by your sides with your palms facing down. As you inhale, engage your back muscles and lift your chest and legs simultaneously. As you exhale, continue to lift your chest and try to lift your hands off the floor completely, keeping your palms facing down. Hold the pose for a few breaths, lengthening your spine and reaching through your fingertips.

Practice with your feet on a chair or blocks to help lift the chest.

Another variation of locust pose involves pressing the tops of the feet into a prop, such as a chair or blocks placed behind you to

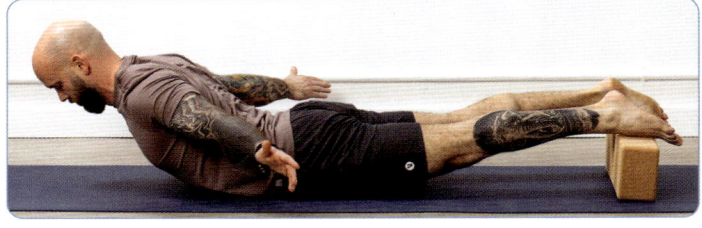

help engage and reinforce the lifting action in the chest. Lie face-down on a yoga mat. Place a chair or blocks behind you and place the tops of your feet on the prop, keeping your toes pointing straight back. Place your hands beside your body, palms down. As you inhale, engage your back muscles and lift your chest, arms, and legs off the floor simultaneously. As you exhale, continue to lift your chest and press the tops of your feet into the prop behind you as if you are trying to lift your chest higher. Hold the pose for a few breaths, lengthening your spine and extending your fingertips. This variation helps strengthen the muscles of the back, shoulders, and legs. It also helps improve posture and can relieve tension and pain in the upper body. By pressing the tops of the feet into the prop behind you, you can engage the leg muscles and reinforce lifting through the chest for a deeper and more effective stretch.

Practice one leg at a time with a wall.

Locust pose is an excellent way to strengthen the muscles of the back and improve posture. However, for individuals who have difficulty getting up from and down on the floor, practicing locust pose can be challenging. You can practice locust pose using a wall as a prop for support and stability. Face a wall with your feet hip-width apart. Place your hands on the wall at shoulder height, with your fingers spread wide. As you inhale, press into the wall with your hands and extend through the spine, creating space across the chest. As you exhale, lift one leg off the floor and extend it back, balancing on your other

The Complete Guide to Yoga Props

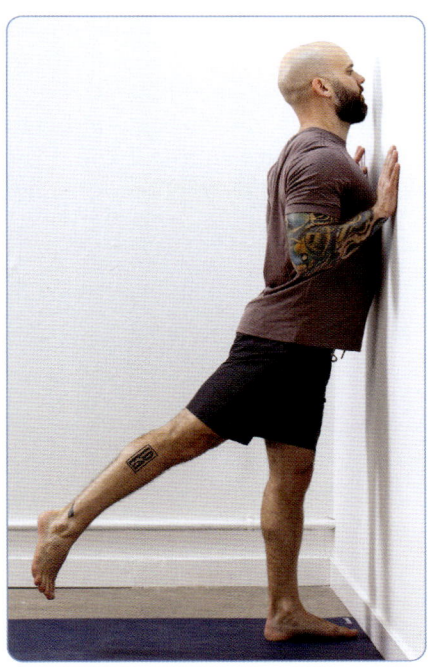

foot. Hold the pose for a few breaths, then release and repeat on the other side. This variation helps strengthen the muscles of the back and legs, while also improving balance and stability. It also allows you to focus on the alignment and engagement of the back muscles without the distraction of trying to balance on the floor.

Practice with a strap.

Here are three ways you can utilize a strap around various parts of the body in this pose. For the first variation, you can loop a strap around the forearms in the superhuman version of locust pose where the arms reach over the head in front of you. While doing so, you still maintain the resistance of the strap. To practice this variation, lie face-down on your yoga mat with your arms in front of you and overhead and a shoulder-width strap looped around your forearms. As you inhale, engage your back muscles and lift your chest, arms, and legs off the floor simultaneously, pressing your forearms into the strap (see figure a). The addition of the strap provides resistance, engaging the muscles of the upper back, arms, and sides of the body, which can improve posture and reduce tension in the upper body over time.

For another variation, as you also see in figure a, looping a strap around the ankles or shins can offer additional benefits for the lower back and hips. Using a strap creates space in the lower back, engages the outer thighs, and aligns the femur bones in the hip sockets. Set up for locust pose with a strap looped around your ankles or shins, adjusted so that it's snug but not too tight. As you enter the pose, press your legs into the strap, working against the strap's resistance and engaging the outer thighs. Using the strap this way helps create space in the lower back and reduce compression in the lower back (lumbar spine), reducing pain or discomfort. Engaging the outer thighs with the strap can also help to stabilize the hips and prevent the legs from splaying too far out to the sides.

For a third variation, loop a strap around your flexed feet to traction the spine. Before you lie down, fold a strap in half at the end of your mat with the free ends pointing to the top corners of the mat. Lie on the mat so that both feet are inside the strap and your hands can reach back for the ends. Tuck your toes under, flexing your feet, and slide the loop up to the arches of your feet. As you inhale, engage your back muscles and lift your chest, arms, and legs off the floor simultaneously. At the same time, press your feet into the strap and pull on it with your hands, lengthening the spine and engaging all the supporting muscles (see photo *b*). This variation can be practiced with the toes grounded to create greater extension through the spine or with the feet lifted off the floor. Either way, the opposing force created by the feet and the hands can help to apply traction, reducing compression in the spinal column.

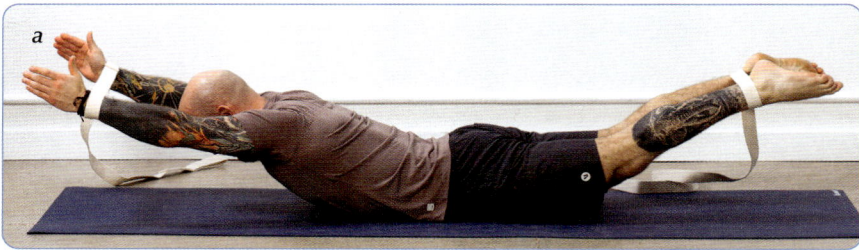

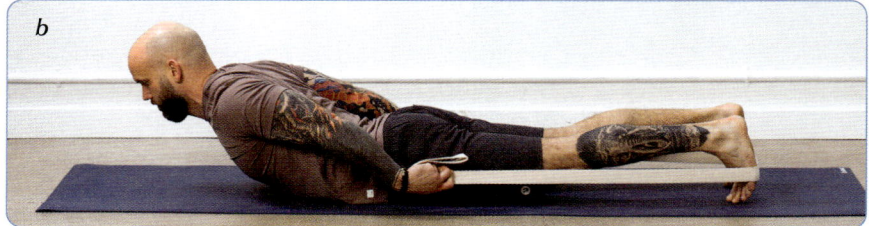

One-Legged King Pigeon Pose (Sleeping Variation)

Eka Pada Rajakapotasana   एक पाद राजकपोतासन

The sleeping variation of one-legged king pigeon pose is a therapeutic yoga posture that invites you to fold over your front leg, deepening the stretch. This variation specifically targets and opens the hips, with a focus on the psoas, thighs, piriformis, and the gluteus muscles. Embracing this pose aids in relieving low back and sciatic pain while promoting relaxation through the pacification of the parasympathetic nervous system. Let's look at a few common variations of the pose using props.

Use a block, bolster, or folded blanket to elevate your hips.

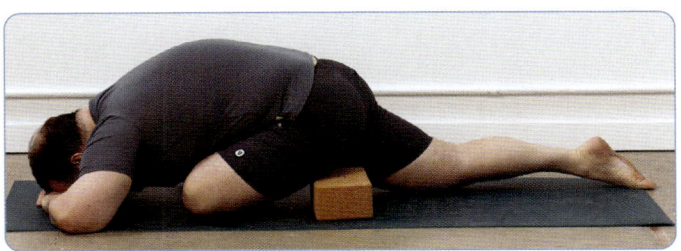

The supported variation of sleeping pigeon pose is particularly beneficial for those looking to level their hips and alleviate pressure on the front knee. In many cases, when the hip and leg muscles are unable to adequately support the demands of the pose, the body may compensate by either resisting gravity or shifting the hips and body weight to one side. By using a block, bolster, or rolled-up blanket as support, practitioners can fully relax into the pose without compromising alignment. This allows for a more comfortable and sustainable practice, regardless of skill level or body type. Blankets and bolsters can slide all the way under the hips, or you could just rest the sitting bone of your front leg on the props.

Place blocks diagonally under your armpits to apply traction to your neck.

Using blocks to support the upper body in sleeping pigeon pose is a wonderful way to alleviate tension and decompress the cervical spine. In addition to reducing strain on the shoulders and upper back, the blocks also promote greater extension in the thoracic spine. Begin in pigeon pose and gradually transition into sleeping pigeon by walking your arms forward. Then place two blocks on the tallest height diagonally in front of your front shin. Rest your armpits on the blocks and allow your chest to soften toward the floor. Finally, release your head and neck, allowing the weight of your head to create a gentle traction on the cervical spine. This modification can be a great option for anyone looking to deepen their yoga practice and experience greater relaxation and release in the upper body.

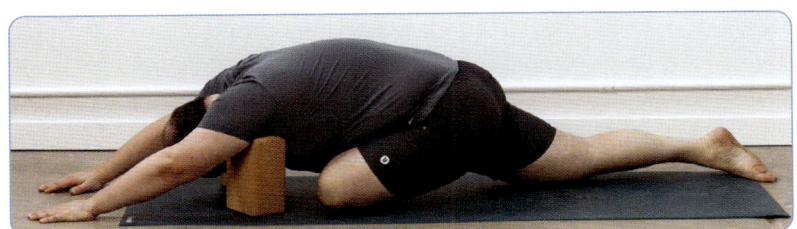

One-Legged King Pigeon Pose
(Sleeping Variation) (continued)

Place blocks under the torso and forehead to support spinal extension.

This variation of pigeon pose is ideal for practitioners who are comfortable with their front shin parallel to the top of the mat. A block supports the torso so you can reinforce the alignment of the shin while elevating and supporting the upper body. A second block under the forehead provides support for the head and neck and facilitates greater extension through the spine. Start in a table top position and bring your left knee toward your left wrist and your left ankle toward your right wrist. Place a block on medium height, lengthwise, under your abdomen, aligning the short edge with your left calf. Extend your right leg straight back and roll your right inner thigh toward the sky while drawing your right hip toward the mat. Draw your left outer hip back and in and release your right thigh toward the floor. Place a second block on medium height under your forehead and extend your arms forward. Relax your head and neck fully and soften your belly into the block. Flex your left toes to protect your left knee. Repeat the sequence on the right side.

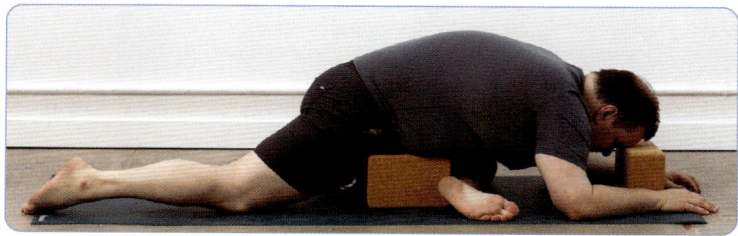

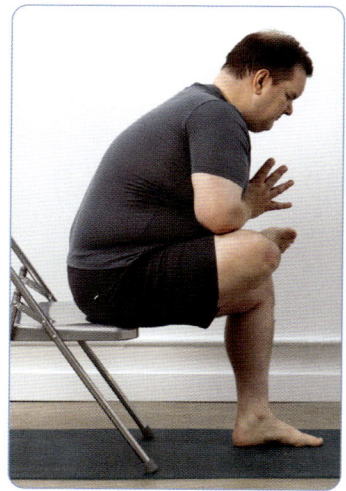

Sit on a chair to take pressure off the joints.

Chair-supported pigeon pose provides similar benefits to traditional pigeon pose. It puts less force on the joints and is great for those who have difficulty getting up from and down on the floor. Sit on a chair with your feet planted firmly on the floor. Cross one ankle over the opposite knee and let your cross-legged knee gently fall to the side. As you inhale, lengthen through your spine, and as you exhale, fold forward over your legs. Rest your forearms on your shin or the chair seat and relax your head and neck. Hold this position for several deep breaths, then switch sides. This variation provides a gentle stretch and a release of tension and tightness in the outer hips and gluteal muscles. This can be especially beneficial for those who sit for long periods or suffer from lower back pain. Chair-supported pigeon pose can also help to improve hip mobility and increase flexibility in the hips and lower back.

Place a block, blanket, bolster, or chair under your forehead to bring the floor to you.

Placing a block, blanket, bolster, or chair under your forehead reduces the distance between you and the floor and it also increases the relaxation in the pose. The different props offer an array of heights and

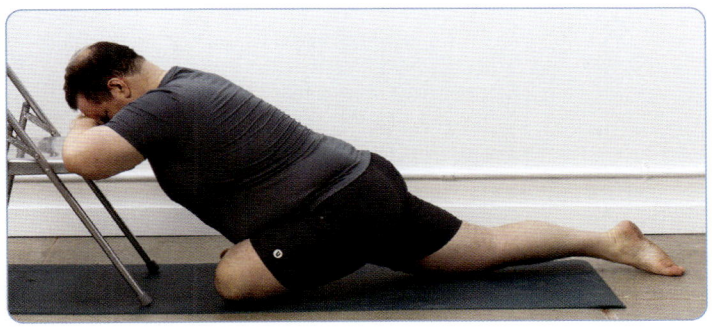

cushioning options. You can always soften some of the harder props with a blanket for added comfort. In addition, placing a block, blanket, bolster, or chair under your forehead in sleeping pigeon pose can help to deepen the stretch in the hips while also providing a gentle release for the neck and shoulders. This can be particularly helpful for those who experience tension in these areas.

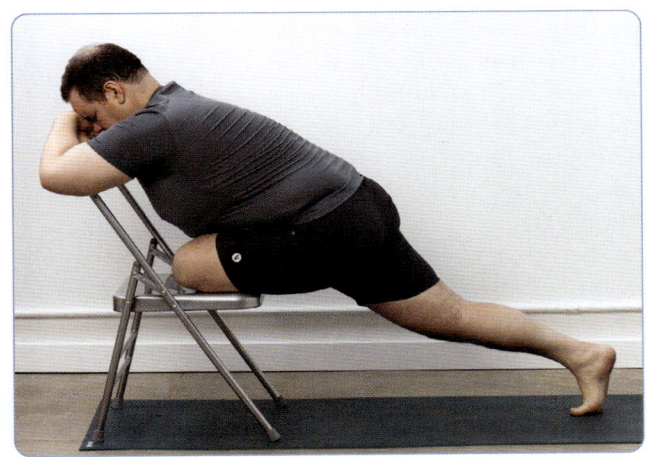

Practice with your front thigh on a chair seat and your forehead on the back rail.

This modified sleeping pigeon pose is a great way to deepen the stretch in the hips and thighs while providing support and stability for the body. Place a chair in front of you and stand facing it. Place the thigh and shin of one leg on the chair seat and slide your back leg back behind you, keeping the back knee lifted and your toes tucked under, pressing into the floor. This action will help to level the hips. Lower your forehead onto

the back rail of the chair to support your upper body. Hold the pose for several breaths, focusing on releasing tension in the hips and thighs and allowing your body to relax, then switch sides. The use of the chair for support can also help to stabilize the body and prevent strain on the lower back or hips. This modification can also be helpful for those with limited mobility or flexibility in the hips and thighs because it is a more accessible version of the pose. Finally, this variation benefits those with injuries or conditions that make it difficult to practice the traditional version of the pose on the floor.

One-Legged King Pigeon Pose
(Sleeping Variation) *(continued)*

Create a bolster ramp to practice restorative pigeon.

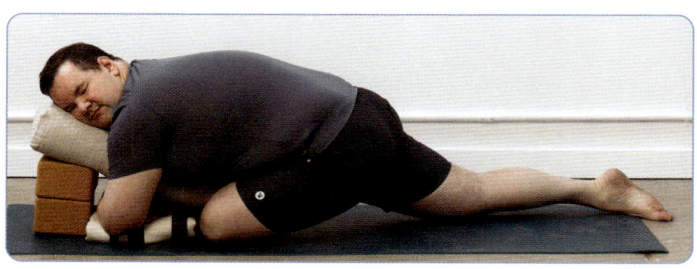

Restorative pigeon pose can be practiced by creating a bolster ramp to support the body. Position the short edge of the bolster in your hip crease and rest the other end on a block or stacked blocks. Fold your body over the bolster, wrapping your arms around it and sliding them through the space underneath it. Let your body fully relax into the support of the bolster, releasing any tension or stress in the hips and thighs. This variation provides many benefits for the body, including deep relaxation and release of tension in the hips and thighs.

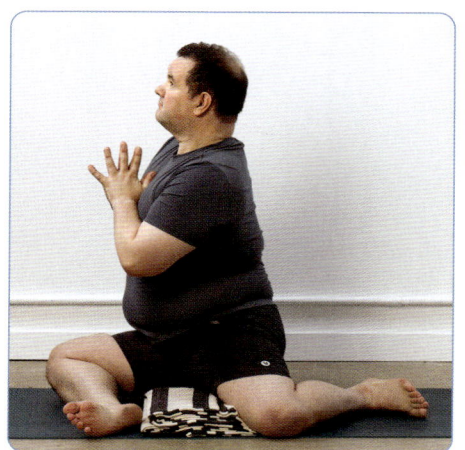

Use a blanket to practice a supported Z-sit variation.

The supported Z-sit variation of pigeon pose is a great way to stretch your hips and entire body more gently than in a traditional or reclined pigeon pose. This variation is especially helpful for those who experience tension in their knees or the rotational muscles of their legs, because it elevates the hips, relieving pressure. This variation also works toward lengthening the psoas but with less intensity than in traditional pigeon pose. Begin in table top position and slide your right knee toward your right wrist. Bring your left knee behind you as far as is comfortable, ranging from pointing to the side of the mat (as shown) or more towards the back of the mat. Your shins can be perpendicular to your thighs, or you can bend your knees and form a less-than-90-degree angle. If you feel tension in your knees or hips, place a rolled blanket under your sitting bones. Work your left hip point forward and down, moving to level your hips to the front of the mat. Your torso can be upright or folding forward.

Bow Pose

Dhanurasana

धनुरासन

Bow pose is a prone heart opener that stretches muscles in the chest, neck, shoulders, abdomen, hips, and the front of the thighs while simultaneously strengthening the back muscles, the backs of the thighs, and the buttocks. Embracing the pose not only promotes spine flexibility, but it also stimulates the adrenal glands, combating fatigue, and it increases blood flow to the digestive system. Let's explore a few common variations of the pose using props.

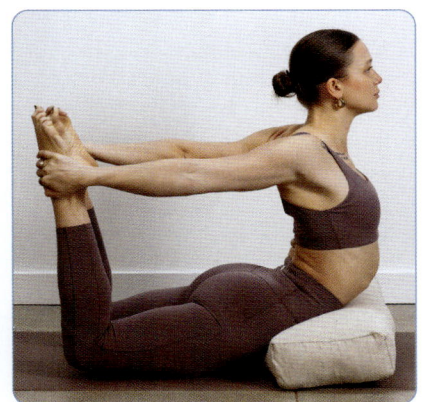

Use a bolster for a supported variation.

Using a bolster in the supported version of bow pose offers several benefits, including elevating your hips to lessen the intensity of the pose and the potential for back strain. The bolster also makes it easier to reach for your ankles and keeps your knees and thighs grounded so that your knees stay together, which can prevent discomfort in the lower back. Using a bolster also takes some weight out of the midsection, allowing you to hold the pose longer. Start in a table top position with a bolster on the floor just behind your wrists. Lower the front of your hips onto the bolster and lift through your chest. Engage your hamstrings and begin to bend at your knees, drawing your heels toward your gluteal muscles. Reach back for your ankles, one hand at a time. Energetically reach toward your ankles, and if you can catch your ankles, kick into your hands to press your thighs into the mat and lift and open through the chest.

Practice reaching back using a strap to bridge the gap.

Bow pose can be modified using a strap to bridge the gap between your hands and your feet, which can help you focus on engaging specific muscles and creating more space in the pose. By modifying the pose using a strap, you can also achieve the benefits of the pose without overexerting yourself or compromising your alignment. Start by lying on your belly and bringing your heels toward your gluteal muscles by engaging your hamstrings. Loop the strap over your ankles or the tops of your feet

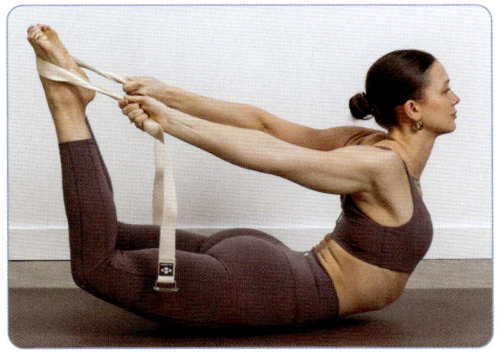

and hold the ends in your hands with your arms by your sides. Make sure the strap is tight so that when you kick into it, you can lift your chest and the tops of your thighs off the mat. If you need more space, you can slide your hands down the strap.

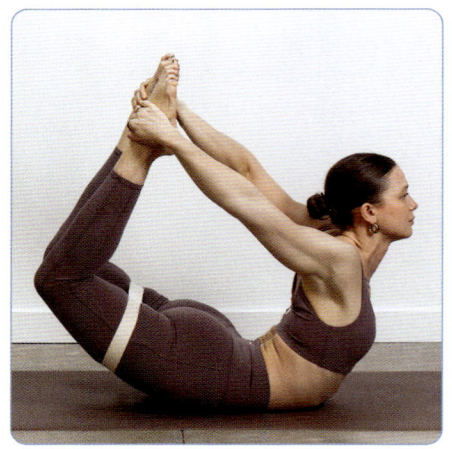

Loop a strap around your thighs to direct the position of the knees and hips.

This variation can help direct the position of the knees and hips, ensuring that the legs are parallel and the heads of the femur bones are resting in a neutral position in the hip sockets. This can help to protect the hip joints and prevent strain or injury. It will also help to widen through the lower back. By using a strap to maintain a healthy alignment of the legs, you can also focus on engaging the muscles in the back and core, which can help to strengthen the spine and improve overall posture. Before getting on your belly and into the pose, loop a strap around your thighs so that the legs are about hip-width apart. As you enter the pose, press your thighs into the strap.

Use a wall to open the chest and spine.

By using a wall for support, you can modify the traditional bow pose to focus on opening the chest and shoulders while extending the thoracic spine, protecting the lumbar spine from compression. Place your knees against or near the wall, to ground the tops of your thighs into the floor. Keep your feet flexed with your toes spread, pressing them into the wall behind you. This will leave some space for your fingers to wrap around your ankles as you kick your shins toward the wall. By using the wall as a support, you can deepen

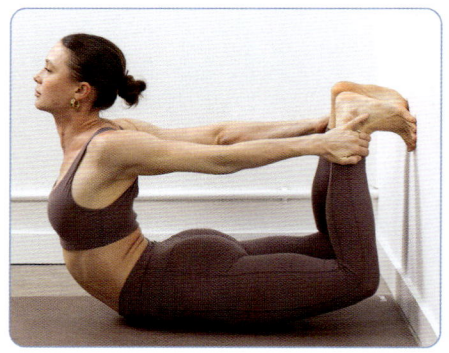

your stretch, maintain alignment, and reduce the risk of injury. This variation can be especially helpful for those who have low back pain or limited mobility in the lumbar spine and hips.

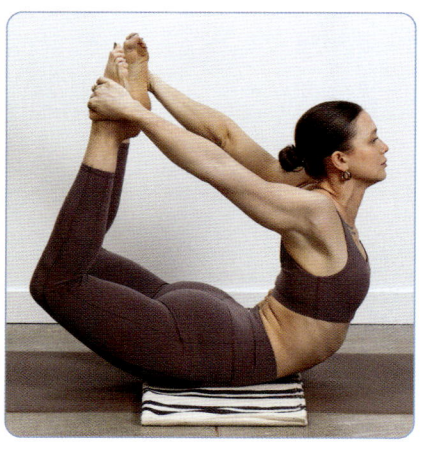

Place a folded blanket under your belly and pelvis to rest on something softer than the floor.

If you the floor is too hard for comfort while doing bow pose, fold a blanket and place it under your pelvis and lower abdomen. This can make the floor feel significantly softer, making the pose more comfortable and accessible. Adding a blanket can also help to provide additional support for the lower back and reduce the risk of injury or strain. This modification is an easy way for you to fully experience the benefits of bow pose without discomfort.

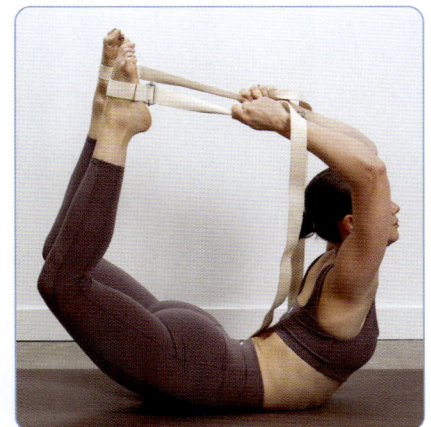

Use straps to practice flipping your grip.

This bow pose variation helps you to work on the mechanics of the challenging grip without risking a shoulder or back injury. Before attempting the full pose, work on improving your shoulder mobility and range of motion in other ways. If you are using two straps looped around the feet, there is less chance of the straps sliding off. But if you only have one strap, you can loop it around both ankles, holding the ends in your hands. Use the strap or straps to draw up through your feet and chest, while your elbows pull down and out to the sides. As you slowly navigate your elbows forward and kick your feet up and back, you can extend further through your arms. If you feel any pain or discomfort in your shoulders while trying this, add more slack to the strap to reduce the intensity.

Use a chair to release into the pose.

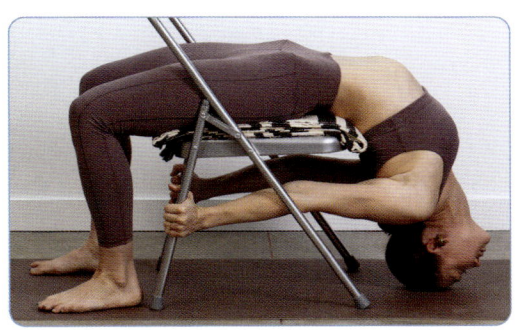

This variation of bow pose is perfect for those with lower back pain and for those who do not have the strength and mobility to reach their ankles and kick into their hands. The chair provides extra support to lengthen the lumbar spine and create a more accessible version of the pose by working with gravity instead of against. Sit with your feet on the floor, hip-width apart, with your legs through the back of the chair. Hold the side rails and lean back until your pelvis and lumbar spine are fully supported by the chair seat. Release your head back and adjust your position so that your shoulder blades rest on the front edge of the seat. If your head doesn't touch the floor, use a prop like a block or rolled blanket to support it. Extend your arms back and reach for the back legs of the chair to deepen the stretch in your chest.

Bow Pose *(continued)*

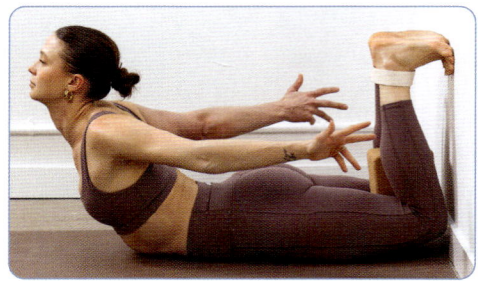

Use a block and strap to practice balanced adduction and abduction.

Achieving balanced adduction and abduction is a fun challenge for overall lower body strength and stability. This is where a block and a strap can come in handy. Place a block on its narrowest width between your thighs. This will help align your knees with your hips and ankles. Loop a strap around your ankles—have a teacher or friend assist you with this step if needed—making sure the loop is about the same distance as your knees. As you come into the pose, focus on two movements: pulling your inner thighs in to keep your legs from moving away from each other and pressing the outer ankles into the strap to abduct the tops of the thighs. This will help keep your low back free from discomfort or compression and ensure that you're engaging the right muscles in all the right places. As shown in the photo, the pose is demonstrated using a wall as you reach back for the feet, but it can also be practiced away from a wall and, if accessible, the hands can grab hold of the feet or ankles.

Kick your heels into blocks to fire up your hamstrings.

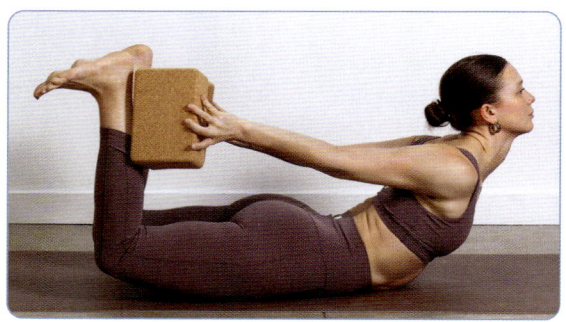

This variation offers a unique twist on a traditional yoga pose by reversing the muscle actions. Instead of kicking up and out, you will be hugging in, engaging your hamstrings. You can change a pose entirely by switching which muscles to turn on or off. This technique strengthens the muscles along your back and lengthens the fronts of your hips and thighs. Hold two blocks and reach them back as if you were trying to grab your feet. Draw your heels to the blocks and press into them to lift through your chest and legs. As you push, resist back, using your arms to create space along your spine. When you are starting, lighter blocks are preferred to prevent any strain or injury.

The Complete Guide to Yoga Props

Sphinx Pose

Salamba bhujangasana सलम्ब भुजङ्गासन

Sphinx pose is a foundational yoga posture that brings strength and balance to the upper body and spine. This pose actively strengthens the arms and shoulders while enhancing the flexibility of the chest and lungs. Simultaneously, it tones the abdomen and back, contributing to improved postural muscles. Let's delve into a few common variations of sphinx pose using props to enrich your practice.

Loop a strap around your arms to inform alignment and open the chest.

Looping a strap around the arms creates a gentle resistance that activates the muscles between the shoulder blades, which can help to counteract rounding of the shoulders. It also helps to prevent the elbows from splaying. As the chest expands and lifts, the strap creates a gentle stretch across the muscles of the chest and shoulders, which can help to release tension and promote a greater sense of relaxation and ease in the upper body. Before entering sphinx pose, loop a strap around your forearms near the wrists, shoulder-width apart or just above your elbows. Play around to see which you prefer! With the help of the strap, lower the hips into sphinx directly from forearm table top or forearm plank.

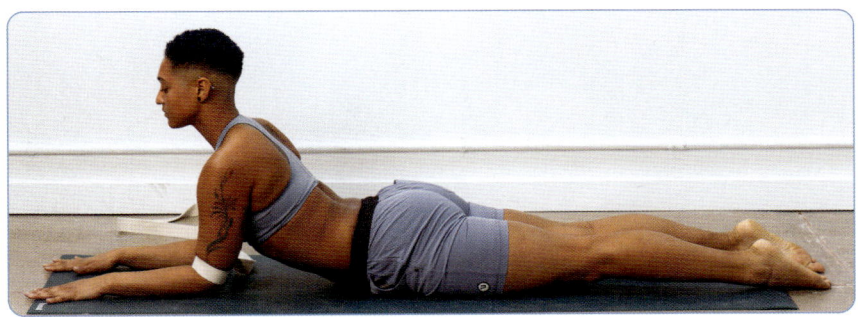

Place a rolled-up blanket under your hips.

Rolling a blanket under your hips to elevate the height of the hips reduces the spinal extension required to lift the chest. Place a rolled-up blanket under your hips so that your pubic bone rests on the blanket. Bring your elbows directly under your shoulders, press your forearms and palms firmly into the floor, and draw your shoulder blades down your back. As you inhale, lengthen your spine and lift your chest away from the floor. Keep the tops of your shoulders relaxed and avoid hunching them up toward your ears. As you exhale, draw your lower ribs in to engage your core muscles and protect the lower back.

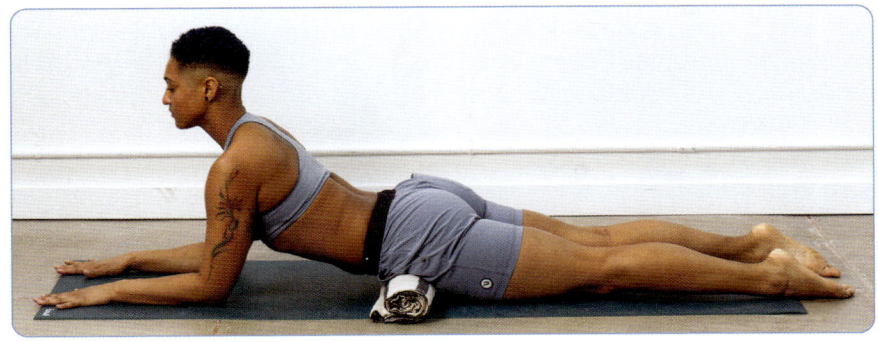

Prop yourself up with a bolster.

One way to use the bolster is by placing it just in front of your lower ribs (see photo *a*). The bolster provides support in lifting the chest, preventing it from collapsing. Your elbows and forearms can come down just in front of the bolster, making the stretch less intense. This variation also helps build muscle memory if you're working on your strength and mobility. Another variation involves angling the bolster into the armpits and under the backs of the arms (see photo *b*), which looks like crocodile pose in yin yoga. You can then cross your arms and release through the head and neck, or stay upright as shown in the photo. If the bolster is too big, roll up a blanket instead. This restorative option, crossing the arms and releasing the head and neck, allows the upper back to release fully as the chest gently opens, providing a more relaxing experience.

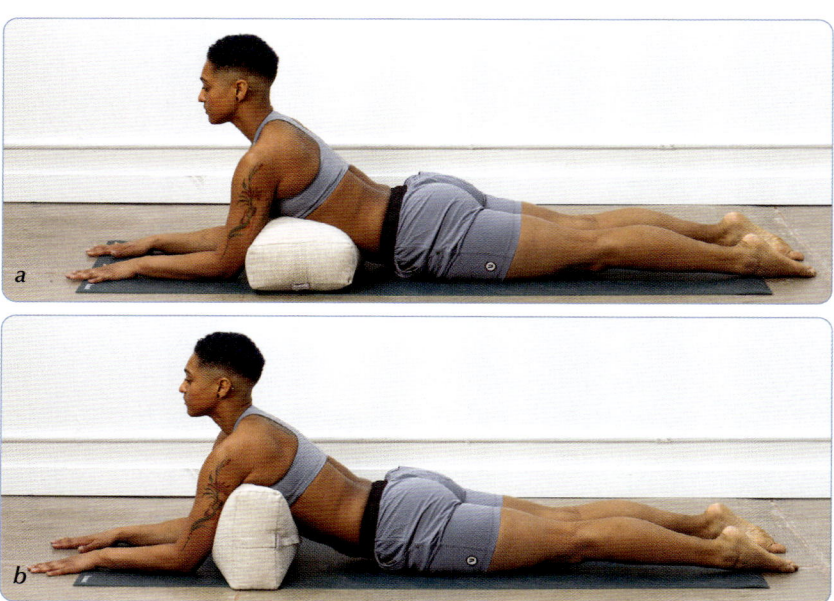

Rest your forehead on a block.

One way to modify sphinx pose is to rest your forehead on a block. This variation offers all the benefits of the traditional version and allows you to release tension in your head and neck. This can be particularly helpful for those with neck strain. After entering sphinx pose, place a block on its tallest height and rest your forehead on it. You have the option to slant the block, as shown, to mirror the natural extension of the spine. If necessary, stack the blocks on their lowest height for additional support or to adjust the height. This modification helps you to extend through your thoracic spine and release tension in your cervical spine through traction.

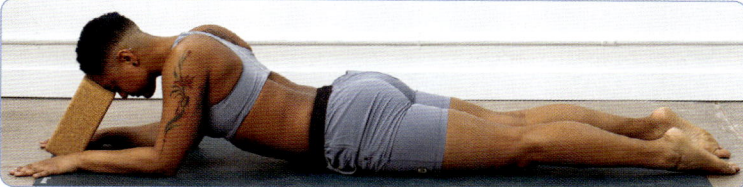

Loop a strap around your ankles to align and strengthen.

Looping a strap around your ankles helps to align your legs and feet. This helps to engage the thighs and create more stability in the pelvis. This alignment can also help to activate the gluteal muscles and lower back muscles, which can help to support the spine and create more length in the lower back. By engaging your legs and feet more actively, you can create space in the back that allows you to lift the chest with more ease. By pressing your outer ankles into the strap, you can create a slight resistance that helps to engage your lower body and activate your core. Before entering sphinx pose, loop a strap around your ankles at no more than hip-width apart.

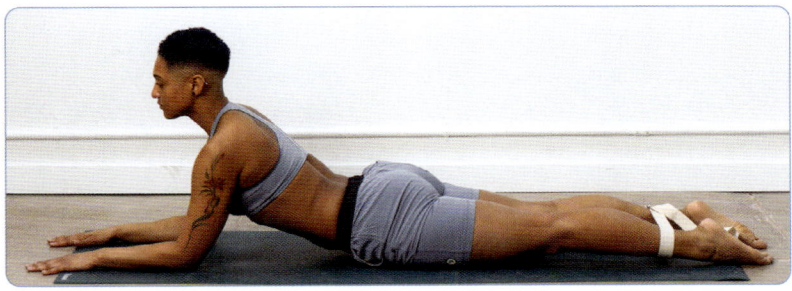

Face a wall to build strength.

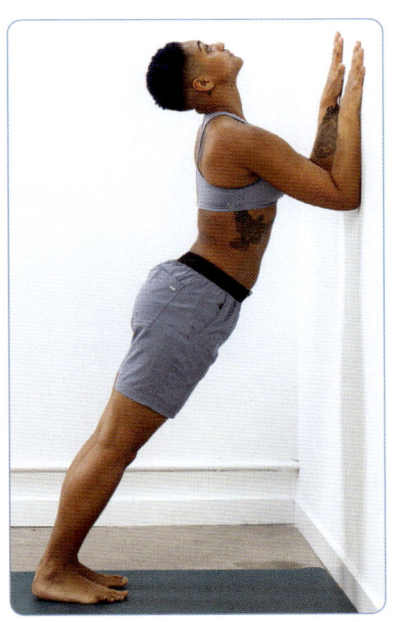

Using a wall for sphinx pose is a great modification for those who have difficulty getting up from and down on the floor or who are building strength and mobility in their upper body. Stand facing the wall and place your forearms on the wall, shoulder-width apart, and walk your feet back a few feet or so from the wall. Lift your chest and gently engage your core while maintaining contact between your forearms and the wall. This variation removes the weight-bearing by the forearms and allows you to focus on strengthening the upper back and shoulder muscles while lengthening the spine. The added support of the wall also allows you to maintain the benefits of the pose, such as improved posture and relief of lower back pain.

Use a chair to practice the pose.

Here are two ways you can use a chair. The first variation can add a little extra challenge to sphinx pose as you enter it from a forearm plank. Position your forearms on the chair seat and walk your feet back into a plank position. To increase support, hold the edge of the chair seat. Lower your hips and broaden your chest (see photo *a*). Since you don't have the floor's support, you'll need to engage your muscles to avoid collapsing through your belly and shoulders. Contract your thighs to lessen the weight on your upper body. Another option is perfect for those who have limited mobility or strength to get up from and down on the floor. Sit on the chair's edge and place a bolster on your thighs. Lower your forearms onto the bolster, shoulder-width apart, and arch your back to mimic sphinx's upper body posture. Lengthen and ground your tailbone on the chair seat (see photo *b*).

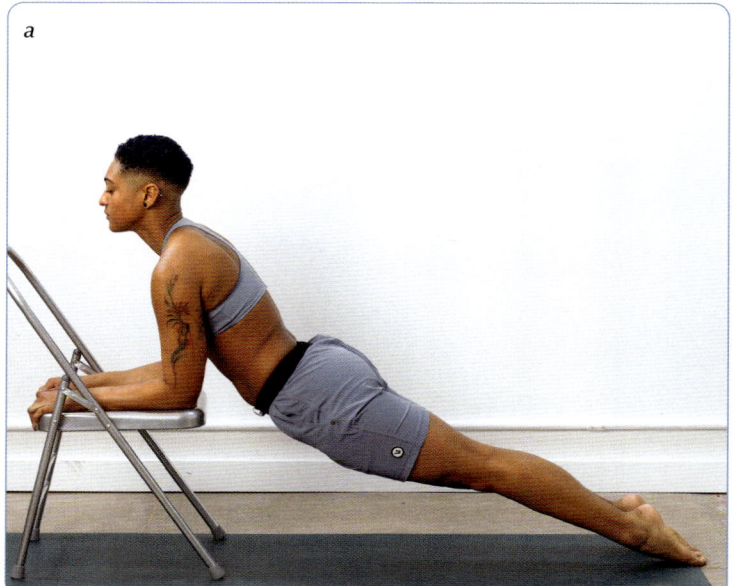

a

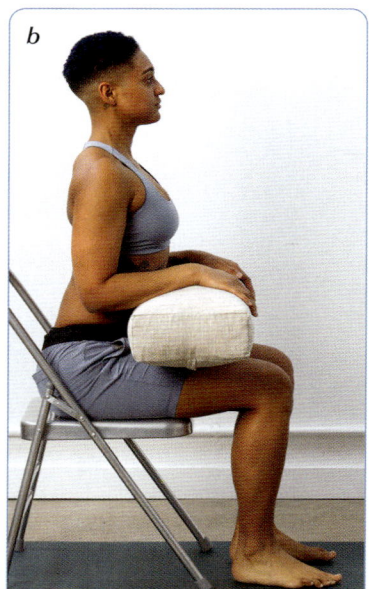

b

Cobra Pose

Bhujangasana   भुजङ्गासन

Cobra pose, a fundamental yoga posture, offers a multitude of benefits for the upper body and spine. This pose actively opens the chest, neck, and shoulders while fostering improved spinal posture and mobility. Cobra pose enhances circulation, opens the lungs, and provides a gentle massage to regulate the adrenal glands. Let's explore a few common variations of the pose using props to enhance your practice.

Sit on a chair to make the pose more accessible.

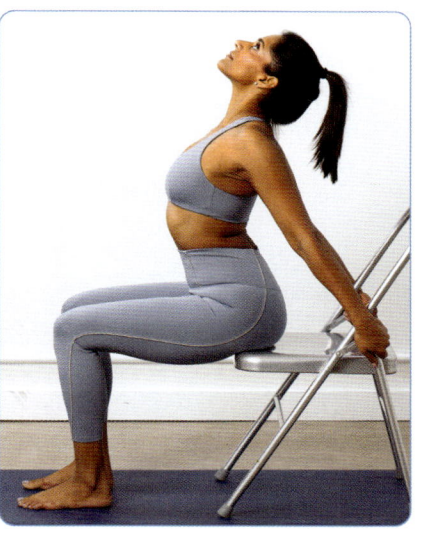

Sit on the chair with your feet planted firmly on the floor. To adjust the degree of stretch, alter the distance of your sitting bones to the front edge of the seat. Reach back for the sides of the back rail of the chair and grab it with your palms facing one another. Extend your chest forward and up, widening across your collar bones. Gently lift your gaze to stretch through your neck as well. The resistance from holding on to the chair should aid in the stretch.

Practice using a wall to reduce wrist tension and flexion.

Here are two ways you can practice this pose using a wall. The first variation begins by standing facing the wall and placing your hands on the wall, just in front of your shoulders. Position your hips as close as comfortable to the wall. Press your hands into the wall to lift your chest and gently engage your core (see photo a). If you can, press your hips into the wall for stability in the

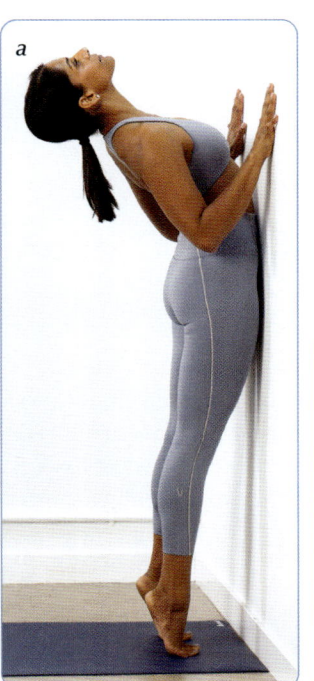

a

lower back. This variation takes the weight-bearing off the wrists, lengthens the spine, and allows you to focus on strengthening the upper back and shoulder muscles. The second variation begins by lying on your stomach in a prone position with your face near a wall. Place your hands on the wall in front of you at shoulder height and shoulder-width apart. Your fingers point toward the ceiling. From here, press into the wall to lift your chest and broaden across your collarbones. Keep your elbows close to your sides if your arms are bent and hug your shoulder blades down and back to support the opening in your chest (see photo b). For a deeper

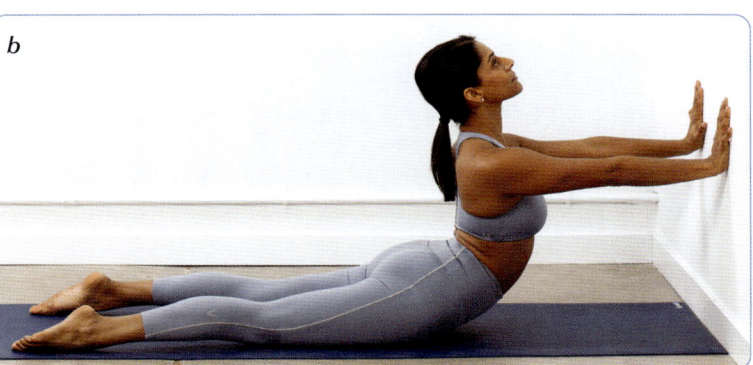

b

stretch, walk your hands farther up the wall. By using the wall for support, you can focus more on the lifting and broadening actions of the chest and shoulders, rather than the weight-bearing aspect of the pose. This variation can also provide a safe and comfortable alternative for those who experience discomfort or pain in their wrists or hands when practicing traditional cobra pose on the floor.

Practice a restorative version of cobra pose to relax and feel ease.

Three props provide benefits in this variation. Fold a blanket and place it under your thighs and ankles. Next, place a bolster just under your chest and ribs, allowing your pelvis to rest heavy on the floor. Place a block at your preferred height under your forehead to support your neck and head. Rest your arms by your sides and allow your muscles to fully let go. This variation of cobra pose allows for a deeper stretch through the spine while promoting relaxation and release. The blanket can help release tension in the hips and legs, while the bolster supports the chest and ribs to allow for a gentle backbend. The block helps to release any tension in the neck and promotes a sense of ease and relaxation.

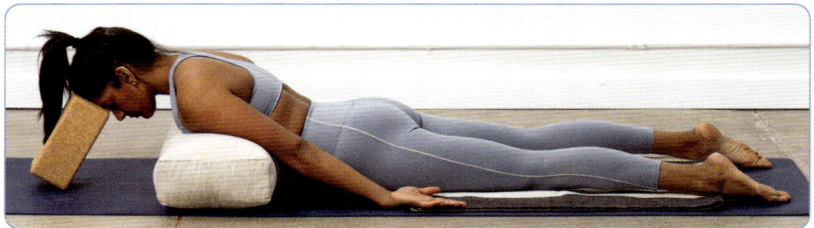

Use a strap around your feet to practice king cobra.

This variation helps you work on increasing flexibility and range of motion without overexerting your hamstrings. Lie on your belly with your knees bent and your heels drawn in toward your buttocks. Place a strap around the tops of your feet, holding the ends of the strap in your hands. Make sure the strap is snug. Place the ends under your hands as you set up for cobra, then press down through your

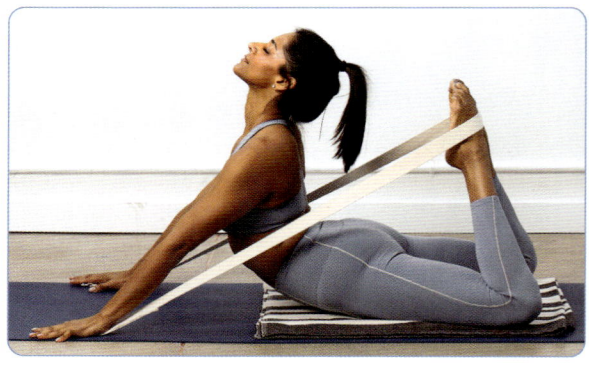

hands to lift the elbows and chest. Use the strap to bring your feet toward your head and adjust the length of the strap so that there is enough tension to assist your hamstrings in comfortably bringing the heels closer. Engage your core muscles to protect your lower back and maintain stability. Hold the pose for several breaths, continuing to lift through the chest and lengthen through the crown of your head.

Practice with either a block between your thighs or a strap around the thighs to engage and align.

Practicing cobra pose with a block between the thighs helps to draw the legs in and align them, which, in turn, helps to support the lower back (see photo a). This alignment can also help to engage the inner thighs and create stability, allowing you to focus on opening the chest and heart. When practicing cobra with a strap just above the knees, the strap can help to align the legs and prevent them from splaying (see photo b). This is especially beneficial in the shins-lifted version of the pose, where the legs can easily slide outward and compress the lower back. The strap helps to maintain space in the lower back and create more stability and can engage the outer hips to create a strong foundation for the pose.

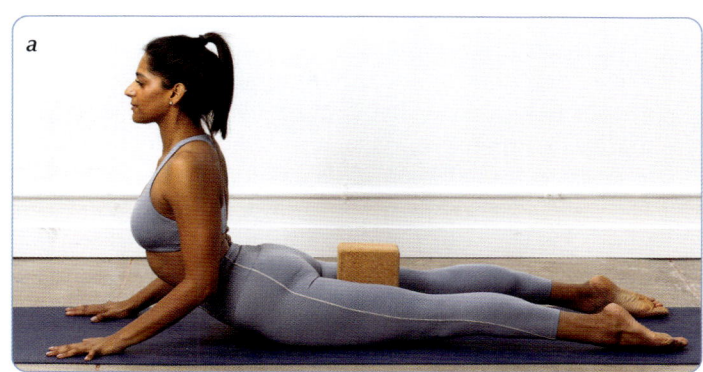

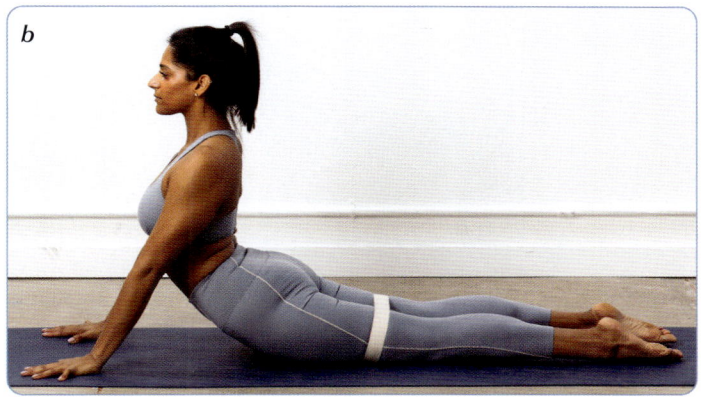

Practice with the backs of your upper arms on a chair to support the wrists.

For a backbend that allows you to deepen your stretch while putting less pressure on your wrists, begin by kneeling facing the front edge of a chair seat. Place your elbows on the chair, sliding them forward until the backs of your arms touch the seat and the front edge of the chair rests in your armpits. Bring your hands together in a prayer position. Walk your legs back to lower your hips, pressing the backs of your arms into the chair to support your weight. If your hips don't reach the floor, support them with blocks, a bolster, or a folded blanket. Lift your chest by pressing down into your elbows. You can also bend your knees and draw your heels toward your gluteal muscles for an extra stretch.

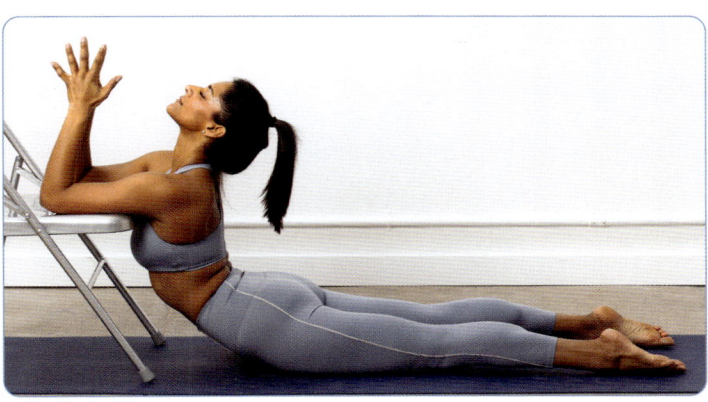

Cobra Pose *(continued)*

Use a looped strap to lift you into the pose.

This variation of cobra uses a strap to help lift the chest and create space in the upper back. Place a strap behind your back, across your shoulder blades. Loop the ends of the strap under the armpits and over the shoulders, securing the ends. The loop should reach your buttocks when you stand. Lie on your belly and bend one knee at a time to draw your heels toward your buttocks, sliding each foot under the loop. Place your hands

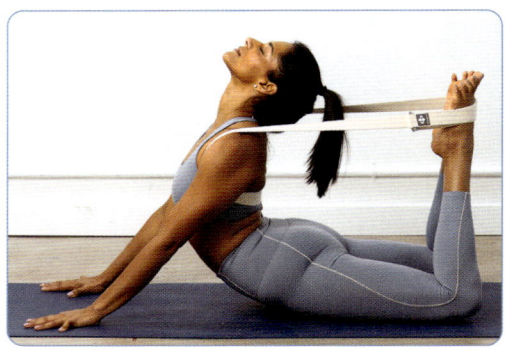

under your shoulders and, on an inhale, straighten through your arms while simultaneously kicking into the strap. This action will lift the chest and create space in the upper back, preventing the shoulder blades from collapsing together.

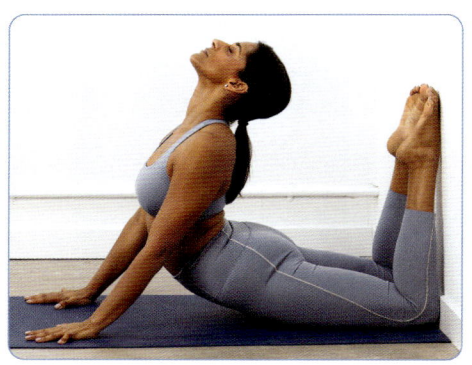

Place your shins on a wall.

This variation helps create space in the lower back for a deeper backbend with less compression in the lumbar spine. The wall will help to align the knees and shins, and the action of pressing the shins into the wall, will offer some relief to the lower back. Lie on your belly near a wall with clear space, with your legs extended behind you toward the wall. Bend your knees and rest your shins on the wall, with your toes pointing toward the ceiling. Adjust your distance from the wall to find a comfortable position. With your shins supported by the wall, you can focus on engaging the back muscles to lift your chest and firm your shoulder blades into the backs of the ribs.

Use a bolster to deepen the stretch.

You can use a bolster in two ways to work on building flexibility in the fronts of your thighs and hips needed for the more challenging king cobra pose. The first variation involves a gentler stretch, which is still deeper than having your legs fully grounded. Place a bolster under your feet, ankles, or shins, and then come into the pose. Press the tops of your ankles or shins into the bolster to lengthen and extend the legs (see photo *a*). In the second variation, place the bolster under your thighs, just above your knees, and keep your hips grounded. As you bend your knees and bring your feet toward your gluteal muscles, engage your hamstrings. The bolster's height will deepen the stretch in your hips and thighs, allowing them to open more. As you press your hands into the floor, lift and broaden across the chest to lift the torso into cobra pose (see photo *b*).

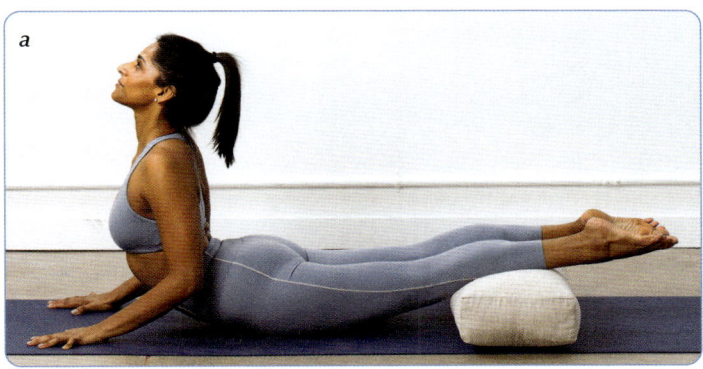

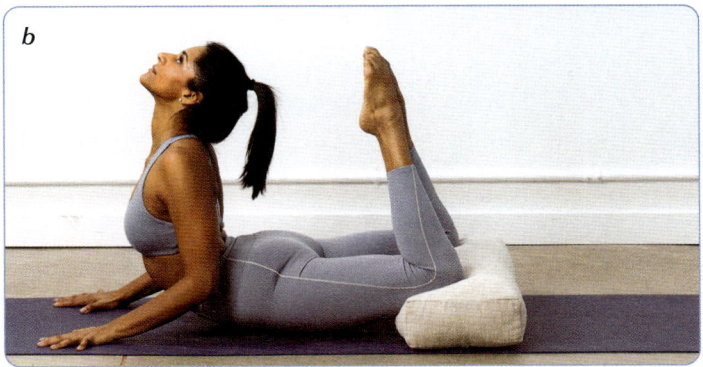

Downward-Facing Twisted Stomach Pose

Adho Mukha Jathara Parivartanasana

अधोम्‌ खजठरपरविर्तनासन

Downward-facing twisted stomach pose is a relieving yoga posture that targets the back and hips. This pose effectively releases tension, creating space between the vertebrae to enhance blood flow. It also opens the intercostal muscles between the ribs and stimulates the digestive organs. Let's explore some common prop-supported variations of downward-facing twisted stomach pose to elevate your practice.

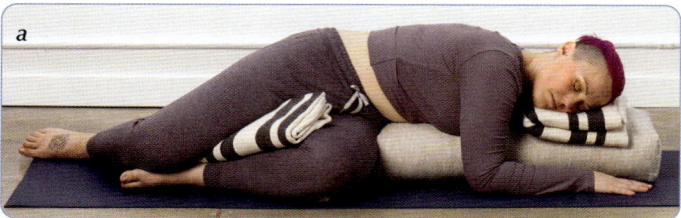

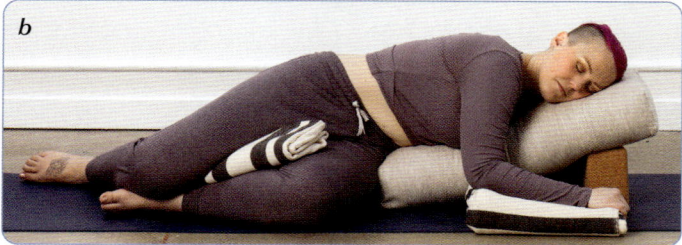

Practice with a bolster and a folded blanket.

A bolster beneath your chest and abdomen can support the spine and open the chest in a prone twist, enabling you to breathe more fully and deeply. Resting your head on the bolster also encourages relaxation of the neck and jaw muscles, which can alleviate headaches and other forms of tension. For more height in the front of the bolster, use a folded-up blanket as a pillow (see photo a). The gentle pressure of the bolster against the belly can stimulate the digestive system. To further support and relax your hips, place a folded blanket between your legs, stacking or staggering them. For a less intense twist, create even more height with a bolster ramp by placing stacked blocks underneath the front end of the bolster (see photo b).

Practice prone dancing shiva variations.

In this twist, the leg closest to the floor will be extended to the side, and the leg farthest from the floor will extend back behind you. The first variation involves using a bolster under the belly with a folded blanket under the head (see photo *a*). This variation can help to improve spinal mobility and create a gentle opening in the chest for easier deep breathing. Resting the head on a bolster or blanket can also help to reduce tension in the neck and jaw muscles. The second variation involves using a strap looped around the foot of the leg extended to the side and held in the hand closest to that foot. As you lower through your chest, place a block under it to bridge the gap between your chest and the floor and another block under your head (see photo *b*). This variation can help to deepen the stretch in the hips and shoulders while improving flexibility and alignment.

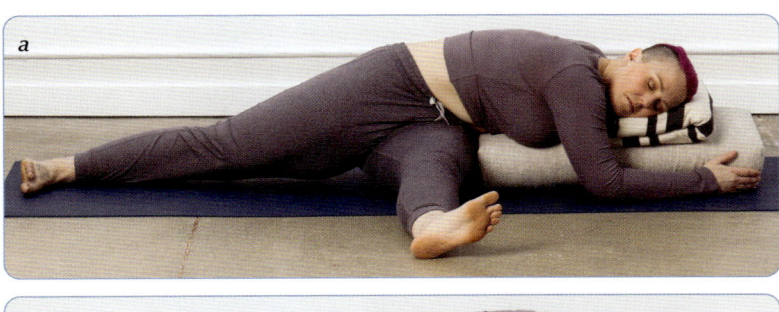

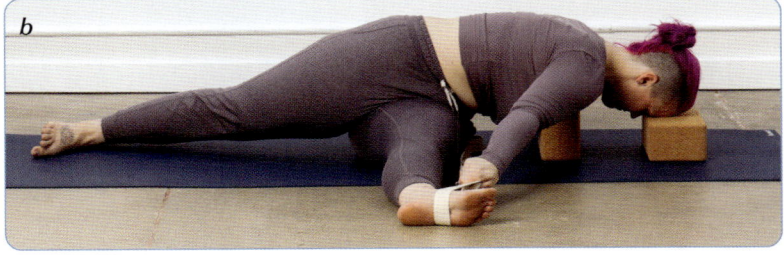

Frog Pose and One-Legged Frog Pose

Mandukasana and Eka Pada Mandukasan

मण्डूकासन and एकपादमण्डूकासन

Frog pose and its one-legged variation are effective yoga postures that focus on stretching the chest, shoulders, and inner thighs. These poses provide a deep stretch in these areas, promoting flexibility and opening through the upper body and inner thigh muscles. Let's explore some common prop-supported variations of frog pose to enhance your practice.

Use a bolster to add height.

Resting the torso on a bolster in frog pose (see photo a) can help release tension in the lower back and hips, provide support for the upper body for deeper relaxation, promote better alignment of the spine, and reduce the risk of strain or injury. If you need additional height, create a ramp by placing stacked blocks underneath the front end of the bolster. You may need need a second bolster to support the hips if you do this (see photo b). If your arms cannot comfortably reach the floor, fold a blanket and slide it under the space between the bolster and the floor to rest your arms. If practicing the one-legged variation, you can use the bolster similarly.

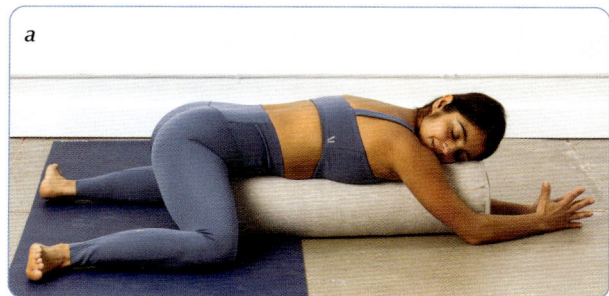
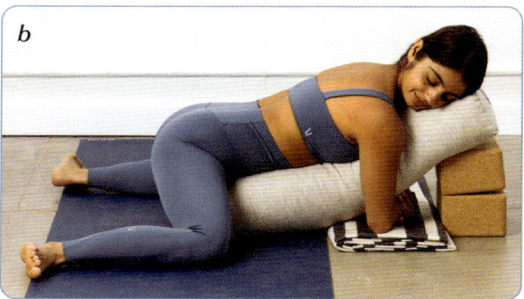

Use blocks and blankets to support your knees, hips, and low back.

Enhance your frog pose practice with supportive props in three ways. One option is resting your knees on folded blankets. Fold blankets to cushion and support your knees, creating a more comfortable foundation for a sustained hip and groin stretch (see photo a). A second option is to elevate the floor's height by placing blocks under your forearms, and to bring your torso in line with or higher than your hips, reducing strain in the stretch (see photo b). This will also help you to more evenly distribute weight between your upper body and your hips, making it easier to keep your hips in the same plane as your knees. Third, for added support in the lower back, introduce a block and a rolled-up blanket. Set the block at its lowest height and place the rolled-up blanket on top, bridging the gap between your hips and the floor (see photo c). This modification promotes lower back lengthening, psoas

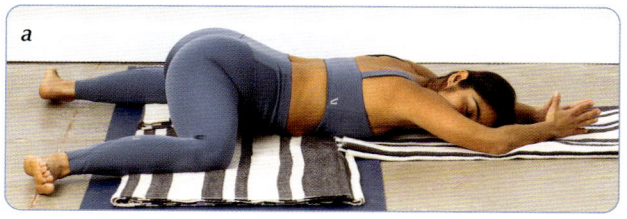

release, and improved circulation and digestion. Align your shoulders with your hips by resting your forearms on the mat. Explore these variations for a well-rounded and comfortable frog pose experience.

The Complete Guide to Yoga Props

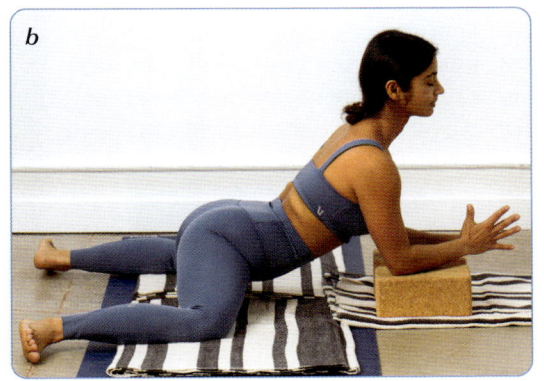

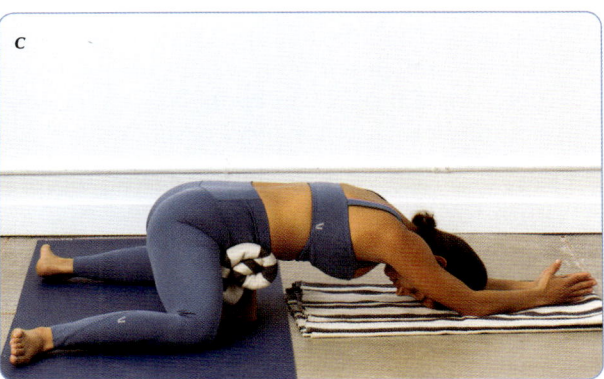

Bring your feet to a wall to encourage knee and ankle alignment.

To encourage stacked knee and ankle alignment in frog pose, use a wall for support. Traditionally, the feet are turned to the sides, shins perpendicular to the thighs, and knees aligned with the hips. However, every body is different and this wall variation should be seen as a suggestion rather than the only correct

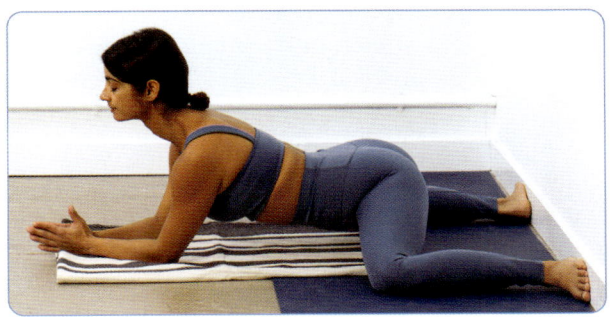

alignment. The wall helps keep the shins and feet stable and allows you to press back into it as you work your hips back to be parallel with your knees. Enter frog pose, facing away from a wall. Walk your feet back to press into the wall. Your heels don't need to reach the mat as long as you press your flexed feet into the wall and activate through the shins to protect the knee joint. If your hips are not all the way to the floor, you can adjust the turnout of the ankles so that the knees don't suffer from the difference in turnout between the knees and the hips.

Place a block, bolster, or blanket under your shin in one-legged frog to deepen the stretch and support your knees.

Lie on your back with a block, bolster, or folded blanket near your left hip on the lowest height. Draw your right knee toward your right armpit, then slowly guide it across your body to the left, contacting the prop. Roll all the way onto your belly from the supine twist, sliding the prop and knee to the right. Use your hands as a pillow for your forehead to rest on and breathe deeply into your lower back and hips, allowing your hip flexors and belly to soften. Repeat on the other side.

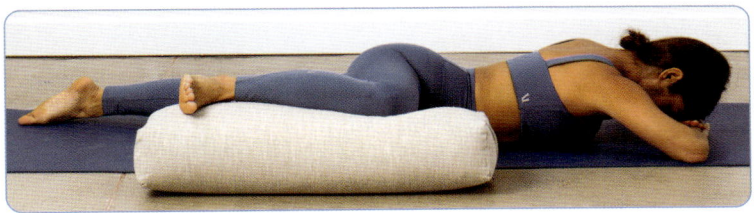

Frog Pose II and Half Frog Pose

Bhekasana and Ardha Bhekasana

भेकासन and अर्ध भेकासन

Frog pose II and its half frog version are dynamic yoga postures that strengthen the back muscles, stretch the hips, thighs, ankles, and shins, and open the chest and shoulders. These poses provide an energizing effect while promoting strength and flexibility. Let's explore some common prop-supported variations of frog pose II to enhance your practice.

Practice with a strap around the thighs to align the knees.

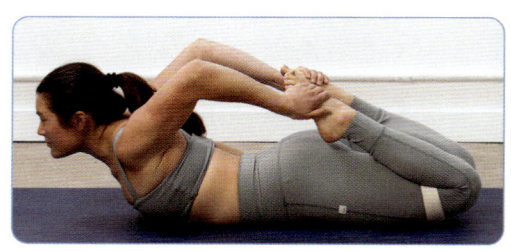

Frog pose II involves lying face-down and bringing the heels toward the buttocks while holding the ankles or pressing on the tops of the feet. Place a strap around the thighs to help align the knees and prevent them from splaying, providing additional support to the lower back. The strap also helps deepen the stretch in the quadriceps and hip flexors and protect the knee joints.

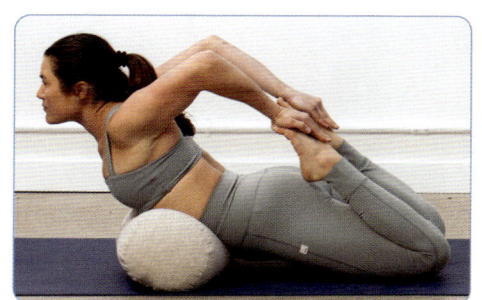

Use a rolled-up blanket or bolster to support your chest and ribs.

This variation of frog pose II benefits practitioners who have limited flexibility or strength in their back or shoulders. Place a rolled blanket or bolster underneath your torso, just below your rib cage. This creates a gentle lift in the chest, making it easier to reach for your feet without straining your back or neck, and it will support you so you can redirect your focus to the lower half of the body.

Use a block to strengthen your hamstrings.

To strengthen the hamstrings, use a block in this variation of half frog. Begin in sphinx pose and place a block between your left heel and buttock. Press firmly into the block with your heel, engaging your

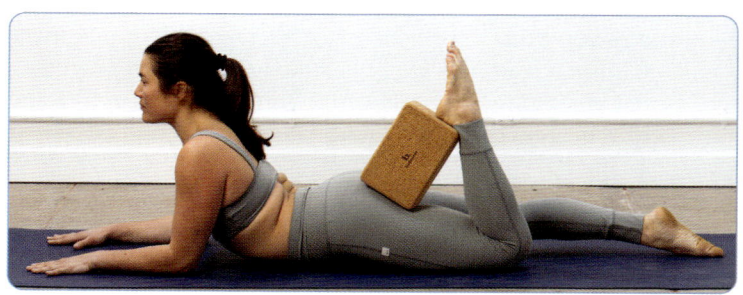

hamstring muscles. For a more intense stretch in your quadriceps, lift your left thigh off the floor and hold for a few breaths. Repeat on the right side.

Sit on a chair if you have difficulty getting up from and down on the floor.

There are two variations of half frog pose that provide the benefits of this pose without the discomfort of getting up from and down on the floor. For the first variation, sit on a chair with your feet planted firmly on the floor. Bend one knee and bring the foot toward the hip, then reach down and hold the foot (see photo a). In the second variation, sit sideways on the chair with one thigh resting on the seat of the chair and the other hanging off the edge with the knee bent and supported by a block. Place a blanket over the block for additional support. Hold the back railing or back edge of the chair seat to help you stabilize and balance as you reach back with your other hand for the foot of the bent knee (see photo b). If reaching the foot is difficult, loop a strap around the foot to bridge the gap between it and your hand. Draw the heel of your foot toward your buttocks, stretching through your quadriceps. Repeat each on the other side.

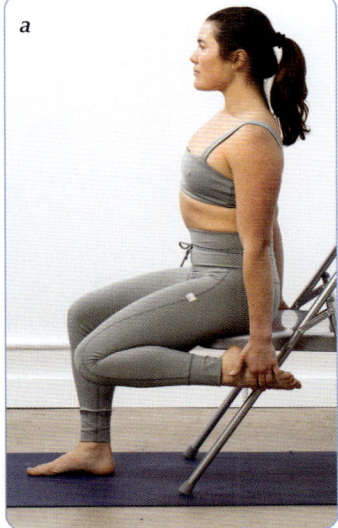
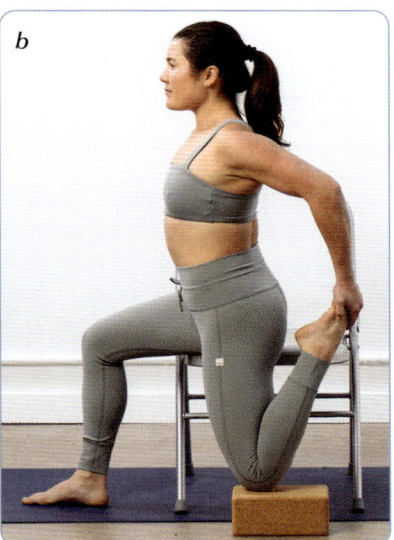

Practice with a strap around your foot to extend your reach.

This variation of half frog pose involves using a looped strap to help extend your

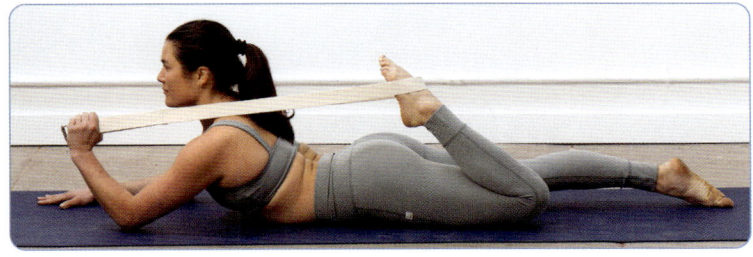

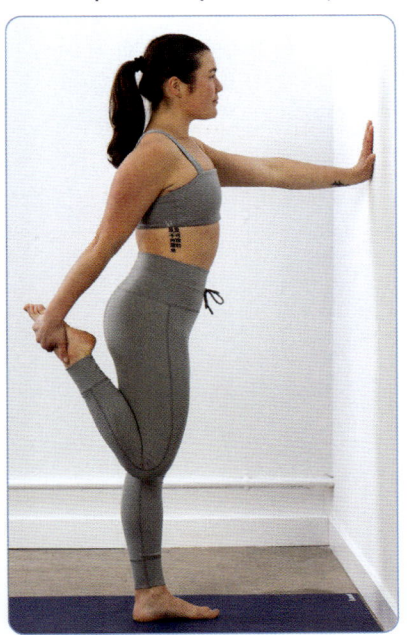

reach if it's difficult to grab your foot. Loop the strap around your foot and gently pull on it to deepen the stretch in the quadriceps and hip flexor muscles. This modification is particularly helpful for those with limited mobility or flexibility in the hips, as well as those who have an injury. Repeat on the other side.

Practice at a wall to assist balance.

By practicing half frog pose at a wall, you can reap the benefits of the pose while standing and using the wall to maintain balance. Stand facing a wall and place the left hand on the wall as you lift the right foot toward your gluteal muscles and reach back to hold it with the right hand. This variation is especially helpful for those who have difficulty getting on the floor or have limited mobility. Repeat on the other side.

Side Corpse Pose

Parshva Savasana   पार्श्व शवासन

Side corpse pose is a restorative yoga posture that offers various benefits, including lowering blood pressure. Lying on the right side takes pressure off the heart, reducing heart rate and calming the nervous system. Lying on the left side increases circulation, improving blood flow to the heart and the fetus for those practicing prenatal yoga. It also enhances lymphatic drainage. Let's explore some variations of side corpse pose with props to enhance your relaxation experience.

Practice with blocks, a blanket, or a bolster between the thighs and a rolled blanket or bolster under the head.

In this variation of corpse pose, you can place a rolled blanket or bolster under your head and rest your top arm on a block overhead, on a block by your chest, or rest the arm on your side. The props help to release tension in the hips and spine while promoting relaxation and deep breathing. This variation is especially beneficial for those who have difficulty lying flat on their back, including pregnant individuals.

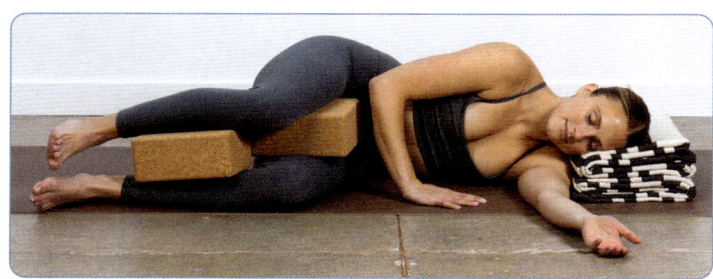

Practice with one leg extended and a bolster under the shin.

This variation helps to release tension in the hip flexors, elongate the spine, and improve overall relaxation. It also stretches and lengthens through the bottom leg and hip, making it a great option for individuals who experience discomfort or tightness in that area. Enter a supine twist with your top shin resting on a bolster, then roll over on to your side, stacking your shoulders. Adjust your bottom arm to rest your head on your biceps or rest your head on blankets as shown.

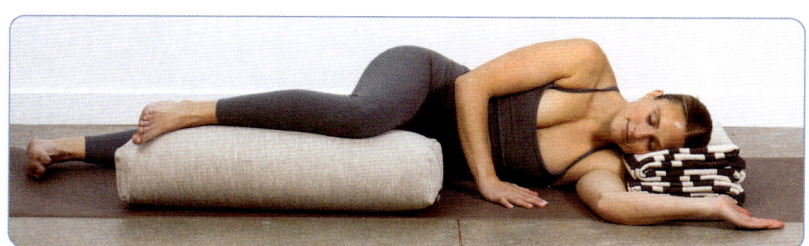

Belly-Down Corpse Pose

Adho Mukha Shavasana   अधोमुखशवासन

Belly-down corpse pose is a therapeutic posture with various benefits. It helps relieve lower back and hip pain, improves diaphragmatic breathing, and stimulates the digestive organs and can improve circulation. This pose provides peace of mind to individuals uncomfortable with the front of the body facing up and can also strengthen the muscles of the back, neck, and shoulders while gently stretching the abdomen and hip flexors. Let's explore some variations of belly-down corpse pose with props to enhance your experience.

Prop yourself up with blankets to support your body and your neck.

Belly-down corpse pose with blanket support can help alleviate stress and tension, improve breathing, and promote relaxation. Here are two variations to try with blankets. The first variation is especially helpful for releasing tension in the lower back and pelvis by placing a folded blanket under your abdomen, allowing your pelvis to release behind it. Alternatively, if you want to lengthen the front of the torso, place the blanket under the thighs up to the hip points as shown in the photo. You can also place another folded blanket under the forehead, which gives your nose enough space to breathe comfortably. Additionally, you can frame your head with your arms on two more folded blankets running from your armpits to your hands. To create more space in your lower back, roll the fronts of your thighs inward and let your heels splay open (see photo *a*).

The second variation involves folding a blanket or two under your torso, stopping just at the front of the pelvis, to lengthen the tailbone, or extending all the way to the thighs for added comfort (as shown). For extra comfort and support, place a rolled blanket under your ankles. This will help to widen the space across your lower back as well as alleviate any discomfort in the ankles. Stack one or two folded blankets under your forehead until you have enough space to comfortably breathe. Bring your arms with palms face-up by your sides or frame your head cactus style (see photo *b*). Take slow, deep breaths as you hold each variation, allowing your body to fully relax into the support of the blankets.

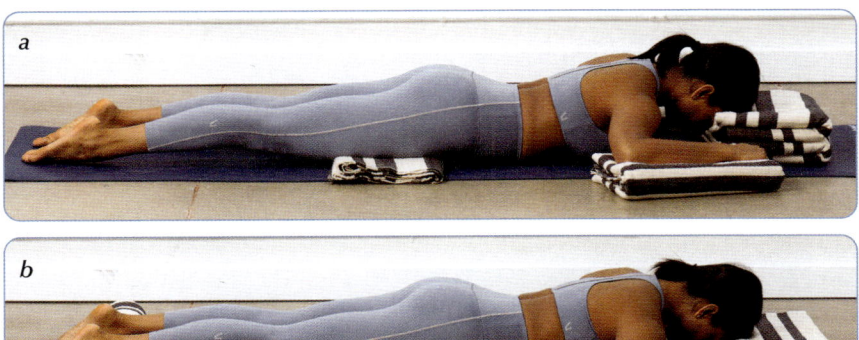

Belly-Down Corpse Pose (continued)

Practice with a weighted blanket on your back.

In this variation, you can use folded blankets or a blanket and a block over your lower back to increase the weight. As you inhale, feel the gentle resistance on your lower back and the resistance from the floor in your belly. This resistance helps to activate and strengthen the muscles that support your breath such as the respiratory diaphragm. As the belly expands into the floor, allow the lower back to rise to accommodate space for the lungs to expand and the diaphragm to release. The added weight helps to deepen your breath and reinforce better diaphragmatic breathing habits. This variation is beneficial for those who want to improve their breath support, strengthen their respiratory muscles, and relieve tension in the lower back.

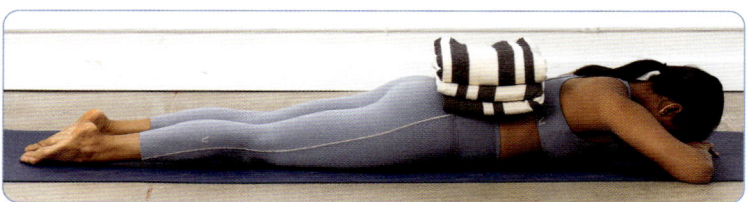

Add a restorative shoulder release.

This restorative shoulder release can help ease upper back, neck, and shoulder tension with the force of gravity. Place a bolster horizontally in the middle of your mat and position a block or rolled-up blanket in front of the bolster for head support. Lie on your belly over the bolster, cross your left arm over your right, reaching your fingertips as far away from each other as you can with your palms face-up. Lean forward, allowing your chin to rest on your arms. Keep your neck elongated. Breathing into the space between your shoulder blades enhances the stretch across your upper back. This pose can help relieve neck and upper back stiffness while gently stretching the spine, sacrum, and lower back. With time, you can progress to removing the bolster and resting your forehead on a folded blanket or the floor. Repeat on the other side.

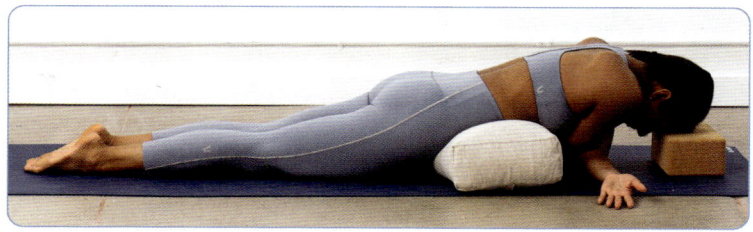

Plank Pose

Phalakasana   फलकासन

Plank pose is a foundational posture with multiple benefits. This pose tones the abdomen, chest, and back, while also strengthening the arms, wrists, and shoulders. Additionally, it provides a gentle stretch to the toes and wrists. Let's explore some variations of plank pose with props to enhance your practice.

Place a block between your thighs to become aware of the pelvis.

A block will help to neutralize the pelvis and help you to notice the direction of the thighs and tailbone. It helps to firm and engage through the thighs, taking pressure off the lower back. Begin in downward dog with a block on the narrowest width placed between your upper thighs. Shift your weight until your shoulders

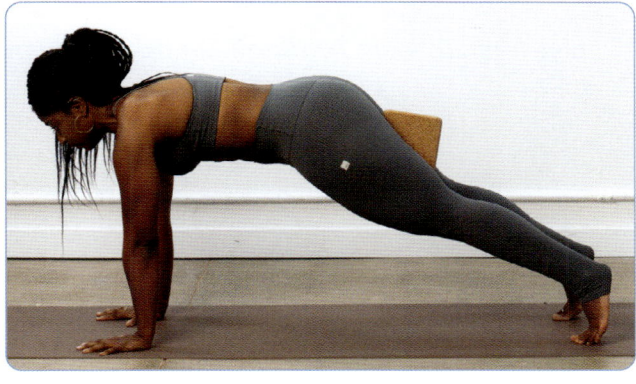

are stacked over your wrists and your heels over the balls of your feet. Squeeze the block toward your pubis and lengthen your tailbone toward your heels. Let the block guide you to ensure that your hips are not tucking or arching too much. Extend your head forward and your heels back as if pressing into a wall behind you.

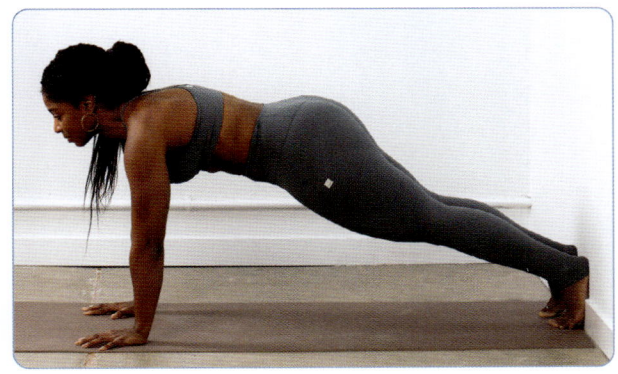

Press your heels into a wall to engage the leg muscles and support the lower back.

Pressing the heels into the wall in plank position helps to engage the leg muscles, particularly the quadriceps and gluteal muscles. This engagement supports the lower back and promotes stability in the core. Align the heels directly over the toes so that the legs are parallel informing alignment in the lower body. This can help to prevent unnecessary strain on the knees and hips.

Practice flying plank with blocks under your shoulders.

This twist on a traditional plank position requires greater engagement of the core and leg muscles to prevent collapsing of the spine. Begin in a table top position with blocks placed lengthwise at medium

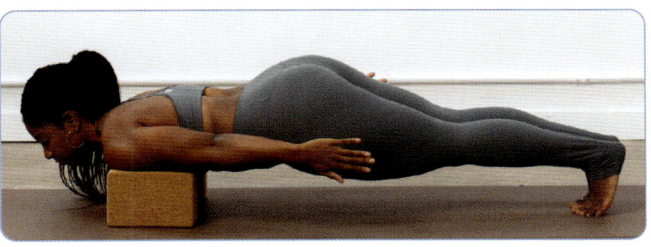

height in front of your fingertips; adjust the height as needed. Bend your elbows as if moving into a knees-chest-chin position and rest the tops of your shoulders on the blocks. Lift your knees off the mat and walk your feet back until your legs are fully extended, like in plank pose. Keep your feet hip-width apart and lift one hand at a time from the mat, extending your arms out to the sides and hugging them in toward your body. Gaze toward the top of the mat, engage your thighs to reduce pressure on your lower back, draw your tailbone toward your heels, and engage your core by drawing your navel toward your spine.

Use a chair, wall, or blocks to modify plank pose.

One way to modify plank pose is by placing the hands on the seat of a chair instead of the floor (see photo *a*). This is particularly helpful for beginners or those with limited upper body strength because it reduces the amount of weight-bearing required of the upper body. It also makes the pose more accessible for those with wrist or shoulder pain or weakness. Another way to modify the plank pose is by placing the hands on a wall instead of the floor (see photo *b*). A third option is to use blocks under your hands, which can move some of the weight-bearing from the upper body to the lower body, making the pose more accessible for those still building upper body strength or with wrist pain (see photo *c*).

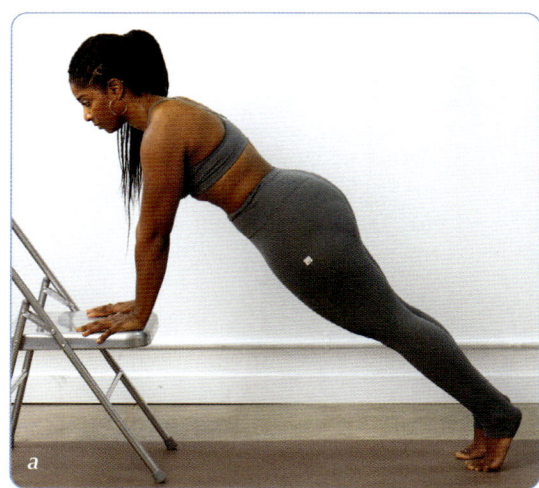

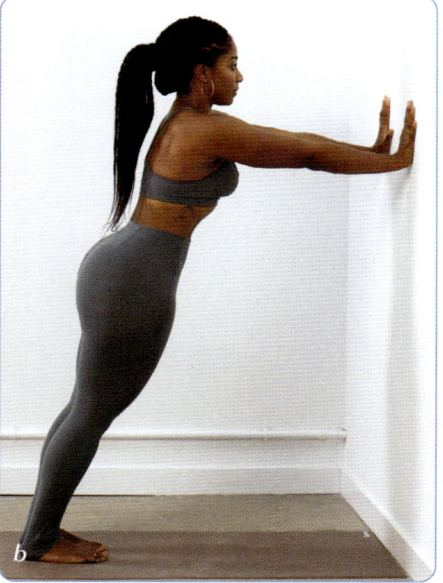

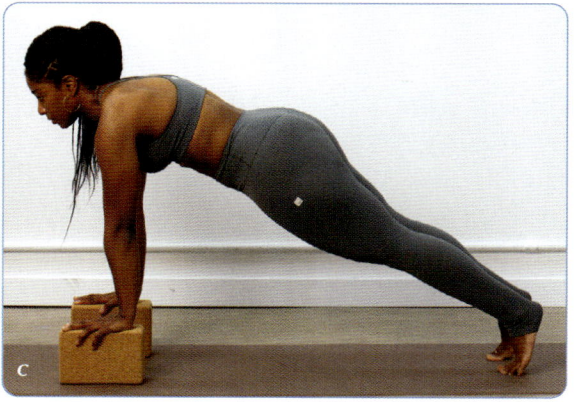

Use a blanket to challenge the core.

To make your plank pose more challenging, replace your yoga mat and use a folded blanket on a hard floor under your feet for added movement. You can slide the blanket forward and back by tucking your knees into your chest

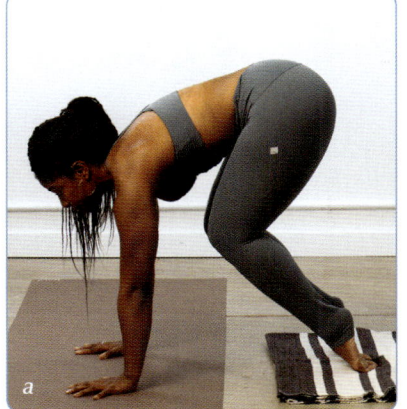

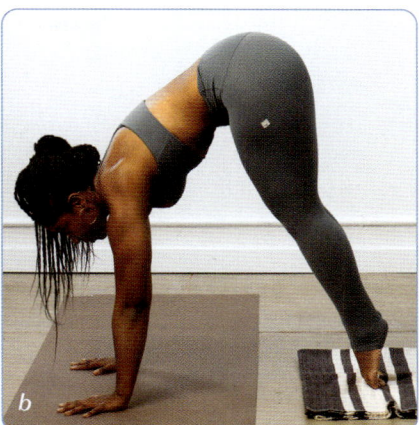

(see photo *a*). Alternatively, you can pike your hips over your shoulders with straight legs (see photo *b*). Another option is to use the blanket under only one foot and slide the knee of that leg toward your triceps and back, then switch sides and repeat (see photo *c*). You can also modify option *c* by shortening your stance as shown. These variations will increase the engagement of your core muscles and add an element of instability, improving balance and stability over time.

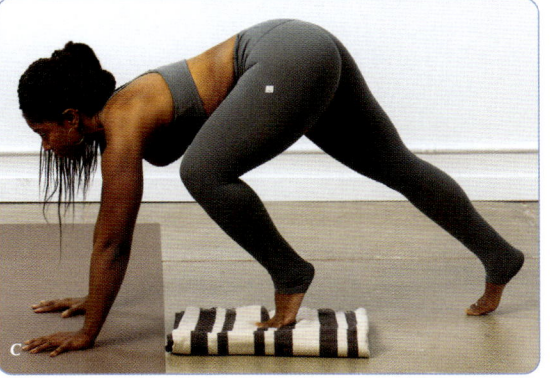

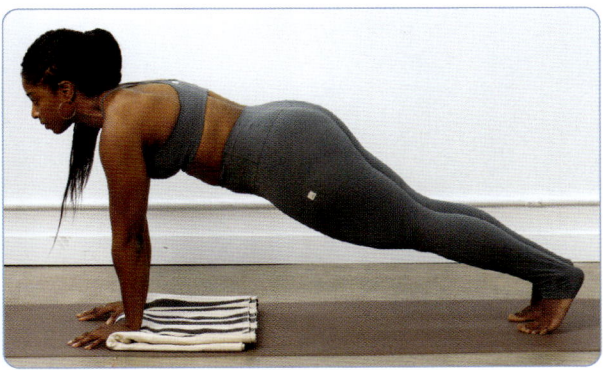

Fold the edge of your mat or a blanket under the heels of your hands to support the wrists.

Adding elevation with a folded mat or blanket under the heel of the hands in plank pose can provide great support to the wrists, especially for those with limited mobility or wrist pain. The elevated prop decreases the angle of flexion in the wrists and the amount of weight-bearing by the wrists. This modification also reduces the pressure on the wrists by engaging the muscles in the forearms and upper arms. This allows for a more stable and aligned plank pose.

Plank Pose (continued)

Use a strap around your upper arms to practice plank or forearm plank.

This variation can help to engage the shoulder blades and upper back muscles more effectively, which can lead to improved posture and reduced upper body tension. It can also help to prevent the shoulders from sinking or rounding, which can lead to strain on the neck and upper back, and build strength and stability in the arms, shoulders, and core muscles. Finally, it can benefit individuals who have limited mobility or injury, because it provides support and stability during the pose. Loop a shoulder-width-size strap around your arms, just above the elbows, and enter plank or forearm plank pose.

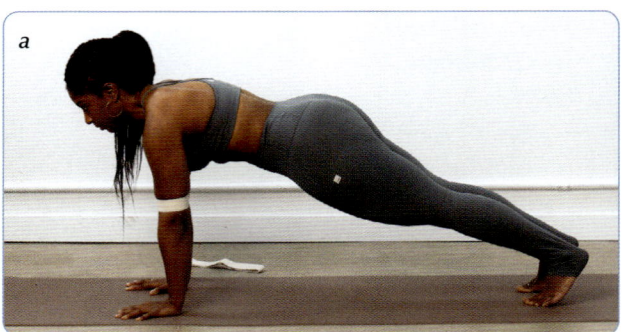

a

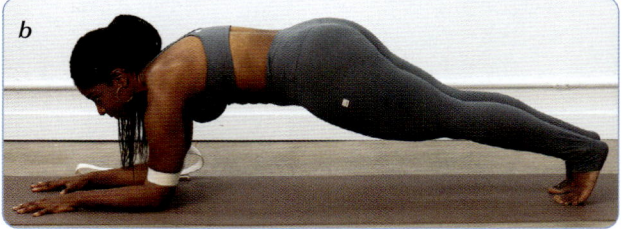

b

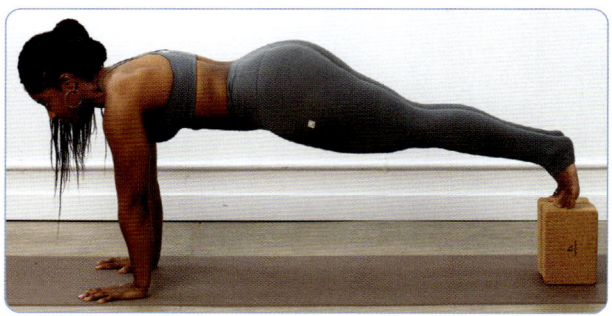

Place blocks under your feet to make the posture more challenging.

Placing blocks under the feet in plank pose shifts more weight onto the upper body, making the posture more challenging. This variation requires greater activation of the core muscles and can help build strength in the shoulders and arms. The added difficulty and slight inversion can also increase the cardiovascular intensity of the pose.

Loop a strap around the ankles to engage both the adductors and abductors.

Looping a strap around the ankles in plank pose can help to engage the abductors. Placing the ankles hip-width apart encourages you to keep the legs parallel and to activate the outer thighs

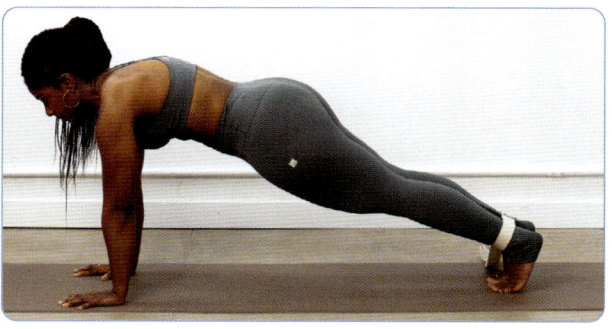

to hold the strap in place. This engagement of the abductors can provide additional stability and support for the plank pose, helping to prevent the legs from splaying and encouraging a stronger, more centered posture. To engage the adductors simultaneously, imagine drawing the inseam of your legs up toward your pubic bones as the ankles press into the strap.

Four-Limbed Staff Pose

Chaturanga Dandasana   चतुरङ्ग दण्डासन

Four-limbed staff pose, sometimes referred to as chaturanga (the shortened version of the sanskrit name), is a foundational posture with several benefits. This pose strengthens the arms, wrists, shoulders, and chest while toning the abdominal muscles. It also serves as excellent preparation for more advanced postures, such as bent-arm arm balances, making it a key element in building strength and stability. Let's explore some variations of four-limbed staff pose with props to enhance your practice.

Practice with blocks to inform alignment.

Using a block or two in four-limbed staff pose helps inform alignment by keeping the chest from dropping too low and reminding you to shift weight forward to stack your elbows over your wrists. Start in the plank position with either one block on the tallest height just in front of and between the hands (or two blocks on the tallest height just in front of the fingertips) and shift your weight forward onto the tiptoes so that the chest or

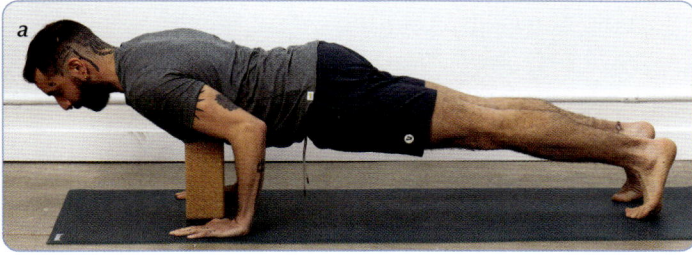

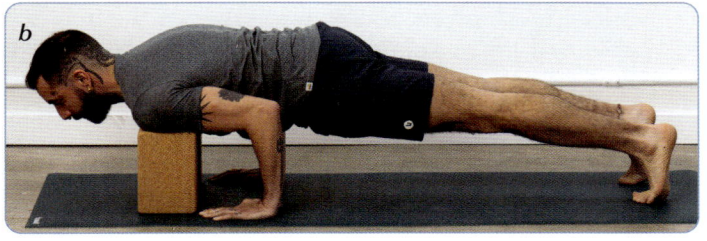

shoulders hover over the blocks. Lower yourself, hugging your elbows into the sides of the ribs and stopping when the chest meets the blocks, ensuring the shoulders are about the same height as the elbows (see photo *a* for an example with one block between the hands and photo *b* for an example with two blocks in front of the fingertips). If your forearm is longer than a block, you will want to hover over the blocks rather than contact them. If your hips are piked or collapsing toward the mat, lengthen the tailbone towards the heels and drive the heels back as the chest extends forward.

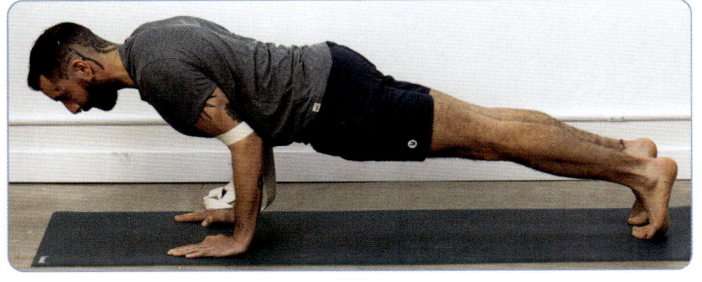

Loop a strap around the arms to support alignment.

This variation can greatly improve alignment and reduce the weight-bearing load on the chest and shoulders. Enter plank with a strap looped around the arms, just above the elbows. The strap acts as a carrier for the ribs, preventing them from going below the elbows while drawing the low ribs into the backside of the body, strengthening your core. This tension from the torso on the strap also helps to keep the elbows in position, pinning them into the sides of the body, reducing the strain on your shoulder girdle. By reducing the weight-bearing load on the chest and shoulders, the strap allows for greater awareness and control of the alignment of the head, neck, hips, and leg muscles. This can be particularly helpful for those with limited upper body strength or shoulder mobility, as well as for those who are working on building four-limbed staff pose alignment.

Place blocks under your thighs to support the lower body.

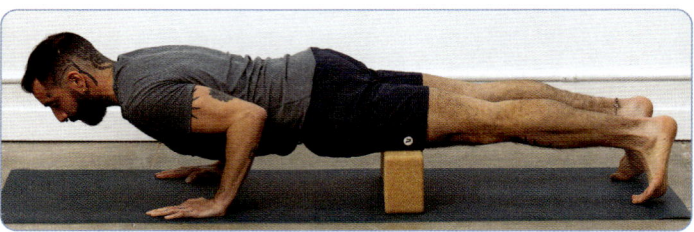

Using blocks in four-limbed staff pose helps keep the hips and lower back from dropping too low. The blocks also support the lower body, allowing you to focus more closely on alignment in the upper body. Place two blocks lengthwise across the middle of your mat on medium height. Then, walk the tops of your thighs over the blocks and enter a plank position. Spread your fingers and ground down through all of the knuckles. Bend the elbows and stop when the tops of your thighs meet the blocks. If your hips are piked or collapsing toward the mat, lengthen your tailbone down to your heels and drive your heels back as your chest extends forward. Broaden through your chest, draw your shoulder blades down the back, and draw your front ribs up and in. Gaze toward the top of the mat in front of you.

Modify using a wall or a chair.

Modifying this pose using a wall helps to avoid pressure on the wrists and allows for easier spinal alignment without risking the collapse of your hips or shoulders. Stand in mountain pose, arm's-length distance from a wall. Place your palms on the wall at shoulder height, fingers spread wide, and wrist creases parallel to the floor. Inhale to lift your heels and

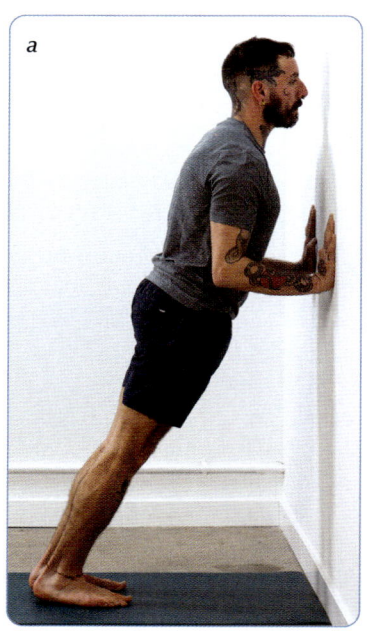

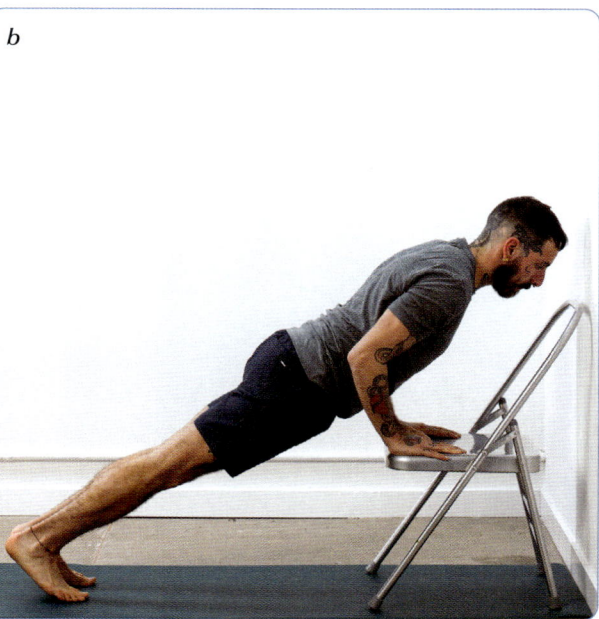

rise onto your tiptoes, then exhale and bend your elbows, stopping before they pass your ribs. Keep your elbows close to your body and point them straight back while lengthening your tailbone down to your heels and drawing your lower-front ribs in toward your spine. Broaden through your chest and draw your shoulder blades down your back, keeping your ears in line with your shoulders (see photo *a*). To add more conditioning, you can incorporate wall push-ups, alternating between straight and bent elbows. To take it up a notch while still bearing less weight than the traditional posture, place the hands on a chair seat rather than a wall (see photo *b*). Ensure the chair is on a sticky mat or against a wall to prevent sliding.

Use a bolster to build strength while maintaining accessibility.

If you're looking for a less challenging way to practice this pose, get into a high plank position with the bolster under your chest, turned lengthwise.

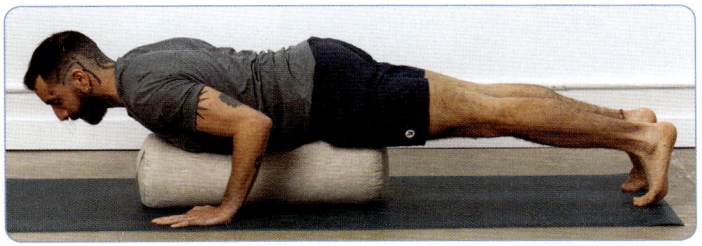

If necessary, stack two bolsters to get them to the height of your forearms. Activate your core and shift your weight forward, then bend at your elbows. As you exhale, lower your body, while continuing to broaden across the chest. Lower your torso until it rests over the bolster. Using a bolster lets you focus on your technique while building strength to stop yourself without a bolster.

Side Plank Pose

Vasishthasana   वसष्ठिासन

Side plank pose offers a myriad of benefits for your practice. This pose enhances balance and concentration while toning the abdominal muscles and strengthening the legs, wrists, and shoulders. When practiced only on the side of a spine with lumbar scoliosis, with the convex curve facing down, it can contribute to strengthening the muscles on that side, potentially aiding in reversing or slowing the progression of the curve. Let's delve into some prop-supported variations to enrich your side plank experience.

Practice with a block between your thighs to become aware of the pelvis.

To neutralize the pelvis and engage the thighs while reducing pressure on the lower back, a block on its narrowest width can be placed between the thighs while in plank pose. To transition into side plank, shift onto the outer edge of one foot and raise the opposite arm with the assistance of the block to maintain the alignment of one hip stacked directly over the other. Repeat on the other side.

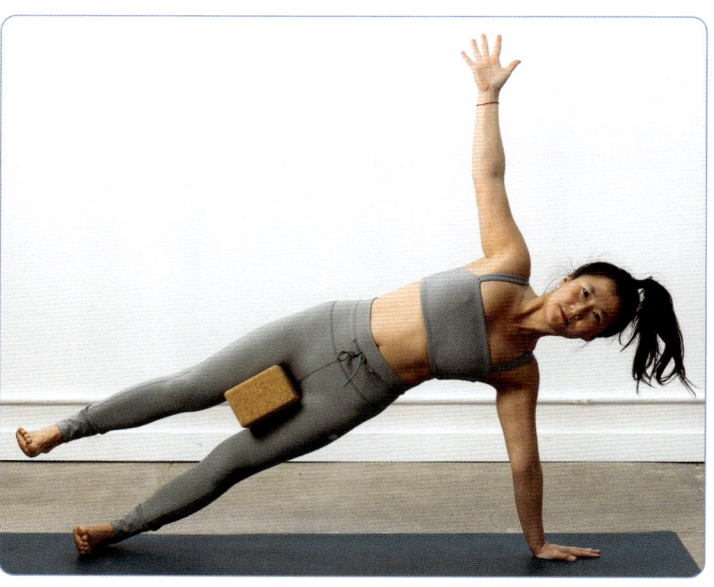

Place a block between your feet or shins.

By placing a block between your feet or shins, you can take your side plank to the next level while ensuring stacked alignment. Enter plank with your feet squeezing a block standing tall between them, then enter side plank. If you are less stable doing side plank on the ankles, opt for the shins rather than the feet. Squeezing the block with your legs will help you develop a greater awareness of your lower body, from your feet to your pelvic floor. This action also activates your inner thighs, while the block ensures that your legs are stacked directly on top of each other for optimal alignment. Repeat on the other side.

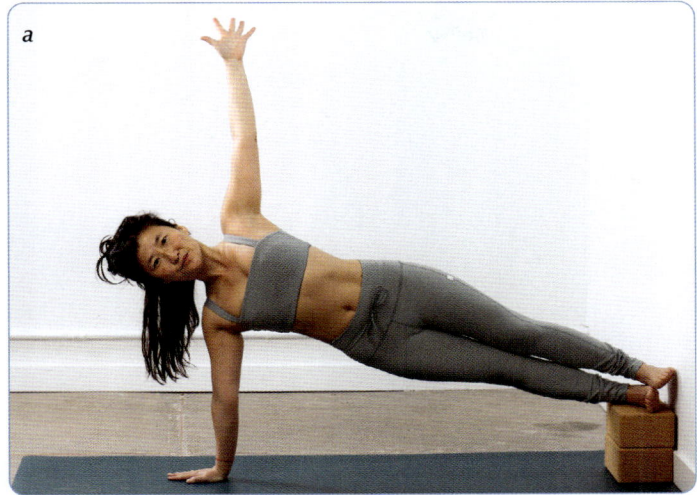

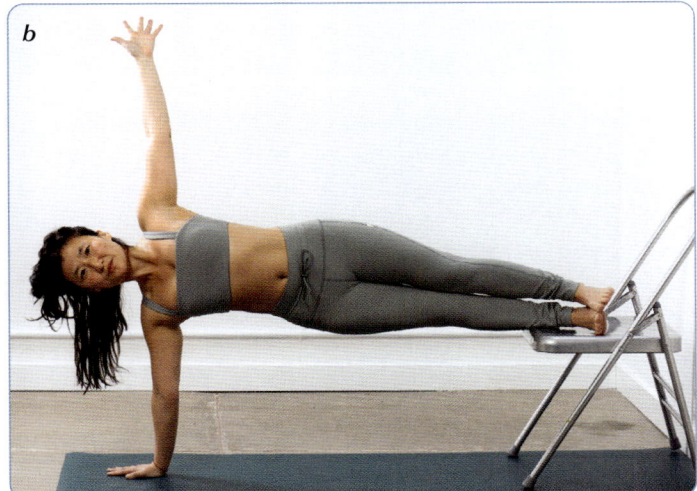

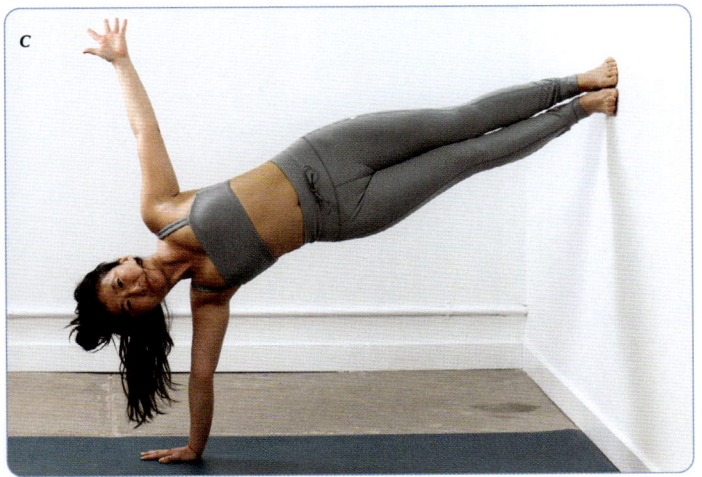

Stack your feet on blocks, a chair, or a wall to challenge your core and shoulder strength.

These three variations challenge your core and shoulder strength while also shifting more weight into the upper body. The first variation involves stacking your feet on blocks, which requires greater stability and balance in the core, hips, and legs (see photo *a*). This variation also requires more engagement in the shoulders and arms to support the weight of the body. By placing the feet on blocks, you also elevate the hips, which creates a deeper stretch in the sides of the body and challenges the oblique muscles. The other variations involve placing the feet on a chair (see photo *b*) or against a wall (see photo *c*) to increase the angle of the body relative to the floor and shift more weight into the upper body. These variations challenge the shoulder girdle and strengthen the arms. They also engage the core muscles. In the wall variation, you need to press into the wall with your feet to prevent them from sliding down. It also leads to a greater stretch in the sides of the body and challenges the oblique muscles. Repeat on the other side.

Side Plank Pose (continued)

Use a strap and your foot to help lift your ribs.

Elevate your one-legged side plank by using a strap to lift your ribs and foot. This variation is perfect for those working toward mastering the one-legged side plank, because the strap helps to stabilize the body and engage leg muscles. To begin, measure the size of your loop by placing the strap around one side of your rib cage and around the ball of the opposite foot in hand-to-big-toe pose. Enter a side plank with the strap resting loosely around the ribs, then draw the knee of your top leg toward your top armpit and grab the strap with your top hand to loop the other end around the ball of your foot. To better support this process, you can rest the hip closest to

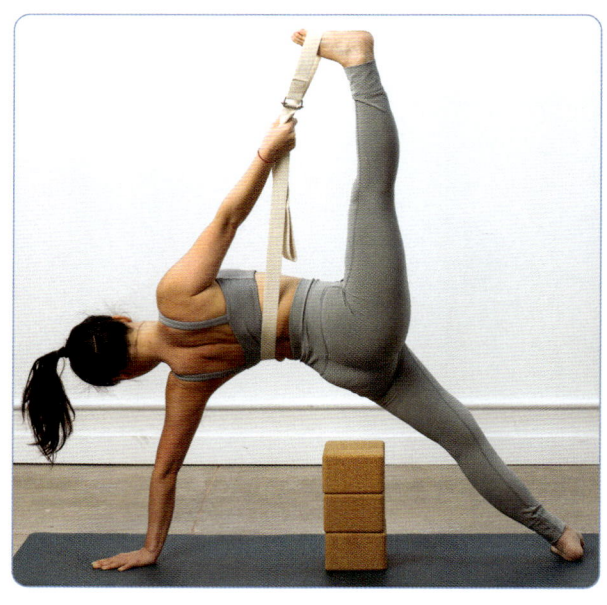

the floor on stacked blocks while looping the strap around your foot. Then lift the hips from this position, as shown in the photo. As you extend your leg, feel the strap gently lifting the rib cage up, creating space in your armpit region. This action helps to improve your posture and prevent slouching. It also challenges your balance. For more support, practice this variation with a wall behind you or with a teacher spotting you. Repeat on the other side.

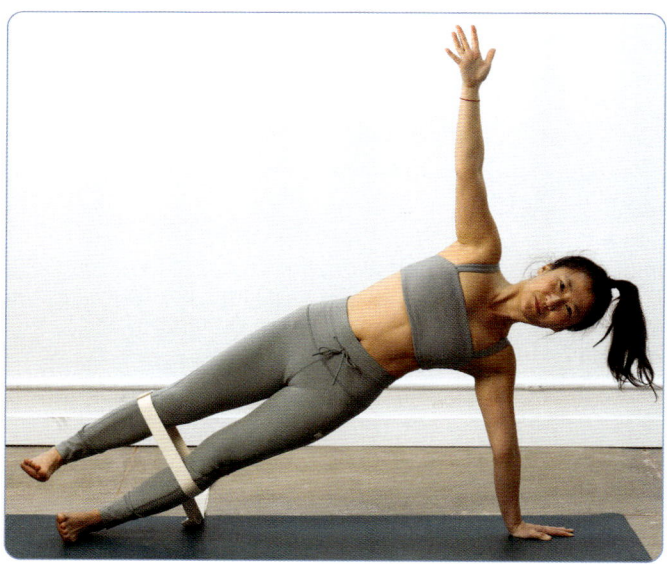

Place a strap around your shins to fire up your abductors.

This variation of side plank involves placing a strap around your shins to activate your abductor muscles. As you transition into your side plank, press the legs away from each other against the resistance of the strap. This action strengthens and tones the outer thighs and hips, while also increasing stability and balance in the pose. The strap can also help to improve alignment and prevent the legs from sinking towards the floor. Repeat on the other side.

The Complete Guide to Yoga Props

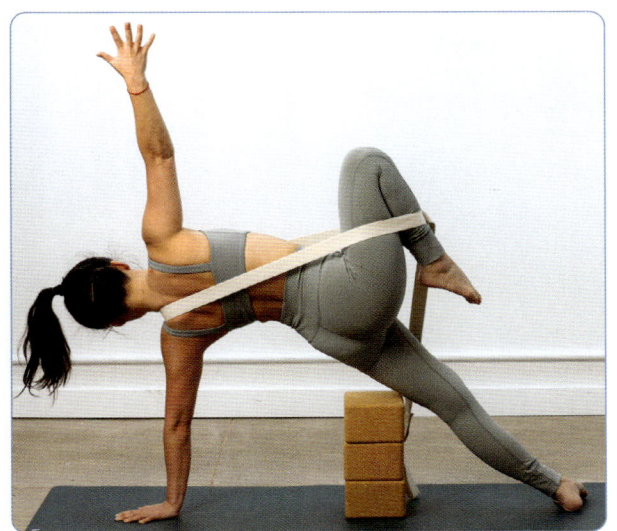

Use a strap to support tree pose variation.

To add support to your tree pose variation of side plank, use a strap to help lift your leg and create a deeper stretch. Start by stacking your lower hip on blocks and loop the strap around your top ankle, bringing it over the opposite shoulder. Tighten the strap to lift your top foot higher, while also drawing your shoulder down away from the ear. Lift your hips off the blocks to find balance in the pose. The foot can rest on the leg or it can be lifted as shown in the photo. Repeat on the other side.

Use a chair to modify and support.

Here are two ways you can use a chair in this pose. In the first variation, place your bottom hand on the chair seat to shift some weight from your upper body to your legs (see photo a). This will also alleviate strain on your wrists. To move closer to the floor, switch to placing your bottom hand on a block. This raises the ground height and shifts weight to the lower body but requires more strength and balance to counteract gravity. In the second variation, try side plank with a chair in front of you for support if you feel unsteady. Place your top hand on the chair to help you find balance and lengthen through the waist (see photo b). Try lifting your top hand overhead, knowing that the chair is there if you need support, and then return your hand to the chair. Repeat on the other side.

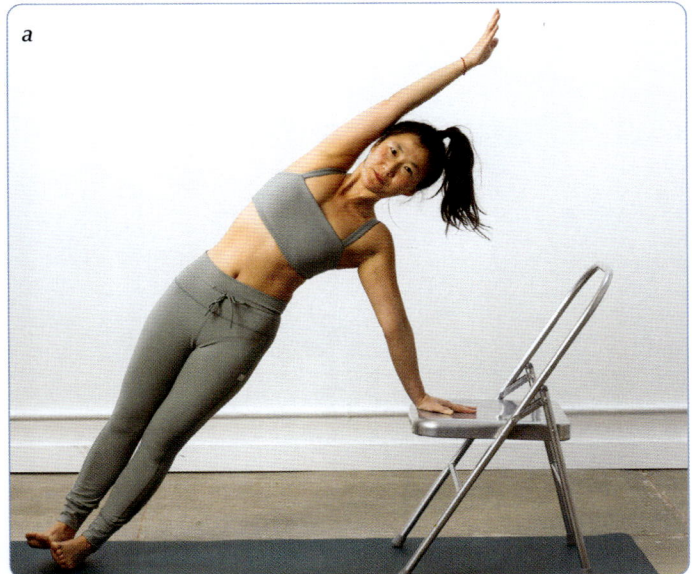

a

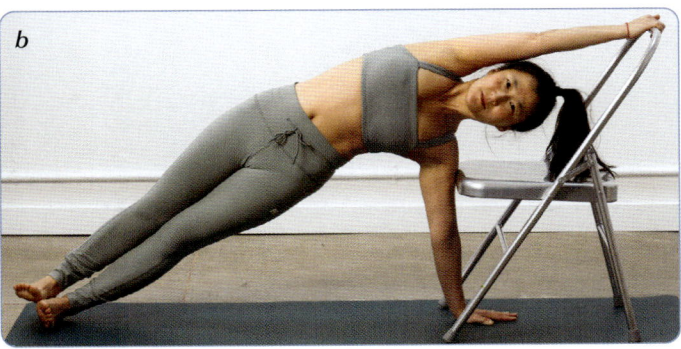

b

Use a blanket to support your joints.

Placing a blanket under the knees or hips in modified side plank provides cushioning and support, helping those with sensitive joints or injuries (see photos *a* through *c*). The extra padding also allows for a greater range of motion and stability, making it easier to maintain alignment and engage the targeted muscles effectively. The blanket can also provide feedback and sensory input to the body, helping to improve body awareness.

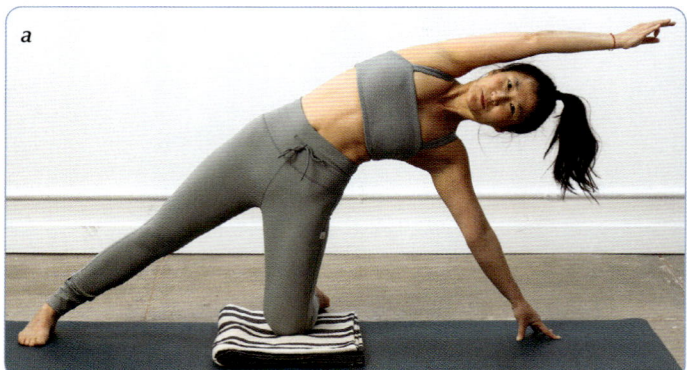

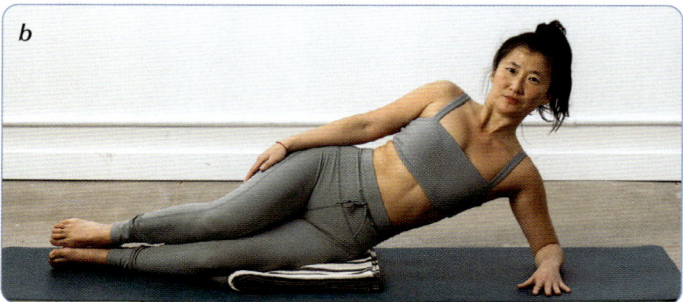

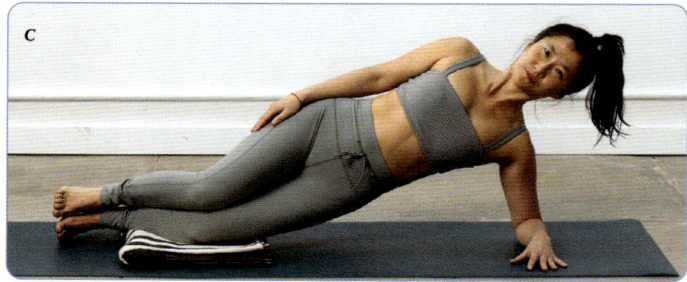

Use a chair to help engage your adductors.

Begin in side plank, then place the top foot on the seat of the chair. Press the inner edge of the flexed top foot into the chair seat to assist in lifting the bottom leg to hover off the floor, just below the chair seat. This will involve adducting through the bottom leg differently, because the top leg is using downward force, and the bottom leg is lifting against gravity. This posture challenges the stability of the supporting leg while also engaging the muscles of the lifted leg. It can be a great way to strengthen and tone the legs and

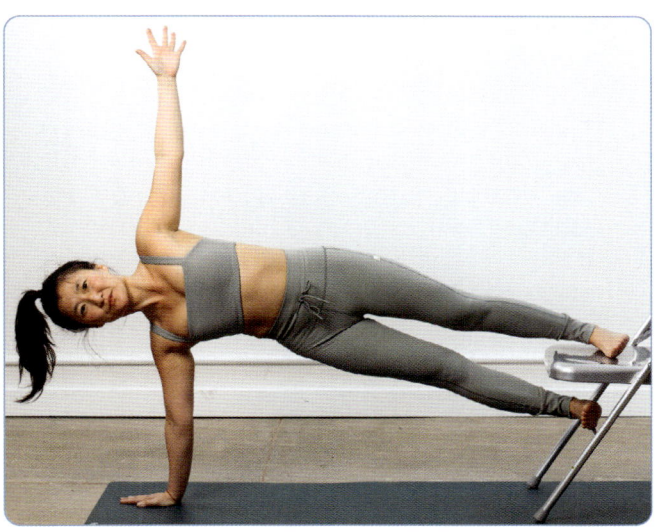

improve balance and stability. Note that you can also practice this in forearm side plank. Repeat on the other side.

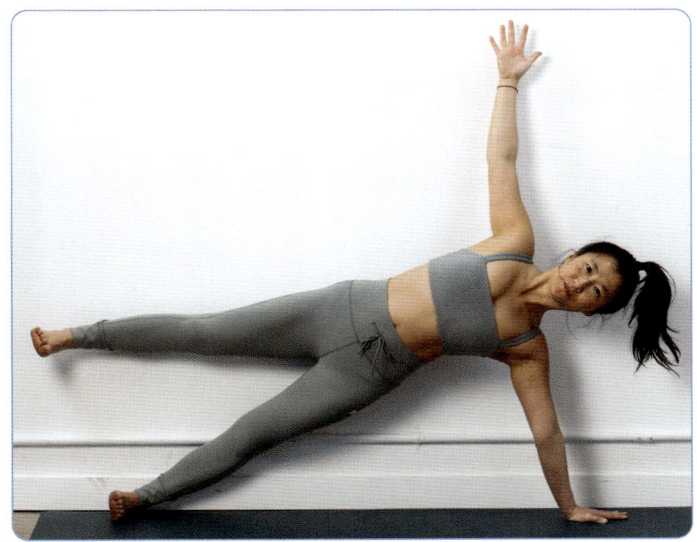

Practice with your back against a wall to inform alignment.

This variation of side plank can be beneficial for those who struggle with balance and alignment in the pose. By placing your back against a wall, you can ensure that your torso is in a straight line and your hips are stacked correctly. This can help to prevent compensations that can lead to discomfort or injury. The support from the wall can help you to hold the pose for longer periods of time. Practice on both sides.

Side Plank Pose (continued)

Stand with your hand on a wall to modify the pose.

This version of modified side plank involves standing with your hand on a wall instead of being on the floor. The main benefit of this modification is that it provides support and stability, making it a great option for beginners or those with wrist or shoulder injuries. You can focus on engaging your core and muscles along the side of the body with less balancing and weight-bearing in your upper body. This variation also lets you adjust the angle of your body in relation to the wall, so you can adjust the level of challenge you want or need. This version of side plank can also help to improve overall posture, because it encourages you to engage your core muscles and stand tall with your shoulders back and down. Practice on both sides.

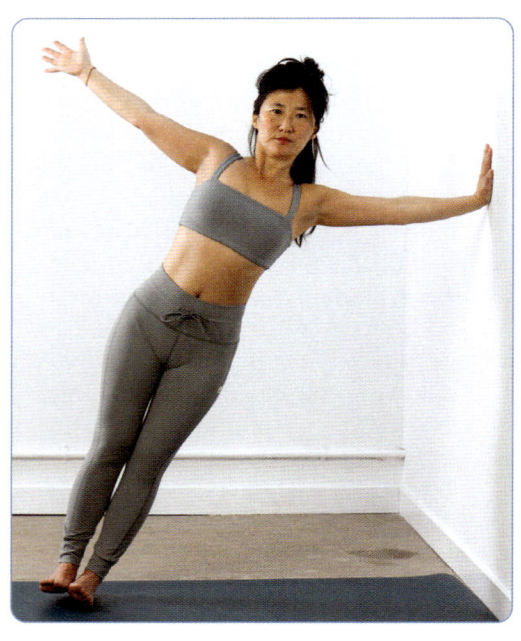

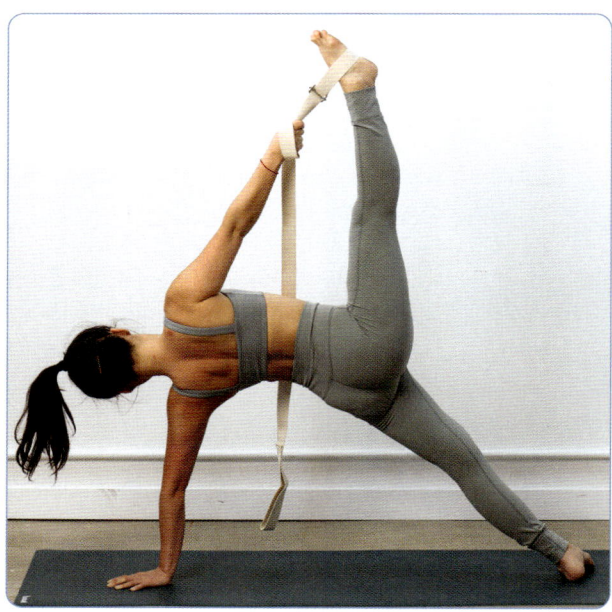

Use a strap in the hand-to-big-toe pose variation to bridge the gap between your foot and hand.

Begin in side plank with your left hand on the floor and your right foot stacked on top of your left foot. Bend your right knee and loop a strap around the ball of your right foot. Hold the other end of the strap in your right hand, extending your arm straight up. Straighten your right leg, using the strap to create tension and bridge the gap between your foot and your hand. This posture helps to stretch and strengthen the leg muscles and improve balance and flexibility. Note that if you want to omit weight-bearing and flexion in your wrists entirely, practice this version with your forearm or hand on a wall. Repeat on the other side.

Sage Visvamitra's Pose

Vishvamitrasana वश्विामत्रिासन

Sage Visvamitra's pose a dynamic and energizing asana that not only improves balance and concentration but also opens the hips and shoulders. It actively tones core muscles and those along the spine, simultaneously strengthening the arms and legs. As a potential peak pose, it shares foundational roots with side plank (vasishthasana) and seated compass pose (parivritta surya yantrasana). Refer to those postures and their variations to see how they may fit into adapting this pose as well, but here is one prop-supported variation unique to the pose.

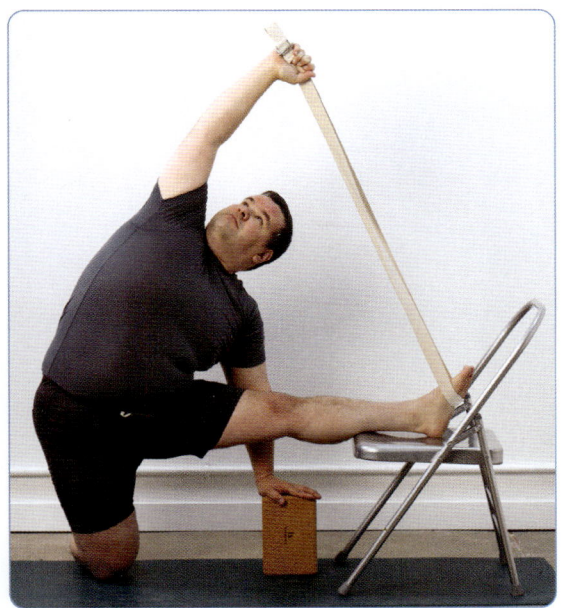

Kneel with your heel on a chair seat and use a block to raise the height of the floor.

Begin by kneeling and placing the heel of your left foot on the front edge of the chair seat with your toes pointing up. Lean your torso to the left, placing your left hand on a block to reduce the distance between you and the floor. With your right arm, reach overhead for the left foot. If needed, use a strap to bridge the gap between your hand and foot. If you would like to intensify the pose, extend the bottom leg fully as if you were in side plank. Repeat on the other side.

Chapter 9

Supine Poses

One should relish the emptiness of the small self
for peace and overwhelming joy. When one disappears,
there is no possibility of being or leaving.

Rodney Yee

In this chapter, we delve into the world of supine postures, offering flexible adaptations achieved with the use of props. These supine postures offer a new way to experience a pose, with your belly toward the sky, allowing you to take in the world from a fresh perspective. Beyond just offering a change in viewpoint, these postures provide opportunities to ground and release, inviting us to surrender to the embrace of gravity. Additionally, some supine poses introduce a playful connection to the ground below, facilitating a novel exploration of our spine's alignment, often fully supported for heightened awareness of posture. Much like prone postures, the floor in supine poses serves as a conduit for deeper breath awareness, acting as a feedback loop for the respiratory diaphragm and lungs. As we ground ourselves further, we open doors to explore our inner landscapes—whether in motion or stillness—within our physical shell. Just as the floor offers support, so do props, which we'll utilize here to enhance comfort, respond to diverse body needs, or even challenge ourselves. From the vantage point of our backs, it becomes clear that the sky is the limit in our exploration of supine yoga. It's important to note that the chapters in part II are organized based on each pose's originally intended form, but in some cases the adaptations alter the orientation of the posture from its initial form. Also, there are a few ambiguous postures (poses in which the individual is in a sideways orientation) that are included here because they flow best with the overall theme of the chapter and because they need a home.

> Mantra: I release, I let go,
> and I find serenity within.

Reclined Bound Angle Pose

Supta Baddha Konasana   सुप्त बद्धकोणासन

Reclined bound angle pose, a soothing and grounding pose, offers a gentle stretch to the inner thigh, groin, and knees and promotes a release of muscle tension. This restorative pose contributes to lowering blood pressure, providing a calming effect. Explore variations and props to enhance your experience of reclined bound angle pose.

Place a block or bolster under your knees to support your joints.

Using blocks or a bolster to support your knees in this pose allows your psoas (hip flexors) to relax and release, reduces strain in your lower back, and minimizes stress on your knee joints. Lie on your back with the soles of the feet together, letting your knees open to the sides. Slide a bolster or blocks, at your preferred height, under your knees (see photos *a* and *b*). You

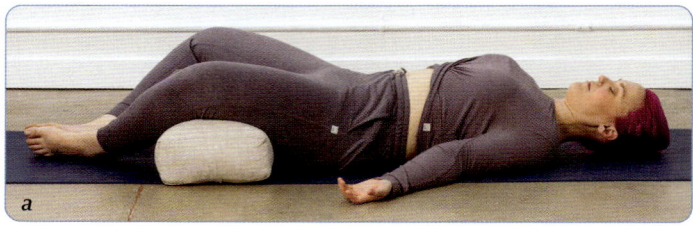

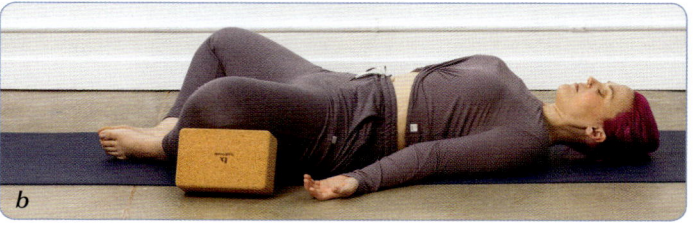

can also slant the blocks so they match the slope of your thighs. Let the outer, upper thighs roll away from the thigh bone toward the mat and roll your shoulders underneath the back of your ribs. Extend your arms to the sides with your palms up and lengthen your tailbone down toward your heels. If you experience any low back pain, bring your heels farther forward, away from the hips. Finally, soften through the belly to fully relax into the pose.

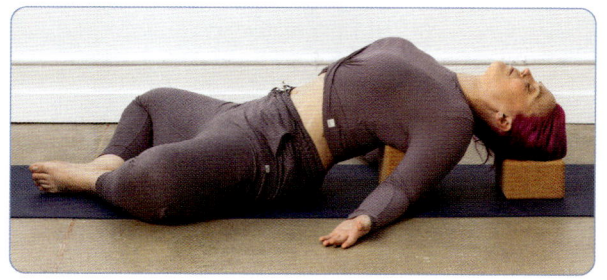

Use two blocks to find a gentle heart opener.

Using blocks to facilitate thoracic spine extension can result in a deeper opening in your chest muscles and thus deeper breathing. Sit with your knees and feet together and the soles of your feet planted on the mat. Turn one block to its medium height and place it about 12 inches (30 cm) behind your seat so that it lines up with your shoulders when you recline. Turn another to its lowest height and place it about 6 inches (15 cm) behind that block to rest your head on. The block under your shoulders can be positioned in a wide (more supported) or narrow (deeper stretch) orientation. Walk your hands behind you and gently lower onto your forearms, then lower your upper back onto the first block so that it rests directly under your shoulder blades. Ease your head back onto the second block, adjusting its height to align with the block height under your upper back if needed. Let your knees open to the sides with the soles of the feet together while entering the pose.

Use a bolster and a strap to apply traction to your spine and open your hips.

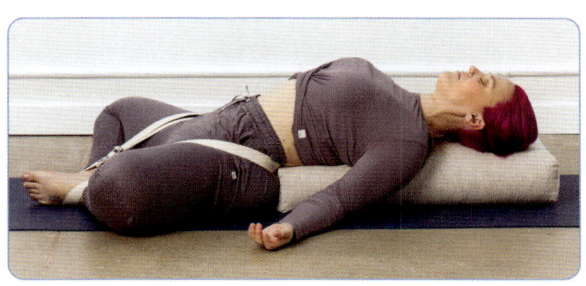

The restorative nature of this position allows you to surrender into deep relaxation and provides a gentle stretch. The strap will hold your feet and legs in position, eliminating the need for muscular effort. The added elevation provided by the bolster reduces tension in the lower back as well—if the back tends to be tight. Assume the starting position of bound angle pose with a strap within reach. Create a large loop with the strap and draw it over your head and torso. Place the back of the loop around the rim of your pelvis or sacrum and position the front of the loop over your ankles and under your feet. The sides of the strap can rest on top of your inner thighs or calves. Gradually tighten the looped strap, gently pulling your feet closer to your pubic bone until you experience a pleasant, strain-free stretch. The increased tension will also encourage you to sit up straighter. Lie back onto the bolster, releasing any tension in your body. Seek a comfortable point with a gentle stretch in your inner thighs, allowing the strap to facilitate traction in your lumbar spine.

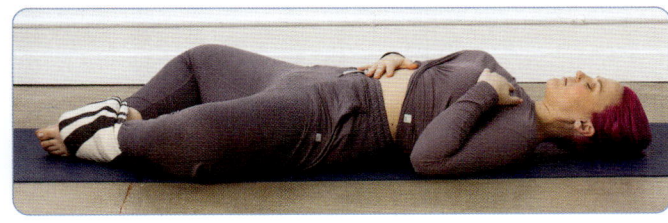

Use a blanket to support your ankles and knees.

This variation supports a neutral ankle position while binding the soles of your feet together and reduces stress on the knees and hips by elevating the knees and shins. Sit in bound angle pose with a rolled or narrowly folded blanket nearby. Place the center of the blanket on the inner edges of your feet and wrap it around your ankles, drawing it under the ankles and calves for support. Walk your arms behind you to slowly lower your spine onto the mat. If you experience lower back discomfort, adjust by sliding your ankles farther away. For added cervical spine (neck) support, place the rolled edge of another blanket behind your neck.

Reclined Spinal Twist and Revolved Belly Pose

Supta Matsyendrasana and Jathara Parivartanasana

सुप्तमत्स्येन्द्रासन and जठर परिवर्तनासन

Reclined spinal twist and revolved belly pose invite a revitalizing twist to your practice. These twists stimulate the abdominal organs, kidneys, and liver, promoting digestion. They enhance the twisting range of motion in the thoracic spine, offering stretches that alleviate pain and stiffness in the chest, shoulders, hips, and the entire back. Explore variations and prop-supported options to deepen your experience of these rejuvenating twists.

Place a bolster, rolled-up blanket, or blocks under your shin to support your lower back.

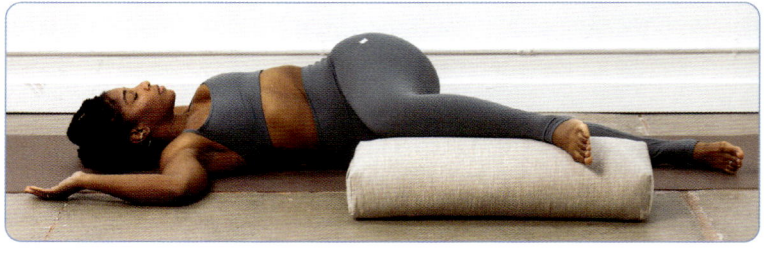

A bolster, blanket, or blocks bring the floor closer to you in reclined spinal twist, reducing strain on the lumbar spine and aiding in healthy spinal alignment. Lie on your back and draw your left knee toward your left armpit, guiding the knee across the body to the right, using a block, blanket, or bolster under your left shin or knee to bridge the gap to the floor when you encounter resistance. Extend your arms out to a *T* shape or goal-post shape, relaxing the chest and moving the left shoulder closer to the mat with each exhalation. Adjust the depth of the stretch by bringing the left knee closer to or further from the torso. As you twist, visualize the left hip point releasing away from the lower left ribs, creating more spinal extension. Repeat the sequence on the other side. Note that you can also use these props for revolved belly pose by drawing both knees into your chest before finishing the twist and resting your shins on the props.

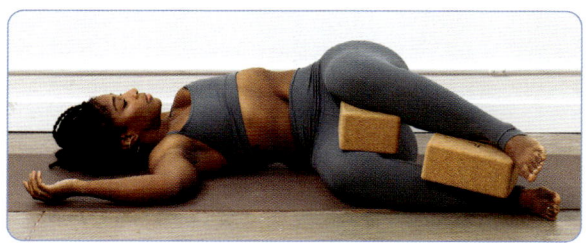

Place a bolster, rolled-up blanket, or block between your thighs and shins to support your hips.

Prop placement between the thighs and shins in revolved belly pose plays a crucial role in neutralizing the pelvis and relieving low back pain. It also helps align the hips, knees, and ankles parallel to each other for stability. Lie on your back and bring both knees into your chest. Bring the legs and hips into 90-degree angles, with the shins parallel to the mat. If you're using blocks, slide one block lengthwise between your upper thighs and another between your shins or ankles. For a bolster or folded blanket, wedge it lengthwise between your thighs and shins. To enter the twist, gently guide both knees over to the right side while hugging the blocks or prop between your legs. Extend your arms out to a *T* shape or goalpost shape, with your arms perpendicular to the body. To release from the twist, gently peel the left hip back toward the mat. Repeat the same sequence on the other side.

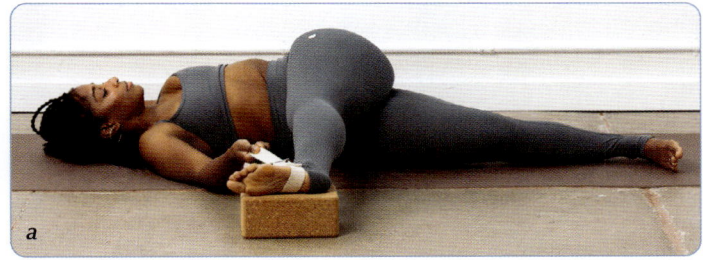

a

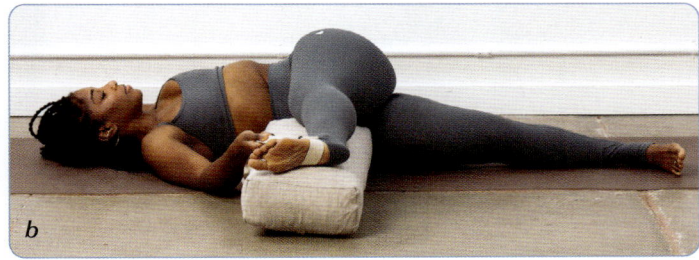

b

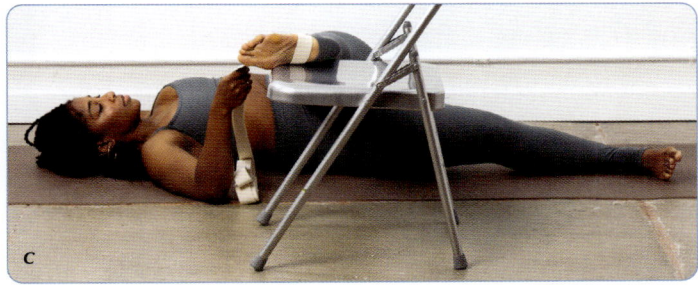

c

Practice a reclined dancing Shiva variation of the pose.

Props brings the floor closer to you, allowing for greater accessibility and support in reclined spinal twist. They can also provide relief from sciatica, lower back discomfort, and tension in the iliotibial band. The strap bridges the gap between your hand and foot, assisting you in reaching the point where you can hook your peace fingers around your big toe or capture your foot in your hand. Lie on your back, keep the right leg extended, and draw your left knee into your chest. Bridge the gap between your hand and your foot by looping a strap over the ball of your left foot and holding the ends in your right hand. To lengthen the spine, hook your left thumb into the left hip crease, gently pulling it down and creating more space along the length of your back. To enter the twist, slowly lower the left leg and right arm to the right side, allowing the left hip to lift off the mat. If you meet resistance, place a block under the left foot (see photo *a*) or a bolster along the length of the leg (see photo *b*). For added height, rest your left ankle on a chair seat (see photo *c*). Cushion with a blanket if needed. With each exhale, encourage the left shoulder to descend toward the mat, gently softening the chest. When you're ready to release from the pose, gently guide the left hip back toward the mat. Repeat the sequence on the right side.

Reclined Spinal Twist
and Revolved Belly Pose *(continued)*

Use a chair to practice a gentler version of the pose.

This revolved belly pose variation provides a gentle, supported twist that helps to release tension and tightness in the spine, hips, and lower back. Resting the legs on a chair allows for more relaxation and a passive stretch, promoting a sense of ease and comfort. As flexibility and comfort increase, you can work your way toward the

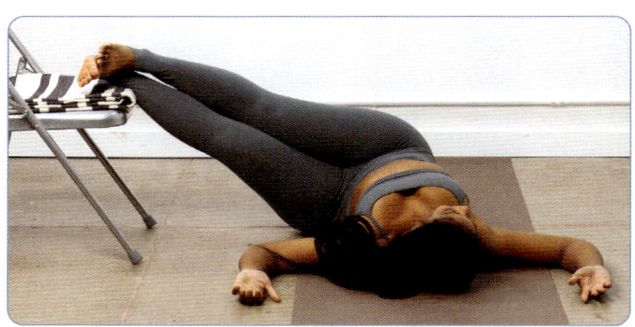

floor by bringing your ankles to a block, blanket, or bolster, allowing for a greater range of motion and a deeper twist. Lie on your back with both legs extended toward the sky, then on an exhale, lower your legs to the left to rest your ankles on the chair seat. Repeat on the other side.

Use a strap to practice cat pulling its tail pose for a gentle stretch.

These variations of reclined spinal twist offer support and enable you to feel a comfortable and rejuvenating twist in your practice and receive a gentle stretch to the hips and quadriceps. If reaching your foot or ankle is challenging, loop a strap around your foot to bridge the gap (see photo *a*). Alternatively, for a hands-free and deeply relaxing option, loop a strap around your hips and your back foot (see photo *b*).

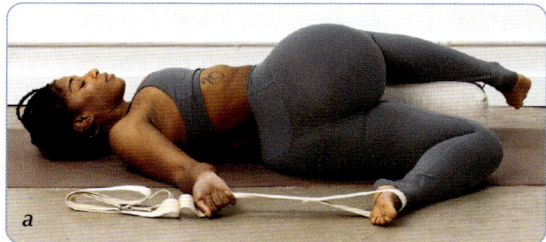
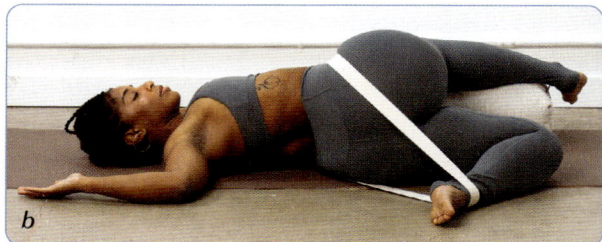

Flex your feet against a wall to ground and stabilize the legs and hips.

Here are two ways you can use a wall in revolved belly pose. In the first variation, enter revolved belly pose with your knees and shins stacked on one another and place both feet firmly against the wall (see photo a). This allows you to adjust the intensity of the stretch by moving your hips closer to or farther from the wall. In the second variation, explore a figure four supine twist. Come into a reclined pigeon pose at the wall, then transition into the twist. With your foot against the wall, the bottom leg stays in place, providing a stable foundation to deepen the hip-opening stretch in the top leg (see photo b). These variations enhance stability and support, allowing you to fully engage in the hip-opening and twisting aspects of the pose.

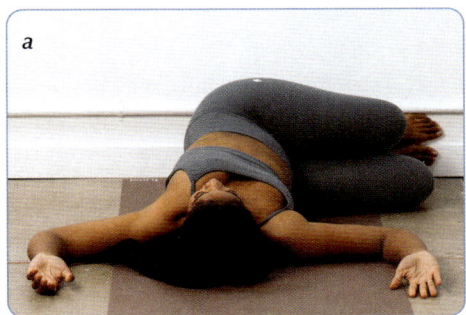 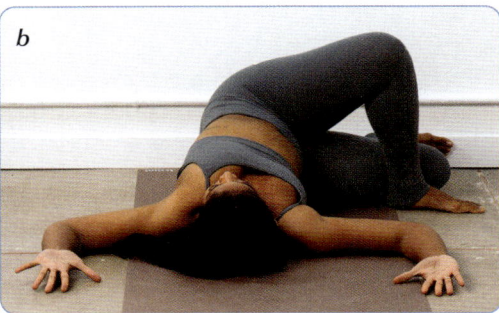

Use a block or blanket to practice a supine windshield wiper variation of the pose.

This variation of revolved belly pose reduces strain on both knee joints as it elevates the height of the top knee, minimizing torque on the knee and hip joints, and alleviates pressure on the bottom knee. Lie on your back with your feet planted about mat-width apart from each other and your knees toward the sky. Lower both knees to the right and hook your right foot over your left thigh, just above the knee joint. Place a block or blanket under one or both knees. This allows for a gentle lengthening sensation through the outer thigh, hip, and waist on the side of the bottom leg.

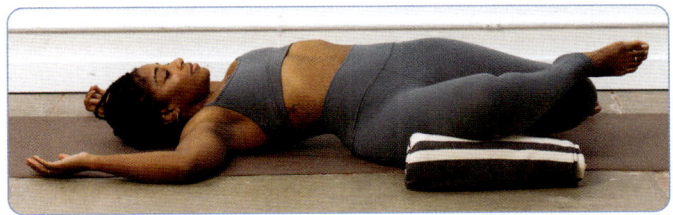

Reclined Hero Pose

Supta Virasana   सुप्त वीरासन

Reclined hero pose unfolds a restorative stretch across the thighs, knees, ankles, abdomen, and hip flexors. Embrace the strengthening benefits it offers to the arches of your feet and experience increased circulation. Explore prop-supported variations to enhance your comfort and deepen the therapeutic effects of this pose.

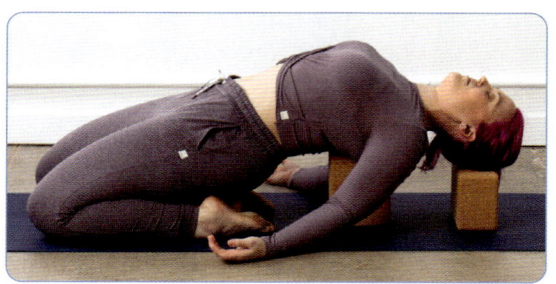

Place blocks under your hips, shoulders, and back of head for opening and support.

By placing blocks strategically, you can enhance your breath capacity and chest expansion, inviting you to relax into the pose. The use of blocks also promotes extension in the thoracic spine and provides relief to the thighs and knees by elevating the floor.

Begin in a supported hero pose with a block at the lowest height under your sitting bones. Position another block, lengthwise, turned to tall or medium height behind your seat, and another block on turned to medium or low height about six inches (15 cm) behind the first block. As you lower onto your forearms and rest your upper back on the first block, align the block directly under your shoulder blades and adjust as needed. Gently rest your head on the second block. If needed, modify the height of the second block to align with the one under your upper back. Rest your arms by your sides with palms facing up or extend them overhead. Roll your inner thighs slightly inward to create more space in the low back and draw your tailbone toward your pubic bone.

Use a block to practice a heart-opening variation.

Begin by kneeling and positioning your pelvis between your feet. Align your knees with your hip sockets to enter hero pose. If sitting on the floor is uncomfortable, sit on a block or a folded blanket. Place a block behind you, turned to tall or medium height.

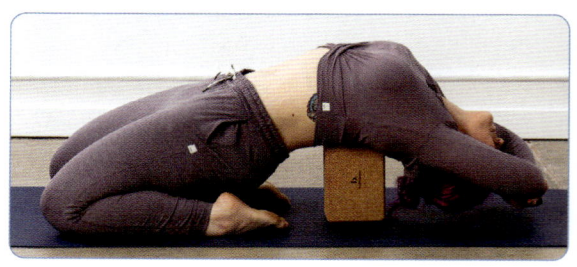

The narrow edge of the block should align with your spine and rest between your shoulder blades. Lower yourself onto the block, allowing the curve of your spine to deepen. Reach your arms overhead and grasp your elbows with the opposite hands. This gesture expands your chest and intensifies the stretch.

Place a block or bolster between your ankles.

Using a block or bolster in reclined hero pose is a great way to reduce pressure on the knee joints and lessen the intensity through the psoas, thighs, ankles, and shins. One option is to place a block between your ankles at the widest width on its lowest or medium height. Place a bolster behind the block and lie back onto it (see figure a). Another option is to do the reverse and sit on the bolster with a block under your head (see photo b). You can use two bolsters by sitting on the front edge of a bolster so that your knees can come together, just in front of it, then stack a second bolster on top of the first behind you. Place a block under the second bolster where it extends off the back edge of the first for optimal support (see photo c).

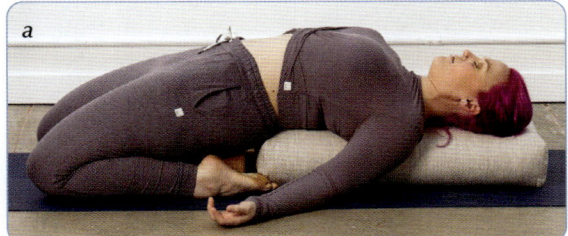

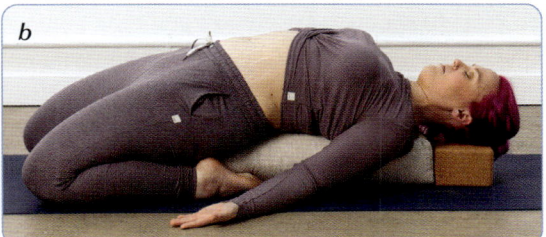

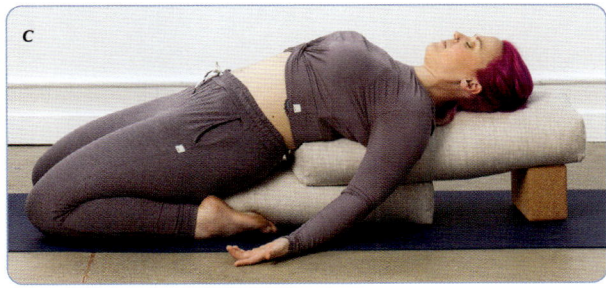

Use a looped strap to support your legs.

Use a strap to hold the legs and knees together. For some variations of reclined hero pose where the hips are elevated away from the floor on a prop, the strap will be looped just around the thighs (see photo a). For all other variations, where the hips are fully grounded on the mat, you can loop the strap around the shins to keep your lower legs from splaying (see photo b).

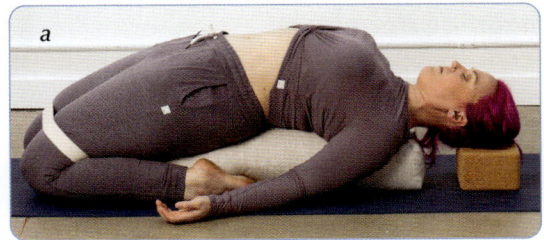

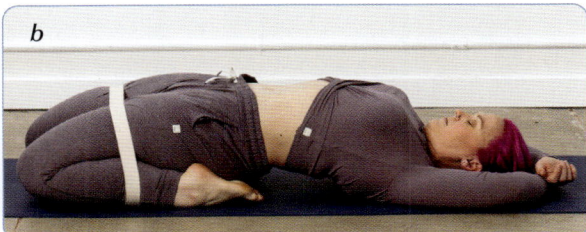

Use a chair to make the pose more accessible.

Using a chair can assist in traction of the spine and promote extension while reducing the intensity of the stretch and minimizing strain on the hips and knees. Sit in hero pose, with your back facing the seat of a chair. For comfortable extension of your back, place a block or two under your sitting bones to

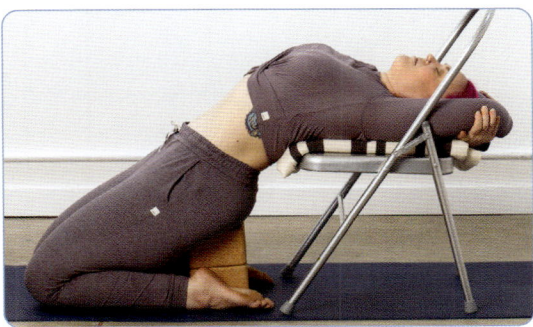

Reclined Hero Pose *(continued)*

elevate your hips. The height of your hips can be adjusted for the depth of the backbend you desire. Place your hands on the soles of your feet and gradually lower the back of your ribs and shoulders onto the chair. For added comfort or elevation, use folded blankets on the chair seat, especially if you wish to further support the cervical spine. As you settle into the pose, extend your arms overhead through the chair's backrest. For enhanced shoulder positioning and external rotation, hold a block between your hands.

Use blocks or a chair to create a bolster ramp.

Using a bolster ramp helps reduce the intensity of the posture, allowing you to stay in the position longer and fully enjoy its benefits. Here are two variations of reclined hero pose for creating a bolster ramp in this pose. In the first variation, set up a bolster ramp by placing blocks under the end of the bolster farthest from you. If you

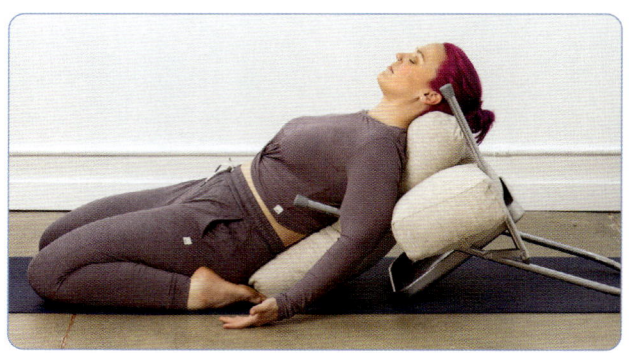

are starting the pose sitting on a block or blanket, raise the end of the bolster closest to you to the same height using a block or blanket. This setup provides a gradual incline for added comfort and support. The second variation involves using a flipped chair. Place the chair on its back, with the seat and backrest resting on the floor. Position one bolster horizontally across the bottom legs of the chair for structural stability. Place a second bolster lengthwise on top of the first bolster, forming a plus sign. This configuration offers a stable and reliable bolster ramp. Once your bolster ramp is ready, gently lean back into it (see photo). Enjoy the deep relaxation and opening this posture provides as you rest into it.

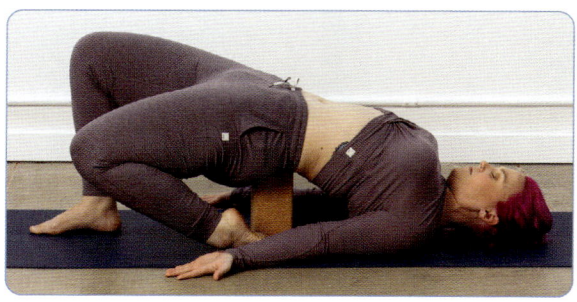

Use a block to practice one-legged reclining hero pose.

This option may enhance the opening in your front thighs and groin. Lie on your back with your feet planted on the floor and knees pointing toward the sky, as in the starting position of bridge pose. Lift your hips slightly and position a block on its medium height or stack two blocks horizontally under your sacrum, creating a

supported bridge. Lift your left knee and foot off the floor and reach for your foot or ankle with your left hand. Point your toes and engage your calf muscles as you gently draw your foot toward your shoulders. Ensure that your left knee points away from you and down toward the mat. Once your leg is in position, release your arms alongside your body and relax into the pose, supported by the block. When you're ready to release, gently bring your left foot back to the floor and repeat the pose on the other side.

Use blankets to support your joints.

Blankets offer cushioning and provide necessary support to enhance your practice, creating a more supportive and comfortable experience for your joints. The blankets aid in reducing pressure, increasing flexibility, and promoting proper alignment for greater ease and relaxation in the pose. The first option of this variation of reclined hero pose focuses on reducing pressure on the knees and shins. You can place one or more folded blankets under your knees and shins, effectively alleviating any discomfort or pain associated with these areas. As you sit between your ankles, gently roll your calves outward, creating space for your hamstrings when you sit back (see photo a).

In the second option of the variation, if you experience tightness in your ankles and struggle to extend them comfortably, you can roll a second blanket or the rolled end of one blanket to your desired thickness for a gentler stretch and support. Place this second blanket or the rolled end of your blanket between your ankles and the floor, allowing your ankles to have something to release into (see photo b). The third option addresses tightness in the hips and thighs, which can inadvertently strain the knee joints. To mitigate this, fold a blanket and position it just under your knees (see photo c). The added elevation reduces the intensity of the stretch and minimizes strain.

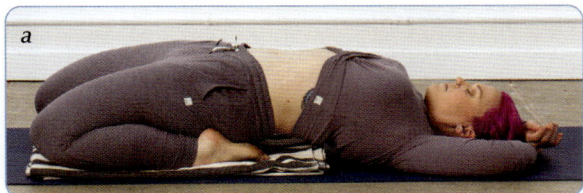 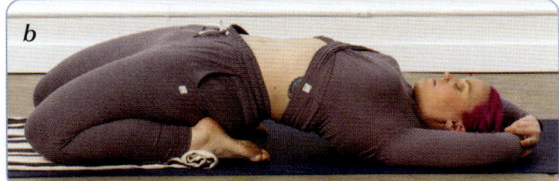

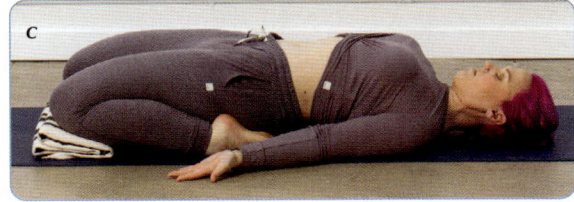

Legs Up the Wall Pose

Viparita Karani

वपिरीतकरणी

Legs up the wall pose invites a gentle stretch to your hamstrings and lower back, fostering a calming effect on the nervous system. This pose facilitates the release of fluid from your legs and feet, reducing edema, while enhancing overall circulation throughout the body. Explore prop-supported variations to tailor this pose to your comfort and maximize its soothing benefits.

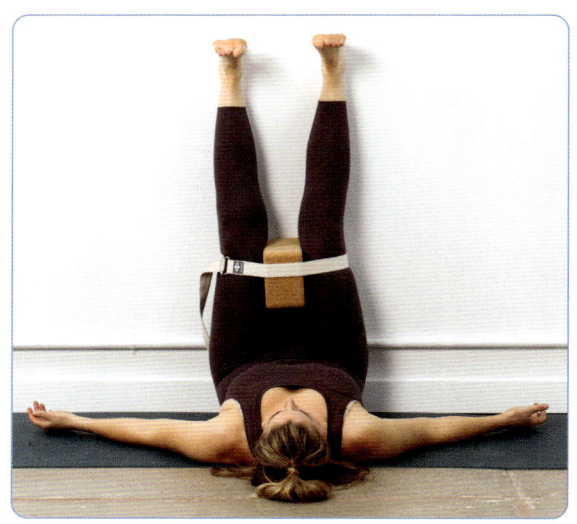

Place a block with a strap between the thighs to align and release.

A strap plays a crucial role in allowing the leg muscles to completely release and relax by promoting even weight distribution in the legs and bringing them into parallel alignment. The strap helps prevent external rotation in the hip sockets. A combination of a block and a strap also helps reduce strain on the lower back by ensuring alignment and support. Find a comfortable, seated position facing a wall. Extend your legs and place a block on its narrowest width between your upper thighs. Loop a strap around the thighs and the block, tightening it enough to hold the block in place without engaging the thighs excessively and avoiding direct contact between the metal part of the strap and your thighs. Scoot your sitting bones against the wall while lying on your side and roll onto your back so that your sacrum rests on the mat and your legs extend up the wall. Allow the thighs to relax into the straps and release any tension in your muscles.

Use a strap to practice a wide-legged variation.

Experience a wide-legged variation with the support of a strap in two different ways, allowing your legs to fully let go and release. The first option of this variation of legs up the wall pose involves sliding a looped strap farther up toward the ankles (see photo a). By doing so, you create more stability as the strap remains secure and prevents the legs from sliding apart. For the second option, looped a longer strap around the sacrum, the outer edges of the legs, and over the tops of the feet (see photo b). This variation offers deep relaxation by relieving tension in the lower back, gently supporting the natural

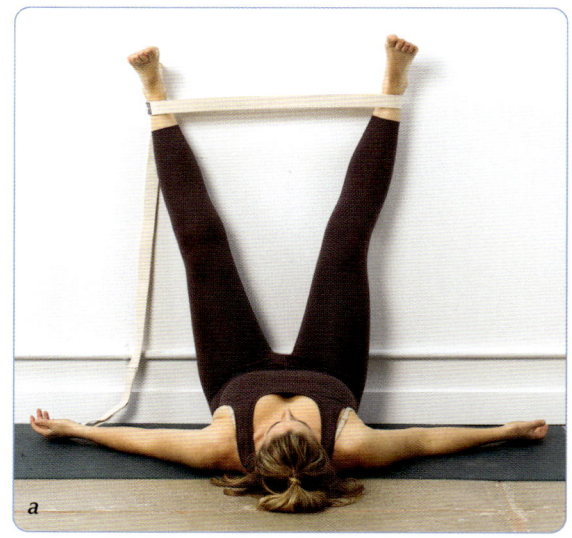

a

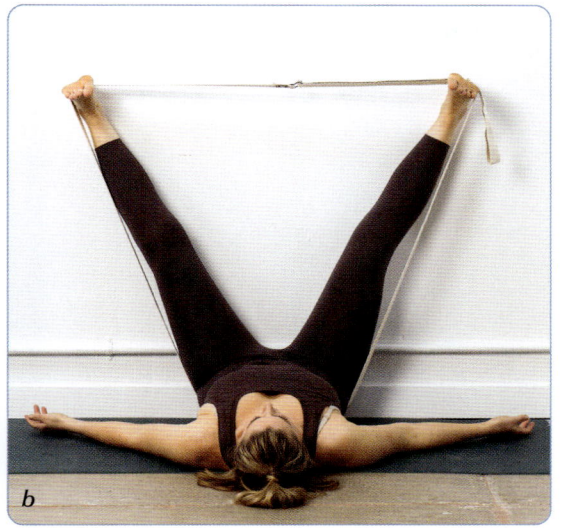

b

curve of your spine, providing a resting place for the legs and knees, and grounding the femur bones into the hip sockets with a gentle pressure on the tops of the feet. Moreover, it aligns the thighs parallel to each other without requiring muscular engagement.

Use a bolster or folded blanket to elevate the hips.

This variation of legs up the wall pose creates a gentle elevation and support for the hips for a more comfortable and sustainable posture. It helps to alleviate potential strain or discomfort in the low back, especially if the psoas or hamstrings are feeling tight. Lifting the hips also encourages a slight tilt of the pelvis, which aids in lengthening the spine. Furthermore, using a bolster or blanket under the hips enhances the passive inversion aspect of the pose

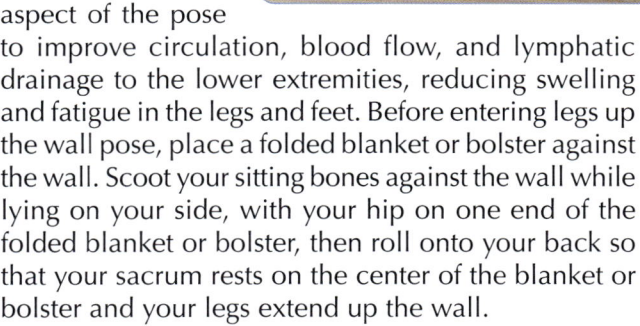

to improve circulation, blood flow, and lymphatic drainage to the lower extremities, reducing swelling and fatigue in the legs and feet. Before entering legs up the wall pose, place a folded blanket or bolster against the wall. Scoot your sitting bones against the wall while lying on your side, with your hip on one end of the folded blanket or bolster, then roll onto your back so that your sacrum rests on the center of the blanket or bolster and your legs extend up the wall.

Use a blanket to tuck yourself in.

Swaddling your legs with a blanket creates a sense of comfort and coziness, allowing you to fully relax without any strain or effort and let go of any tension in your body. Swaddling the legs with a blanket can help to calm the nervous system and reduce stress and

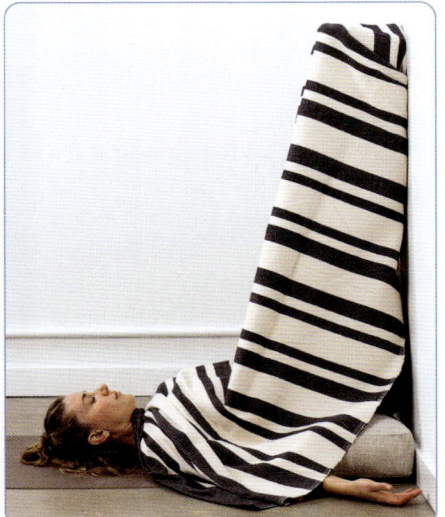

anxiety, like the feeling of being hugged. After entering the pose, bend your knees, slide your feet down the wall, and wrap a blanket over your heels. Then slide your legs back up the wall, tucking yourself in with the blanket around your legs. You can also ask someone else to tuck you in if necessary.

Place a bolster or weighted blankets on your feet to ground and release.

The added weight and pressure on the feet in this variation provide a grounding sensation, promoting a sense of stability and relaxation throughout the body. This can help to calm the nervous system and reduce feelings of anxiety or restlessness. The weight of the blankets gently stretches the muscles in the legs, promoting a deeper release and increased blood circulation and lymphatic flow. This can help to alleviate tension and fatigue in the lower body. The blankets also create a comforting sense of swaddling or cocooning. After coming into legs up the wall pose, bend your knees, sliding your feet down the wall so you can place your prop of choice above the feet, then extend the legs again. This might be easier with someone to help place the prop over your feet while the legs are still extended.

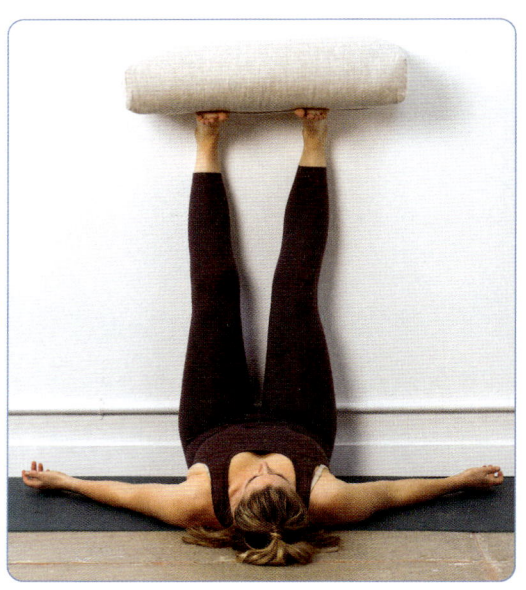

Practice with legs on a chair to make the pose more accessible.

Lying on your back with your calves and ankles releasing onto the chair seat allows your legs to rest upon a supportive platform while still enjoying the benefits of inversion. This variation helps to alleviate pressure and strain on the lower back and hips, allowing for a gentle release of tension and promoting relaxation. Bending the knees also makes it a suitable option for those with tight hamstrings or limited flexibility. The elevated position of the legs can improve blood circulation, reducing swelling and fatigue in the lower extremities. The support of the chair allows for a deeper sense of grounding and stability, making it a more comfortable and relaxed posture that may be easier to sustain for longer periods of time. Set up how you would for legs up the wall, but lying on your side in front of a chair with the seat facing you. Roll onto your back with your legs up, then lower your calves onto the chair seat.

Create a bolster ramp if your legs hyperextend or you want less of an angle.

A bolster ramp can reduce the strain on your legs and allow a more comfortable and supported stretch, alleviating the pressure on hyperextended legs. The ramp also allows you to customize the angle of the

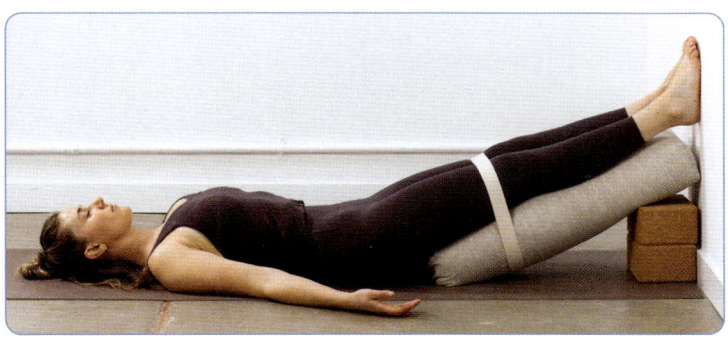

pose, creating a gentler incline that is better suited for your body. This can be particularly helpful for individuals who have limited flexibility, injuries, or specific comfort preferences. A bolster ramp also provides added stability that supports the weight of your legs and allows you to relax fully into the pose without worrying about maintaining the position. To enter this variation, create a bolster ramp against the wall. Support the end of the bolster closest to the wall with either stacked blocks or a block wedged at an angle at the junction of the wall and floor, as shown in the photo. Loop a strap around your thighs to hold the legs together, then come into the pose using the ramp just as you would the wall.

Reclined Pigeon Pose

Supta Kapotasana

सुप्त कपोतासन

Reclined pigeon pose gracefully opens the hips, offering relief from sciatica while stretching the piriformis muscle. This pose enhances blood flow to the pelvis, promoting the optimal function of synovial fluid in the hips by facilitating joint movement. Embrace the improved circulation in the hips through the calming and therapeutic benefits of this pose. Dive deeper into your practice by exploring prop-supported variations tailored to your comfort and needs.

Practice with your foot on a wall to stabilize and release.

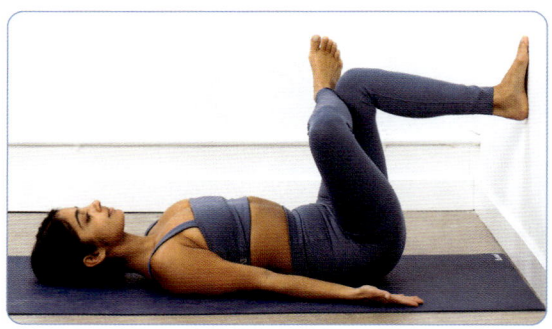

This variation of reclined pigeon pose allows you to focus on stretching the hips while disengaging the upper body as you relax and hold the pose for a longer duration, facilitating deeper hip opening and release. This setup eliminates the need to round the spine or strain to reach your leg and pull it toward your body, enabling a more comfortable and accessible stretch. A foot against the wall helps to stabilize the hips. To practice reclined pigeon pose at a wall, lie on your back with your feet facing the wall. Scoot your hips close enough to the wall that you can enter a supine table top position with your feet placed hip-width apart on the wall. Stack your knees over your hips and level your ankles with your knees. Cross one ankle over the other knee, creating a figure four with your legs. If this is too intense, scoot your hips farther from the wall. Rest your arms by your sides, palms up, while opening your chest and heart space. Relax the muscles of your face, neck, and shoulders and release any tension held in your jaw. As you progress in your practice, gradually move your hips closer to the wall, deepening the stretch.

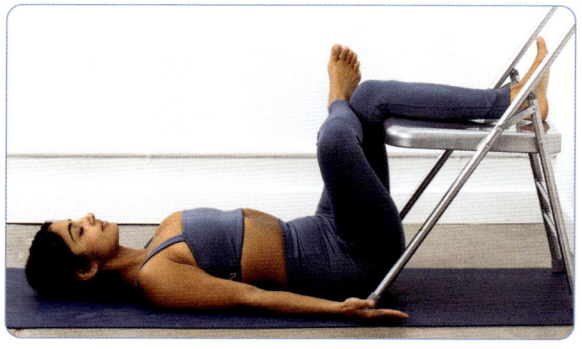

Practice with your calf on a chair to ground and relax.

One of the key benefits of this variation of reclined pigeon pose is the relaxation it offers to the upper body. By resting on the floor and elevating the calf on the chair, you can disengage the upper body and focus solely on the hips and lower body. This relaxation promotes a sense of ease and allows you to hold the pose longer. This variation also helps to stabilize the hips and lifted leg, minimizing strain on the knee joint and promoting stability throughout the pose. Practicing reclined pigeon pose with the calf on the chair also allows for a more accessible experience. This is especially beneficial for individuals with limited flexibility or those recovering from injury, because it reduces the strain while still offering the benefits of the pose. Begin in the chair-supported version of legs up the wall pose, then cross your right ankle over your left knee. Scoot your hips closer to, or farther from the chair to adjust the intensity of the stretch accordingly. Repeat on the other side.

The Complete Guide to Yoga Props

Thread a strap around your thigh so you can relax your head, shoulders, and neck.

This variation of reclined pigeon pose allows you to avoid straining your neck and shoulders off the floor to reach for your thigh. The strap assists in maintaining alignment and ease in the pose, and by wrapping the strap around your thigh, you can gently draw your leg closer to your torso without exerting unnecessary effort in your upper body. The strap offers support

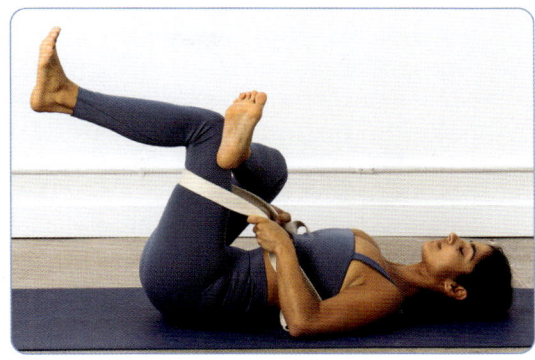

and stability, allowing you to find a comfortable position and hold the pose longer. This can deepen the stretch in the hip and gluteal muscles, promoting increased flexibility and releasing tightness. Remember to adjust the strap's tension to your comfort level and maintain a relaxed state throughout the pose.

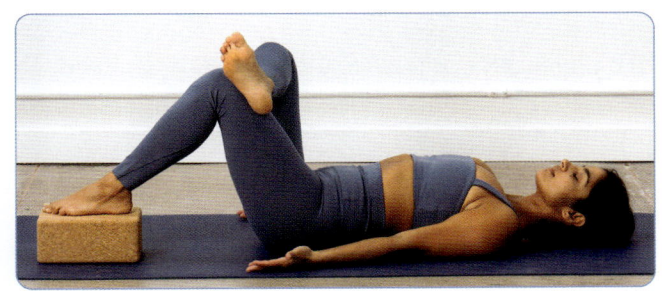

Use a block to elevate your bottom foot and ease into the stretch.

You can find a midway step between having the bottom foot grounded on the floor and lifting it completely off the floor with this variation. It offers additional support and stability, allowing you to maintain a balanced and controlled position throughout the pose. This can be especially helpful if you're working on deepening the stretch but can't yet bring your knees all the way over your hips. This variation also helps to create a gentle stretch in the hip and gluteal muscles. By elevating the foot, you can increase the degree of hip flexion and external rotation. This can be particularly beneficial if you want to gradually improve your flexibility and range of motion in the hips. Using a block to elevate the bottom foot makes the pose more accessible. Lie on your back with your feet planted on blocks, hip-width apart and knees toward the sky. Cross your right ankle over your left knee. Repeat on the other side.

Place a bolster or folded blanket under your hips to lessen strain in the hamstrings and hips.

The elevation provided by the prop allows for a slight release of the hamstrings, reducing the risk of straining them. It promotes a safer and more supportive alignment, making the pose more accessible for practitioners with tight hamstrings or limited flexibility. Secondly, this variation of

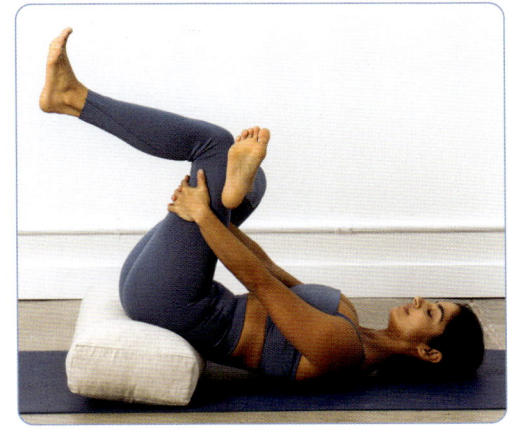

reclined pigeon pose offers relief and support for the hips by raising them slightly, creating a sense of space and ease in their joints. This can be particularly beneficial for those who experience discomfort or sensitivity in the hips or lower back during the pose. Lie on your back with your feet firmly planted and your knees toward the sky. Press your feet into the mat to lift your hips and slide your folded blanket or a bolster under the hips. Cross your right ankle over your left knee, then draw the left knee in toward your body, as shown in the photo. As you practice this variation, you can adjust the height and thickness of the bolster or folded blanket as needed. Repeat on the other side.

Find a deeper stretch with the help of a strap.

For this version of reclined pigeon pose, explore extending your bottom leg and using a strap to bridge the gap in space between your hands and find a bind. In the non–strap-supported version of this pose, the top arm supports the back of your head like a hammock, and then it holds onto the bottom hand. The bottom elbow crease is wrapped over the ankle. To modify this, enter a reclined pigeon pose, with your right ankle over the left knee, then loop a strap around the right foot. Hold the ends of the strap in your leg hand and find a crunch or curl to lift your shoulders off the mat. Reach your right arm overhead and bend at the elbow as if you were doing a half cow face arm pose, then use your left hand to assist the transfer of the strap ends into your right hand. Hold under the ankle with the left hand, as shown in the photo, and extend your left leg. Release your head into your right arm. Repeat on the other side.

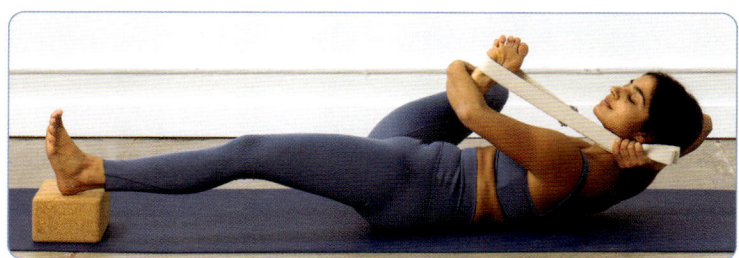

Half Wind-Relieving Pose

Ardha Pavana Muktasana अर्धपवनमुक्तासन

Half wind-relieving pose gently stretches the hips, groin, hamstrings, and gluteal muscles, providing relief from lower back pain. By lengthening the spine, this pose becomes a gentle facilitator of improved digestion and elimination. Embrace the nourishing benefits of this posture and explore variations with the support of props to deepen your practice and enhance its therapeutic effects.

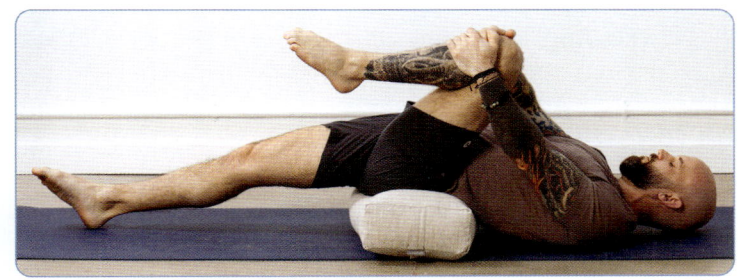

Place a block, bolster, or blanket under the hips to deepen the stretch.

By placing a block, bolster, or blanket under your hips, you create a supportive foundation that allows for a more profound and effective stretch. If using blocks, one block is suitable, but two blocks side by side give you a wider surface to rest your hips on. Place the blocks on their lowest height, under your sacrum, to maintain stability and alignment. Draw one knee toward your chest while simultaneously extending and reaching through the opposite leg. This movement engages the hip flexors and facilitates a deep stretch in the iliopsoas muscle group. As you bring your knee in, you can feel the opening and release along the front of your body, creating space and length in the hip area. Remember to listen to your body and adjust the height and support of the prop according to your comfort level and needs.

Loop a strap around your thigh to bring your leg to you.

This variation of the half wind-relieving pose, particularly beneficial for individuals with tight hamstrings or hips, provides a supported approach to deepen the stretch while promoting relaxation in the upper body.

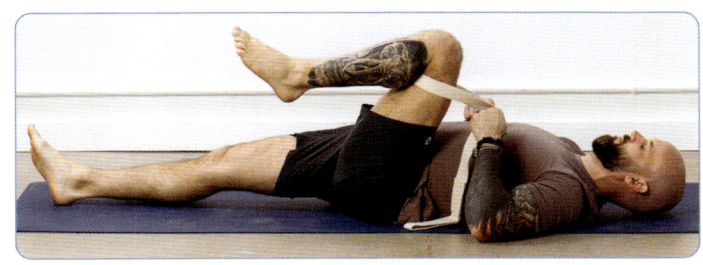

Loop the strap around the back of your thigh, holding the ends, and bend your knee. As you gently draw your knee closer to your chest using the strap, focus on fully letting go of tension in the upper back, head, and neck, allowing these areas to rest and relax. Adjust the tension of the strap according to your comfort level, gradually exploring deeper stretches as your body allows. With this modification, you can experience the benefits of a more open and relaxed lower body while nurturing the well-being of your upper back, head, and neck.

Loop a strap around your shin and upper back for a hands-free variation.

Begin this variation of half wind-relieving pose by looping the strap around your shin and upper back, creating a secure connection. As you draw your leg toward your chest using the strap, you can feel a gentle opening in the hips and a lengthening sensation in the hamstrings. Adjust the tension of the strap according to your comfort level, ensuring that it allows for a gentle stretch without causing any discomfort or strain. Repeat on the other side.

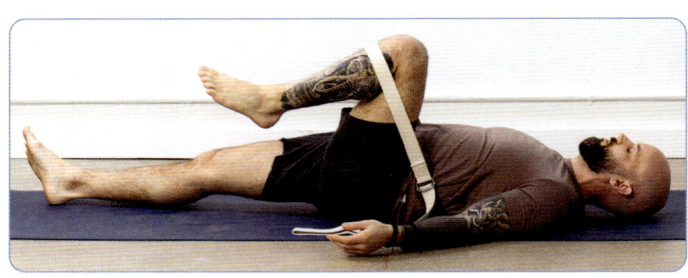

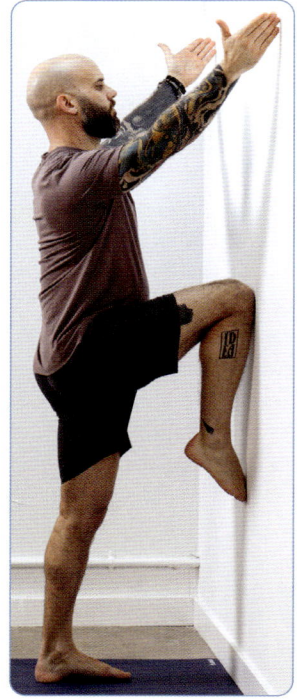

Stand with your shin against a wall.

By placing your shin against the wall, you can enhance the stretch while simultaneously incorporating an element of balance into your practice. This variation of half wind-relieving pose is particularly beneficial for individuals seeking to deepen the stretch in their hips and legs. Face a wall in a one-legged mountain pose. Rest your shin against the wall with your toes pointing down toward the floor. For added support and stability, place your hands on the wall to help level your hips and find balance. Gradually lean your hips forward toward the wall and simultaneously bring your lifted heel closer to your gluteal muscles. As you lean into the wall, you will feel a gentle stretch in the ankle of your standing leg, enhancing the overall benefits of the pose. This variation allows for a deeper stretch and offers an opportunity to cultivate and refine your sense of balance. Engaging with the support of the wall lets you focus on grounding through your standing leg and finding stability in your posture. Repeat on the other side.

Sit in a chair for a more accessible option.

This variation of half wind-relieving pose is helpful for those with mobility limitations, those who find it challenging to transition between floor and standing positions, or those who just prefer a seated option. By incorporating the chair into your seated practice, you can reap the benefits of hip flexor release, improved spinal alignment, enhanced core engagement, and increased accessibility. Sit in the chair with an upright and elongated spine, maintaining your posture throughout the practice. As you draw one knee into your chest, focus on lifting through your chest to prevent any rounding or collapse in the spine. This is especially important for individuals with conditions such as osteopenia or osteoarthritis, because maintaining a tall spine helps protect the integrity of the vertebrae and supports overall spinal health. Repeat on the other side.

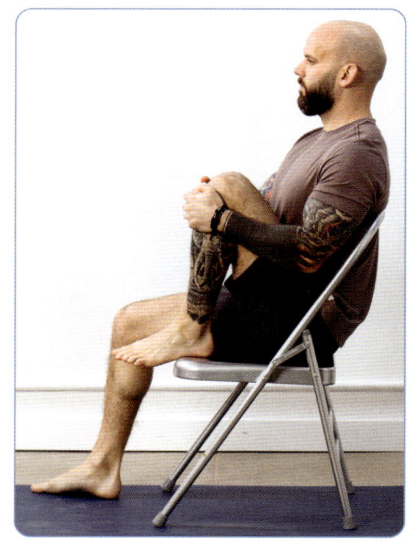

Reclined Hand to Big Toe Pose I and Pose II

Supta Utthita Hasta Padangushthasana I and II

सुप्त उत्थति हस्त पादाङ्ग्ष्ठासन I and II

Reclined hand to big toe pose I and pose II, as supine postures, gracefully stretch the ankles, calves, hamstrings, hip flexors, and groin, fostering improved circulation. Embrace the potential relief from lower back pain that these poses can offer. Let's explore some variations supported by props, allowing you to experience the full therapeutic benefits of these reclined poses.

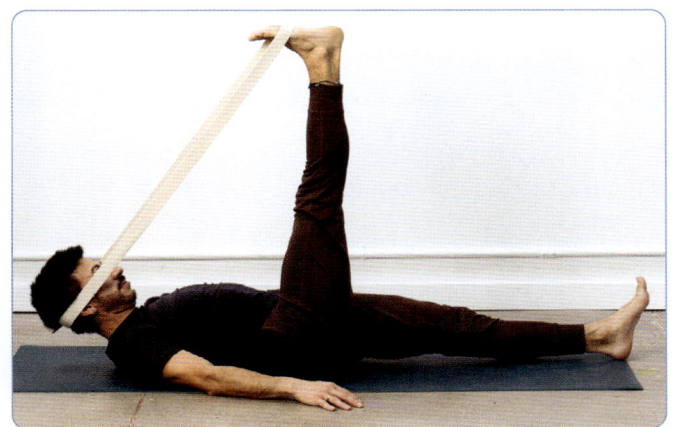

Loop a strap around your head and foot to apply traction to your neck.

This variation is particularly beneficial for individuals seeking to create space and alleviate tension in the cervical spine in reclined hand to big toe pose I. The strap acts as a gentle hammock for the head, lifted by the extended leg. Create a large loop with the strap. While lying on your back, position the strap around the base of your head where it meets the spine. Then, loop the other end of the strap loop around the ball of your extended leg's foot. Find a comfortable position for your lifted leg, allowing the foot to be slightly below perpendicular to your body. This positioning adds a natural weighted pull on the head, aiding in the traction effect. For a more active variation, tighten the strap's loop and gently reach your leg away from your face, engaging the muscles on the back of the leg. The pull created by the lifted leg provides a beneficial traction effect on the back of the neck, which can help relieve head and neck tension and allows for decompression in the cervical spine, promoting the release of any accumulated stress or discomfort. Repeat on the other side.

Use a strap to bridge the gap in space between your hand and foot.

When you can't reach your big toe, usually bending the knee is the next best option. If you have a strap, though, you can loop it around your foot, holding both ends in the same-side hand of the lifted leg. Once the leg is extended, move your hip and shoulder back so that they are level with the hip and shoulder on the opposite leg

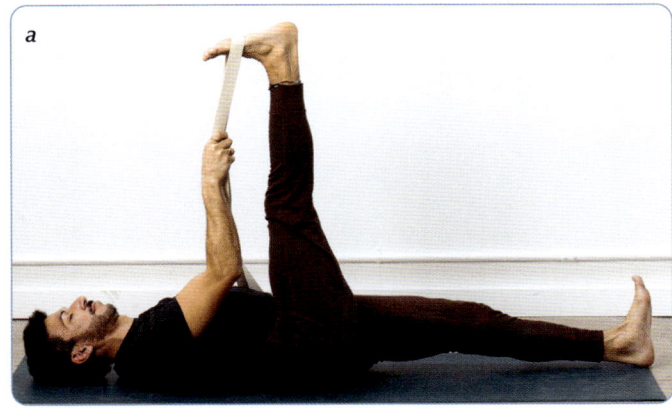

a

Reclined Hand to Big Toe
Pose I and Pose II (continued)

side. See photo *a* for an example of reclined hand to big toe pose I and photo *b* for an example of reclined hand to big toe pose II. Repeat on the other side.

Loop a strap around your foot and your upper back for a hands-free option.

These variations of the reclined hand

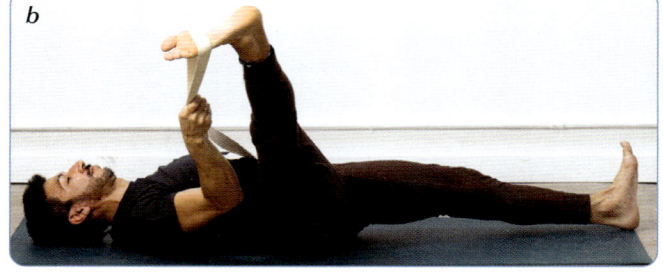

to big toe poses offer a convenient and effective way to deepen the stretch while providing support to different areas of the body. Loop the strap around your foot and position the other side of the strap loop behind your back wherever you prefer between the lower ribs and the shoulder blades. Find a placement that allows you to comfortably engage with the strap and maintain a sense of stability throughout the pose. As you settle into reclined hand to big toe pose I, focus on pressing the back of your body into the strap (see photo *a*). This action helps to lengthen the spine, engage your core muscles, and gently deepen the stretch. By grounding your shoulders and hips into the strap, you enhance stability and create a solid foundation for the pose. This hands-free variation can be applied to both reclined hand to big toe pose I and pose II.

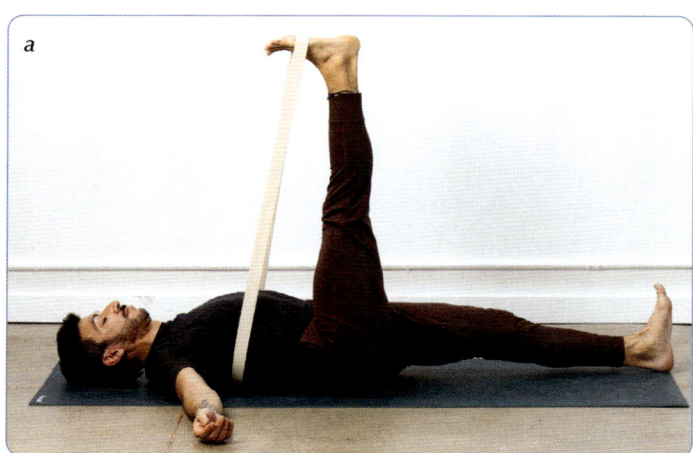

In the second variation, the strap serves the additional purpose of preventing the ribs from arching away from the foot, maintaining alignment and engagement in reclined hand to big toe II. As you extend your leg out to the side in reclined hand to big toe pose II, pressing into the strap provides a grounding sensation, ensuring stability in the shoulders and hips (see photo *b*). The support of the strap helps you feel a greater sense of control and depth in the pose, allowing you to explore and expand your flexibility and maintain proper alignment. Repeat on the other side.

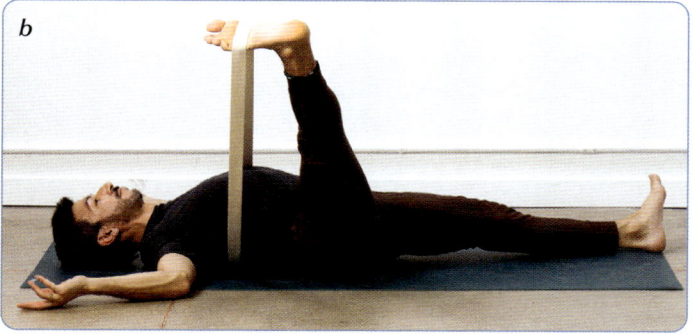

Ground your bottom leg foot against a wall to engage and align.

As you position yourself for either reclined hand to big toe pose I or pose II, ensure that your bottom leg is extended along the floor, with the sole of the foot pressing firmly against the wall (see photo *a* for an example of reclined hand to big toe pose I and photo *b* for an example of reclined hand to big toe pose II). Repeat on the other side. The simple action of pressing the foot against the wall activates the leg muscles, promoting stability and engagement throughout the pose. Furthermore, it helps to lengthen the spine, creating a sense of extension and openness in the posture. This contributes to better alignment and a more effective stretch. Focusing on

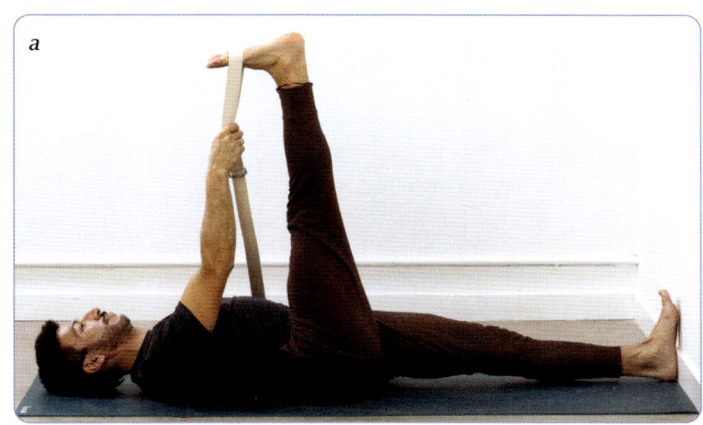

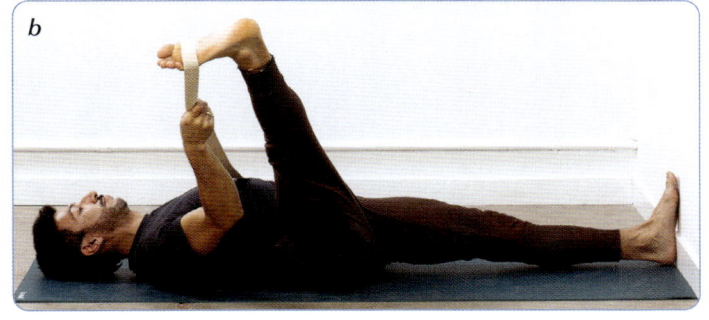

aligning your toes to point up while grounding the foot against the wall helps to maintain proper leg positioning. By avoiding rotation of the thigh in the hip socket, you can guard against unnecessary strain and ensure a more balanced and supportive alignment.

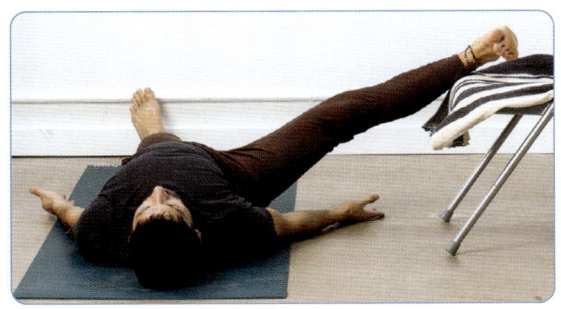

Use a wall, chair, or bolster for a gentler version.

This variation of reclined hand to big toe pose II provides a gentle and supported hip opening that helps to release tension and tightness in the spine, hips, and lower back. Resting the leg on an elevated surface also allows for a deeper relaxation and passive stretch, promoting a sense of ease and comfort. Start with the wall; as flexibility and comfort increase over time, you can work your way toward the floor by bringing your ankle to the chair or bolster, allowing for a greater range of motion and a deeper hip opening. Repeat on the other side.

Reclined Hand to Big Toe
Pose I and Pose II *(continued)*

Loop a strap around your leg, thigh, and foot to engage and align.

This strap variation, used for both reclined hand to big toe pose I and pose II, takes a little bit of strap measuring in advance, but it is so worth it! The strap simultaneously encourages leveling the hips, anchoring the lifted thigh back, and engaging through the leg muscles and core stabilizing muscles. By pressing the foot into the strap, you also reinforce lengthening in the spine, creating space from your tailbone to the crown of your head, and lengthening through your waist. Loop a strap around the ball of your grounded foot, then over the lifted thigh so that it rests in the hip crease. There should be enough tension in the

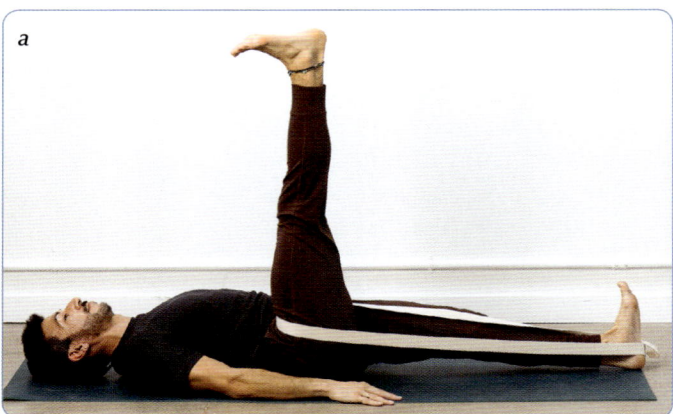

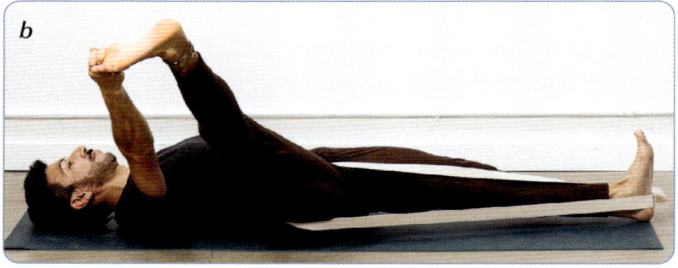

strap that the hips remain level as you draw your lifted leg toward you or to the side (see photo *a* for an example of reclined hand to big toe I and photo *b* for an example of hand to big toe II). Repeat on the other side.

Happy Baby Pose

Ananda Balasana आनन्द बालासन

Happy baby pose, a delightful asana, playfully stretches the hamstrings, inner thighs, hips, and groin, while gracefully lengthening the spine. Beyond its physical benefits, this pose invites playfulness and acts as a calming tonic for the nervous system, offering a reprieve from stress and anxiety. Explore variations with props to enhance your experience and deepen the therapeutic effects of this joyful pose.

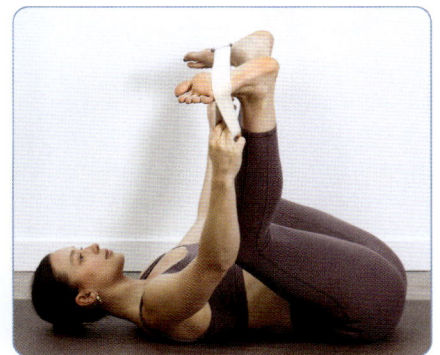

Use a strap if your feet are out of reach.

When you place the strap across the soles of your feet, it becomes an extension of your hands, allowing you to contact your feet even if you can't reach them directly. This variation of happy baby pose also helps release tension in your shoulders by allowing them to fully relax on the floor, without straining to reach your feet or ankles. To try it, slide the strap over the soles of your flexed feet and gently pull down, drawing your knees toward your armpits.

Use a strap around your feet and behind your ribs for a hands-free option.

This modification of happy baby pose allows you to deepen the stretch without the need to actively hold your feet. Lie with your shoulder blades or the backs of your ribs on a strap turned into a large loop. Securely place the other side of the strap around the arches of your feet. As you draw your knees toward your armpits, tighten the strap so that it maintains tension. The strap provides gentle support, enabling you to relax and release tension in your upper body. The strap also helps maintain alignment by preventing the rounding of your upper back, promotes flexibility in the hips and groin, and relieves lower back discomfort.

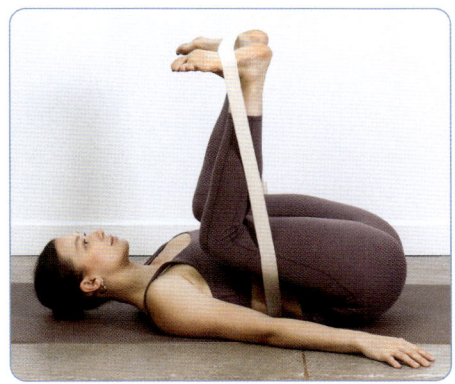

Happy Baby Pose *(continued)*

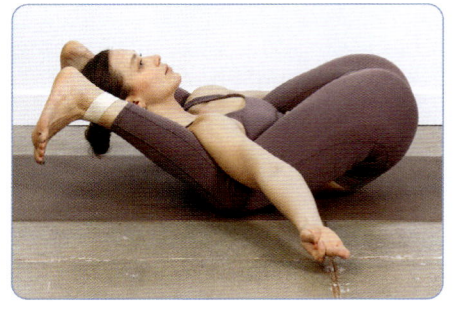

Use a strap to practice yogic sleep pose (yoganidrasana) variation for added support and progression.

This variation of happy baby pose serves as a stepping stone to bringing your feet behind your head while providing cervical spine support through the use of the strap, which acts like a comfortable head hammock. The strap allows you to experience the benefits without crossing your feet. It is essential, though, that you do not force the pose before you're ready. Begin in happy baby pose and create a loop with the strap, placing your feet inside the loop. Adjust the size of the loop according to your comfort and flexibility. Position the other side of the loop behind your head. Lengthen the back of your neck as you lean into the strap while gently pulling your knees down to stretch through the hips. With consistent practice, you can gradually make the loop smaller, bringing your feet closer to your head. As you progress, your legs will naturally rotate externally.

Use a bolster or blanket to stretch and support your lower back.

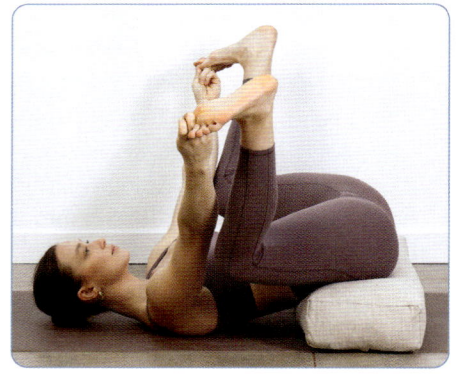

Unlike the traditional happy baby posture, in which you lengthen through the tailbone and ease the hips toward the mat, this variation focuses on finding a gentle flexion in the lower back. If you have any contraindications or discomfort in your low back, avoid this variation. However, if you experience tightness in the lumbar spine or have lordosis, this variation can offer a beneficial alternative. By using a bolster or blanket, you can bring the knees closer to your armpits and bridge the gap between your hips and the floor, providing increased stability and a grounded sensation. Enter a supported bridge pose with a bolster or folded blanket under your sacrum. Then draw your knees toward your armpits and point your feet toward the sky, reaching for the outer edges of your feet, ankles, or the backs of your knees with your hands.

Practice seated in a chair.

This first option of this variation of happy baby pose is for added ease and spinal support. It is particularly beneficial for individuals who find it challenging to transition between the floor and standing positions or for those seeking to avoid rounding of the spine due to spinal conditions like osteoporosis, osteopenia, or disc herniations. Sit upright in a chair and engage your core (or use a strap around your left foot to assist) to lift your left knee toward your chest. For increased stability, hold the edge of the chair seat with your right hand, which allows you to press down and promote lengthening through your spine. Once in position, you can choose to grasp the leg behind the left knee or reach for your outer ankle or foot with your left hand. As you lift through your chest and sternum, draw the left knee toward your left armpit for a gentle stretch while maintaining proper alignment and stability. Repeat on the other side (see photo *a*).

The second option of this variation aims to facilitate hip opening and spinal release by incorporating a distinctive stretch. This gentle rounding of the spine not only imparts a beneficial traction effect on the spine but also creates space and openness in the hips, contributing to a profound sense of relaxation. Sit on the edge of a sturdy chair. Place your feet wider than shoulder-width apart, ensuring a comfortable stance. Gradually fold forward, guiding your hands down to blocks or the floor for support. Once you have fully surrendered into the forward fold, transition your hands behind your ankles and place them just outside your feet (see photo *b*). If you are using blocks, feel free to bring them along to maintain the desired height.

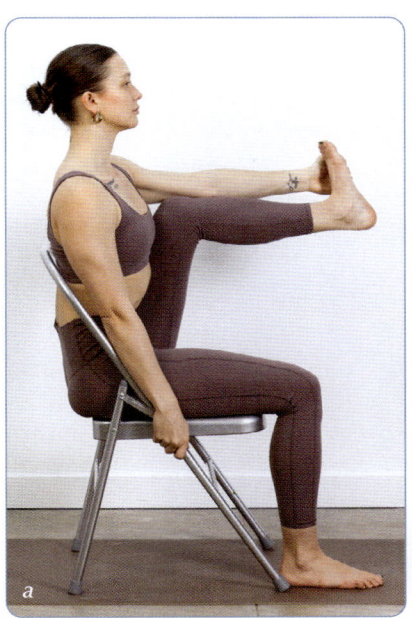
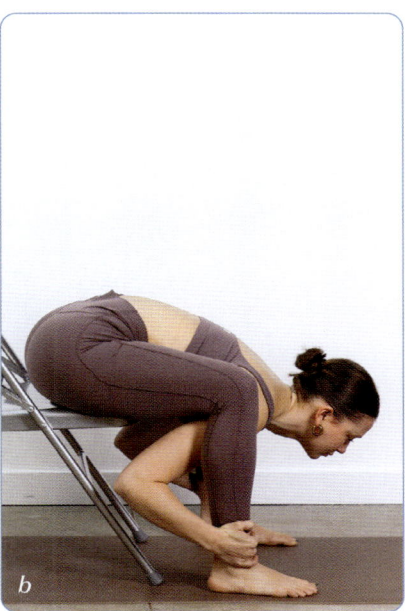

Sleeping Vishnu Pose

Anantasana

अनन्तासन

Sleeping Vishnu pose, also known as Vishnu's couch pose or side-reclining leg lift, unfolds as a serene stretch for the hips, calves, pelvis, and groin. While you are toning the abdominal muscles, it elegantly enhances balance and hip mobility. With its therapeutic touch, this pose may even alleviate the discomfort of sciatica. Experience both the beneficial and challenging nuances of this pose by exploring prop-supported variations for an enriched practice.

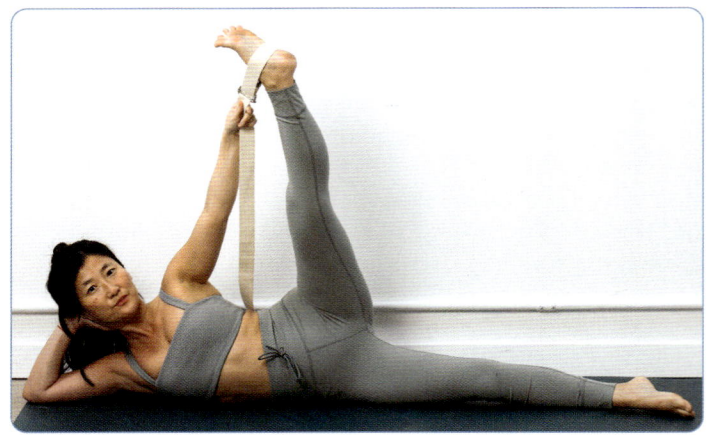

Use a strap for a longer reach.

The strap acts as a helpful tool in this variation of sleeping Vishnu, allowing you to reach your foot with ease and deepen the stretch along the sides of the body. Lie on your right side with your legs extended straight. Place your right arm out long, in the same line as your body, to provide support or bend your elbow to rest the side of your head in your hand. Bend your left knee and draw it in. Secure a strap around the arch of your left foot and hold the strap with your left hand. On an exhale, extend your left leg toward the ceiling, keeping it straight. As you do so, feel the gentle opening along the left side of your body. Find a comfortable position for your head, resting it on your right arm, hand, or a folded blanket for added support. Take several deep breaths, stretching deeper with each exhale. Repeat on the other side.

Use a strap around your ribs and foot for a hands-free option.

By securing the strap around your ribs and lifting your leg, you create a stable and secure connection that allows you to fully relax your upper body. This means you can let go of any tension or strain in your shoulders, neck, and arms, enabling a more profound and focused experience. The strap in this variation of sleeping Vishnu acts as an extension of your hands, providing a traction that deepens the stretch. It allows you to focus

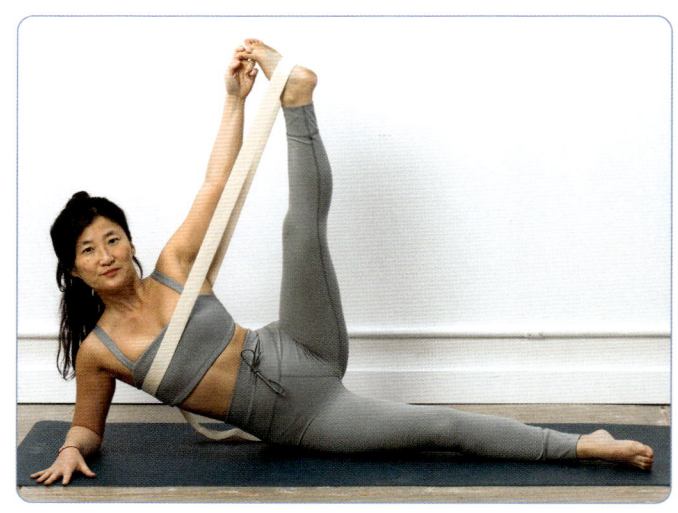

on the alignment and engagement of your core and lower body without the worry of maintaining a grip or balance. Using the strap in this way helps to improve your body awareness and proprioception. As you explore the stretch, you can pay attention to the subtle shifts in your alignment, the engagement of your muscles, and the opening of your hips. Lie on your right side, with a looped strap around your ribs and your legs extended straight. Place your right arm out long, in the same line as your body to provide support, or bend your elbow to rest your head in your hand. For a more engaged variation, you can come onto your forearm as shown in the photo. Bend your left knee and draw it toward your chest. Secure the other end of the loop around the arch of your left foot and extend your leg. Adjust the tension on the strap so that there is tension and support once the leg is fully extended. Gently press the opposite end of the strap loop into the floor with the right side of your rib cage. Repeat on the other side. While she is holding her foot in the photo, the strap gives the option to let go.

Place a bolster or rolled-up blanket under your ribs and armpit.

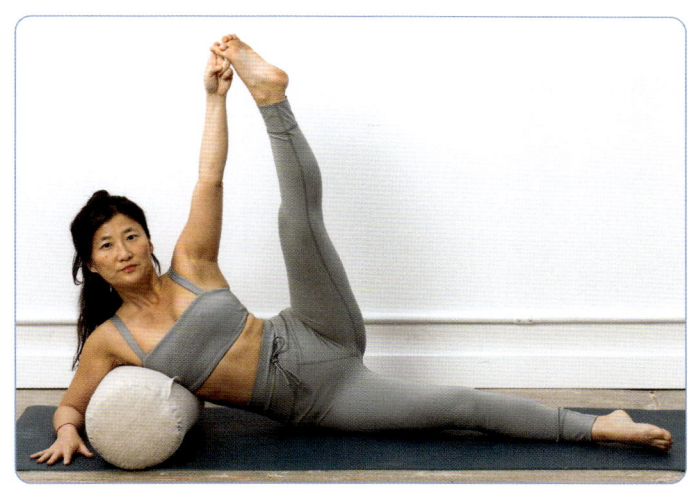

This variation of sleeping Vishnu bridges the gap between your armpit and the floor when supporting your head in your hand or resting on your forearm. This addition not only offers a comfortable surface for you to release into, providing greater stability, but it also gently stimulates and massages the lymph nodes under the armpit, possibly promoting immune-boosting effects. It is particularly beneficial for individuals with limited mobility in the shoulders and sides of the body, because it helps create a safe and accessible space to explore the pose with increased comfort and ease. Repeat on the other side.

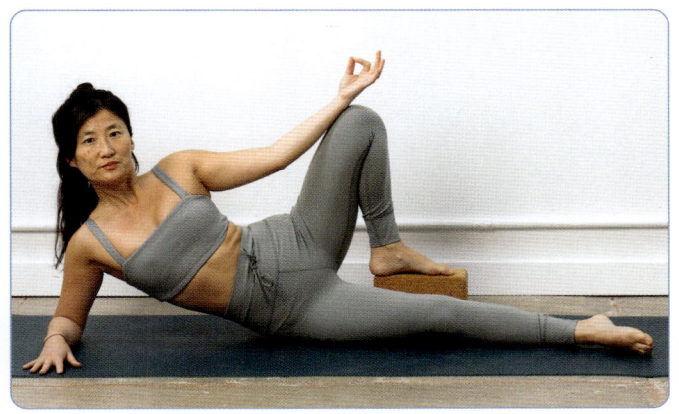

Use a block to support your foot.

Placing your foot on a block provides support and helps you maintain the sleeping Vishnu posture with greater ease. Additionally, the use of the block gently stretches the hips, promoting flexibility and releasing tension in the hip joint. To enter this variation, start by bending your left knee and bringing it toward your chest. Then, place your left foot on the floor behind your right knee, with the foot resting on the block. Repeat on the other side.

Sleeping Vishnu Pose (continued)

Practice against a wall to prevent rolling backward.

When you lean your back against the wall while reclining in sleeping Vishnu, you can stay grounded and balanced throughout the pose, focusing on the alignment of your body and engaging the necessary muscles without the worry of losing your balance. By maintaining contact with the wall, you can develop a deeper sense of body awareness and proprioception, enhancing your overall stability and control. The wall serves as a tactile reminder, guiding you to maintain posture and alignment, preventing any excessive backward movement. This variation is especially beneficial if you have limited balance or stability, allowing you to build confidence and gradually progress in your practice. Repeat on the other side.

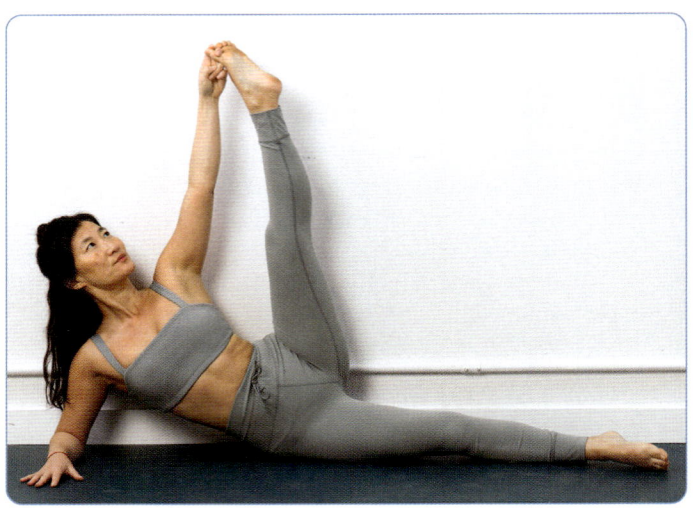

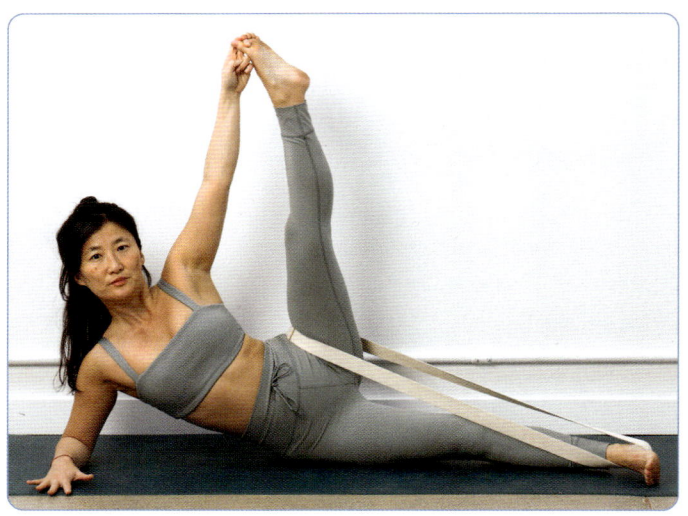

Use a strap to lengthen through your waist and enhance the stretch.

Looping a strap around the foot of your grounded leg and the hip crease of your lifted leg in sleeping Vishnu pose offers several benefits, particularly in lengthening through your waist and enhancing the stretch in the hips. The strap helps create gentle traction to elongate and release tension in the waist area. The strap acts as a bridge between the grounded leg and the lifted leg, allowing you to maintain alignment while deepening the stretch in the hips. This lengthening effect can help improve flexibility, relieve tightness, and promote a greater range of motion in the lower body. The strap also provides support and stability, allowing you to comfortably explore the pose without straining or compromising your balance.

Supine Table Top Pose

Supta Bharmanasana

सुप्त भरमानासन

Supine tabletop pose, also called reverse table top, emerges as an effective alternative to tabletop pose that strengthens the chest, arms, psoas, and deep core muscles. Remarkably, it achieves this without exerting any pressure on the wrist and knee joints. Explore prop-supported variations to enhance your experience and discover the subtle benefits of this nurturing pose.

Use blocks to work your core.

You can use blocks in two ways to work your core in supine table top pose. The first way strengthens the rectus abdominis, training the body to engage the core by drawing in a flat belly instead of rounding and tensing it. Lie on your back with your feet on the floor and knees bent. Press the heels of your feet into the mat, lengthening the tailbone toward your feet, creating a scoop in the low belly and ensuring the lower back remains in contact with the mat. Keep the low back engaged as you lift your shins perpendicular to the mat, aligning your knees directly over your hips. Position blocks against your thighs. Press into one side of the blocks with your hands and press your thighs into the opposite, maintaining the position of your knees (see photo a). Engage your deep core muscles by drawing your navel toward

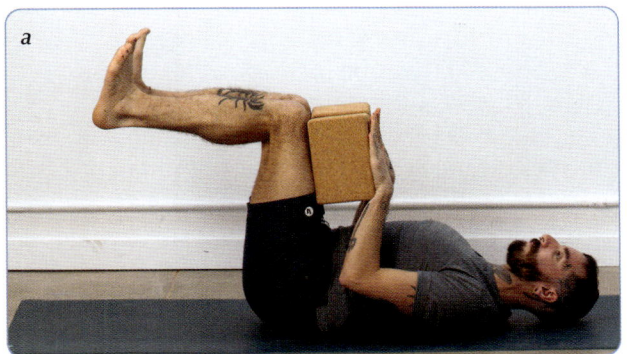

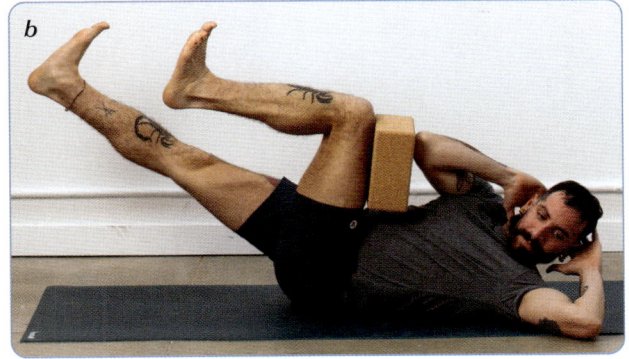

your spine. Relax your head, neck, and facial muscles. Remember to breathe throughout the exercise. To release, allow the belly to soften and gently lower your feet to the mat.

The second way to work the core involves adding a twist and leg extensions to your block-supported supine table top. In this variation, the block provides strengthening for the muscles of the rectus abdominis, as well as the internal and external obliques. It reinforces the importance of drawing in the belly during core exercises instead of allowing it to round and become rigid, making it a valuable preparation for plank pose. Set up in the previous supine core exercise position, with one block this time. Place the block against your left thigh and position your right elbow on the block. Interlace your hands behind the base of your skull. Extend your right leg toward the sky, and then slowly lower it toward the mat. Stop lowering when you feel arching of the back occurring. Lift your right shoulder off the mat. Eventually, and with practice, you can aim to lift the left shoulder as well. Press your elbow into the block and the thigh into the opposite side of the block to stabilize the pelvis and prevent the block from dropping. Draw your pubic bone toward your navel and your navel toward your spine (see photo b). You have the option here to continuously lift and lower the left leg if desired. Hold the twist for 5 to 10 breaths, maintaining stability and control, and then repeat the exercise on the other side.

Use a strap to encourage spinal alignment and test your abdominal strength.

This variation of supine table top pose specifically targets the rectus abdominis muscles, providing a focused activation of your core. It helps refine the alignment of your spine and pelvis, which support the stability of your lower back during core work. The strap also prevents arching in the lower back, promoting a controlled and effective movement. Lie on your back with the strap on

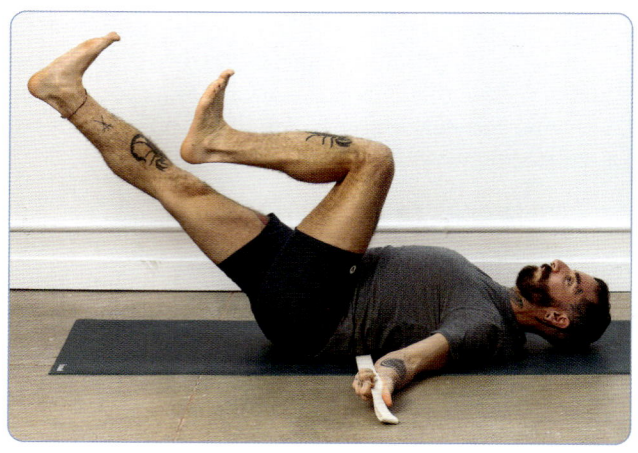

the floor behind your waist. Hold both ends of the strap with both hands, gently lifting to add resistance and create awareness of the counteraction needed in your spine and pelvis. Draw your navel toward your spine, pressing your low back onto the strap, and maintain this pressure. Move into the supine table top position with your knees over your hips. Experiment by extending one leg while keeping the alignment of your spine intact, then alternate sides. For an added challenge, hold the strap in just one hand and pull on it, aiming to keep it pinned down with your lower back, preventing it from sliding out.

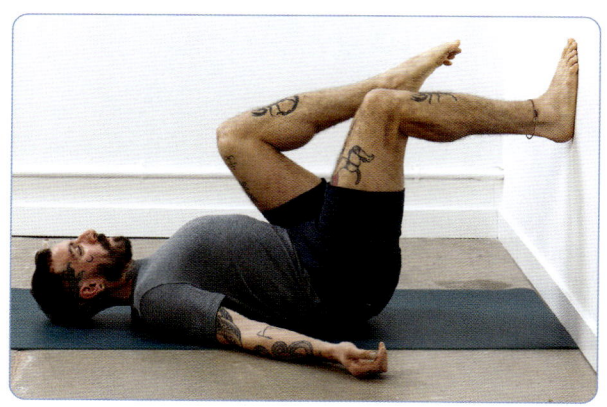

Use a wall or chair to practice supine table top to engage your core and target your abdominal muscles.

This exercise challenges your stability and strengthens your abdominal muscles. To perform the movement, lie on your back with your arms resting by your sides. Position yourself close to a wall or a chair so that you can reach the surface with your feet while having your knees stacked directly over your hips. Maintaining a strong core, draw one knee into your chest. Do not rely on excessive support from the chair or wall. As you bring your knee in, focus on keeping your navel scooped toward your spine, which helps maintain alignment and prevents arching the spine. Continue the exercise by alternating legs, ensuring each repetition is performed with controlled movements and minimal reliance on external support.

Use a wall to practice bird dog on your back.

Lying on your back allows you to reap all the core-strengthening benefits of the supine table top pose without putting excessive pressure on the wrists and knees, which can be especially beneficial if you have joint sensitivities. If you struggle with balancing on your hands and knees, the wall provides additional support and stability. It also helps to support spinal alignment by keeping it in contact with the mat, reducing the likelihood of developing excessive lordosis or collapsing in the shoulders as seen more often in the traditional pose. Additionally, practicing bird dog against a wall aids in achieving square hip alignment by minimizing the risk of rotation of the extended leg. To measure the distance from the wall, lie on your back with your legs extended at around a 45-degree angle to the floor, pressing both feet into the wall in front of you. Release your feet from the wall and plant both feet firmly on the floor with knees bent. Engage your core by drawing your tailbone toward the backs of your knees and hollowing out your abdomen. Lift your shins to a position parallel to the mat, ensuring that your knees are stacked directly over your hip points. Extend your arms toward the sky, aligning your wrists with your shoulders. On an inhale, extend your left leg forward, placing your foot against the wall, while simultaneously reaching your right arm overhead. Exhale and return to the supine table top position. Repeat this, alternating sides, for 5 to 10 repetitions.

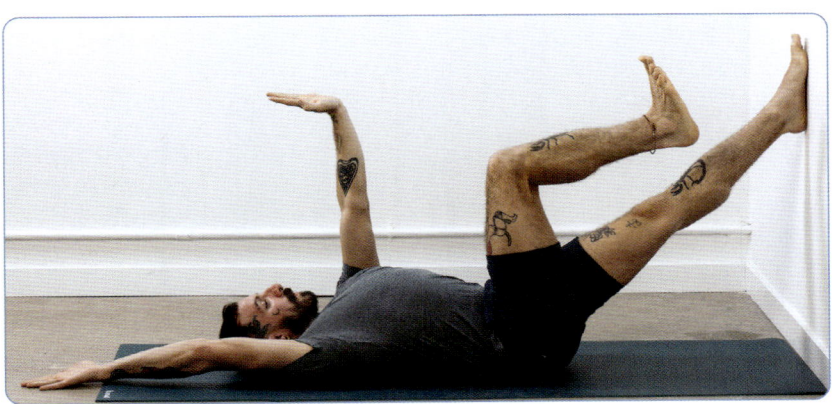

Use a strap to reset your sacroiliac joint.

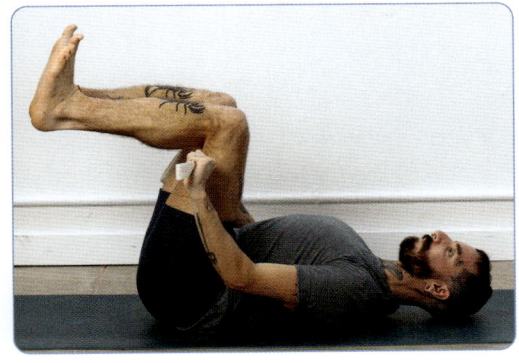

This variation provides a challenging core workout and the benefit of relieving discomfort in the sacroiliac area. Assume a supine table top position, lying on your back with your knees bent and feet flat on the floor. Slide a strap over your left thigh, then under your right thigh, ensuring that you have a firm grip on both ends of the strap with your hands positioned close to the sides of your thighs (the farther away, the more you may end up pulling the strap back toward your upper body). Lift your shins so they are parallel to the mat, entering a supine tabletop position. Then, holding the strap tightly out to the sides, press your thighs into the strap, with your left thigh drawing toward you and your right thigh moving away from you. Repeat this sequence on the other side to balance the exercise.

Corpse Pose

Shavasana   शवासन

Corpse pose, the epitome of relaxation, offers a complete release for both body and mind. It is a powerful practice that unwinds the entire being, alleviates stress, diminishes fatigue, and fosters a state of deep calmness. By lowering blood pressure and promoting better digestion and immune response, this pose becomes a surrender of the ego, unraveling neurological, emotional, and physical patterns. Allow yourself to fully embrace the serenity of corpse pose and experience the profound benefits it provides with the aid of props.

Use a block, bolster, or blanket to support your lumbar spine.

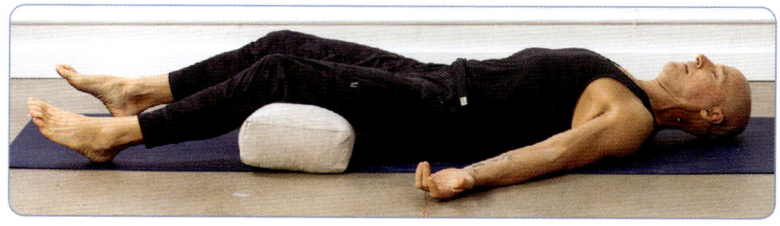

By placing a prop under your knees in corpse pose, you can alleviate pressure in the lumbar spine and the psoas muscles. This gentle support encourages a more neutral alignment in the lower back and releases tension and tightness in the lower back, promoting a deeper state of relaxation and ease. As you settle into this supported position, focus on your breath, allowing it to flow naturally and deeply, further enhancing the relaxation response.

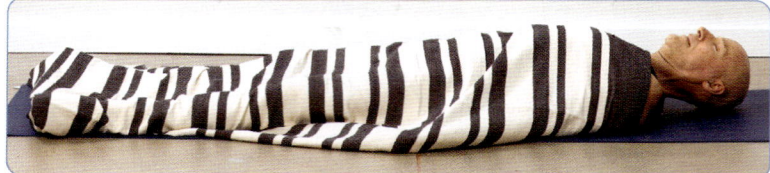

Place a blanket over your body to provide comfort.

Covering yourself with a blanket in corpse pose provides a comforting and grounding sensation, as well as a sense of security and relaxation. The weight of the blanket can also promote a deeper release of tension in the muscles and a feeling of being held and supported. The blanket helps to maintain warmth, which is especially beneficial during longer periods of relaxation. This allows the body to remain cozy and comfortable throughout the practice.

Use a blanket to support your cervical spine.

This variation of corpse pose is especially beneficial if you experience "tech neck" or have a kyphotic spine. Roll the edge of a blanket to a thickness of two to three inches (5-8 cm) and place it under your neck, creating a gentle curve. Place the blanket behind your head so that your chin is the same height as your forehead, allowing for a slight tucking of the chin. You can wrap the excess blanket around your head for added comfort or leave it as is. Take deep breaths and remain in this position for 5 to 10 minutes, experiencing the relaxing and supportive effects.

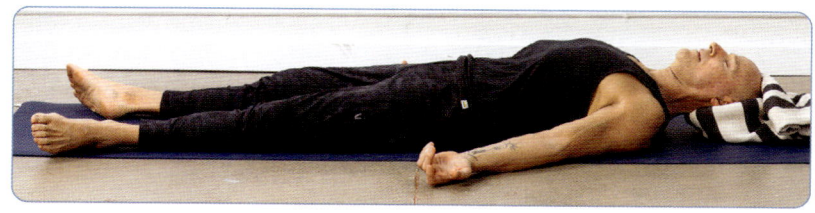

Use a strap to release your legs and hips.

Tying your legs together in corpse pose helps to cultivate a sense of stability and grounding, allowing you to relax more deeply into the pose. It encourages a symmetrical alignment of the body for balance and harmony. This practice also helps to release tension in the hip area and encourages a deeper release of muscles throughout the body. You can practice this variation with your legs on the floor (see photo *a*), or for a restorative twist, loop the strap around both legs and a bolster, lengthwise, underneath your legs (see photo *b*). The added elevation will provide a calming effect and will alleviate tension in the lumbar spine. Finally, for optimal lower back widening and support, you can modify this by practicing constructive rest instead by looping the strap just above the knees. In this final variation, have your feet wide and knees resting inward on one another (see photo *c*). If your lower back still feels strained, walk your feet forward a little, farther from the hips.

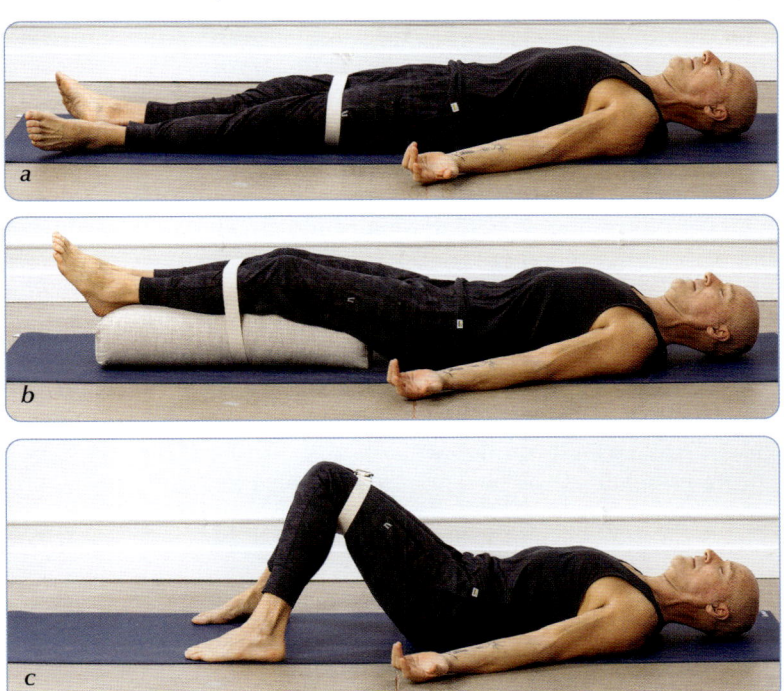

Use blocks and a bolster to practice Stonehenge for low back pain relief.

The Stonehenge variation of corpse pose provides specific benefits for low back pain relief. By creating a structure with two blocks and a bolster, this variation helps to elevate the legs and support the lower back, promoting alignment and reducing strain on the lumbar region. If a bolster is not available, stacked, folded blankets can be used instead.

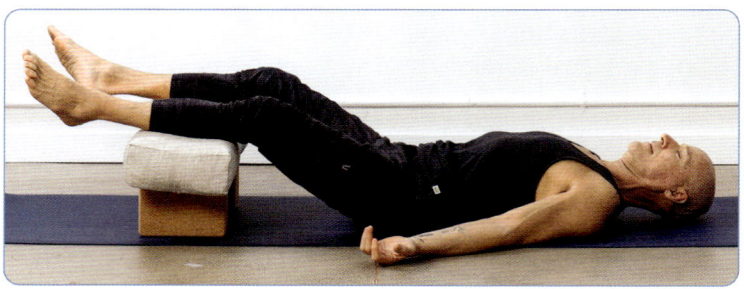

Use a block, bolster, blanket, or strap to practice supine diaphragmatic breathing.

Here are a few breathing techniques that can be practiced while in the corpse pose body position. The first variation involves placing a block, bolster, or folded blanket over the belly, providing gentle reinforcement for the breath (see photo *a*). The weight of the prop helps guide the movement of the diaphragm, allowing for a deepening of the breath as the low belly rises on the inhale and releases on the exhale. The second option focuses on the movement of the ribs during the breath. Loop a strap around the back of the rib cage, crossing the ends over the front of the rib cage, and gently pull it out to the sides to engage the intercostal (inner rib) muscles (see photo *b*). This helps to expand the ribs outward on the inhale and return them to a neutral position on the exhale, facilitating a circular breath that expands the circumference of the ribs and waist as you inhale and gradually contracts as you exhale.

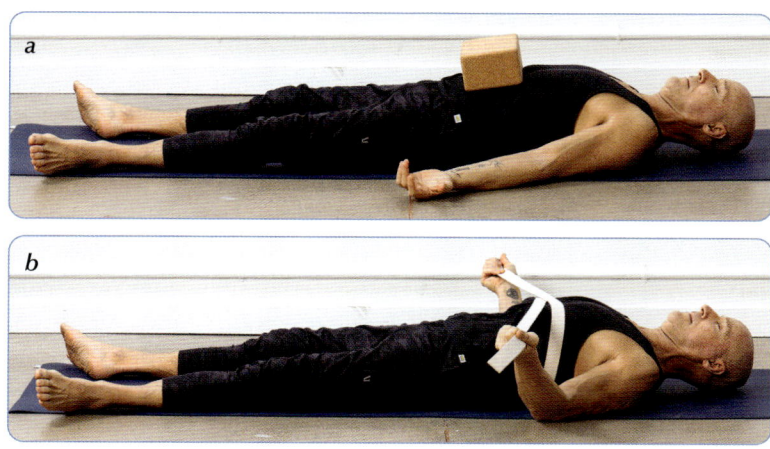

Appendix: Pose Transliteration and Sanskrit Guide

Before delving into the Sanskrit chart, it's important to note that there exist various acceptable English transliterations, particularly concerning the multiple sounds that correspond to the *s*, *c*, and *r* letters found in Latin script (the alphabet that English employs). In the IAST schema for transliterating Sanskrit to the Latin alphabet, different *s* sounds are indicated by using diacritics such as ś or ṣ. When transliterating to English without using diacritics, consistency is maintained by using a *sh* spelling consistently. This may diverge slightly from spellings commonly seen for words such as *parshva*. An example is the Sanskrit name for corpse pose, for which both *savasana* and **sh**avasana are accepted transliterations, with the latter spelling better reflecting the correct pronunciation of the sound represented in the IAST schema as ś. Similarly, the Sanskrit name for camel pose is often written in English as *ustrasana*, yet *u***sh**trasana more accurately represents the pronunciation of the sound represented in IAST as ṣ. Likewise, *padangu***sh**thasana is sometimes spelled without the *h*, but including it better reflects the pronunciation of the sound represented in IAST as ṣ. I have chosen English transliterations that best convey the retroflex vowel ṛ nature, where the tongue rolls back behind the teeth: such as in the word *parivṛtta*. The IAST character *c* is pronounced as *ch*; hence I have opted for this spelling in English transliterations, such as **ch**aturanga (spelled in the IAST schema as *caturaṅga*) or *brahma***ch**aryasana (spelled in the IAST schema as *brahmacaryāsana*).

Posture	Sanskrit	English transliteration	IAST transliteration	Page number
Baby crow pose	बाला काकासन	Bala kakasana	Bālā kākāsana	198
Balancing table pose	दण्डायमान भरमानासन	Dandayamana bharmanasana	Daṇḍāyamāna bharmanāsana	89
Belly down corpse pose	अधोमुखशवासन	Adho mukha shavasana	Adho mukha śavāsana	331
Big toe pose (half-lotus tip toe pose)	अर्ध बद्ध पद्म पादाङ्गुष्ठासन	Ardha baddha padma padangushthasana	Ardha baddha padma pādāṅguṣṭhāsana	98
Bird of paradise	स्वर्ग द्वजिसन	Svarga dvijasana	Svarga dvijāsana	88
Boat pose	नावासन	Navasana	Nāvāsana	142
Bound angle pose	बद्धकोणासन	Baddha konasana	Baddhakoṇāsana	113
Bow pose	धनुरासन	Dhanurasana	Dhanurāsana	311
Bridge pose	सेतुबन्ध सर्वाङ्गासन	Setu bandha sarvangasana	Setu bandha sarvāṅgāsana	164
Camel pose	उष्ट्रासन	Ushtrasana	Uṣṭrāsana	170
Celibate's pose	ब्रह्मचर्यासन	Brahmacharyasana	Brahmacaryāsana	211
Chair pose	उत्कटासन	Utkatasana	Utkaṭāsana	30
Child's pose	बालासन	Balasana	Bālāsana	296
Cobra pose	भुजङ्गासन	Bhujangasana	Bhujaṅgāsana	319
Corpse pose	शवासन	Shavasana	Śavāsana	382
Cow face pose	गोमुखासन	Gomukhasana	Gomukhāsana	121
Crane pose	बकासन	Bakasana	Bakāsana	194
Crow pose	काकासन	Kakasana	Kākāsana	194
Dancer pose	नटराजासन	Natarajasana	Naṭarājāsana	76
Dolphin pose	अर्ध पञ्च मयूरासन	Ardha pincha mayurasana	Ardha piñca mayūrāsana	254
Downward-facing dog pose	अधोमुखश्वानासन	Adho mukha shvanasana	Adho mukha śvānāsana	248
Downward-facing tree pose	अधोमुखवृक्षासन	Adho mukha vrikshasana	Adho mukha vṛkṣāsana	288
Downward-facing twisted stomach pose	अधोमुखजठरपरिवर्तनासन	Adho mukha jathara parivartanasana	Adho mukha jaṭhara parivartanāsana	324
Eagle pose	गरुडासन	Garudasana	Garuḍāsana	73
Ear pressure pose	कर्णपीडासन	Karnapidasana	Karṇapīḍāsana	286

Posture	Sanskrit	English transliteration	IAST transliteration	Page number
Easy pose	सुखासन	Sukhasana	Sukhāsana	94
Eight-angle pose	अष्टावक्रासन	Ashtavakrasana	Aṣṭāvakrāsana	214
Extended hand to big toe pose I	उत्थिति हस्त पादाङ्गुष्ठासन I	Utthita hasta padangush-thasana I	Utthita hasta pādāṅguṣṭhāsana I	78
Extended hand to big toe pose II	उत्थिति हस्त पादाङ्गुष्ठासन II	Utthita hasta padangush-thasana II	Utthita hasta pādāṅguṣṭhāsana II	78
Extended side angle pose	उत्थिति पार्श्वकोणासन	Utthita parshvako-nasana	Utthita pārśvakoṇāsana	56
Extended triangle pose	उत्थिति त्रिकोणासन	Utthita trikonasana	Utthita trikoṇāsana	47
Fallen star pose	पतति तारासन	Patita tarasana	Patita tārāsana	181
Feathered peacock pose	पञ्चि मयूरासन	Pincha mayurasana	Piñca mayūrāsana	275
Firefly pose	टिट्टिभासन	Tittibhasana	Ṭiṭṭibhāsana	205
Fire log pose	अग्निस्तिम्भासन	Agnistambhasana	Agnistambhāsana	116
Fish pose	मत्स्यासन	Matsyasana	Matsyāsana	167
Flying lizard pose	उदयन उत्थान पृष्ठासन	Udayana utthan prishthasana	Udayana utthan pṛṣṭhāsana	245
Flying pigeon pose	एकपाद गलवासन	Eka pada galava-sana	Eka pāda galavāsana	200
Formidable face pose	गण्डभेरुण्डासन	Ganda bherun-dasana	Gaṇḍabheruṇḍāsana	216
Four-limbed staff pose	चतुरङ्ग दण्डासन	Chaturanga dan-dasana	Caturaṅga daṇḍāsana	337
Frog pose II and half frog pose	भेकासन and अर्ध भेकासन	Bhekasana & ardha bhekasana	Bhekāsana & ardha bhekāsana	328
Frog pose and one-legged frog pose	मण्डूकासन and एकपाद-मण्डूकासन	Mandukasana & eka pada mandu-kasana	Maṇḍūkāsana & eka pāda maṇḍūkāsana	326
Garland pose	मालासन	Malasana	Mālāsana	110
Gate pose	परिघासन	Parighasana	Parighāsana	91
Goddess pose	उत्कट कोणासन	Utkata konasana	Utkata koṇāsana	86
Half lord of the fishes pose	अर्ध मत्स्येन्द्रासन	Ardha matsyen-drasana	Ardha matsyendrāsana	135
Half moon pose	अर्ध चन्द्रासन	Ardha chandrasana	Ardha candrāsana	65

Posture	Sanskrit	English transliteration	IAST transliteration	Page number
Half wind-relieving pose	अर्धपवनमुक्तासन	Ardha pavana muktasana	Ardha pavana muktāsana	367
Happy baby pose	आनन्द बालासन	Ananda balasana	Ānanda bālāsana	373
Head to knee pose	जानुशीर्षासन	Janu shirshasana	Jānu śīrṣāsana	123
Hero pose	वीरासन	Virasana	Vīrāsana	106
Heron pose	क्रौञ्चासन	Kraunchasana	Krauñcāsana	108
High crescent lunge pose	अष्ट चन्द्रासन	Ashta chandrasana	Aṣṭa candrāsana	59
Humble warrior pose	बद्ध वीरभद्रासन	Baddha Virabhadrasana	Baddha vīrabhadrāsana	40
Intense side stretch pose	पार्श्वोत्तानासन	Parshvottanasana	Pārśvottānāsana	51
King pigeon pose	एक पाद राजकपोतासन	Eka pada rajakapotasana	Eka pāda rājakapotāsana	178
Legs up the wall pose	विपरीतकरणी	Viparita karani	Viparīta karaṇī	360
Lizard pose	उत्थान पृष्ठासन	Utthan prishthasana	Utthan pṛṣṭhāsana	35
Locust pose	शलभासन	Shalabhasana	Śalabhāsana	302
Lotus pose	पद्मासन	Padmasana	Padmāsana	131
Low lunge pose	अञ्जनेयासन	Anjaneyasana	Añjaneyāsana	33
Melting heart pose	अनाहतासन	Anahatasana	Anāhatāsana	148
Monkey pose	हनुमानासन	Hanumanasana	Hanumānāsana	118
Mountain pose	ताडासन	Tadasana	Tāḍāsana	26
One-legged crow pose	एक पाद काकासन	Eka pada kakasana	Eka pāda kākāsana	240
One-legged king pigeon pose (sleeping variation)	एक पाद राजकपोतासन	Eka pada rajakapotasana	Eka pāda rājakapotāsana	307
One-legged mountain pose	एक पाद ताडासन	Eka pada tadasana	Eka pāda tāḍāsana	28
Partridge pose	कपिञ्जलासन	Kapinjalasana	Kapiñjalāsana	185
Peacock pose	मयूरासन	Mayurasana	Mayūrāsana	222
Pendant pose	लोलासन	Lolasana	Lolāsana	209
Pigeon pose	कपोतासन	Kapotasana	Kapotāsana	174

Posture	Sanskrit	English transliteration	IAST transliteration	Page number
Plank pose	फलकासन	Phalakasana	Phalakāsana	333
Plow pose	हलासन	Halasana	Halāsana	283
Pose dedicated to the sage Koundinya I and II	एक पाद कौण्डिन्यासन I and II	Eka pada Kaundinyasana I & II	Eka pāda Kauṇḍinyāsana I & II	229 and 233
Pose dedicated to the sage Marichi I II, III, and IV	मरीच्यासन I, II, III, and IV	Marichyasana I, II, III, & IV	Maricyāsana I, II, III, & IV	137
Reclined bound angle pose	सुप्त बद्धकोणासन	Supta baddha konasana	Supta baddha koṇāsana	350
Reclined hand to big toe pose I and II	सुप्त उत्थिति हस्त पादाङ्गुष्ठासन I and II	Supta utthita hasta padangushthasana I & II	Supta utthita hasta pādāṅguṣṭhāsana I & II	369
Reclined hero pose	सुप्त वीरासन	Supta virasana	Supta vīrāsana	356
Reclined pigeon pose	सुप्त कपोतासन	Supta kapotasana	Supta kapotāsana	364
Reclined spinal twist and revolved belly pose	सुप्तमत्स्येन्द्रासन and जठर परिवर्तनासन	Supta matsyendrasana & jathara parivartanasana	Supta matsyendrāsana & jaṭhara parivartanāsana	352
Revolved crescent lunge pose	परिवृत्त अञ्जनेयासन	Parivritta anjaneyasana	Parivṛtta añjaneyāsana	61
Revolved half moon pose	परिवृत्त अर्ध चन्द्रासन	Parivritta ardha chandrasana	Parivṛtta ardha candrāsana	69
Revolved hand to big toe pose	परिवृत्त हस्त पादाङ्गुष्ठासन	Parivritta hasta padangushthasana	Parivṛtta hasta pādāṅguṣṭhāsana	82
Revolved head to knee forward bend pose	परिवृत्त जानु शीर्षासन	Parivritta janu shirshasana	Parivṛtta jānu śīrṣāsana	126
Revolved side angle pose	परिवृत्त पार्श्वकोणासन	Parivritta parshvakonasana	Parivṛtta pārśvakonāsana	61
Revolved triangle pose	परिवृत्त त्रिकोणासन	Parivritta trikonasana	Parivṛtta trikoṇāsana	53
Sage Visvamitra's pose	वश्विामित्रासन	Vishvamitrasana	Viśvāmitrāsana	347
Scorpion pose	वृश्चकिासन	Vrishchikasana	Vṛścikāsana	226
Seated compass pose	परिवृत्त सूर्य यंत्रासन	Parivritta surya yantrasana	Parivṛtta sūrya yantrāsana	133
Seated forward bend	पश्चिमोत्तानासन	Pashchimottanasana	Paścimottānāsana	100

Posture	Sanskrit	English transliteration	IAST transliteration	Page number
Seated side stretch pose	पार्श्व उपवष्टि कोणासन	Parshva upavishtha konasana	Pārśva upaviṣṭa koṇāsana	129
Shoulder-pressing pose	भुजपीडासन	Bhujapidasana	Bhujapīḍāsana	203
Side arm staff pose	पार्श्वभुजदण्डासन	Parshva bhuja dandasana	Pārśva bhuja daṇḍāsana	237
Side corpse pose	पार्श्व शवासन	Parshva savasana	Pārśva śavāsana	330
Side crow pose	पार्श्व काकासन	Parshva kakasana	Pārśva kākāsana	218
Side plank pose	वसिष्ठासन	Vasishthasana	Vasiṣṭhāsana	340
Simple sitting twist pose I and II	भरद्वाजासन I and II	Bharadvajasana I & II	Bharadvājāsana I & II	140
Sleeping Vishnu pose or Vishnu's couch pose	अनन्तासन	Anantasana	Anantāsana	376
Sphinx pose	सलम्ब भुजङ्गासन	Salamba bhujangasana	Sālamba bhujaṅgāsana	315
Staff pose	दण्डासन	Dandasana	Daṇḍāsana	96
Standing forward bend pose	उत्तानासन	Uttanasana	Uttānāsana	257
Standing half forward bend pose	अर्ध उत्तानासन	Ardha uttanasana	Ardha uttānāsana	262
Standing splits pose	उर्ध्व प्रसारति एक पादासन	Urdhva prasarita eka padasana	Ūrdhva prasārita eka pādāsana	85
Supine table top pose	सुप्त भरमानासन	Supta bharmanasana	Supta bharmanāsana	379
Supported headstand pose	सालम्ब शीर्षासन	Salamba shirshasana	Sālamba śīrṣāsana	272
Supported shoulder stand pose	सालम्ब सर्वाङ्गासन	Salamba sarvangasana	Sālamba sarvāṅgāsana	279
Table top pose	भरमानासन	Bharmanasana	Bharmanāsana	89
Thunderbolt pose	वज्रासन	Vajrasana	Vajrāsana	112
Tiger pose	व्याघ्रासन	Vyaghrasana	Vyāghrāsana	182
Tree pose	वृक्षासन	Vrikshasana	Vṛkṣāsana	74
Tripod headstand pose	मुक्तहस्त शीर्षासन	Mukta hasta shirshasana	Mukta hasta śīrṣāsana	270
Twisted chair pose	परिवृत्त उत्कटासन	Parivritta utkatasana	Parivṛtta utkaṭāsana	32

Posture	Sanskrit	English transliteration	IAST transliteration	Page number
Twisted lizard pose	परविृत्त उत्थान प्ृष्ठासन	Parivritta utthan prishthasana	Parivṛtta utthan pristhāsana	37
Two-legged inverted staff pose	द्वपिाद वपिरीत दण्डासन	Dwi pada viparita dandasana	Dwi pāda viparīta daṇḍāsana	159
Upward-facing bow pose	ऊर्ध्व धनुरासन	Urdhva dha-nurasana	Ūrdhva dhanurāsana	154
Upward-facing dog pose	ऊर्ध्व मुख श्वानासन	Urdhva mukha shvanasana	Ūrdhva mukha śvānāsana	151
Upward plank pose	पूर्वोत्तानासन	Purvottanasana	Pūrvottānāsana	190
Warrior I pose	वीरभद्रासन I	Virabhadrasana I	Vīrabhadrāsana I	38
Warrior II pose	वीरभद्रासन II	Virabhadrasana II	Vīrabhadrāsana II	42
Warrior III pose	वीरभद्रासन III	Virabhadrasana III	Vīrabhadrāsana III	44
Wide-angle seated forward bend	उपवष्ठि कोणासन	Upavishtha kona-sana	Upaviṣṭa koṇāsana	103
Wide-legged for-ward bend pose	प्रसारति पादोत्तानासन	Prasarita padotta-nasana	Prasārita pādottānāsana	265
Wild thing pose	चमत्कारासन	Chamatkarasana	Camatkārāsana	188

Bibliography

"About Lakshmi Voelker—Lakshmi Voelker Chair Yoga." 2021. Web.archive.org. Get Fit Where You Sit. March 10, 2021. https://web.archive.org/web/20210310040428/https://getfitwhereyousit.com/about-lakshmi-voelker.

Amin, Daniel James, and Maureen Goodman. 2014. "The Effects of Selected Asanas in Iyengar Yoga on Flexibility: Pilot Study." *Journal of Bodywork and Movement Therapies* 18, no. 3: 399-404. https://doi.org/10.1016/j.jbmt.2013.11.008.

Christensen, Alice, and David Rankin. 1979. *Easy Does It Yoga for Older People*. New York, NY: Harper Collins.

Clark, Bernie. 2015. "The Why, What & How behind Using Yoga Props." *Elephant Journal* (blog). January 7, 2015. www.elephantjournal.com/2015/01/the-why-what-how-behind-yoga-props.

Desikachar, T. K. V. 1995. *The Heart of Yoga: Developing a Personal Practice*. Rochester, VT: Inner Traditions International.

Iyengar, Bellur K. S. 2013. *B.K.S. Iyengar Yoga, the Path to Holistic Health*. London, England, UK: Penguin.

Koletsou, Alexia. 2020. "How Old Is Yoga? (plus a Yoga History Timeline)." Yoga My Old Friend. May 29, 2020. https://yogamyoldfriend.com/how-old-is-yoga-a-brief-history-plus-a-timeline-of-key-events.

Lacerda, Daniel. 2015. *2,100 Asanas: The Complete Yoga Poses*. New York: Black Dog & Leventhal.

Lasater, Judith Hanson. 2011. *Relax and Renew: Restful Yoga for Stressful Times*. Berkeley, CA: Rodmell Press.

Lu, Yi-Hsueh, Bernard Rosner, Gregory Chang, and Loren M. Fishman. 2016. "Twelve-Minute Daily Yoga Regimen Reverses Osteoporotic Bone Loss." *Topics in Geriatric Rehabilitation* 32, no. 2: 81-87. https://doi.org/10.1097/TGR.0000000000000085.

Mehta, Silva, Mira Mehta, and Shyam Mehta. 1990. *Yoga*. New York, NY: Alfred A. Knopf.

Monier-Williams, Monier, Ernst Leumann, and Carl Cappeller. 2005. *A Sanskrit-English Dictionary: Etymologically and Philologically Arranged With Special Reference to Cognate Indo-European Languages*. Delhi: Motilal Banarsidass.

Moosbrugger, Ashlee. 2015. "Then + Now: 40 Years of Yoga Gear." *Yoga Journal*. July 14, 2015. www.yogajournal.com/lifestyle/fashion-beauty/yoga-gear/40-years-yoga-gear.

Nhất Hạnh, Thích. 2005. *Being Peace*. Berkeley, CA: Parallax Press.

Parker, Gail. 2020. *Restorative Yoga for Ethnic and Race-Based Stress and Trauma*. Philadelphia, PA: Singing Dragon.

Powell, Seth. 2018. "The Ancient Yoga Strap." *The Luminescent*. June 18, 2018. www.theluminescent.org/2018/06/the-ancient-yoga-strap-yogapatta.html.

Singh Khalsa, Sat Bir, Lorenzo Cohen, Timothy McCall, and Shirley Telles. 2016. *Principles and Practice of Yoga in Health Care*. London, England, UK: Handspring.

Sircar, Dineschandra. 1966. *Indian Epigraphical Glossary*. New Delhi, India: Motilal Banarsidass.

Sivaramakrishnan, Divya, Claire Fitzsimons, Paul Kelly, Kim Ludwig, Nanette Mutrie, David H. Saunders, and Graham Baker. 2019. "The Effects of Yoga Compared to Active and Inactive Controls on Physical Function and Health Related Quality of Life in Older Adults—Systematic Review and Meta-Analysis of Randomised Controlled Trials." *The International Journal of Behavioral Nutrition and Physical Activity* 16, no. 1: 33. https://doi.org/10.1186/s12966-019-0789-2.

Wile, Nancy. 2012. "Yoga Teacher Training Sanskrit Words and Pronunciation Sanskrit Words and Pronunciation for Yoga Teachers." https://yogaeducation.org/wp-content/uploads/2019/05/sanskrit-1.pdf.

Wren, Anava A., Melissa A. Wright, James W. Carson, and Francis J. Keefe. 2011. "Yoga for Persistent Pain: New Findings and Directions for an Ancient Practice." *Pain* 152, no. 3: 477-480. https://doi.org/10.1016/j.pain.2010.11.017.

Tolle, Eckhart. 2016. *A New Earth: Awakening to Your Life's Purpose*. London, UK: Penguin Books.

About the Author

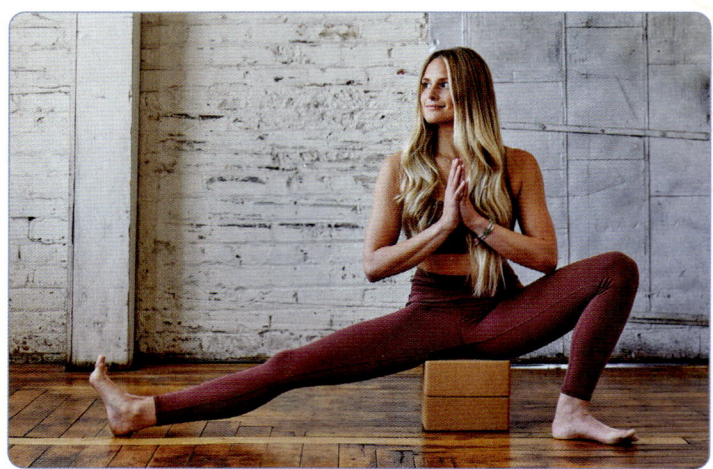

©Ty Milford

Jenny Clise is a certified yoga therapist (C-IAYT) with over 1,000 hours of training, and she has been teaching yoga since 2012. She completed her yoga therapy training at Prema Yoga Institute and integrates therapeutic principles into her practice, making yoga accessible and inclusive for all students. Jenny's approach prioritizes individual needs and encourages self-discovery through mindful movement, breath work, and props.

Her teaching style emphasizes building from a strong foundation, finding alignment based on individual needs, and safely guiding students through more challenging postures. Jenny believes in cultivating an intentional practice that nurtures both physical and mental strength. By offering her students and clients personalized guidance and encouragement, Jenny helps them find their own paths to wellness.

Beyond the studio, Jenny is an avid traveler who leads yoga retreats in beautiful locations worldwide. Her love for adventure complements her teaching, offering students unique experiences to deepen their practice in nature. As an experienced writer, she regularly contributes to *Yoga Journal*, sharing insights on yoga, meditation, and wellness.

Jenny began sharing her passion for yoga props with her ebook *Blockasanas*. She has now channeled her expertise into writing this comprehensive book. These works demonstrate her commitment to educating and empowering others in their yoga journey.